Medical Management of Heart Disease

Clinical Guides to Medical Management

Consulting Editor

BURTON E. SOBEL, M.D.

Department of Medicine
The University of Vermont College of Medicine
and Fletcher Allen Health Care
Burlington, Vermont

Medical Management of Heart Disease, *edited by Burton E. Sobel*

Additional Volumes in Preparation

Medical Management of Heart Disease

edited by

Burton E. Sobel

*University of Vermont College of Medicine
and Fletcher Allen Health Care
Burlington, Vermont*

Associate Editors

Michael E. Cain
Paul R. Eisenberg
*Washington University School of Medicine
St. Louis, Missouri*

Marcel Dekker, Inc.   **New York • Basel • Hong Kong**

Library of Congress Cataloging-in-Publication Data

Medical management of heart disease / edited by Burton E. Sobel ;
  associate editors, Michael E. Cain, Paul R. Eisenberg.
    p. cm.
  Includes index.
  ISBN 0-8247-9315-3 (alk. paper)
  1. Heart — Diseases. I. Sobel, Burton E. II. Cain, Michael E.
(Michael Edwin). III. Eisenberg, Paul R.
  [DNLM: 1. Heart Diseases — therapy. 2. Heart Diseases — diagnosis.
WG 210 M489 1996]
RC681.M44 1996
616.1'2—dc20
DNLM/DLC
for Library of Congress
                                                96-4747
                                               CIP

The publisher offers discounts on this book when ordered in bulk quantities. For more information, write to Special Sales/Professional Marketing at the address below.

This book is printed on acid-free paper.

MARCEL DEKKER, INC.
270 Madison Avenue, New York, New York 10016

Current printing (last digit):
10 9 8 7 6 5 4 3 2 1

PRINTED IN THE UNITED STATES OF AMERICA

Preface

The treatment of heart disease is demanding but gratifying. The methods are often sophisticated, and extensive knowledge based on past and recent advances is required for optimal patient care. Because patients with heart disease are encountered by physicians from diverse disciplines and because medical management is so critical, this book was written to serve as a clinician's consultant to practicing physicians, students, and fellows.

The format is straightforward but not simplistic. Information is presented in terms of both cardinal manifestations of disease and specific etiologies. The book is organized into five major sections. Parts I and II explore the cardinal manifestations of heart disease, including the symptoms and signs that bring the patient to the physician's attention. In each case, underlying conditions responsible for cardinal manifestations are differentiated in terms of the essential observations that must be made. Treatment strategies are provided for each.

Medical students have long been taught that the patient writes the chief complaint; the physician writes the present illness—an epigram underscoring the primacy of the chief complaint in leading the astute observer to a specific diagnosis and treatment. We have emphasized cardinal manifestations of heart disease to the same end. Sometimes, however, patients, when first seen, are already known to harbor a specific disorder. Part III, on treatment, is designed to help the physician identify optimal therapeutic approaches when the starting point is an already established diagnosis. The chapters in this part are extensively cross-referenced to those in Parts I and II.

Part IV addresses manifestations of heart disease in special settings, such as pregnancy, high risk of coronary disease, and in patients harboring antiarrhythmia devices.

Part V considers several classes of pharmacological agents used in the treatment of patients with heart disease.

The authorities selected to contribute to this book have extensive clinical experience, have contributed to new knowledge in their fields, are committed to teaching, and have been willing to take unambiguous positions based on current information in serving as the clinician's consultant. It is hoped that cardiologists, cardiothoracic surgeons, internists, and primary care physicians, as well as generalists and specialists from diverse disciplines who encounter patients with heart disease, can benefit from the concise, pragmatic, and rigorous presentations of the treatment and medical management of heart disease.

Burton E. Sobel

Contributors

W. Kemper Alston, M.D.   Assistant Professor of Medicine, Department of Medicine, University of Vermont College of Medicine, Burlington, Vermont

J. Thomas Bigger, Jr., M.D.   Professor of Medicine and Pharmacology, Division of Cardiology, Department of Medicine, Columbia University College of Physicians and Surgeons, New York, New York

Stephen P. Bradley, M.D.   Chest and Critical Care Medicine, Scripps Clinic and Research Foundation, La Jolla, California

Michael E. Cain, M.D.   Tobias and Hortense Lewin Professor of Medicine and Director, Cardiovascular Division, Department of Medicine, Washington University School of Medicine, St. Louis, Missouri

A. John Camm, M.D., F.R.C.P.   Professor of Clinical Cardiology, Department of Cardiological Sciences, St. George's Hospital Medical School, London, England

Jack L. Clausen, M.D.   Clinical Professor of Medicine, Division of Pulmonary and Critical Care, Department of Medicine, University of California, San Diego, School of Medicine, San Diego, California

James Coromilas, M.D.   Associate Professor of Clinical Medicine, Division of Cardiology, Department of Medicine, Columbia University College of Physicians and Surgeons, New York, New York

Paul R. Eisenberg, M.D., M.P.H.   Associate Professor of Medicine and Director, Cardiac Care Unit, Cardiovascular Division, Department of Internal Medicine, Washington University School of Medicine, St. Louis, Missouri

Uri Elkayam, M.D.   Professor of Medicine; Director, Heart Failure Program; and Physician in Charge, Cardiology High-Risk Obstetric Clinic; Department of Medicine, University of Southern California, School of Medicine, Los Angeles, California

v

Perry M. Elliott, M.B., B.S., M.R.C.P. Research Fellow, Department of Cardiological Sciences, St. George's Hospital Medical School, London, England

Kevin J. Ferrick, M.D., F.A.C.C., F.A.C.P. Associate Professor of Medicine and Director, ECG and Holter Division, Montefiore Medical Center, Albert Einstein College of Medicine, Bronx, New York

John D. Fisher, M.D., F.A.C.C. Professor of Medicine and Director, Cardiology and Arrhythmia Services, Montefiore Medical Center, Albert Einstein College of Medicine, Bronx, New York

Bernard J. Gersh, M.B., Ch.B., D.Phil., F.R.C.P. W. Proctor Harvey Teaching Professor of Cardiology and Chief, Division of Cardiology, Georgetown University Hospital, Washington, D.C.

Elsa Grace V. Giardina, M.D. Professor of Clinical Medicine, Division of Cardiology, Department of Medicine, Columbia University College of Physicians and Surgeons, New York, New York

James A. Goldstein, M.D. Cardiovascular Division, William Beaumont Hospital, Royal Oak, Michigan

Christopher J. Grace, M.D. Associate Professor of Medicine, Department of Infectious Diseases, University of Vermont College of Medicine, Burlington, Vermont

Jay N. Gross, M.D., F.A.C.C. Associate Professor of Medicine and Director, Intercampus Pacemaker Service, Montefiore Medical Center, Albert Einstein College of Medicine, Bronx, New York

William E. Hopkins, M.D. Associate Professor of Medicine, Cardiology Unit, Department of Medicine, University of Vermont College of Medicine, Burlington, Vermont

Allan S. Jaffe, M.D. Professor and Director, Division of Cardiology, Department of Medicine, State University of New York Health Science Center at Syracuse, Syracuse, New York

Mark E. Josephson, M.D. Professor of Medicine, Harvard Medical School, and Director, Harvard-Thorndike Electrophysiology Institute and Arrhythmia Service, Beth Israel Hospital, Boston, Massachusetts

David M. Kaufman, M.D. Professor of Neurology and Psychiatry, Department of Neurology, Montefiore Medical Center, Albert Einstein College of Medicine, Bronx, New York

Josef Kautzner, M.D. Cardiology Registrar, Department of Cardiological Sciences, St. George's Hospital Medical School, London, England

Soo G. Kim, M.D., F.A.C.C., F.A.C.P.   Professor of Medicine and Director, Electrophysiology Laboratory, Montefiore Medical Center, Albert Einstein College of Medicine, Bronx, New York

John C. LaRosa, M.D.   Chancellor and Professor, Department of Medicine, Tulane University Medical Center, New Orleans, Louisiana

Bruce D. Lindsay, M.D.   Associate Professor of Medicine and Director, Clinical Electrophysiology Laboratory, Cardiovascular Division, Washington University School of Medicine, St. Louis, Missouri

William J. McKenna, M.D.   Professor of Cardiac Medicine, Department of Cardiological Sciences, St. George's Hospital and Medical School, London, England

Kenneth M. Moser, M.D.   Professor of Medicine, University of California, San Diego, School of Medicine, San Diego, California

Robert A. O'Rourke, M.D.   Charles Conrad Brown Distinguished Professor in Cardiovascular Disease, Division of Cardiology, Department of Medicine, The University of Texas Health Science Center at San Antonio, San Antonio, Texas

James A. Reiffel, M.D.   Professor of Clinical Medicine, Division of Cardiology, Department of Medicine, Columbia University, College of Physicians and Surgeons, New York, New York

Stuart Rich, M.D.   Professor of Medicine and Chief, Section of Cardiology, University of Illinois at Chicago Medical Center, Chicago, Illinois

Robyn A. Schaiff, Pharm.D., B.C.P.S.   Clinical Pharmacist, Critical Care Medicine, Barnes Hospital, St. Louis, Missouri

Joseph M. Smith, M.D., Ph.D.   Assistant Professor of Medicine; Associate Director, Clinical Electrophysiology Laboratory, Cardiovascular Division; and Assistant Professor of Biomedical Computing, Institute for Biomedical Computing at Washington University, Washington University School of Medicine, St. Louis, Missouri

Burton E. Sobel, M.D.   Amidon Professor and Chair, Department of Medicine, The University of Vermont College of Medicine; and Physician-in-Chief, Fletcher Allen Health Care, Burlington, Vermont

Allen J. Solomon, M.D.   Assistant Professor of Medicine, Division of Cardiology, Department of Medicine, Georgetown University Medical Center, Washington, D.C.

Jay M. Sullivan, M.D., F.A.C.C.   Professor of Medicine and Chief, Division of Cardiovascular Diseases, Department of Medicine, The University of Tennessee, Memphis, Tennessee

Matthew W. Watkins, M.D.   Assistant Professor of Medicine and Associate Director, Cardiac Catheterization Laboratory, Cardiology Unit, Department of Medicine, The University of Vermont College of Medicine, Burlington, Vermont

Ronald Wharton, M.D.   Assistant Professor of Medicine, Emergency Department, Montefiore Medical Center, Albert Einstein College of Medicine, Bronx, New York

Contents

Preface   iii
Contributors   v

Part I   CARDIAC SYMPTOMS
Evaluation and Treatment of Patients Organized
According to Presenting Cardiac Symptoms   1

1. **Chest Pain**   3
   Diagnostic Approach to the Patient with Chest Pain Compatible
   with Definite or Suspected Angina Pectoris   4
   Robert A. O'Rourke

   Unstable Angina with ST-Segment Elevation   22
   Paul R. Eisenberg

2. **Shortness of Breath/Dyspnea on Exertion/PND/Orthopnea/**
   Platypnea/Orthodeoxia   37
   Evaluation and Treatment of Patients with Shortness of Breath   38
   Stephen P. Bradley, Jack L. Clausen, and Kenneth M. Moser

   Dyspnea as a Manifestation of Pulmonary Vascular Disease   51
   Stuart Rich

   Dyspnea and Congenital Heart Disease   56
   William E. Hopkins

3. **Other Cardinal Manifestations of Heart Disease: Evaluation**
   and Treatment of Patients with Cough   59
   Stephen P. Bradley, Jack Clausen, and Kenneth M. Moser

4. Palpitations   **61**
Michael E. Cain

5. Syncope and Presyncope   **79**
*John D. Fisher, Soo G. Kim, David M. Kaufman, Kevin J. Ferrick,
Jay N. Gross, and Ronald Wharton*

**Part II   CARDIAC SIGNS
Evaluation and Treatment of Patients
with Signs of Cardiovascular Disease**   **95**

6. General Observations   **97**
William E. Hopkins

7. Hypertension   **101**
Jay M. Sullivan

8. Shock   **145**
James A. Goldstein and Burton E. Sobel

**9. Suspicions of Cardiovascular Disease Raised by Results of
"Routine" Diagnostic Tests**   **161**
Allan S. Jaffe

**Part III   CARDIAC TREATMENT
Management of Specific Cardiac Problems**   **167**

10. Management of Patients with Chest Pain of Cardiac Origin   **169**
Allen J. Solomon and Bernard J. Gersh

11. Management of Patients with Acute Myocardial Infarction   **189**
Paul R. Eisenberg

12. Management of Patients with Congestive Heart Failure   **221**
James A. Goldstein

13. Management of Patients with Pulmonary Vascular Diseases   **235**
Stuart Rich

14. Management of Patients with Valvular Heart Disease   **239**
Burton E. Sobel, Matthew W. Watkins, and James A. Goldstein

15. Management of Patients with Pericardial Diseases   267
James A. Goldstein

16. Management of Patients with Supraventricular Arrhythmias   285
Management of Patients with Cardiac Arrhythmias   286
James A. Reiffel, James Coromilas, J. Thomas Bigger, Jr.,
and Elsa Grace V. Giardina

Intraatrial Reentrant Arrhythmias   299
Joseph M. Smith

Atrioventricular Nodal Reentrant Tachycardia   311
Michael E. Cain

Accessory Pathway–Mediated Tachycardias   318
Bruce D. Lindsay

17. Management of Patients with Ventricular Arrhythmias   333
Ventricular Premature Complexes   333
J. Thomas Bigger, Jr.

Ventricular Tachycardia   343
Mark E. Josephson

18. Management of Patients with Bradycardias   373
Abnormalities of Impulse Formation and Atrioventricular
Conduction   373
A. John Camm and Josef Kautzner

Intraventricular Conduction Abnormalities   393
A. John Camm and Josef Kautzner

19. Cardiac and Pulmonary Arrest   397
Allan S. Jaffe

**20. Evaluation and Management of the Survivor of Cardiac
Arrest**   403
Mark E. Josephson

Part IV   Heart Disease in Special Settings   421

21. Cardiac Findings in Athletes with and without Heart Disease 423
A. John Camm and Josef Kautzner

22. **Pregnancy** 433
   Management of Cardiac Disease in Pregnancy 434
   Uri Elkayam

   Management of Arrhythmias in Pregnancy 443
   A. John Camm and Josef Kautzner

23. **Chronic Pulmonary Disease** 455
   A. John Camm and Joseph Kautzner

24. **Diagnosis and Management of Arrhythmias in Patients with Cardiomyopathy** 461
   William J. McKenna and Perry M. Elliott

25. **Management of Congenital Heart Disease in Adults** 467
   William E. Hopkins

26. **Evaluation and Management of Patients with Ischemic Heart Disease Undergoing Noncardiac Surgery** 481
   Allan S. Jaffe

27. **Preventive Cardiology** 489
   John C. LaRosa

28. **Infective Endocarditis** 509
   W. Kemper Alston and Christopher J. Grace

29. **Management of Patients with Antiarrhythmic Devices** 519
   Bruce D. Lindsay

Part V   Medications 527

30. **Use of Common Medications in the Treatment of Patients with Heart Disease** 529
   Robyn A. Schaiff, Paul R. Eisenberg, and Burton E. Sobel

Index 551

I

CARDIAC SYMPTOMS

Evaluation and Treatment of Patients Organized According to Presenting Cardiac Symptoms

Most approaches to descriptions of cardiovascular disease and its management begin with specific disease entities and consider them in terms of etiology, diagnosis, pathophysiology, and treatment. The clinician, however, is confronted with the need for a different sequence of epistemology in evaluating a patient with specific symptoms to provide the foundation for optimal treatment. All too often, symptoms can be misinterpreted because of preconceptions about the disease entity or the failure of the clinician to heed Osler's mandate that we first "listen to the patient."

Cardinal symptoms of cardiovascular disease include chest pain, difficulty in breathing, fatigue, palpitations, loss of appetite, awareness of atypical pulsations, or discomfort from edema. The astute clinician will truly listen to the patient, thereby being better able to differentiate intermittent from waxing and waning yet constantly present pain, pain with a quality of pressure as opposed to burning or stabbing, and pain in one locus as opposed to pain with a migratory pattern. Such a clinician will differentiate fatigue (often a sign of pulmonary hypertension) from shortness of breath (often a sign of pulmonary venous congestion and left atrial hypertension) and will elucidate the nature of palpitations by having the patient simulate the rhythm by "tapping it out." Remarkably, patients can often provide accurate simulations of sudden as opposed to gradual onset of arrhythmia, the rate of a tachycardia, regularity or irregularity of rhythm, the nature of offset, and the presence or absence of compensatory pauses. Without knowing the definition of any of the terms, the patient can simply but elegantly replicate experience.

The cardinal symptoms of heart disease are discussed in the part that follows, along with diagnostic implications and the company they keep. The material is cross-referenced extensively to salient signs, pathophysiological features underlying both signs and symptoms, and treatment with an emphasis on correction of underlying pathophysiological abnormalities. This format is consistent with the way a patient presents to a physician.

Among the most frequently encountered symptoms and signs of heart disease, none is more significant to the patient and to the physician than chest pain. As the first symptom to be presented, it is considered with respect to typical angina pectoris and its differential diagnosis, unstable angina, and myocardial infarction. Physical findings and objective diagnostic criteria are covered in the same sequence.

1

Chest Pain

Diagnostic Approach to the Patient with Chest Pain
Compatible with Definite or Suspected Angina Pectoris   **3**
    I.   Terminology   4
    II.   Characteristics of Angina Pectoris   5
    III.   Associated Symptoms   7
    IV.   Cardiac Risk Factors   9
    V.   Differential Diagnosis   9
    VI.   Chest Pain: Physical Findings in Patients with Angina
        Pectoris and Conditions Simulating It   14
    VII.   Electrocardiography   16
    VIII.   Chest Radiography   16
    IX.   Additional Initial Tests Likely to Be Helpful in
        Patients with Chest Pain   17
    X.   Noninvasive Testing for Detection of Myocardial
        Ischemia   17

Unstable Angina with ST-Segment Elevation   **22**
    XI.   General Principles   22
    XII.   Clinical Presentations Associated with ST-Segment
        Elevation Not Caused by Myocardial Infarction   22
    XIII.   Initial Evaluation and Management of Patients with
        Myocardial Infarction and ST-Segment Elevation   25
    XIV.   Reperfusion in Patients with Acute Myocardial
        Infarction and ST-Segment Elevation   26
    XV.   Selection of Patients   27
    XVI.   Selection of Fibrinolytic and Conjunctive Agents   30

    Suggested Reading   34

Diagnostic Approach to the Patient with Chest Pain Compatible with Definite or Suspected Angina Pectoris

Robert A. O'Rourke

I. TERMINOLOGY

Angina pectoris (literally "strangling in the chest") is repetitive chest discomfort or pain associated with myocardial ischemia and dysfunction but without myocardial necrosis. Characteristically, the chest pain is retrosternal, induced by exertion and relieved promptly by rest or nitroglycerin.

Angina pectoris is classified as *stable* when its subjective characteristics have not changed over the previous 60 days. *Unstable angina* involves a distinctive increase in the number, severity, or duration of episodes—that is, it is angina occurring at decreasing levels of exercise, sometimes at minimal exercise, or at rest.

An increase in myocardial oxygen demand (demand ischemia), a decrease in or inadequate coronary blood flow (supply ischemia), or their combination may be responsible for the chest pain. The former is more likely in patients with chronic stable angina. Diminished coronary blood supply (attributable to absolute or relative coronary vasoconstriction or thrombosis) is more likely when unstable angina or acute myocardial infarction is present.

Episodes of chest pain usually resolve within 5–10 min in patients with stable angina. Chest discomfort may persist much longer in patients with unstable angina or myocardial infarction. Criteria of myocardial necrosis are the only definitive means for separating patients who have unstable angina with prolonged episodes of chest pain from those with acute myocardial infarction.

The mechanisms responsible for pain of cardiac origin are not yet clearly understood. Nonmedullated small sympathetic nerve fibers that parallel the coronary arteries are thought to serve as the afferent sensory pathway for angina and enter the spinal cord in the C8-T4 segments. Impulses are transmitted to corresponding spinal ganglia and then through the spinal cord to the thalamus and cerebral cortex. Angina pectoris, like other pain of visceral origin, is often poorly localized and commonly referred to the corresponding segmental dermatomes. Often, it originates or is localized outside the chest.

II. CHARACTERISTICS OF ANGINA PECTORIS

The *quality* of the chest discomfort is usually described in such words as "tightness," "pressure," "burning," "heavy," "aching," "strangling," or "compression." Usually the patient perceives a deep rather than a superficial origin of the pain. The description of the pain is affected greatly by the patient's intelligence, education, and social/cultural background. Other features besides the qualitative nature of the chest pain often provide useful information including the location of the chest discomfort, precipitating factors, mode of onset, duration, and mode of disappearance.

The *location* of chest pain provides information that is important in determining etiology. Angina is ordinarily retrosternal or felt slightly to the left of the midline, beside or partly under the sternum. Usually, it is *not* isolated to the cardiac apex in the inframammary region. The chest pain of myocardial ischemia tends to radiate bilaterally across the chest into the arms (left more than right) and into the neck and lower jaw. Occasionally radiation to the back or occiput is noted. In the arms, the pain typically passes down the ulnar and volar surfaces to the wrist and then only into the ulnar fingers, not into the thumb or down the lateral surface of the arm—areas associated with different dermatomes. Sometimes pain may be felt only in the arm or may begin in the arm and radiate to the chest. The patient's gestures used in describing and localizing the pain may be helpful in determining its etiology. One or two clenched fists held by the patient over the sternal area (Levine's sign) much more likely indicates angina pectoris than does a finger pointed to a small, circumscribed area in the left inframammary region.

Precipitating factors are important. Angina pectoris is often induced by exercise, emotions, eating, or cold weather. A recognizable pattern of reproducibility of chest pain with certain activities is an important feature of angina for which the patient must be questioned specifically. Angina often occurs with exertion after meals and tends to be precipitated more readily by arm exercise (e.g., lifting or carrying), which involves a greater element of isometric exercise. Chest pain occurring only after exercise has been concluded or at the end of the day rarely is attributable to myocardial ischemia. However, nocturnal angina is common in patients with severely depressed cardiac function. Exertional angina is more likely to occur when the patient is outdoors, especially when the temperature is extremely high or low and when the patient is walking uphill against the wind in cold weather. Angina occurs commonly after the patient has eaten a heavy meal or when the patient is excited, angry, or tense.

Angina pectoris characteristically has a *crescendo pattern* at the onset of pain peaks and diminishes abruptly. Pains often described as "shooting" or "stabbing" that reach their maximum intensity virtually instantaneously are usually musculoskeletal or neurological in etiology. Angina is usually relieved within 5–10 min by rest with or without the use of vasodilator drugs such as nitroglycerin, although nitroglycerin often hastens relief. Failure to obtain relief with rest or nitroglycerin suggests another cause of pain or impending myocardial infarction. The reproducible relief of chest pain in an appropriate time frame (1–10 min) provides strong evidence favoring myocardial ischemia as the etiology. However, nitroglycerin can relieve the pain of esophogeal or other visceral spasm as well. A trial of nitroglycerin can be a useful diagnostic strategy. Patients with angina pectoris are often classified functionally depending upon the amount of activity necessary to induce pain (Table 1). The morbidity and mortality of patients with chronic ischemic heart disease is generally inversely related to the exercise workload necessary to produce angina.

The answers to three questions are critical in determining whether chest pain is angina pectoris: (a) Is the chest pain substernal in location? (b) Is it precipitated by exercise? (c) Is it relieved within 10 min by rest or nitroglycerin? If all three answers are positive, the designation of *typical angina pectoris* can be made based on the history. If two of three answers are positive, *atypical angina* describes the symptom complex. If only one of the three answers is positive, the pain is likely to be *nonanginal chest pain.* Myocardial ischemia (detectable by noninvasive testing) is decreased and important coronary artery stenosis (detectable by coronary arteriography) is diminished in patients depending on the category of the symptom complex defined in this manner (Table 2). In each category, the incidence of significant coronary artery disease is greater in older patients, males, and patients with two or more coronary artery risk factors.

Angina pectoris rarely lasts less than 1 min or more than 15 min in the

Table 1   Canadian Cardiovascular Society Functional Classification of Angina Pectoris

I.   Ordinary physical activity, such as walking and climbing stairs, does not cause angina. Angina results from strenuous or rapid or prolonged exertion at work or recreation.

II.   Slight limitation of ordinary activity. Walking or climbing stairs rapidly, walking uphill, walking or stair climbing after meals, in cold, in wind, or when under emotional stress, or only during the few hours after awakening. Walking more than two blocks on the level and climbing more than one flight of ordinary stairs at a normal pace and under normal conditions.

III. Marked limitations of ordinary physical activity. Walking one to two blocks on the level and climbing more than one flight under normal conditions.

IV.   Inability to carry on any physical activity without discomfort—anginal syndrome may be present at rest.

Source: Modified from Campeau L: Letter to the editor. *Circulation* 1976; 54:522. Reproduced with permission from the American Heart Association, Inc., and the author.

Table 2 Pretest Likelihood of Coronary Disease According to Age, Sex, and Symptoms[a,b]

Age, Years	Nonanginal chest pain (%)		Atypical angina (%)		Typical angina (%)	
	Men	Women	Men	Women	Men	Women
35–45	10.5 ± 6.3	2.7 ± 2.4	42.8 ± 14.4	15.5 ± 11.1	80.9 ± 10.4	45.4 ± 18.6
45–55	20.6 ± 9.0	6.9 ± 5.1	60.1 ± 12.9	31.7 ± 16	90.7 ± 4.9	67.7 ± 16.7
55–65	28.2 ± 1	12.7 ± 8.0	69 ± 10.6	46.5 ± 17.4	93.9 ± 2.9	83.9 ± 10.8
65–75	28.2 ± 10	17.1 ± 9.7	70 ± 1.3	54.1 ± 16.9	94.3 ± 2.6	94.7 ± 5.7

Source: Modified from Diamond GA: A clinically relevant classification of chest discomfort. *J Am Coll Cardiol* 1983; 1:574. Reproduced with permission from the author and the American College of Cardiology.
[a]Each value represents the percentage ± standard error of the percentage.
[b]Assessment of anginal symptoms: (a) Is chest pain substernal? (b) Is it precipitated by exertion? (c) Is it relieved within 10 min by rest or nitroglycerin? "Yes" to three questions = typical angina. "Yes" to two of three questions = atypical angina. "Yes" to one of three questions = nonanginal chest pain.

absence of myocardial infarction or persistent arrhythmias. Most patients with angina pectoris report prompt relief in less than 5 min after cessation of activity or with the use of sublingual nitroglycerin. Delayed relief of chest pain by nitroglycerin for over 15–20 min is inconsistent with the drug's rapid onset of action and may be ascribed to a placebo effect.

Carotid sinus massage by the physician will frequently relieve chest pain indicative of angina because of the reflex induction of a relative bradycardia and a decrease in systolic blood pressure, with consequent reduction of myocardial oxygen demand. Carotid sinus massage should be performed only in the absence of extracranial occlusive cerebrovascular disease as manifested by carotid bruits or decreased carotid arterial pulsations and with careful monitoring of the heart rate by auscultation. The Valsalva maneuver may relieve the pain as well, by decreasing myocardial wall tension secondary to the reduced venous return and left ventricular volume induced by the increase in intrathoracic pressure.

III. ASSOCIATED SYMPTOMS

Nausea, vomiting, faintness, fatigue, or diaphoresis often accompany severe episodes of myocardial ischemia. Patients with stable angina may have episodes of myocardial ischemia that are asymptomatic or silent. In addition, patients may then have episodes of myocardial ischemia that result in symptoms from either systolic or diastolic left ventricular dysfunction but are not associated with chest discomfort or symptoms characteristic of angina pectoris. As with other types of angina, *angina equivalent* symptoms are usually associated with exertion and are relieved by rest and nitroglycerin. The most common such symptoms are (a) exertional dyspnea, which is probably related to pulmonary venous hypertension resulting from ischemia-induced left ventricular diastolic dysfunction, and (b) exertional fatigue or exhaustion, likely to be caused by an acute decrease in cardiac output because of decreased left ventricular systolic function or associated mitral regurgitation from transient papillary muscle dysfunction.

A. Unstable Cardiac Chest Pain (Unstable Angina) Without ST-Segment Elevation

Cardiac chest pain is defined as unstable if it is new, occurs at rest, or changes in frequency or severity. It comprises a spectrum between stable angina and acute Q-wave myocardial infarction. Both unstable angina pectoris and non-Q-wave myocardial infarction share similar pathophysiological features, consisting of fixed atherosclerotic coronary artery disease with superimposed plaque rupture, platelet activation, and thrombus formation. Thus, the clinical presentations and treatment of each are similar. The distinction between the two probably depends on the extent and duration of compromised coronary blood flow and the presence or absence of collateral vessels. Differentiation may not be possible until sufficient time has elapsed to allow laboratory criteria of infarction to evolve and results of assays of cardiac enzymes have become available.

Recent guidelines from the Agency for Health Care Policy and Research define stratification of patients with unstable angina pectoris and will have a major impact upon decisions regarding hospitalization, angiography, and noninvasive testing. Once a diagnosis of unstable cardiac chest pain has been made, the patient should be stratified into a low, intermediate, or high-risk subgroup. Low-risk patients are defined as those with recent-onset angina (greater than 2 weeks), or increasing frequency, severity, or duration of angina with a normal or unchanged electrocardiogram (ECG). Such patients can usually be managed as outpatients. High-risk patients have at least one of the following features: prolonged chest pain, pulmonary edema, rest angina with dynamic ECG changes, a new or worsening murmur of mitral regurgitation, or hemodynamic instability. Such patients, and those with intermediate risk (i.e., manifesting a syndrome with severity of signs and symptoms between low and high risk), require immediate hospitalization and with cardiac monitoring to reduce mortality and prevent or limit myocardial necrosis. Initial therapy consists of bed rest, oxygen, and sedation. Subsequent therapy consists of aspirin, heparin, nitrates, beta blockers or calcium channel antagonists, and coronary revascularization (percutaneous or surgical). All high-risk patients should be evaluated early for the presence of precipitating factors such as anemia, hyperthyroidism, pulmonary disease with hypoxemia, infection, uncontrolled hypertension, arrhythmias, valvular heart disease, or hypertrophic cardiomyopathy.

IV. CARDIAC RISK FACTORS

No consideration of myocardial ischemia as a likely cause of chest discomfort is complete without careful deliberation of the context of known risk factors for coronary artery disease. Established independent coronary risk factors— including increasing age, male gender, hypercholesterolemia, cigarette smoking, diabetes, hypertension, and a family history of premature coronary artery disease— increase the likelihood of coronary artery stenosis. The probability of significant coronary artery stenosis increases markedly when the risk factors are present in addition to a history of chest pain consistent with angina pectoris.

V. DIFFERENTIAL DIAGNOSIS

Chest pain due to myocardial ischemia must be differentiated from chest pain attributable to other cardiac causes and chest pain of noncardiac etiology. Table 3 lists the differential diagnosis of chest pain according to major diagnostic categories.

Chest pain attributable to other cardiac diseases includes *ischemic chest pain not due to coronary atherosclerosis* or nonischemic chest pain resulting from pericarditis, aortic dissection, or mitral valve prolapse. In the first case, angina is attributable to hemodynamic changes associated with an inadequate myocardial oxygen supply in relation to a normal or increased myocardial oxygen demand. Cardiac causes include aortic valve stenosis, hypertrophic cardiomyopathy, and systemic arterial hypertension in which left ventricular systolic pressure and left ventricular wall tension are greatly increased or left ventricular hypertrophy is present. Chest pain attributable to myocardial ischemia also occurs with severe aortic regurgitation secondary to increased ventricular volumes, a resulting increase in myocardial oxygen demand, and a decrease in diastolic perfusion pressure in the coronary arteries. Occasionally, very severe anemia or hypoxia may produce myocardial ischemia caused by inadequate oxygen supply even in the absence of associated coronary artery disease.

Nonischemic chest pain of cardiac origin is usually attributable to pericarditis, aortic dissection, or mitral valve prolapse. The chest pain of *pericarditis* is most often sharp and penetrating in quality and relieved when the patient sits up and bends forward. The cardinal diagnostic feature of pericardial pain is its frequent worsening by changes in body position, with deep inspiration, and occasionally with swallowing. Radiation of the chest discomfort may involve the shoulders, upper back, and neck because of irritation of the diaphragmatic pleura, which is innervated through the phrenic nerve by fibers originating in cervical sympathetic ganglia C3 to C5. The chest pain associated with pericarditis is caused predominantly by parietal pleural irritation. A careful history and physical examination as well as noninvasive testing as indicated usually establish the correct diagnosis.

Table 3 Differential Diagnosis of Chest Pain

1. Angina pectoris/myocardial infarction
2. Other cardiovascular causes
   a. Likely ischemic in origin
      (1) Aortic stenosis
      (2) Hypertrophic cardiomyopathy
      (3) Severe systemic hypertension
      (4) Severe right ventricular hypertension
      (5) Aortic regurgitation
      (6) Severe anemia/hypoxia
   b. Nonischemic in origin
      (1) Aortic dissection
      (2) Pericarditis
      (3) Mitral valve prolapse
3. Gastrointestinal
   a. Esophageal spasm
   b. Esophageal reflux
   c. Esophageal rupture
   d. Peptic ulcer disease
4. Psychogenic
   a. Anxiety
   b. Depression
   c. Cardiac psychosis
   d. Secondary gain
   e. Chest wall pain
5. Neuromusculoskeletal
   a. Thoracic outlet syndrome
   b. Degenerative joint diseases of cervical/thoracic spine
   c. Costochondritis (Tietze's syndrome)
   d. Herpes zoster
6. Pulmonary
   a. Pulmonary embolus with or without pulmonary infarction
   b. Pneumothorax
   c. Pneumonia with pleural involvement
7. Pleurisy

Aortic dissection can be misdiagnosed as an acute myocardial infarction. Myocardial infarction is, of course, a recognized complication of aortic dissection. However the pain of dissection per se is usually of sudden onset compared with the pain of myocardial ischemia, which builds in intensity over time. Patients frequently characterize the pain of dissection as excruciating, the most severe discomfort that they have ever experienced, and tearing in quality. With the exception of patients with Marfan's syndrome or idiopathic cystic medial necrosis, most patients with aortic dissection will have a history of long-standing systemic arterial hypertension or its manifestation, evident on physical examination or by results of electrocardiography, chest radiography, or echocardiography.

Patients with *mitral valve prolapse* often present with atypical chest pain. In many, the pain appears to be phsychogenic in nature. In some, the chest discomfort reflects palpitations attributable to premature ventricular contractions. In most patients with mitral valve prolapse, myocardial perfusion imaging after exercise demonstrates no evidence of myocardial ischemia.

The major noncardiac etiologies of chest pain include phsychogenic causes of chest pain; chest pain caused by gastrointestinal tract disease; neuromuscular-skeletal causes of chest pain; and pulmonary causes of chest pain.

A. Psychogenic Causes of Chest Pain

Recurrent chest discomfort of psychogenic origin is often difficult to distinguish from angina pectoris, particularly in patients with multiple risk factors for coronary artery disease or in otherwise asymptomatic patients with well-documented coronary artery disease. Anxiety is the most common phychogenic cause. Although anxiety can coexist with and often aggravates chest pain attributable to myocardial ischemia, several characteristics of the pain help to differentiate the two. Psychogenic chest pain is often described as sharp or stabbing, commonly localized to the left inframammary area, and usually sharply circumscribed. Terms such as "stabbing" or "lighteninglike" may be used to describe extremely short (less than 1 min) episodes of pain. At times, the pain may persist for many hours or several days, in contrast to pain caused by myocardial ischemia, which characteristically persists for shorter periods of time. Psychogenic pain is usually not related to exercise. Often, nonvocal activities by the patient, such as a worried facial expression, retarded motor activity, and hand wringing may indicate an underlying depression. Observation of the patient during spontaneous or exercise-induced pain frequently suggests a psychogenic etiology. Often the pain is atypical, the patient's emotional response inappropriate, and no other evidence for myocardial ischemia apparent. Patients with anxiety often have multiple complaints such as breathlessness, giddiness, and palpitations. Associated symptoms, such as air hunger, circumoral paresthesias, globus hystericus, and multiple somatic complaints may suggest a neurasthenic personality or hyperventilation syndrome. Sometimes, voluntary forced hyperventilation will reproduce the chest pain complaint exactly.

Many patients with mitral valve prolapse have atypical chest discomfort and often complain of chronic fatigue as well. On careful physical examination (see Chapter 2), the presence of a midsystolic click or late systolic murmur indicates that the atypical chest pain may be related to the mitral valve prolapse leaflet syndrome.

B. Chest Pain Attributable to Gastrointestinal Disease

Pain originating from gastrointestinal tract disturbances, particularly that of esophageal origin, is commonly confused with angina pectoris. *Diffuse esophageal spasm*, a neuromuscular motor disorder of the esophagus causing chest pain, is the extracardiac condition that is most frequently misdiagnosed as symptomatic coronary artery disease. Esophageal spasm can occur at any age but is more common in individuals in the fifth decade. The pain is usually retrosternal; may be burning, squeezing, or aching in quality; and often radiates to the back, arms, and jaw. It usually begins during or after a meal and can last for minutes or hours. In some patients, the pain may be precipitated or worsened by exercise, and relief may be obtained with nitroglycerin, which also relaxes esophageal smooth muscle. Useful features distinguishing the pain of diffuse esophageal spasm are its frequent occurrence during swallowing, its association with dysphagia, and the associated regurgitation of gastric contents. Episodes of pain often are precipitated either by extremely hot or cold drinks or an emotional upset. The diagnosis of diffuse esophageal spasm is based on the history, the exclusion of cardiac and musculoskeletal causes of chest pain, and the demonstration of abnormal esophageal motility on cine-esophagrams or by esophageal manometry.

Reflux esophagitis results from mucosal irritation caused by lower esophageal sphincter dysfunction and the regurgitation of highly acidic gastric contents into the distal esophagus. The epigastric or retrosternal pain is usually burning in quality and is commonly initiated by the assumption of a recumbent position or by bending over. The "heartburn" and regurgitation often occur after meals, after the ingestion of coffee, or after postural changes. Patients may be awakened by the chest discomfort caused by acid reflux that occurs with the recumbent position. Affected patients are often obese and report relief of chest pain by food, antacids, and elevation of the head of the bed. Stricture formation secondary to long-standing esophageal reflux may cause dysphagia. A report of "heartburn" related to meals and posture and relieved with antacids suggests the correct diagnosis. An upper GI series may demonstrate hiatal hernia, but this finding is common and does not necessarily indicate the presence of esophagitis or esophageal reflux. Esophagoscopy and esophageal biopsy may demonstrate mucosal lesions and are useful for assessing the severity of inflammation and for excluding malignancy. Sphincter incompetence may be documented by the use of esophageal manometry. Esophageal acid perfusion testing (the Bernstein test) will often invoke the patient's usual symptoms, and distal esophageal pH monitoring will indicate gastroesophageal reflux.

Acute esophageal rupture, an often catastrophic event, causes severe retrosternal pain attributable to the chemical mediastinitis produced by acidic gastric contents. Spontaneous rupture may follow a prolonged bout of vomiting or retching after a heavy meal. Rupture occurs also as an iatrogenic complication of esophageal instrumentation. The pain varies in location depending on the site of rupture and position of the patient. Diagnosis is based on symptoms and signs of mediastinal air following vomiting or esophageal instrumentation.

C. Neuromuscular-Skeletal Causes of Chest Discomfort

Diseases affecting the neuromuscular-skeletal systems often produce pain distributed in dermatome patterns similar to those occurring with angina pectoris. In the *thoracic outlet syndromes,* diverse neural and vascular structures are compressed, producing discomfort or pain that sometimes resembles angina pectoris. Although pressure on the neurovascular bundle by a cervical rib or the scalenus anterior muscle may cause discomfort radiating to the head and neck, the shoulder region, or the axilla, most patients develop pain in the upper extremity secondary to somatic nerve compression, usually in the distribution of the ulnar nerve. The existence of associated paresthesias, presence of pain unrelated to physical exercise, and worsening of discomfort or its aggravation by assumption of certain body positions are useful differentiating features. The diagnosis of thoracic outlet syndrome can be confirmed in most patients by careful physical and neurological examination.

Tietze's syndrome, or *idiopathic costochondritis,* may cause anterior chest wall pain aggravated by movement and deep breathing. The initiation of the chest pain by direct pressure over the involved costochondral junction or its disappearance after local infiltration with lidocaine are helpful diagnostic maneuvers. *Degenerative arthritis* of the cervical and thoracic vertebrae may cause bandlike pain confined to the chest, neck, or back that often radiates to the arms. Because radiographic changes of degenerative arthritis affecting the cervical and thoracic vertebrae are often found in asymptomatic elderly patients, the production or exacerbation of pain by assumption of various postures, movement, sneezing, or coughing is more useful for attributing chest pain or arm discomfort to vertebral disease.

In its preeruptive stage, *herpes zoster* may cause bandlike chest pain over one or more dermatomes. Advanced age in the patient; additional symptoms of malaise, headache, and fever; the presence of hyperesthesia of the involved area on physical examination; and the subsequent eventual appearance of typical lesions 4 or 5 days after the beginning of symptoms will indicate the correct diagnosis.

Chest wall pain and tenderness may occur for unknown reasons. The discomfort may be reproduced by pressure over the painful area and by movements of the thorax such as bending, twisting, or turning. The variable duration of the pain and the lack of relief by nitroglycerin differentiate it from angina. Rarely, pectoral lymphadenopathy may be responsible.

D. Pulmonary Causes of Chest Pain

Acute massive *pulmonary embolism*, with its associated acute pulmonary hypertension and low cardiac output, may occasionally simulate acute myocardial infarction, and myocardial ischemia may be present in both conditions. The quality of chest pain may be identical to that observed in patients with acute coronary syndromes or may be pleuritic, as described below. However, the accompanying signs of severe dyspnea, tachypnea, and intense cyanosis—associated with considerable, profound anxiety and agitation—indicate a high likelihood of pulmonary embolism. Physical examination often reveals evidence of pulmonary hypertension, tricuspid regurgitation, and acute right heart failure.

The clinical setting may suggest the diagnosis because of the known increased incidence of pulmonary embolism occurring during long trips, in the postpartum or postoperative state, in patients with congestive heart failure and peripheral edema, and in those with deep vein thrombophlebitis. Arterial blood gases, pulmonary-perfusion ventilation scans, and, if needed, pulmonary arteriography will establish the correct diagnosis.

Other pulmonary conditions causing chest pain, such as *pneumothorax*, are rarely confused with symptomatic coronary artery disease because of characteristic clinical features. Spontaneous pneumothorax usually occurs in young, otherwise healthy males in the third and fourth decades. It is characterized by the abrupt onset of agonizing unilateral pleuritic chest pain associated with severe shortness of breath. the plain or expiratory chest radiograph provides the definitive diagnosis. The discomfort of *pleuritis* caused by pneumonia or pulmonary infarction is sharp, varies acutely with breathing, and is commonly accompanied by a reduced inspiratory effort. Associated signs of pulmonary parenchymal infection or infarction—such as fever, cough and sputum production, or hemoptysis—usually indicate the underlying diagnosis.

VI. CHEST PAIN: PHYSICAL FINDINGS IN PATIENTS WITH ANGINA PECTORIS AND CONDITIONS SIMULATING IT

The physical examination is often entirely normal in patents presenting because of angina pectoris. This is particularly true when the patient is examined between episodes of chest discomfort. The physical examination may indicate the presence of predisposing risk factors for coronary artery disease such as hypertension, diabetes, or hyperlipidemia (xanthomata), or it may indicate other evidence of cardiac disease such as the presence of congestive heart failure or the likelihood of a prior myocardial infarction.

At times, the clinical evaluation will suggest a noncardiac origin of chest pain. For example, diffuse wall tenderness or tenderness over a specific costochondral junction indicates a likely neuromusculoskeletal etiology of chest pain, as do zones of hyperesthesia over the dermatome areas affected by disease of the cervical or thoracic vertebrae. Physical findings of pulmonary consolidation or pulmonary infarction suggest the possibility of recurrent pulmonary emboli, as does evidence of thrombophlebitis. During inspiration, a pleural friction is often associated with characteristic chest pain confined to the area with positive physical findings.

In patients with chest pain not attributable to coronary atherosclerosis, the presence of a two- or three-component pericardial friction rub indicates the likely diagnosis of pericarditis. Unequal arterial pulses and different blood pressures in the two arms suggest the possibility of aortic dissection.

The most common physical findings in patients with angina pectoris, including those without a previous myocardial infarction, is a fourth heart sound or presystolic low-pitched gallop sound heard best over the apex of the left ventricle with the patient on his or her left side during auscultation with the bell piece of the stethoscope. In patients with sinus rhythm this finding is present at rest or with handgrip exercise in a high percentage of patients with ischemic heart disease. An accentuated systolic impulse at the apex or along the left sternal border frequently indicates regional wall motion abnormality from a previous myocardial infarction. Bibasilar pulmonary rales with or without evidence of pleural effusion indicate the likelihood of pulmonary congestion due to heart failure.

The physical examination of the patient during an episode of angina may reveal clues to the diagnosis that were not present in the absence of the chest discomfort (Table 4). However, the physical examination conducted while the patient is experiencing pain is often normal in patients in the absence of a previous myocardial infarction. During an episode of angina, the systolic and diastolic blood pressures are often significantly elevated; occasionally, hypotension results when the ischemia is extensive. A mild tachycardia is often present, but bradycardias may appear instead. Abnormal systolic bulges (indicative of dyskinesis) may be present at the apex or ectopic precordial areas. The presence of a new fourth or

Table 4 Clinical Findings During Chest Pain Due to Myocardial Ischemia

Increase or marked decrease in systolic blood pressure
Relative tachycardia or bradyarrhythmia
Palpable left ventricular asynergy
New S_4 or S_3 heart sounds
Reversed splitting of S_2 heart sound
Murmur of papillary muscle dysfunction
Bibasilar pulmonary rales

third heart sound associated with pain, reverse splitting of the second sound, a murmur of mitral regurgitation, or bibasilar pulmonary rales suggests that angina pectoris is the correct diagnosis.

VII. ELECTROCARDIOGRAPHY

The resting ECG is normal in 25–50% of patients with stable angina. Evidence of prior myocardial infarction or the ST-T–wave changes of myocardial ischemia increase suspicion that a patient's chest pain is angina pectoris. The presence of arrhythmias on the resting ECG—such as atrial fibrillation or ventricular tachyarrhythmias—increase the likelihood of underlying coronary artery disease, as do ECGs demonstrating atrioventricular block or bundle branch block. Evidence of left ventricular hypertrophy increases the probability of a cardiac source for the chest discomfort.

An ECG attained while chest pain is present reveals ischemic changes in approximately 50% of patients with a normal resting ECG. ST-segment elevation or depression establishes a high likelihood of angina and indicates ischemia at a low workload, portending a poorer prognosis. Most such patients need no further noninvasive cardiac testing. Coronary arteriography defines the severity of coronary stenoses and the desirability of myocardial revascularization. The induction of tachyarrhythmias, atrioventricular block, or bundle branch block concomitantly with chest pain increases the probability of ischemic heart disease as well and usually leads to coronary arteriography.

VIII. CHEST RADIOGRAPHY

The chest roentgenogram is often normal in patients with stable angina pectoris. It is more likely to be abnormal in patients with previous or acute myocardial infarction, those with a non–coronary artery cause of cardiac chest pain, and those with noncardiac chest discomfort. Cardiac enlargement may be attributable to previous myocardial infarction, acute left ventricular failure, pericardial effusion, or chronic volume overload of the left ventricle (aortic regurgitation, mitral regurgitation). Abnormal physical findings, associated chest x-ray findings (e.g., pulmonary venous congestion), and abnormalities with noninvasive testing (echocardiography) usually indicate the correct etiology. Coronary artery calcification increases the likelihood of symptomatic coronary artery disease.

Enlargement of the upper mediastinum often results from an ascending aortic aneurysm with or without dissection. Pruning or cutoffs of the pulmonary arteries or areas of segmental oligemia may indicate pulmonary infarction/embolism. A chest x-ray may provide evidence of previous cardiac surgery, including sternal markers, coronary vein bypass graft markers, pacemaker leads, and valvular prostheses.

IX. ADDITIONAL INITIAL TESTS LIKELY TO BE HELPFUL IN PATIENTS WITH CHEST PAIN

Patients with unstable or prolonged chest discomfort should undergo measurement of activity in blood of specific cardiac enzymes, such as MB creatine kinase, to determine whether or not myocardial necrosis is present. Other early markers of myocardial necrosis such as plasma MB or MM creatine kinase isoforms and troponin T or I are measured in some laboratories. Enzymes such as aspartate transaminase (AST; previously called serum glutamic-oxaloacetic transaminase, or SGOT) or lactate dehydrogenase (LDH) and its isoenzymes are less specific. Arterial blood gases should be obtained in patients who appear to be hypoxic or at high risk of pulmonary embolism as the cause of chest discomfort.

In the emergency room assessment of patients presenting with chest pain that may be attributable to myocardial ischemia, various algorithms are used in an effort to "rule out" acute myocardial infarction at the earliest time possible. In addition to serial ECGs and isoenzyme measurements, two-dimensional (2D) echocardiography is useful for the detection or exclusion of regional wall motion abnormalities. Myocardial perfusion imaging with thallium or technetium sestamibi can determine the presence or absence of a myocardial perfusion defect. Ready access to a catheterization laboratory is available at some facilities, with diagnostic coronary arteriography being performed when clinical suspicion of early infarction is high and the ECG is normal or nondiagnostic. However, if the clinical suspicion of infarction is high, negative test results at any single time cannot and should not be the basis for exclusion of the diagnosis. Sequential evaluation is essential.

X. NONINVASIVE TESTING FOR DETECTION OF MYOCARDIAL ISCHEMIA

Most special tests in patients with suspected angina pectoris are performed either to establish the diagnosis or to obtain prognostic information. In general, men with a history of classic angina pectoris have a higher probability of having significant coronary artery disease recognized by coronary arteriography than do women. The gender difference is even greater for patients with atypical angina pectoris. Table 2 in this chapter outlines the likelihood for each gender by age and characteristics of the chest discomfort. It also illustrates one reason why women have more false-positive responses to ECG exercise testing than do men. Bayes' theorem states that the pretest prevalence of disease influences the posttest likelihood of significant disease. A nondiagnostic test for myocardial ischemia may be of limited *additional diagnostic value* in patients with either a very high or very low pretest risk for coronary artery disease. On the other hand, an exercise test may give *important prognostic information*, and nuclear scintigraphy or echocardiography may provide valuable information about the functional aspects of the coronary circulation. For example, a 55-year-old man with hypertension and a family history of premature coronary artery disease who has chest pain at rest that is typical of angina pectoris and is associated with ECG ST-T–wave depression needs no further testing before initiation of treatment and referral for coronary arteriography. If the same patient had atypical chest pain, no associated cardiac risk factors, and a normal ECG at the time of chest discomfort, noninvasive testing for myocardial ischemia might provide important information regarding the likelihood of the presence or absence of important coronary artery disease and the need for coronary arteriography.

Noninvasive tests for detecting myocardial ischemia are based on documenting myocardial ischemia at a time when myocardial oxygen demand is increased by exercise, pacing-induced tachycardia, or administration of drugs that either cause coronary artery vasodilation or increase myocardial contractility (Table 5). The usefulness of such tests depends upon the patient population considered, the sensitivity and specificity of the test used, the accuracy of the laboratory performing the test, and the resources available.

A. Exercise Electrocardiography

Exercise electrocardiography is the most commonly used test for obtaining objective evidence of myocardial ischemia and determining the probability of important coronary artery disease. It is performed also to obtain prognostic information regarding ventricular function in patients with known coronary artery disease. The sensitivity and specificity of exercise ECG testing are 55–70% and 85–90% respectively. The sensitivity and specificity in diverse reports varies depending upon the patient population; whether the patient had an abnormal resting electrocardiogram; whether single-, two-vessel, or more extensive coronary artery stenoses were considered to make up a positive arteriographic result; and whether the patient was able to obtain at least 85% of the age-predicted heart rate during exercise. Additional important indications of coronary disease include the devel-

Table 5 Detection of Myocardial Ischemia

Methods
    Electrocardiography
    Myocardial perfusion imaging (thallium-201, technetium sestamibi)
    Assessment of wall motion (echocardiography, radionuclide ventriculography)
Stress testing
    Exercise
    Coronary vasodilators (dipyridamole, adenosine)
    Positive inotropes (dobutamine)
    Pacing

opment of symptoms or new physical findings (bibasilar rales, S_4 sound) during exercise testing, a lack of the normal increase in systolic blood pressure, and symptom system-limited duration of the exercise.

Exercise ECG testing is of greatest *diagnostic value* in the assessment of middle-aged men with atypical angina pectoris and a pretest likelihood of significant coronary artery disease of 30–70%. Results of exercise ECG testing for diagnosis are somewhat more ambiguous and hence controversial in women with typical or atypical angina; men with atypical chest pain and complete right bundle branch block; apparently healthy men more than 40 years old in special occupations; and asymptomatic men with two or more major risk factors for coronary disease. Exercise ECG testing for diagnostic purposes is not indicated in asymptomatic men and women who are apparently healthy or who have chest pain that is definitely due to another cause.

The *prognostic significance* of exercise testing has been well documented. In the normotensive patient with a normal resting ECG who can achieve the target heart rate, positive ECG results and physical findings during exercise testing often indicate significant left main coronary artery disease, severe three-vessel coronary artery disease or extensive two-vessel disease with severe stenosis of the proximal left anterior descending, particularly when the coronary artery stenoses are associated with depressed left ventricular systolic function. Patients with ECG ST-segment depression at low workloads (< 5 METS), in five or more ECG leads or ST-segment depression persisting for several minutes after the cessation of exercise have a worse prognosis than do individuals with transient ST-segment depression obtained only at high levels of exercise and confined to one or two ECG leads. A negative ECG stress test performed to near maximum exercise is associated with an excellent long-term prognosis.

B. Ambulatory ECG Recordings

Ambulatory ECG (Holter) recordings for 24 or 48 hr are less sensitive than ECG recordings during exercise for detecting myocardial ischemia. Although ambulatory ECG recordings may provide evidence of ST-segment depression attributable to ischemia in one or more ECG leads in patients who at the time are not having symptoms, the presence of such "asymptomatic" or "silent" myocardial ischemia is seen primarily in patients who have positive ECG exercise tests, particularly if they are being assessed for angina pectoris. Except in patients with variant or Prinzmetal's angina attributable to coronary artery spasm, the ambulatory ECG recording is *not* a diagnostic procedure of choice for assessing the probability of coronary artery stenosis as the cause of chest pain. The advent of pharmacological stress combined with the noninvasive assessment of regional left ventricular function or myocardial perfusion imaging has minimized the usefulness of ambulatory ECG recordings for the diagnosis of angina pectoris in patients unable to perform sufficient exercise.

C. Stress Myocardial Perfusion Scintigraphy

Although more expensive, exercise myocardial perfusion (thallium 201) images obtained early after exercise and 3 hr later provide greater sensitivity and specificity for the diagnosis of coronary artery disease than exercise ECG testing. Accuracy may be less dependent upon the level of exercise achieved. Some of the findings that indicate a poor prognosis include increased thallium-201 intake in the lung, extensive myocardial perfusion defects, and postexercise transient left ventricular dilation. In general, normal thallium-201 rest and redistribution perfusion scans indicate a probability of the patient experiencing a cardiac event similar to that in the general population, even if the patient has known coronary artery disease.

Pharmacological stress testing—usually with dipyridamole, adenosine, or dobutamine—and thallium 201 can be used in patients unable to exercise because of peripheral vascular disease, poor exercise tolerance, arthritis, neurological disorders, or other limitations or contraindications. Stress scintigraphy is useful in the evaluation of selected patients with chronic stable angina, those with suspected coronary artery disease before noncardiac surgery, and those who have sustained acute myocardial infarction. The use of technetium-99m sestamibi and other recently introduced agents may significantly improve imaging capabilities but requires two injections of isotope, one during exercise and the other at rest.

D. Positron Emission Tomography

Positron emission tomography (PET) imaging is not available in most institutions. However, it has been useful for the assessment of myocardial viability and can identify segments of myocardium distal to severe coronary artery stenoses with limited coronary blood flow but persistent myocardial viability reflected by metabolic activity. It provides a quantitative estimate of coronary blood flow and coronary flow reserve as well as myocardial viability.

Patients with stable angina may have persistent defects in 3-hr redistribution images obtained with thallium 201. As many as 30–40% of such patients may exhibit improved perfusion and function after revascularization. Although the use of PET is not recommended as an initial test for the detection of myocardial ischemia in patients with chest pain likely to be due to coronary artery disease, its value in determining which patients with known coronary artery disease are likely to benefit from myocardial revascularization has been well demonstrated, particularly in patients with markedly depressed left ventricular systolic function.

E. Radionuclide Ventriculography

Radionuclide ventriculography (RVG) with determination of peak exercise left ventricular ejection fraction has been used to detect coronary artery disease. The results are more specific for coronary disease when the presence of stress-induced regional left ventricular wall motion abnormalities is demonstrated with bicycle egrometry. The presence of irregular heart rhythms, left bundle branch block, or marked left ventricular dysfunction limits the diagnostic value of RVG.

F. Stress Echocardiography

Two dimensional echocardiography at the time of exercise or pharmacological stress (dobutamine) is useful for the detection of new or worsening regions of segmental systolic wall motion as indicators of myocardial ischemia. The sensitivity and specificity of exercise and dobutamine echocardiography are similar to those of thallium redistribution imaging in the large majority of patients with chronic stable angina in whom good echocardiographic recordings can be obtained before, and during, or immediately after stress.

Doppler echocardiography—transmitral valve velocity recordings—have been used before and after stress to detect the presence of abnormalities in diastolic left ventricular compliance due to myocardial ischemia. Specificity of abnormal test results remains controversial.

G. Coronary Arteriography

Not all patients with coronary artery stenosis have myocardial ischemia resulting from the stenosis. Other cardiac disorders may result in a disparity between myocardial oxygen demand and supply and therefore myocardial ischemia. Not every patient with "possible angina pectoris" needs coronary arteriography, particularly if the pretest likelihood of significant coronary disease is extremely low and the patient has no evidence of myocardial ischemia with noninvasive testing despite adequate stress.

Whether or not all patients with stable angina pectoris should undergo coronary arteriography remains controversial. Arteriography is certainly useful for all patients with angina pectoris at a low workload, those with evidence of extensive myocardial ischemia shown by noninvasive testing, and those with associated moderate to severe left ventricular systolic dysfunction. Some cardiologists recommend cardiac catheterization and coronary arteriography routinely to estimate left ventricular regional and generalized wall motion and evaluate the extent and location of coronary artery disease. Others are more selective and obtain coronary arteriograms only if the diagnosis is in question or if revascularization by coronary artery bypass surgery or coronary angioplasty is contemplated. In general, patients whose symptoms are well controlled by medication; who, with treatment, no longer exhibit noninvasive criteria of myocardial ischemia; and who demonstrate a good exercise tolerance are less likely to benefit significantly from revascularization. Other factors such as patient's age, comorbidity, and desired lifestyle must be considered as well as the response to medical therapy.

Unstable Angina
with ST-Segment Elevation

Paul R. Eisenberg

XI. GENERAL PRINCIPLES

Documentation of ST-segment elevation in a patient presenting with unstable chest pain mandates rapid evaluation to determine whether immediate intervention for an evolving acute myocardial infarction is necessary. Chest discomfort lasting longer than 30 min that does not respond to treatment with sublingual nitroglycerin suggests the diagnosis of acute infarction. Often, chest discomfort is associated with dyspnea, diaphoresis, and, less frequently, nausea with or without vomiting. Atypical clinical presentations of acute infarction, such as epigastric discomfort or atypical chest, neck, or upper extremity discomfort can usually be clarified by prompt evaluation with an ECG.

Acute myocardial infarction can usually be differentiated from pericarditis, coronary vasospasm, myocarditis, or ST-segment changes due to other causes on the basis of the history, a prompt yet thorough physical examination, and serial ECGs.

Posterior wall infarction in patients who present with anterior precordial lead ST-segment depression (i.e., V_1–V_3) must be recognized. Posterior wall infarction can often be distinguished from ST-segment depression secondary to anterior wall ischemia on the basis of electrocardiographic criteria, including the presence of associated ST-segment elevation in inferior limb leads (i.e., II, III, aV_F), tall, upright T waves in association with anterior ST-segment depression, and tall and slightly widened R waves in V_1 and V_2. If necessary, immediate echocardiography may help in distinguishing posterior infarction from anterior ischemia.

Once the diagnosis of myocardial infarction has been established, recanalization of the infarct-related artery with fibrinolytic agents or primary angioplasty should be initiated rapidly.

XII. CLINICAL PRESENTATIONS ASSOCIATED WITH ST-SEGMENT ELEVATION NOT CAUSED BY MYOCARDIAL INFARCTION

A. Coronary Vasospasm

Although patients with coronary vasospasm may present with chest discomfort at rest, many have exertional symptoms as well. A distinguishing feature compared with unstable angina is the lack of an acceleration in the pattern of chest discomfort. Although most episodes resolve spontaneously, chest discomfort may be prolonged and associated with myocardial infarction or arrhythmias. Electrocardiograms obtained while chest discomfort is present demonstrate ST-segment elevation that may mimic changes with acute myocardial infarction. However, coronary vasospasm generally responds to sublingual nitroglycerin, with resolution of ST-segment elevation and chest pain. Thus, in patients with vasospasm, the lack of evolution of Q waves, and chest discomfort that responds to nitrates, serial ECGs are of value to document resolution of ST-segment elevation. Typically, patients with coronary vasospasm have minimal obstructive atherosclerotic coronary disease; in some cases, angiograms are interpreted as normal. Nonetheless, abnormal vasomotor reactivity can often be demonstrated with provocative testing with pharmacological agents such as ergonovine maleate or acetylcholine.

Episodes of chest pain caused by coronary vasospasm can usually be managed with sublingual nitrates. Refractory or recurrent coronary vasospasm should be managed with intravenous nitrates and calcium channel blocking agents. Long-acting nitrates or calcium channel antagonists effectively reduce the frequency of episodes of chest pain in patients with coronary vasospasm.

In some patients with acute coronary thrombosis, coronary vasospasm may be present as well. It can be responsive to nitrates in this setting. If so, ST-segment elevation may decrease following administration of sublingual nitroglycerin. However, only rarely is the resolution of ST-segment elevation complete, as it is in patients with coronary vasospasm. Immediate recanalization is indicated in such patients unless resolution of ST-segment elevation is complete.

B. Pericarditis

Chest pain associated with pericarditis may be relatively acute in onset and prolonged, mimicking the pain of an acute myocardial infarction. Distinguishing features include exacerbation of pain in the supine position with relief when the patient is upright or leaning forward. Occasionally, the pain of pericarditis is pleuritic in nature, but it is only infrequently associated with marked dyspnea. The electrocardiogram often shows diffuse ST-segment elevation with flat depression of the PR segment. Detection of a pericardial friction rub is often the initial key to the diagnosis of pericarditis. Pericarditis may complicate an acute myocardial infarction occurring 24 hr or more earlier. If so, ST-segment elevation and new Q waves may appear on the ECG and a pericardial friction rub may become audible.

C. Myocarditis

Unstable chest discomfort, dyspnea, diaphoresis, and ECG features mimicking those of acute myocardial infarction may occur in patients with myocarditis. This diagnosis should be suspected particularly in patients less than 30 years of age who present with unstable chest discomfort and ST-segment elevation, especially if drug abuse with agents that induce coronary spasm, such as amphetamines or cocaine, can be excluded. Immediate echocardiography may be of value in differentiating acute myocardial infarction from acute myocarditis that is typically manifest by global left and/or right ventricular dysfunction, although only focal wall motion abnormalities may be present. Elevation of cardiac enzymes in plasma occurs with myocarditis. Diagnosis often requires myocardial biopsy and demonstration of lack of coronary artery disease by coronary angiography.

D. Unstable Chest Discomfort in Patients with History of Drug Abuse

The need for evaluation of chest discomfort in patients who have abused drugs is increasing. Electrocardiographic findings of ST-segment elevation indicative of early repolarization rather than acute infarction are frequent, particularly in young, inner-city black males. The most common presentation is acute chest discomfort several hours after cocaine use, especially inhalation of crack cocaine; this occurs in some patients as late as 24 to 48 hr after the last use or exposure. When typical ST-segment elevation and tall, peaked, symmetrical T waves (i.e., hyperacute T waves) are present, acute myocardial infarction is usually the cause. Although chest discomfort may decrease in response to nitrates, coronary thrombolysis or coronary angioplasty are needed in patients with evolving infarction. Immediate echocardiography or coronary angiography may be necessary when the ECG is not conclusive.

E. Pulmonary Embolism

Infrequently, patients with acute pulmonary embolism present with unstable chest discomfort, dyspnea, and an ECG pattern of ST-segment elevation, often in the inferior leads and occasionally in leads V_1 and V_2. A history of pleuritic chest discomfort and sudden onset of dyspnea suggests the diagnosis of pulmonary embolism. An increased alveolar-to-arterial oxygen gradient recognized by arterial blood gas measurements associated with clear lung fields on chest examination and a lack of pulmonary infiltrates on the chest x-ray suggest pulmonary embolism. The diagnosis may be particularly difficult in patients with hemodynamic instability. Uncertainty can often be reduced by acquiring a careful history of risk factors likely to predispose to acute pulmonary embolism, such as immobility, malignancy, use of birth control pills, or a previous history of venous thromboembolic disease. Immediate echocardiography may be of value in demonstrating right ventricular dilatation. However, dilatation must be distinguished from that seen when inferior wall infarction is accompanied by right ventricular infarction. Perfusion and ventilation scintigraphy is often helpful in establishing the diagnosis.

XIII. INITIAL EVALUATION AND MANAGEMENT OF PATIENTS WITH MYOCARDIAL INFARCTION AND ST-SEGMENT ELEVATION

Patients who present with accelerating or prolonged chest pain should be evaluated rapidly with an ECG. Initial management is directed to reducing symptoms, establishing venous access for drug administration, and determining whether the patient is a candidate for treatment with either fibrinolytic agents or primary angioplasty. In critically ill patients, treatment of hypo- or hypertension, pulmonary edema, or life-threatening ventricular arrhythmias may be necessary first. Accordingly, initial management should proceed as follows:

1.   After assessment of blood pressure and pulse, 0.4 mg sublingual nitroglycerin should be given to patients with systolic blood pressure greater than 100 mmHg and repeated every 5 min up to three doses if symptoms persist. Intravenous saline should be administered in patients with borderline low blood pressure or if blood pressure decreases in response to intravenous nitrates. Hypotension in response to nitroglycerin may be a particular problem in patients with inferior wall myocardial infarction and right ventricular involvement. Therefore, when right ventricular involvement is suspected on the basis of either physical signs (e.g., elevation of the jugular venous pulsation) or electrocardiographic criteria (e.g., ST-segment elevation lead V_{4R}) and blood pressure is low, saline should be administered promptly and nitrates used cautiously if at all.

Pain associated with acute myocardial infarction is rarely relieved or markedly improved by administration of sublingual nitroglycerin. Therefore, intravenous morphine sulfate at doses of 2–4 mg should be given every 5–10 min until chest pain is relieved. In addition to its analgesic effects, morphine decreases anxiety and modestly decreases preload by inducing venodilatation. It is the drug of choice for the initial management of acute pulmonary edema. Ultimately, the best treatment for chest pain is prompt coronary recanalization with either fibrinolytic agents or primary angioplasty.

2.   Intravenous access, preferably with two 21-gauge or larger intravenous catheters, should be established rapidly in all patients presenting with unstable chest pain and ST-segment elevation. Oxygen should be administered at 2–4 L/min by nasal cannula, even in patients without obvious respiratory distress. In patients in respiratory distress, oxygen should be administered by face mask at concentrations of 60–100%. Patients in severe respiratory distress should be intubated promptly and ventilated mechanically to reduce the work of breathing. Arterial blood gas measurements should be deferred in patients who are candidates for thrombolytic agents, particularly when oxygenation can be monitored transcutaneously. Continuous ECG monitoring should be established, preferably with a defibrillator in close proximity to the patient.

3.   Hemodynamic stability should be assessed frequently by measurement

of the blood pressure and observing the general appearance of the patient. Obtundation or confusion, poor peripheral perfusion, or cyanosis often indicates the presence of cardiogenic shock. Respiratory distress suggests pulmonary edema, usually secondary to extensive left ventricular dysfunction or acute mitral regurgitation. A rapid evaluation of central and peripheral pulses should be performed to detect potential inequalities suggesting aortic dissection or poor perfusion that might limit acquisition of arterial access needed for invasive procedures. The chest examination should identify inspiratory crackles suggestive of pulmonary edema, bronchospasm, or inequality of breath sounds. The cardiovascular examination should include palpation of the heart to identify cardiomegaly and dyskinesis consistent with left ventricular dysfunction. Often, in patients with acute myocardial infarction, the palpable maximal impulse will be difficult to feel or localize because of anterior wall hypokinesis. The jugular venous pulse should be assessed. In patients with inferior wall infarction, its elevation will often be indicative of right ventricular infarction. Auscultation will generally detect an S_4 gallop in patients with acute myocardial infarction. An S_3 gallop implies considerable left ventricular dysfunction. An S_3 is unlikely unless the heart rate exceeds 100 beats/min. The intensity of the gallop should be noted on both inspiration and expiration; increases in the intensity of an S_4 or S_3 gallop with inspiration suggest right-sided pathology (e.g., right ventricular infarction, acute pulmonary embolism). The presence of murmurs and their quality and radiation should be delineated. (See Chapter 12, on myocardial infarction, for a discussion of the management of specific valvular problems in such patients.)

The abdominal examination should be brief but thorough. Acute cholecystitis can mimic acute myocardial infarction.

Examination of the extremities should focus on the potential presence of peripheral edema (suggesting chronic left ventricular dysfunction), clubbing (suggesting chronic pulmonary disease), and cyanosis. In patients with a questionable history of peptic ulcer disease or gastrointestinal bleeding, a rectal examination and assay of stool for occult blood should be performed before administering antithrombotic or thrombolytic agents. The objective of the initial physical assessment is to define overall stability of the patient, exclude causes of chest discomfort and ST-segment elevation other than acute myocardial infarction, and acquire the information needed for the selection of initial definitive treatment as rapidly as possible.

XIV. REPERFUSION IN PATIENTS WITH ACUTE MYOCARDIAL INFARCTION AND ST-SEGMENT ELEVATION

Immediate initiation of therapy to induce myocardial reperfusion should be considered in all patients who present within the first hours of myocardial infarction.

Accordingly, once the patient has been stabilized hemodynamically and sufficient information is available to establish the diagnosis of acute infarction with ST-segment elevation, additional history should be obtained immediately to determine whether contraindications to thrombolysis exist. Absolute contraindications are active bleeding, recent major trauma or invasive procedures, and specific risk factors for intracerebral hemorrhage (see Table 6). In patients with absolute contraindications to thrombolysis, primary angioplasty should be performed whenever possible. In patients with relative contraindications to thrombolysis, the decision to treat with fibrinolytic agents as opposed to primary angioplasty should be based on the extent of infarction, the potential for complications accompanying primary angioplasty, and the potential risk of bleeding with thrombolysis as opposed to the extent of delay, the disadvantages of the anticipated late restenosis (approximately 40%) associated with primary angioplasty. Ideally, coronary recanalization should be initiated as promptly as possible and certainly within 60 min following presentation of a patient with acute myocardial infarction. In general, the best current approach to accomplish this objective is treatment with front-loaded tissue plasminogen activator (t-PA) with immediate conjunctive anticoagulation and aspirin (see Table 6 for drug dose) or primary angioplasty if thrombolysis is contraindicated.

XV. SELECTION OF PATIENTS

A. Timing of Reperfusion

The benefits of reperfusion are directly related to the rapidity and extent to which infarct-related artery patency is induced. Myocardial salvage is greatest when reperfusion occurs within 4–6 hr of the onset of symptoms, ideally within the first 1–2 hr. Results of recent studies indicate that front-loaded infusions of t-PA (accelerated dose regimen in Table 6) induce reperfusion rapidly, resulting in a lower mortality compared with administration of intravenous streptokinase (see Table 1 for dose) in patients treated within the first 6 hr after the onset of symptoms. Primary angioplasty performed in the same time frame is associated with a high rate of patency and should result in a similar survival benefit.

Some patients who present more than 6 hr after the onset of symptoms may benefit from reperfusion. Treatment with a 3-hr infusion of t-PA has been shown to be associated with improved survival in patients treated between 6 and 12 hr after the onset of symptoms. Benefit may reflect misclassification of the actual time of onset of infarction in some patients, stuttering infarction with prolonged viability of some jeopardized myocardium in others, and advantages of a patent vessel independent of myocardial salvage in others. Regardless, benefit is quantitatively much greater with early compared with later reperfusion. The benefits of reperfusion between 12 and 24 hr after onset of pain are dubious. However, it is

Table 6 Dosage Regimens of Fibrinolytic Agents for Treatment of Myocardial Infarction

Streptokinase	1.5 million units IV over 60 min
Anistreplase	30-U IV bolus over 2 min
Alteplase	100 mg IV over 3 hr, given as initial 6-mg bolus followed by 60 mg over 1 hr and then 40 mg over 2 hr
	"Accelerated dose regimen": 100 mg over 90 min given as 15-mg bolus, followed by 0.75 mg/kg (up to 50 mg) IV over 30 min, and then 0.5 mg/kg (up to 35 mg) IV over 60 min[a]
	An investigational double-bolus regimen (50 mg twice separated by a 30-min interval) is promising but not yet extensively studied or approved by the FDA

[a]Extensively tested but not approved by the FDA.

reasonable to consider treatment with either fibrinolytic agents or coronary angioplasty in patients with ongoing chest pain after 12 hr, particularly when ST-segment elevation persists and Q waves have not evolved (presumably all indicative of persistently viable but jeopardized myocardium). Patients with extensive infarction complicated by cardiogenic shock or marked hemodynamic instability should be treated with primary angioplasty.

B. Age-Related Risk-Versus-Benefit of Different Strategies

Mortality in patients with acute myocardial infarction increases dramatically with age above 70 years and is reduced in all age groups by treatment with fibrinolytic agents. Accordingly, no absolute age-related restriction applies to the use of thrombolytic therapy. However, older patients are at higher risk for intracerebral hemorrhage. Therefore, in selected patients, primary angioplasty may be preferred to thrombolysis if both can be accomplished in the same time frame. Both thrombolysis and angioplasty may be deferred in patients with a small, uncomplicated myocardial infarction who have relative contraindications to treatment with either or both modalities.

C. Treatment of Patients with Hypertension

Patients who present with marked hypertension (e.g., diastolic blood pressure $\geq$ 110 mmHg) often have a considerable decrease in blood pressure after initial treatment with nitrates and morphine. Such patients are candidates for thrombolytic therapy and should be treated promptly. Patients with a history of marked and long-term hypertension are at greater risk for intracerebral hemorrhage with thrombolytic agents and can be referred for primary angioplasty when facilities are available. It is probably the hypertensive vascular disease rather than the hypertension per se that is the determinant of increased risk in most instances. Therefore, the selection of a strategy in patients with persistent and marked hypertension should be dictated in part by the rapidity with which primary angioplasty can be accomplished.

Patients with long-term hypertension should be treated with intravenous beta-blocking agents as well as a fibrinolytic drug in the absence of contraindications (see Table 7). Intravenous nitroglycerin or intravenous nitroprusside can be used in patients whose conditions are refractory to beta blockers and those with contraindications to their use. Arterial vasodilators (e.g., hydralazine, dihydropyridine, other calcium channel antagonists) should be avoided because of the potential to induce reflex tachycardia and precipitous hypotension.

D. Thrombolytic Therapy Compared with Primary Angioplasty

Long-term improvements in left ventricular function and improved survival are dependent on induction of a patent infarct-related artery within 90 min of initiation

Table 7 Contraindications to Thrombolytic Therapy

Absolute contraindications
Active bleeding
Major trauma, particularly head trauma (within 6 weeks)
Invasive procedure or surgery (within 10 days)
Neurosurgical procedure (within 2 months)
History of cerebral tumor, aneurysm, arteriovenous malformation (AVM) or intracerebral hemorrhage
Stroke or transient ischemic attack (TIA) (within 6 months)
Suspected aortic dissection
Known bleeding disorder
Active cavitary lung disease
Pregnancy
Previous treatment with streptokinase or anistreplase (a contraindicator only for use of the same two agents)
Relative contraindications
Systolic blood pressure $\geq$ 180 mmHg, especially if the hypertension has been prolonged
Diastolic blood pressure $\geq$ 100 mmHg, especially if the hypertension has been prolonged
Current treatment with anticoagulants
Stroke or TIA (within 6 months)
Hemorrhagic diabetic retinopathy or history of intraocular bleeding
Brief cardiopulmonary resuscitation (CPR) of $\leq$ 10 min duration
Severe renal or liver disease
Hypermenorrhea
Bacterial endocarditis

of treatment in patients who present within 6 hr of the onset of symptoms of acute myocardial infarction. Large-scale studies have demonstrated the success of coronary thrombolysis in conferring benefit. Primary angioplasty may provide similar benefits with a lower risk of intracerebral bleeding. Thus, it is a reasonable alternative when patency of the infarct artery can be induced within 90 min after the onset of chest pain in institutions with skilled operators. Late restenosis, occurring in as many as 40% of patients, is a limitation. Facilities should be available for immediate surgery should angioplasty be technically not feasible or should it fail. In patients with absolute contraindications to coronary thrombolysis, primary angioplasty should be performed as rapidly as possible, even if referral to another institution is necessary. Primary angioplasty may be preferable to thrombolysis in patients who present with pulmonary edema, cardiogenic shock, previous coronary surgery, or acute severe mitral regurgitation and in hemodynamically or electrically unstable patients in whom multiple invasive intravascular procedures are likely to be performed.

XVI. SELECTION OF FIBRINOLYTIC AND CONJUNCTIVE AGENTS

A. Fibrinolytic Agents

The currently available fibrinolytic agents differ substantially with respect to (a) selectivity for activating plasminogen bound to fibrin compared with circulating plasminogen; (b) potential for inducing allergic reactions or hypotension; and (c) rapidity with which they induce coronary recanalization. Streptokinase binds to circulating plasminogen, with the resulting streptokinase-plasminogen complex inducing activation of both fibrin-bound and circulating plasminogen. Thus, administration of intravenous streptokinase is associated with rapid, extensive degradation of circulating fibrinogen and numerous other proteins. Urokinase and acylated streptokinase-plasmin complexes (anistreplase) directly activate both circulating and fibrin-bound plasminogen, thereby inducing a systemic lytic state similar to that induced by streptokinase. Recombinant tissue plasminogen activator (t-PA, alteplase) preferentially activates plasminogen bound to fibrin. However, in doses used for treatment of myocardial infarction, it modestly activates circulating plasminogen as well, but much less than is the case with nonselective agents.

Coronary recanalization is induced more rapidly by t-PA than by streptokinase or anistreplase. It is accelerated by administration of t-PA in a 90-min dosing regimen compared with a 3-hr infusion. In the GUSTO trial, treatment of patients with a 90-min infusion of t-PA was associated with an improvement in survival compared with treatment with intravenous streptokinase. A marked survival advantage was associated with treatment with t-PA compared with anistreplase in the Thrombolysis in Myocardial Infarction—4 study. The benefits of more rapid coronary recanalization with t-PA are more prominent in patients treated within the first 4 hr of symptoms and in those with larger infarctions.

The most common complication associated with administration of fibrinolytic agents is bleeding. Although rare among all bleeding episodes, intracerebral bleeding is the most serious. In the GUSTO trial, administration of t-PA was associated with approximately a 0.2% greater incidence of hemorrhagic stroke compared with streptokinase and with a slightly lower incidence of other bleeding complications. However, the combined endpoint of death or disabling stroke favored treatment with t-PA compared with streptokinase. Administration of streptokinase is associated with complications that are infrequent in patients treated with t-PA, including allergic reactions, anaphylaxis, and hypotension.

Although controversy persists regarding the cost:benefit ratios of different fibrinolytic agents, t-PA treatment with front-loaded infusions is associated with improved survival and a lower incidence of side effects than is intravenous streptokinase treatment. The benefits of treatment are most marked in high-risk patients and in those treated early after the onset of infarction.

B. Conjunctive Agents

Aspirin

Conjunctive treatment with aspirin decreases mortality in patients treated with streptokinase and is likely to be of value in patients treated with t-PA as well. Aspirin should be administered initially as 160 mg orally. If enteric-coated aspirin is used, the first tablet should be chewed to increase the rapidity of onset of action. Subsequently, aspirin can be continued at oral doses of 160 mg daily. The value of higher or lower doses of aspirin over long intervals has not been clarified.

Conjunctive Anticoagulation

Conjunctive treatment with intravenous heparin increases late coronary artery patency in patients treated with t-PA, but not 90-min patency with either t-PA or streptokinase. Thus, heparin appears to prevent early thrombotic reocclusion. In patients treated with streptokinase in the GUSTO trial, conjunctive intravenous heparin compared with 12,500 U subcutaneous heparin twice daily did not reduce the incidence of reocclusion or improve survival. Nevertheless, intravenous heparin appears to be beneficial as judged from other endpoints in GUSTO and results in several other smaller studies. Heparin should be administered as an intravenous bolus of 5000 U at the time of initiation of infusion of the fibrinolytic agent followed by a 1000 U/hr infusion. Higher doses of heparin have recently been shown to increase bleeding complications and should generally be avoided in patients treated with fibrinolytic agents. The dose of heparin should be adjusted to a target-activated partial thromboplastin time (aPTT) of 60 to 85 sec. It should be lowered promptly in patients with aPTTs of greater than 90 sec because of the high risk of serious bleeding complications otherwise. The aPTT should be measured every 6 hr during the first 48 hr in patients treated with intravenous heparin after coronary thrombolysis. Treatment with intravenous heparin should be continued for at least 3 days, with the duration generally determined by the need for invasive procedures.

Beta-Adrenergic Blocking Agents

In patients who have been given thrombolytic drugs and who have no contraindications to beta blockers, initial intravenous and subsequent oral administration of beta-blocking agents may decrease the incidence of recurrent ischemic events. Beta blockers should not be administered to patients with marked sinus bradycardia (heart rate < 50 beats/min), marked first-degree AV block (PR interval > 0.24 sec), second- or third-degree AV block, hypotension (BP < 90 mmHg), a history of reactive airways disease, evidence of bronchospasm on examination, or heart failure. Metoprolol or propranolol are the most commonly administered agents given intravenously to patients with acute myocardial infarction. Metoprolol is administered as 15 mg and propranolol as 0.1 mg/kg intravenously, each in divided doses 5 to 10 min apart. The subsequent oral dose of metoprolol is 25 to 100 mg every 12 hr or 10 to 40 mg of propranolol every 6–8 hr. Beta blockers should be discontinued in patients who develop bronchospasm or worsening dyspnea.

Nitroglycerin

Intravenous nitroglycerin decreases infarct size; however, recent data do not suggest that intravenous nitrates in conjunction with fibrinolytic agents improve survival. Furthermore, intravenous nitroglycerin may indirectly decrease peak t-PA levels and thereby impair rapid coronary recanalization. Accordingly, intravenous nitroglycerin should not be administered initially to patients with acute myocardial infarction who are being treated with fibronolytic agents, although it may be useful later.

Lidocaine

Prophylactic lidocaine does not improve survival in patients with acute myocardial infarction or prevent arrhythmias associated with reperfusion. Therefore it should be restricted to treatment of potentially life-threatening ventricular arrhythmias (see Chapter 17).

Calcium Channel Antagonists

Calcium channel antagonists should not be administered initially to patients treated with fibrinolytic agents. In particular, the dihydropyridines (e.g., nifedipine) may promote reflex tachycardia and hypotension, exacerbating ischemia.

C. Monitoring of Thrombolytic Agents

aPTT

The aPTT should be measured every 6 hr after initiation of fibrinolytic agent and intravenous heparin. In patients treated with streptokinase, the aPTT may be prolonged 6 hr after initiation of treatment by the agent itself (because of its effects on the endpoint of the assay in vitro and generation of fibrinogen degradation fragments in vivo). Therefore, the heparin dose should not be decreased at this time based on prolongation greater than 90 sec. However, prolongation of the aPTT of 12 hr or more after the initiation of therapy should prompt an immediate decrease in the dose of heparin. The dose of heparin should be titrated to maintain the aPTT at approximately two times the control. A protocol-based approach to treatment should be used to avoid under- or overdosing of patients.

Fibrinogen

Fibrinogen decreases markedly in blood in patients treated with streptokinase and in some patients treated with t-PA. However, the extent of fibrinogen degradation does not predict bleeding in an individual patient. Accordingly, routine measurement of fibrinogen or fibrinogen degradation product levels is unnecessary.

D. Complications Associated with Thrombolytic Agents

Hypotension

Hypotension in response to administration of fibrinolytic agents is most common in patients treated with streptokinase and is often related to the rapidity of infusion of the drug. Should hypotension occur, the infusion should be discontinued briefly and restarted at a lower rate if the hypotension resolves in response to conservative management, including volume expansion. Persistent hypotension in patients treated with streptokinase warrants discontinuation of the infusion. In high-risk patients, alternative means of inducing reperfusion should be reconsidered, including administration of t-PA or immediate angioplasty.

Allergic Reactions

Minor allergic reactions may occur in patients treated with streptokinase; they include rash, fever, and chills. These can be treated with diphenhydramine and acetaminophen. More severe reactions, including anaphylaxis, although rare, may be fatal and are difficult to manage in the setting of acute infarction.

Bleeding

Significant bleeding is more likely to develop when invasive procedures are performed. Minor bleeding at sites of vascular access occur in 40–50% of patients and require transfusion in 10–20%. If invasive procedures are avoided, bleeding occurs in less than 6%. Accordingly, arterial puncture for blood gas analysis should be avoided and early cardiac catheterization reserved for patients in whom reperfusion is thought to have failed (see Chapter 11, on infarction).

Central venous catheterization should be avoided, if possible, in patients treated with fibrinolytic agents. If absolutely necessary, it should be limited to the femoral vein, a readily compressible site if bleeding should occur. However, retroperitoneal hemorrhage remains a risk.

Should uncontrolled hemorrhage occur, fresh-frozen plasma can be given to attenuate a systemic lytic state. Cryoprecipitate can be used to replete fibrinogen and factor VIII. In patients with a prolonged bleeding time, platelet transfusions may be of value.

Failed Thrombolysis

Failure to induce reperfusion may be associated with a rapid decline in hemo-dynamic stability in patients with acute myocardial infarction. Early coronary angioplasty and angioplasty of occluded infarct-related arteries, when necessary, appears to improve survival. Early coronary angiography increases the risk of bleeding and should be avoided as a routine practice. However, in patients with extensive infarction in whom reperfusion cannot be induced pharmacologically and in those with hemodynamic or electrical instability attributable to failed coronary thrombolysis, salvage angioplasty should be considered. (See Chapter 11 for a discussion on the subsequent management of patients with myocardial infarction.)

SUGGESTED READING

Diagnostic Approach to the Patient with Chest Pain Compatible with Definite or Suspected Angina Pectoris

Beller, GA, Kaul S. Cardiac noninvasive techniques. IN: Stein JH, ed. Internal Medicine. 4th ed. Boston: Mosby-Year Book, 1994:55–74.

Dell'Italia LJ. Chest pain. In: Stein JH, ed. Internal Medicine. 4th ed. Boston: Mosby-Year Book, 1994:86–92.

Dell'Italia LJ, O'Rourke RA. Evaluation of the patient with signs and symptoms of ischemic heart disease. In: Chatterjee K, Parmley WW, eds. Cardiology. Philadelphia: Lippincott 1991:1–19.

Diamond GA, Forrester JS. Analysis of probability as an aid in the clinical diagnosis of coronary artery disease. N Engl J Med 1979; 300:1350–1358.

O'Rourke RA. Chest pain. In: Schlant RC, Alexander RW, O'Rourke RA, Roberts R, Sonnenblick EH, eds. The Heart. 8th ed. New York: McGraw-Hill, 1994:459–467.

Schlant RC, Alexander RW. Diagnosis and management of chronic ischemic heart disease.

In: Schlant RC, Alexander RW, O'Rourke RA, Roberts R, Sonnenblick EH, eds. The Heart, 8th ed. New York: McGraw-Hill, 1994:1055–1082.

Verani MS. Pharmacologic stress myocardial perfusion imaging. Curr Probl Cardiol 1993; 18:481–528.

Unstable Angina with ST-Segment Elevation

Anonymous. Indications for fibrinolytic therapy in suspected acute myocardial infarction: collaborative overview of early mortality and major morbidity results from all randomised trials of more than 1000 patients: Fibrinolytic Therapy Trialists' (FTT) Collaborative Group. Lancet 1994; 343:311–22.

Braunwald E, Jones RH, et al. Diagnosing and managing unstable angina. Circulation 1994; 90:613–622.

Grines C, Browne KF, et al. A comparison of immediate angioplasty with thrombolytic therapy for acute myocardial infarction: The Primary Angioplasty in Myocardial Infarction Study Group. N Engl J Med 1993; 328:673–679.

National Heart Attack Alert Program Coordinating Committee 60 Minutes to Treatment Working Group. Emergency department: Rapid identification and treatment of patients with acute myocardial infarction. Bethesda, MD: National Heart, Lung and Blood Institute, 1993.

Sane DC, Califf RM, et al. Bleeding during thrombolytic therapy for acute myocardial infarction: Mechanisms and management. Ann Intern Med 1989; 111:1010–1022.

Sobel BE. Coronary thrombolysis: Editorial overview. Coron Artery Dis 1990; 1:3–7.

The GUSTO angiographic investigators. The effects of tissue plasminogen activator, streptokinase, or both on coronary artery patency, ventricular function, and survival after acute myocardial infarction. N Engl J Med 1993; 329:1615–1622.

The GUSTO angiographic investigators. An international randomized trial comparing four thrombolytic strategies for acute myocardial infarction. N Engl J Med 1993; 329: 673–682.

2

Shortness of Breath/Dyspnea on Exertion/PND/Orthopnea/ Platypnea/Orthodeoxia

Evaluation and Treatment of Patients with Shortness of Breath   **38**
  I.   Onset and Pattern of Dyspnea   38
  II. Distinction of Cardiovascular Causes of Dyspnea from Pulmonary Disease   41
  III. Key Physical Findings   42
  IV. Initial Diagnostic Tests   43
  V. Specialized Diagnostic Tests: Indications and Selection   46
  VI. Strategies for the Management of Patients with Dyspnea   50

Dyspnea as a Manifestation of Pulmonary Vascular Disease   **51**
  VII. Primary Pulmonary Hypertension   51
  VIII. Pulmonary Embolism   54

Dyspnea and Congenital Heart Disease   **56**
  IX. Specific Entities that May Cause Dyspnea   56

    Suggested Reading   57

Evaluation and Treatment of Patients with Shortness of Breath

Stephen P. Bradley, Jack L. Clausen, and Kenneth M. Moser

Dyspnea can be defined as the symptom of uncomfortable or difficult breathing and is a common reason for patients to seek medical attention. However, identification of its cause is often difficult, for several reasons: (a) because dyspnea is a symptom, it cannot be *measured* or *monitored,* and individual variability in perception of the symptom is wide; (b) dyspnea is normal under certain circumstances; (c) the list of potential causes of dyspnea is long (Tables 1 and 2) and the pathophysiology complex; (d) in many cases, as when dyspnea is related to pulmonary hypertension or shock, the specific pathophysiology remains poorly explained. Despite all of these difficulties, however, careful history taking and physical examination as well as selective use of tests can identify the cause of dyspnea in most patients.

I. ONSET AND PATTERN OF DYSPNEA

The differential diagnostic possibilities in the patient who presents with *acute* dyspnea are modest in number (Table 2) and the need for therapy is usually urgent. In these patients, the urgency of the situation often dictates that only a brief history and physical examination (vital signs and cutaneous, cardiac, and pulmonary examinations) and a few diagnostic tests (usually arterial blood gases, chest x-ray, electrocardiography, and hematocrit) be performed before appropriate therapy is instituted.

The patient with less severe or more chronic dyspnea can be approached more systemically. Determining the onset and rate of progression of the symptom is critical. Patients will often minimize their complaint or deny that they have symptoms until they are essentially incapacitated. Therefore it is important to define what *specific activities* induce dyspnea, when the limitation first appeared, and how the patient has progressed. Often, the spouse or "significant other" is a better source of such information because the patient has adjusted by gradually eliminating those activities that cause shortness of breath. Comparison with other individuals of similar age and extent of physical fitness is essential in determining whether the amount of dyspnea experienced is appropriate for the level of exertion, whether it represents deconditioning, or whether it is secondary to a significant pathological process.

Table 1 Causes of Chronic Dyspnea

Pulmonary disorders	Pleura
Airway	Effusion (fluid, blood, chyle)
Laryngeal	Pneumothorax
Localized foreign body, mass, or	Fibrosis
stenosis	Tumor
Asthma, chronic bronchitis, or	Respiratory musculature
emphysema	Malnutrition
Secretions	Thyroid disease
Bronchiolitis	Phrenic nerve, accessory muscle nerve
Parenchyma	dysfunction
Pneumonitis	Systemic neuromuscular disease
Infectious agents	Respiratory muscle dyskinesia
Allergic reaction	Thoracic cage
Injury (e.g., due to bleomycin,	Injury (e.g., flail chest)
paraquat, cadmium exposures)	Deformity (e.g., kyphoscoliosis)
Unknown origin (diffuse interstitial	Abdominal "loading" (e.g., obesity,
pneumonitis)	pregnancy, ascites, tumor)
Pulmonary edema	Abnormalities in inspired gases
Cardiogenic	Low inspired oxygen concentration
Noncardiogenic (e.g., due to	(high altitude)
neurogenic, induced by high	Significant concentration of carbon
altitude, reexpansion)	dioxide or carbon monoxide
Tumor	Cardiac dysfunction
Primary	Inadequate cardiac output
Metastatic (e.g., discrete masses,	Valvular disease
lymphangitic spread)	Pericardial disease
Vasculature	Ventricular dysfunction
Intravascular obstruction	Other, less common causes (e.g., left
Thromboemboli	atrial myxoma, septal defects)
Tumor	Hypoxemia secondary to right-to-left
Fat	shunt
Foreign body	Anemia (severe)
Septic emboli	Shock
Parasitic disease	Metabolic causes (e.g., metabolic
Venoocclusive disease	acidosis, hyperthyroidism, obesity,
Vasculitis	pregnancy)
AVM	Deconditioning
	Psychological factors (e.g., pain, anxiety)

Table 2   Common Causes of Acute Dyspnea

Airway obstruction (laryngospasm, foreign body, bronchospasm)
Pulmonary edema (cardiogenic and noncardiogenic)
Fulminant bacterial pneumonia
Pulmonary emboli
Pneumothorax
Hemothorax
Shock
Acute hemorrhage
Adult respiratory distress syndrome
Acute cardiac disease with left ventricular dysfunction (with or without pulmonary edema)
Metabolic acidosis

The presence of *associated symptoms* is often useful in identifying the cause of dyspnea. Symptoms of typical or atypical angina suggest underlying cardiovascular disease. Pleuritic chest pain suggests pleural involvement, either as the primary cause of dyspnea (e.g., pleural effusion) or as a concomitant symptom of another process (e.g., pulmonary embolus, parapneumonic effusion).

The *position* of the patient when dyspnea occurs often helps narrow the differential diagnosis. *Paroxysmal nocturnal dyspnea* (PND) (sudden onset of dyspnea after lying flat for some length of time) suggests left-heart cardiac conditions resulting in high pulmonary venous ("capillary wedge") pressures, such as left ventricular dysfunction or mitral stenosis. If volume overload (fluid retention) accompanies these conditions, PND is particularly likely.

Orthopnea (dyspnea immediately upon lying flat) is most commonly due to the same cardiac causes as PND; however, both obstructive airways disease (chronic obstructive pulmonary disease, or COPD; asthma) and respiratory muscle weakness from any cause may present in this fashion. Indeed, patients with bilateral diaphragmatic paralysis develop *severe* dyspnea quite rapidly after lying flat.

Platypnea (dyspnea in the upright position) with or without orthodeoxia (arterial oxygen desaturation when upright) may be due to intracardiac shunts, such as atrial septal defects. Other causes include intrapulmonary shunts such as congenital pulmonary arteriovenous malformations (AVM) as either an isolated finding or in association with Osler-Weber-Rendu disease. Acquired AVM as well as dilated pulmonary capillary and precapillary beds occur in patients with cirrhosis and may cause severe platypnea (and orthodeoxia) in those patients. Platypnea occurs infrequently in various forms of severe parenchymal lung disease, including COPD, interstitial fibrosis, and adult respiratory distress syndrome (ARDS), as well as in autonomic failure. *Trepopnea* (dyspnea in one lateral position but not the other) can occur with unilateral disease of the lung parenchyma, airways, or pleura. For example, with congenital absence of one pulmonary artery or unilateral emphysema (the Swyer-James syndrome), dyspnea often occurs when the patient lies with the "good lung" down, thereby diminishing its ventilatory contribution.

Obtaining a history of dyspnea that occurs intermittently, especially in certain environments, may be helpful. Exposure to specific agents causes dyspnea in patients with both extrinsic asthma and hypersensitivity pneumonitis. However, over time, a chronic component develops that can mask the association between the inciting agent and the symptoms. In addition, the symptoms of hypersensitivity pneumonitis classically occur several hours after exposure. Accordingly, unless a careful exposure history is taken, the association is often missed.

Patients with sleep apnea may present with dyspnea associated with recurrent arousals from sleep. Further clues to this diagnosis include obesity (or recent weight gain), daytime sleepiness, snoring, and witnessed apneas.

II. DISTINCTION OF CARDIOVASCULAR CAUSES OF DYSPNEA FROM PULMONARY DISEASE

A history of significant cardiac or pulmonary disease is often the most important information obtained. Symptoms of angina or myocardial infarction direct one toward cardiovascular disease, with the moderating recognition that esophageal and multiple other disorders may suggest angina and that massive pulmonary embolism can mimic myocardial infarction. Similarly, orthopnea is consistent with (but not diagnostic of) elevated pulmonary venous pressure from any cause. Palpitations suggest underlying cardiac disease as the cause of dyspnea. Cardiac conditions leading to high pulmonary venous pressures are the most common cause of right heart failure; therefore, cardiovascular disease must be considered in any patient with symptoms and signs consistent with right ventricular volume overload, such as hepatomegaly, elevated jugular venous pressure, ascites, or pedal edema.

A cardiac cause for dyspnea is often missed in patients who do not present with the classic symptoms of angina despite having significant coronary artery disease. These patients may present with episodic dyspnea as their "anginal equivalent." Others present with wheezing and are diagnosed as having asthma or COPD. High left atrial filling pressures and wedge pressures induce bronchial edema as well as bronchospasm that may respond to bronchodilators. Thus, a cardiac cause for dyspnea must be considered in any patient with significant cardiovascular risk factors, including those with obstructive lung disease. Delineation of this rather "tricky" differential (i.e., left ventricular failure in a patient with COPD) is vital because the therapeutic approach will differ. For example, a beta$_2$ agonist that induces tachycardia would not be a wise choice if coronary artery disease is the primary problem; conversely, an angiotensin converting

41

enzyme (ACE) inhibitor prescribed to "unload" the left ventricle might exagge-rate cough and bronchospasm if COPD rather than the cardiac dysfunction is the basis of the patient's symptoms.

III. KEY PHYSICAL FINDINGS

Physical examination of the dyspneic patient centers on evaluation of the cardiac and pulmonary systems. Some of the most important points are outlined below.

Listening with the stethoscope placed over the neck—not a "standard" practice—is often critical for recognition of inspiratory stridor due to upper airway obstruction, since auscultation limited to the chest may result in misinter-pretation of the origin of "wheezing." Common causes of inspiratory stridor include foreign-body aspiration, epiglottitis, and vocal cord paralysis, all of which can be life-threatening if not identified and treated rapidly. Focal wheezing limited to one area of the lung fields implies a local area of airway narrowing, as from a tumor or aspirated foreign body. Often, a faint focal "wheeze" during quiet breathing can be exaggerated by deep, rapid breathing. Obstructive lung disease (COPD, asthma) typically presents with diffuse wheezing; however, a patient with depressed ventilation and therefore poor air movement may have little or no wheezing. Thus, the most severely compromised asthmatic ("status asthmati-cus") may present with an ominously nearly "quiet" chest—hyperinflated to nearly full inspiration. "No airflow, no wheezing" is the relevant clinical pearl.

Rales, best heard in the bases, are often described as "wet" (as in congestive heart failure or volume overload) or "dry" (as in interstitial lung disease) and can be elicited often only after the patient is encouraged to take deeper breaths. Bronchial breath sounds imply underlying consolidated lung and are frequently recognized because of asymmetry in the quality of breath sounds. Conversely, a unilateral decrease in breath sounds may be noted in patients with a pneumothorax (with associated hyperresonance to percussion), pleural effusion (dullness to percus-sion), or an obstructed bronchus (normal resonance or dullness to percussion).

Elevated jugular venous pressure (JVP) is an important diagnostic (and prognostic) sign in patients with right ventricular failure. It is simply a reflection of an elevated right atrial pressure. In turn, except in rare instances, right atrial pressure reflects right ventricular end-diastolic pressure. Thus, an elevated JVP usually tells the physician that the right ventricle has failed. The most common cause of right ventricular failure is pulmonary venous hypertension secondary to disorders of the left-sided cardiac chambers.

However, patients with normal wedge pressures can develop right ventricu-lar dysfunction because of extensive constriction, obstruction, or destruction of the pulmonary arteries (e.g., caused by severe interstitial fibrosis or COPD); "primary" pulmonary hypertension; or embolic obstruction of the pulmonary arteries. The presence of peripheral edema implies right ventricular failure in the absence of other chronic volume overload states (e.g., cirrhosis, renal insufficiency). Other useful signs of right heart failure are ascites, hepatomegaly, and hepatojugular reflux.

A vigorous cardiac examination for evidence of either right- or left-sided cardiac dysfunction is an essential element in the evaluation of the dyspneic patient. Careful auscultation for third and fourth heart sounds, recognition of the intensity of pulmonic valve closure and its "splitting" behavior, feeling for a right ventricular (parasternal) heave or pulmonary artery closure tap in the right second intercostal space, and enhancing the holosystolic murmur of tricuspid regurgitation by deep inspiration—all are simple, instructive components of the physical examination that should be part of the diagnostic armamentarium of physicians who evaluate patients presenting with dyspnea.

Despite the widespread availability of high-tech diagnostic tests, nothing substitutes for a good history and adequate physical examination in approaching the diagnosis of the cause of dyspnea.

For example, a 63-year-old woman reported that while hiking through a forest of pine trees at sea level, she developed diffuse wheezing and dyspnea. Over a 2-day period, despite a physician's diagnosis of acute asthma and prescription of prednisone, an antibiotic, and an inhaled beta$_2$ agonist, she worsened. The physician felt she had status asthmaticus and referred her for hospital admission. Physical examination at the hospital disclosed a cyanotic, very dyspneic woman with elevated JVP. She stated that she was a nonsmoker who had never had asthma or any other lung problems and that the dyspnea and wheezing had come on "just like that" during her hike. She had hiked that same pathway many times before without similar symptoms. Auscultatory examination of the lungs revealed diffuse wheezing but also diffuse wet rales. Cardiac examination was significant for the classic systolic murmur of wide open mitral regurgitation. The patient said she had never had a heart murmur before. An echocardiogram confirmed the presence of a ruptured mitral valve and severe mitral regurgitation. She underwent successful mitral valve repair. The rupture of her chordae was "idiopathic."

IV. INITIAL DIAGNOSTIC TESTS

Diagnostic tests are performed in patients presenting with dyspnea either to confirm a diagnosis suspected on the basis of the history and physical examination or to help select more specialized examinations. The four tests used most commonly in patients with dyspnea are chest x-ray, electrocardiogram (ECG), spirometry, and hemoglobin or hematocrit.

Perhaps the most important caveat about the chest x-ray is that several causes of acute dyspnea present typically with a *normal* chest x-ray. In acute pulmonary embolism, roentgenographic clues such as atelectasis, regional oligemia due to decreased blood flow, Hampton's hump (a pleural-based infiltrate in an area of lung infarction), and pleural effusion are unusual. Similarly, the chest x-ray in acute ischemic left ventricular dysfunction lags behind the clinical picture by up to several hours; therefore, early in the course, it will be normal. In the patient with asthma, the chest x-ray will appear normal between acute exacerbations and may show only mild hyperinflation or peribronchial cuffing when the patient is acutely ill. Routine chest x-ray is an insensitive method of detecting central airway obstruction. Neuromuscular disorders, sepsis, and severe anemia are further examples of processes that may cause dyspnea with a normal chest x-ray. Early in the course of primary or chronic thromboembolic pulmonary hypertension, the chest x-ray is usually deceptively normal. Even processes that affect lung parenchyma primarily may not be evident on the routine chest films; for example, in idiopathic pulmonary fibrosis, the chest x-ray is normal in at least 10% of patients with biopsy-proven disease.

Nevertheless, some abnormality on chest x-ray is seen with most cardiac and pulmonary processes that cause significant dyspnea. The roentgenographic pattern seen in pulmonary edema is described in Chapter 14. However, differentiation between pulmonary edema attributable to high pulmonary venous pressure (hydrostatic edema) and that due to acute lung injury (ARDS, high-permeability edema) is not easy. Both cardiogenic and noncardiogenic pulmonary edema may exhibit similar patterns. Such clues as a lack of pulmonary vascular redistribution, a normal-sized heart, an asymmetrical or peripheral pattern, and early development of alveolar filling all may suggest noncardiogenic pulmonary edema, but none can be relied upon. Other, nonradiographic information is often required.

Furthermore, because pulmonary edema may begin with interstitial edema before alveolar edema develops, the interstitial infiltrates associated with lung *parenchymal* disease—such as idiopathic pulmonary fibrosis, pneumoconiosis, sarcoidosis, and lymphangitic spread of tumor—may be confused with early cardiogenic pulmonary edema. In most lung diseases, the infiltrates tend *not* to be perihilar (they may be peripheral or upper- or lower-lobe predominant, depending on the process), and there is no clinical or radiographic evidence of volume overload. The presence of honeycombing (thick-walled cystic areas, most commonly in the bases) is pathognomonic for interstitial lung disease.

Cardiomegaly is present when the cardiothoracic ratio (the ratio between the heart width and the internal diameter of the thorax on routine posteroanterior chest x-ray) exceeds 50%. Certain patterns of cardiac enlargement may be useful in leading toward a diagnosis. A globular or "water bottle" appearance to the cardiac silhouette suggests pericardial effusion or severe cardiomyopathy. On the lateral film, filling of the usually clear anterior (substernal) space by the heart shadow suggests right ventricular enlargement; whereas posterior enlargement suggests left-sided cardiac disorders. Valvular heart disease, atrial and ventricular septal defects, and other forms of heart disease often exhibit distinctive roentgenographic patterns, as noted in Chapters 12, 14, and 25.

Careful review of the chest x-ray will often reveal enlargement of the pulmonary arteries in patients with pulmonary hypertension from any cause. Right ventricular enlargement may also be present. In patients with primary pulmonary hypertension, peripheral pruning of the pulmonary arterial tree may be evident. Marked asymmetry of the central pulmonary arteries (main, lobar) suggests chronic, major-vessel thromboembolic obstruction.

Electrocardiography is most useful in patients with history, symptoms, or signs consistent with underlying cardiac disease. The value of the ECG in patients with myocardial ischemia and infarction, arrhythmias, chamber enlargement, and pericardial disease is discussed in Chapters 11 and 15–18. The physician should be familiar with ECG patterns seen with acute and chronic cor pulmonale, both to

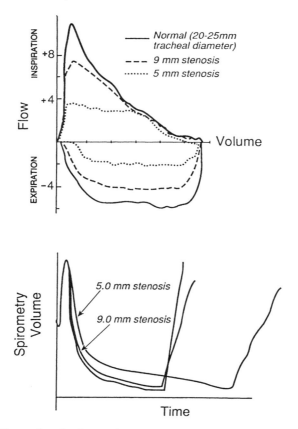

Figure 1 Effects of tracheal stenosis.

avoid overlooking subtle clues to the diagnosis and, in the case of acute cor pulmonale, to avoid attributing the changes to ischemic heart disease.

Spirometry is a rapid and inexpensive means of detecting either obstructive or restrictive lung disease. The usual finding in obstructive disease is a low ratio of forced expiratory volume in 1 sec to forced vital capacity (FEV_1/FVC). Measurements during the middle portion of the forced expiratory flow ($FEF_{25-75\%}$, $FEF_{50\%}$) are more sensitive than the FEV_1/FVC ratio for detecting mild obstruction but must be interpreted with caution given the wide range of normal values. Displaying the output of a spirometer as a flow-volume plot rather than a volume-time graph makes it easier to recognize the flow patterns typical of less common obstructive airway disorders such as tracheal stenosis, vocal cord paralysis, or aspirated foreign body (Figure 1). However, the insensitivity of this test means that a normal flow-volume loop does not exclude significant localized airway obstruction. In restrictive disease, the typical finding is a low FVC and normal or high FEV_1/FVC ratio. Because reductions in vital capacity can occur in both restrictive disorders and diffuse obstructive airway disease, one should always recognize that if both the FVC and expiratory flow rates are reduced, the cause can be either obstructive airway disease or combined restrictive and obstructive disease.

Hemoglobin and hematocrit measurements should be considered early in the evaluation of the dyspneic patient. Although anemia is rarely the sole cause of dyspnea, it will exacerbate dyspnea attributable to any other cause.

V. SPECIALIZED DIAGNOSTIC TESTS: INDICATIONS AND SELECTION

Approximately two-thirds of patients with chronic shortness of breath are found to have either asthma, COPD, interstitial lung disease, or cardiac diseases as the cause. In most, as well in most patients presenting with acute dyspnea (Table 1), a diagnosis can be made based on the history, physical examination, and initial diagnostic tests. In some patients, further evaluation is required to confirm the diagnosis, determine the extent of physiological impairment, or follow response to therapy. For those patients in whom the cause remains uncertain, selective use of additional diagnostic tests (selected on the basis of data gained from the earlier evaluation) may yield a diagnosis.

Measurement of arterial blood gases at rest is invaluable in patients with significant lung disease or suspected acid-based abnormalities. The presence of hypoxemia and/or hypercapnia confirms that a problem exists with gas exchange or ventilation. The pH and Pa_{CO_2} are necessary for interpretation of acid-base disorders. In addition, the values may have both prognostic and therapeutic significance, as in patients with hypoxemia secondary to COPD. Unfortunately, in most forms of pulmonary disease, significant pathological derangement occurs before resting arterial blood gases become abnormal. In addition, resting values predict abnormalities occurring during exercise only poorly. For both reasons, arterial blood gas analysis during exercise is often indicated in patients with normal or minimally abnormal resting values. Testing during exertion is essential also in patients who have dyspnea *only* during exertion. Obviously, studying such patients only at rest does not replicate the condition under which their dyspnea occurs.

Pulse oximetry at rest and with exercise is being used with increasing frequency as a measure of arterial oxygenation. The availability, lower cost—in comparison with serial arterial blood gas (ABG) analyses, and noninvasive nature of this test makes it an attractive substitute for measurement of the Pa_{O_2}. In several settings, this may be appropriate—for example, to titrate oxygen therapy in patients with known reduction of Pa_{O_2} from a prior ABG and as a continuous "trend monitor" in the intensive care unit or operating room. However, three points should be remembered in interpreting the Sa_{O_2} obtained from cutaneous oximeters: (a) it can be dangerous to ignore the pH and Pa_{CO_2}, as when titrating oxygen therapy in patients with hypercarbia; (b) factors that alter the association between Pa_{O_2} and Sa_{O_2} (such as pH and temperature) can lead to inappropriate management decisions; and (c) technical limitations of pulse oximetry can lead to erroneous values. The most important limitation is that the 95% confidence interval for the accuracy of Sa_{O_2} by pulse oximetry is only ± 4–5%. In addition, poor peripheral perfusion, abnormal hemoglobin, hyperbilirubinemia, and dark skin pigmentation can all lead to falsely high or low values.

Cardiopulmonary exercise testing is often used to evaluate patients who on initial evaluation do not appear to have evidence of cardiac, pulmonary, or other organ system disease sufficient to account for their symptoms. The normal response to exercise requires integrated functioning of the lungs, pulmonary circulation, heart, systemic circulation, and skeletal muscles. By placing the patient in conditions that reproduce his or her symptoms (typically progressively increasing, symptom-limited exercise), observations can be made that relate to the level of conditioning, specific organ system affected, and the extent of disability. Careful questioning often reveals that exercise is limited by fatigue, leg pain, or chest discomfort rather than by dyspnea itself.

Measurements obtained during exercise testing can range from simple to complex. In addition to its clear role in evaluating patients with ischemic heart disease, the exercise ECG is often helpful in patients with dyspnea of uncertain etiology. Patients with myocardial dysfunction (or severe deconditioning) will respond to exercise with an inappropriate increase in pulse, thus attaining a maximum predicted heart rate at low levels of exercise. Other patients with cardiac disease will have a blunted heart rate response to exercise.

Arterial blood gas analysis during exercise can provide invaluable information. A decrease in Pa_{O_2} and a widening of the arterial-alveolar oxygen gradient are extremely sensitive indicators of disease involving the lung parenchyma and pulmonary circulation and often more sensitive than cutaneous oximetry, especially for patients with early or mild dysfunction. An increase in Pa_{CO_2} with exercise strongly suggests severe limitations in respiratory function. A decrease in pH occurs when patients reach the anaerobic threshold (the point at which peripheral muscles switch from predominantly aerobic to predominantly anaerobic metabolism); this is useful both as a measure of physical fitness and in determining whether the level of exercise during testing represented the patient's maximal effort.

Measurement of expired gas volumes during exercise requires sophisticated equipment but provides valuable information in some patients. In normal individuals at peak exercise, minute ventilation is 60–80% of maximal voluntary ventilation (MVV) measured at rest. In patients with lung dysfunction, minute ventilation may equal or surpass the MVV, whereas in patients with cardiac disease (or deconditioning), the maximum minute ventilation is usually normal. Oxygen consumption (V_{O_2}) is the best quantitative measurement of the amount of work performed and is particularly valuable in disability assessments. Expired CO_2 is produced as a byproduct of aerobic metabolism and from bicarbonate buffering of lactic acid; analysis of V_{CO_2} allows noninvasive measurement of the anaerobic threshold.

Additional pulmonary function tests are useful in evaluating selected patients with suspected pulmonary dysfunction. A low carbon monoxide diffusing capacity (DLCO) is often more sensitive than the chest x-ray in detecting interstitial lung disease. However, an abnormal result must be interpreted with caution because so many disorders can be responsible. Emphysema, pulmonary embolism, chronic congestive heart failure, anemia, and high carboxyhemoglobin levels (as occur with smoking) all commonly cause a decrease in the DLCO. Increased DLCO may be seen in early congestive heart failure, asthma, and pulmonary hemorrhage.

Measurement of lung volumes by body plethysmography or gas dilution (nitrogen washout or helium dilution) will demonstrate the extent of hyperinflation in obstructive lung disease and also detect superimposed restriction in patients with COPD. Body plethysmography is the preferred method, because dilution techniques may underestimate lung volumes in patients with poorly communicating air spaces, as occurs in bullous emphysema or severe obstructive disease.

Measurement of maximal inspiratory and expiratory pressures (MIP, MEP) is often more sensitive than the vital capacity in the detection of neuromuscular disorders. These tests are particularly useful in evaluating patients with otherwise unexplained restrictive defects evident on spirometry (Table 3).

Bronchial provocation testing is a sensitive method of detecting occult reactive airways disease in patients with a suggestive history but negative spi-

Table 3 Causes of Restrictive Lung Disease

Pleural disease: Effusion, fibrothorax, etc.
Alveolar filling: Pneumonia, congestive heart failure, etc.
Interstitial processes: Idiopathic pulmonary fibrosis, etc.
Neuromuscular disorders: Guillain-Barré syndrome, muscular dystrophy, etc.
Thoracic cage disorders: Kyphoscoliosis, etc.
                    Also: thromboembolic disease (chronic)

rometry. It usually entails having the patient perform spirometry after inhaling a nonspecific reagent (histamine or methacholine) in escalating doses. The dose that induces significant bronchospasm (e.g., 20% reduction in FEV_{10}) is recorded. Having the patient perform spirometry before and after exercising or inhaling cold air can detect cold-induced asthma, as often occurs with some cases of exercise-induced asthma. Rarely, performing bronchial provocation with a specific antigen is helpful, especially in determining occupational or environmental causes of asthma.

Ventilation-perfusion scanning is the diagnostic procedure of first choice in patients with suspected acute or chronic pulmonary embolism. Much confusion regarding the interpretation of this test is avoided if the results are listed as normal (no segmental perfusion defects), diagnostic (multiple unmatched segmental perfusion defects in areas clear by chest x-ray), or non-diagnostic (any other finding). Nondiagnostic scans require further evaluation with lower-extremity studies (impedance plethysmography or venous ultrasound) and/or pulmonary arteriography.

Two additional points require emphasis regarding pulmonary embolism. The first is that a significant number of pulmonary emboli go undetected; thus, a high index of suspicion is needed, especially in patients with the classic risk factors of venous stasis, venous injury, or hypercoagulability. The second is that both the ventilation-perfusion scan and pulmonary arteriographic findings in chronic thromboembolic pulmonary hypertension are quite different from those in acute pulmonary embolism. Proper interpretation often requires an experienced reader.

The use of echocardiography with Doppler to detect and evaluate pericardial disease, left ventricular dysfunction, valvular heart disease, and intracardiac shunts is well recognized. In patients with pulmonary hypertension, right-sided chamber size and function can be evaluated and the extent of pulmonary hypertension estimated based on measurement of the tricuspid regurgitant jet. Increasingly, echocardiography is performed during or after exercise to identify ischemic left ventricular dysfunction or to detect exercise-induced pulmonary hypertension.

Cardiac catheterization may be valuable in some patients in whom cardiac disease is the suspected cause of dyspnea. The role of the left heart catheterization in patients with defined cardiac conditions such as ischemia or arrhythmias is outlined in Chapters 10, 16, and 17. Right heart catheterization is often performed in patients with left ventricular disease to assess the amount of dysfunction and measure filling pressures. In addition, right heart catheterization is indicated in most patients with evidence of pulmonary hypertension (not clearly attributable to cardiac or parenchymal lung disease) to measure pulmonary artery pressures, rule out intracardiac shunt or left ventricular dysfunction as the etiology, and, sometimes, to measure a response to therapy. In an occasional patient, exercise is performed with a right heart catheter in place to assess either increases in pulmonary hypertension or left ventricular dysfunction during exercise. In primary pulmonary hypertension, testing the vasodilator response to various agents (particularly prostacyclin or inhaled nitric oxide) is useful in therapeutic decision making.

High-resolution computed tomography (HRCT) of the lung parenchyma is most useful in evaluating patients with known or suspected chronic interstitial lung disease. It is more sensitive than routine chest x-rays in identifying early or mild involvement in idiopathic fibrosis. Although many disease processes appear to have characteristic patterns on HRCT, at present the diagnosis should be based on additional criteria, such as results of pathological or microbiological studies.

Assessment of respiratory function during sleep is indicated in patients with a history suggestive of sleep apnea. In addition, many patients with CHF have associated sleep apnea for which treatment with continuous or biphasic positive airway pressure or oxygen can lead to improvement in CHF independent of other measures. Another group of patients with underrecognized sleep disorders and breathing abnormalities are those with systemic hypertension. Thus, a history suggestive of sleep apnea should be sought in all hypertensive patients; if indicated, studies of sleeping respiratory function should be performed.

VI. STRATEGIES FOR THE MANAGEMENT OF PATIENTS WITH DYSPNEA

In most patients, a careful evaluation will lead to a specific diagnosis and therapy can then be directed at the underlying cause. It is important to follow not only the patient's symptomatic response but also the physiological response to therapy. Apparent symptomatic improvement without objective confirmation may suggest an unsuspected, alternative cause.

Occasionally, a patient's dyspnea cannot be explained on physiological grounds; some such patients will suffer from psychogenic dyspnea. Frequently, they complain of dizziness, faintness, chest pains, anxiety, and numbness and tingling of the fingers, toes, and perioral areas. Further clues to this syndrome include a normal chest radiograph, a decreased Pa_{CO_2}, and a normal alveolar-arterial oxygen difference. Therapy is directed toward treating the underlying psychogenic disorder. However, a psychogenic cause should be accepted only after a detailed evaluation has been completed. A mildly reduced Pa_{CO_2} (e.g., 26–36) is observed in many patients with lung disease (e.g., interstitial fibrosis or chronic pulmonary emboli).

One of the difficulties in dealing with dyspneic patients is that, even when a cause for dyspnea is found, the response to therapy may be suboptimal and the patient may remain short of breath. Numerous strategies have been tried for these patients, from pharmacological therapy with benzodiazepines, narcotics, and phenothiazines to resection of the carotid body in patients with intractable dyspnea. The results of drug treatment have been mixed. Carotid body removal presents hazards and is of unproven efficacy. Pulmonary rehabilitation—through a process of education, lifestyle modification, and cardiopulmonary conditioning—improves both exercise tolerance and dyspnea in selected patients. However, a maintenance program is needed to sustain the gains over time.

Dyspnea as a Manifestation of Pulmonary Vascular Disease

Stuart Rich

Dyspnea is the most common presenting symptom in patients who have pulmonary hypertension as a result of pulmonary vascular disease. Although lung function is intrinsically normal, the pulmonary hypertension causes patients to hyperventilate to compensate for arterial hypoxemia caused by both reduced cardiac output and ventilation/perfusion inequalities in the lung. Initially the hyperventilation is most notable with exercise; thus a patient's earliest complaint may be dyspnea with marked physical activity. As the disorder progresses, dyspnea can occur at rest.

VII. PRIMARY PULMONARY HYPERTENSION

Primary pulmonary hypertension is almost always manifest by dyspnea. When a patient presents with dyspnea and presumed pulmonary hypertension, it is critical that the etiology of the pulmonary hypertension be ascertained, because its impact on both prognosis and treatment is major. The causes of dyspnea are outlined in Table 4, and the tests necessary to permit elucidation of the etiology of the pulmonary hypertension are listed in Table 5.

Table 4 Causes of Dyspnea Related
to Pulmonary Hypertension

Lung diseases
    Parenchymal lung disease
    Disorder of ventilation
    Hypoxemia
Heart disease
    Disorders of left heart filling
    Systemic-to-pulmonary shunts
Pulmonary vascular obstruction
    Chronic thrombeombolism
    Mediastinal fibrosis
    Foreign-body embolization
    Hemoglobinopathies
Collagen vascular disease and vasculitides
Primary pulmonary hypertension

An open lung biopsy is not necessary to ascertain the etiology of pulmonary hypertension. If interstitial lung disease is suspected and yet not obvious on a standard chest x-ray, a thin-slice high-resolution chest scan by computed tomography (CT) is likely to be helpful. Perfusion lung scans should be obtained for every patient, regardless of whether or not pulmonary embolism has been documented. Lung scans may, of course, be abnormal in patients with primary pulmonary hypertension, but the abnormality is generally one of nonsegmental, patchy uptake. A pulmonary angiogram may not be needed to exclude the diagnosis of

Table 5 Evaluation of Pulmonary Hypertension

Test	Diagnosis to be considered
Chest x-ray	Interstitial lung disease, congenital anomalies
Perfusion lung scan	Pulmonary thromboembolism
Pulmonary angiogram	Chronic thromboembolic pulmonary hypertension
Pulmonary function tests	Obstructive airways disease, restrictive lung disease
Echocardiography	Congenital heart disease, valvular heart disease, myocardial disease
Antinuclear antibodies	Collagen vascular disease
Liver function tests	Chronic liver disease
Right heart catheterization	Documentation of cause and severity of pulmonary hypertension

pulmonary thromboembolism. In patients in whom large-vessel thromboembolism is suspected, however, a pulmonary angiogram is required to ascertain the correct diagnosis. Pulmonary function tests are indicated as well. Those indicative of a restrictive abnormality are typical in patients with pulmonary hypertension of all etiologies and do not necessarily imply underlying restrictive lung disease. The diffusing capacity for carbon monoxide may be quite low in both primary and secondary forms of pulmonary hypertension.

The echocardiogram is very helpful in identifying abnormalities in left ventricular systolic and diastolic function, abnormalities of the cardiac valves, and congenital left-to-right shunts. It may be difficult, however, to accurately detect the presence of an atrial septal defect (ASD) or differentiate an ASD from a patent foramen ovale with standard transthoracic echocardiography. In patients in whom congenital heart disease is a possible cause of the pulmonary hypertension, a transesophageal echocardiogram is indicated. The Doppler assessment of the tricuspid regurgitant jet is helpful to characterize the severity of the pulmonary hypertension. It does not, however, provide an accurate assessment of left ventricular end-diastolic filling pressure, nor is it sensitive enough to detect modest changes in hemodynamics resulting from drug therapy.

For these reasons, cardiac catheterization with documentation of pulmonary artery pressure and cardiac output is essential in every patient with pulmonary hypertension. If catheterization reveals an underlying atrial septal defect, the amount of left-to-right and right-to-left shunting should be quantified. Pulmonary hypertension is not an expected consequence of left-to-right shunting from an atrial septal defect and should be considered a reflection of underlying pulmonary vascular disease unless proven otherwise.

A. Pharmacological Therapy of Primary Pulmonary Hypertension

Patients with primary pulmonary hypertension require long-term pharmacological therapy. The major goals of treatment are to reduce the level of pulmonary artery pressure, maintain or increase cardiac output, and preserve right ventricular function as reviewed in Chapter 2.

The life expectancy of patients with primary pulmonary hypertension of New York Heart Association functional class IV is less than 6 months. Thus, consideration should be given to lung transplantation with the hope of increased survival as well as reduced symptoms. Lung transplantation alone (either single or bilateral) appears to be adequate for most patients with primary pulmonary hypertension and has become the procedure of choice for transplant patient. Patients with coexistent congenital heart disease may be benefited by either a primary repair simultaneously or combined heart and lung transplantation. The optimal timing for transplantation is difficult to define, but transplantation should be strongly considered in any patient with pulmonary hypertension who develops right ventricular failure.

VIII. PULMONARY EMBOLISM

A. Acute Pulmonary Embolism

Although an acute pulmonary embolism is the third most common cardiovascular disease, many instances remain incorrectly or inadequately undiagnosed. Most acute pulmonary emboli arise from deep vein thrombosis as a result either of an underlying predisposing condition (such as cancer, pregnancy, heart failure, or oral contraceptive use) or of an underlying primary hypercoagulable state. The classic symptoms of acute pulmonary embolism are acute shortness of breath associated with chest pain. However, the clinical presentation is so variable that many other conditions are mimicked.

The diagnosis of acute pulmonary embolism is often suggested by results of measurement of arterial blood gases with the patient breathing room air. A normal A-a gradient, associated with a P_{O_2} on room air of greater than 95 mmHg, makes an acute pulmonary embolism highly unlikely. If either the A-a gradient or P_{O_2} is abnormal, a lung scan is indicated.

In instances in which the lung scan is highly suggestive of pulmonary embolism, definitive therapy can be undertaken immediately. In patients with a lung scan of intermediate or low probability, anticoagulation should be initiated first and a pulmonary angiogram obtained subsequently.

There is often great reluctance to obtain a pulmonary angiogram in a patient with suspected pulmonary embolism and cardiovascular compromise. However, the need for an accurate diagnosis, which often can be made only on the basis of the pulmonary angiogram, generally outweighs the low morbidity associated with this procedure. Thus, pulmonary angiography is indicated in any patient in whom the diagnosis remains in doubt.

The mainstay of therapy of pulmonary embolism is anticoagulation. However, this intervention prevents future emboli without modifying already existent insults. If there is no contraindication, heparin should be initiated immediately, using a loading dose followed by a maintenance infusion to achieve a partial thromboplastin time (PTT) of 1.5 times control. Because long-term anticoagulation must be maintained, patients should be tested with warfarin beginning on the first day, with a titration to induce an INR of two to three times control. Heparin and warfarin should be overlapped for approximately 5 days. Warfarin should be maintained for at least 3 months if the source of the pulmonary embolism has been identified and is reversible. In patients in whom the predisposition for recurrent pulmonary embolism is irreversible, anticoagulation should be maintained indefinitely.

Novel thrombolytic agents have been evaluated extensively for treatment of acute pulmonary embolism. By and large they facilitate more rapid resolution of perfusion defects on lung scans and normalization of hemodynamics. However, they do not generally improve outcome and thus are not indicated for use in all patients. In the patient presenting with hemodynamic compromise and hypotension, thrombolytics may be of value. Patients with cardiovascular collapse manifest by hypotension and elevated venous pressure require vasopressors to support blood pressure immediately. If thrombolysis cannot be instituted immediately, emergency pulmonary angiography and embolectomy should be considered, despite the high mortality of surgical embolectomy.

Inferior vena cava interruption with percutaneously placed filters has prevented recurrent embolization in patients with documented deep vein thrombosis. It is indicated when long-term anticoagulation is too risky and in patients who have had recurrent pulmonary embolism despite vigorous and apparently adequate anticoagulant therapy. The Gianturco-Roehm "bird's nest" filter and the Greenfield filter are the most popular devices used.

In a small subset of patients, the initial pulmonary embolism is either unrecognized or inadequately treated and progresses to chronic proximal pulmonary thromboembolism associated with pulmonary hypertension. Recurrent pulmonary embolization is not the presenting problem. Instead, an insidious onset of right ventricular failure supervenes, which is often confused with primary pulmonary hypertension. The diagnosis becomes apparent only after a perfusion lung scan is obtained, which invariably shows multiple perfusion defects. Because many of the occlusions are subtotal, the perfusion lung scan generally underestimates the extent of the thrombotic pulmonary vascular disease. Pulmonary angiography is needed to outline the extent and location of chronic thromboembolism and identify patients who are good candidates for a surgical thromboendarterectomy.

An operative candidate is a patient with documented pulmonary thromboembolism associated with pulmonary hypertension unresponsive to anticoagulant therapy for a minimum of 3 months. The thromboemboli must be rather proximal (at lobar bifurcations) and accessible surgically. Although the operation is associated with a high mortality, experienced centers have reported figures as low as 10%. Fortunately, patients who survive the operation invariably have dramatically improved functional capacity and hemodynamics that cannot be attained with medical therapy alone.

Dyspnea and Congenital Heart Disease

William E. Hopkins

Dyspnea in patients with congenital heart disease can result from generalized deconditioning, ventricular dysfunction with pulmonary edema, decreased systemic cardiac output due to valvular dysfunction, ventricular failure or cardiac shunts, and/or hypoxemia.

IX. SPECIFIC ENTITIES THAT MAY CAUSE DYSPNEA

A. Atrial Septal Defect/Anomalous Pulmonary Venous Connection

The congenital cardiac defects most likely to cause physiologically important left-to-right shunts in adults are atrial septal defects and anomalous pulmonary venous connections. In both, the most common complaints in adults presenting with the disorder for the first time are dyspnea, fatigue, and palpitations. Both an atrial septal defect and anomalous pulmonary venous connection result in shunting of pulmonary venous blood into the right heart. In patients with an atrial septal defect, the shunt occurs via a communication in the atrial septum. The magnitude of the shunt is determined by the relative compliance properties of the left and right ventricles. Because the right ventricle is usually considerably more compliant than the left ventricle, the shunt is most often left-to-right. Anomalous pulmonary veins connect directly to the right atrium or to a systemic vein (most commonly the superior vena cava). Both atrial septal defect and anomalous pulmonary venous connection result in volume loading of the right ventricle (hence right ventricular dilatation) and increased circulation through the lungs (hence shunt vascularity on chest x-ray). The left-to-right shunt results in an underfilled left ventricle and decreased systemic cardiac output. The decrease in systemic cardiac output is more apparent with exercise and therefore is manifest as exertional fatigue and dyspnea. Pathological processes that reduce the compliance of the left ventricle—such as fibrosis associated with previous myocardial infarction, hypertrophy with systemic hypertension, or tachyarrhythmias such as atrial fibrillation—result in an augmentation of the left-to-right shunt and progressive symptoms. Pulmonary hypertension can then develop and result in a significant reduction in the compliance of the right ventricle. If marked enough, the shunt can become a right-to-left shunt and result in systemic hypoxemia (Eisenmenger syndrome) and further dyspnea.

SUGGESTED READING

Evaluation and Treatment of Patients with Shortness of Breath

Altose MD. Assessment and management of breathlessness. Chest 1985; 88:77S–82S.

Clausen J. Pulmonary Function testing. In: Nellis WN, ed. Textbook of Internal Medicine. 2d ed. Philadelphia: Lippincott, 1992:1823–1827.

DePaso WJ, Winterbauer RH, Lusk JA, et al. Chronic dyspnea unexplained by history, physical examination, chest roentgenogram, and spirometry: Analysis of a seven-year experience. Chest 1991; 100:1293–1299.

Dupuis C, Charaf LAC, Breviere G, et al. The "adult" form of the scimitar syndrome. Am J Cardiol 1992; 70:502–507.

Killian KJ, Jones NL. Respiratory muscles and dyspnea. Clin Chest Med 1988; 9:237–248.

Mahler DA. Positional dyspnea. In: Mahler DA, ed. Dyspnea. Mt. Kisco: Futura, 1990: 145–163.

Pratter MR, Curley FJ, Dubois J, et al. Cause and evaluation of chronic dyspnea in a pulmonary disease clinic. Arch Intern Med 1989; 149:2277–2282.

Ries AL. The role of exercise testing in pulmonary diagnosis. Clin Chest Med 1987; 8: 81–89.

Sweer L, Zwillich CW. Dyspnea in the patient with chronic obstructive pulmonary disease: Etiology and management. Clin Chest Med 1990; 11:417–445.

Tobin MJ. Dyspnea: Physiologic basis, clinical presentation, and management. Arch Intern Med 1990; 150:1604–1613.

Wasserman K, Casaburi R. Dyspnea: Physiological and pathophysiological mechanisms. Annu Rev Med 1988; 39:503–515.

3

Other Cardinal Manifestations of Heart Disease

Evaluation and Treatment of Patients with Cough

Stephen P. Bradley, Jack L. Clausen, and Kenneth M. Moser

Cough is a common presenting symptom that can be due to a wide variety of underlying disorders. Involvement of the upper respiratory tract (sinusitis, rhinitis), lower respiratory tract (asthma, bronchitis, bronchiectasis and others), gastrointestinal tract (gastroesophageal reflux, aspiration), and cardiovascular system (left ventricular dysfunction, mitral valve disease) may all present with cough as the primary or sole manifestation of disease.

A careful history will identify patients with acute respiratory tract infections, in whom cough is typically self-limited. Symptoms of sinusitis (sinus fullness, purulent nasal discharge) or rhinitis (clear nasal discharge, frequent throat clearing) are more suggestive of upper respiratory tract causes. Recurrent wheezing suggests asthma, although it should be remembered that congestive heart failure, bronchitis, and, rarely, tracheal or bronchial obstruction may mimic the cough and wheezing of asthma. In addition, wheezing may be absent in patient with "cough-variant" asthma. Chronic bronchitis and bronchiectasis usually present with purulent sputum production, which is greatest in the morning. Heartburn, changes in the voice, and a sour taste in the mouth suggest gastroesophageal reflux as the etiology.

Patients with pulmonary venous congestion on the basis of left ventricular dysfunction or mitral valve disease often present with cough in addition to more typical symptoms of heart failure. Patients may complain of paroxysmal cough—which either occurs when the patient is lying flat or awakens the patient several hours later—instead of the more typical symptoms of orthopnea and paroxysmal nocturnal dyspnea, respectively. The cough due to chronic pulmonary venous hypertension is typically nonproductive. In contrast, in acute pulmonary edema, the sputum is often described as pink and frothy.

Hemoptysis due to hypertrophy and subsequent rupture of bronchial veins is a well-described complication of long-standing pulmonary venous hypertension, most commonly seen in mitral stenosis. Although rarely seen in the United States, rheumatic heart disease remains common in the developing world, and hemoptysis may be the presenting complaint in affected patients. The typical patient is a young adult with a history of rheumatic fever who presents after producing either blood-tinged sputum or a moderate amount of frank blood. The hemoptysis may be recurrent but is rarely massive. There may be no other evidence of heart failure by history or physical examination, although a careful physical examination will usually reveal evidence of mitral stenosis with or without concomitant regurgitation or other valvular lesions. Other common causes of hemoptysis—such as bronchitis, bronchiectasis, bacterial pneumonia, and bronchogenic carcinoma—are usually suggested by a careful history, physical examination, and chest roentgenography.

A dry, nonproductive cough is the most common side effect due to angiotensin converting enzyme (ACE) inhibitors, developing in approximately 10–15% of patients taking these medications. With the increasing use of these medications for hypertension and left ventricular failure, cough has become a frequently seen complication. The cough improves after discontinuation of the drug, and a 4-day trial off medication is sufficient to allow differentiation between cough due to the ACE inhibitor and worsening heart failure or other causes. Occasionally, the cough improves despite continuation of the medication; dose reduction is also effective in some patients. Limited studies suggest a potential role for nonsteroidal anti-inflammatory drugs or calcium channel blockers in alleviating cough; antitussives and antihistamines are rarely effective. Angioneurotic edema is a rare but more serious side effect of ACE inhibitors that calls for immediate medical attention and lifelong avoidance of these medications.

SUGGESTED READING

Hodes RM. Hemoptysis in rheumatic heart disease. Trop Geogr Med. 1992; 44:328–330.

Irwin RS, Curley FJ, French CL. Chronic cough: The spectrum and frequency of causes, key components of the diagnostic evaluation, and outcome of specific therapy. Am Rev Respir Dis 1990; 141:640–647.

Israili ZH, Hall WD. Cough and angioneurotic edema associated with angiotensin converting enzyme inhibitor therapy: A review of the literature and pathophysiology. Ann Intern Med 1992; 117:234–242.

4

Palpitations

I.	Medical History	61
II.	Physical Examination	63
III.	Documentation of the Heart Rhythm During Palpitation	65
IV.	Initial Assessment of the Heart Rhythm	69
V.	Initial Management of Sustained Arrhythmias	74
	Suggested Reading	78

Michael E. Cain

Palpitation is a common symptom defined as an unpleasant awareness of the rapid or the forceful beating of the heart. It may occur because of changes in heart rhythm, heart rate, or stroke volume. This chapter reviews the general principles involved in the initial evaluation of patients with palpitations due to cardiac arrhythmia. The recognition and management of specific cardiac arrhythmias is detailed in Chapter 17, on the management of patients with cardiac arrhythmias.

Optimal evaluation of patients with palpitations begins with accurate documentation and analysis of the heart rhythm during symptoms. This goal is best achieved by the integration of information acquired from the medical history, physical examination, and judicious use of diagnostic tests.

I. MEDICAL HISTORY

A direct dialogue between the patient, a family member or other individual who has witnessed the patient during palpitations, and the physician provides invaluable information on the presence and type of arrhythmia, the factors associated with its initiation and termination, and its severity.

A. Presence and Type of Arrhythmia

Although patients use different terms to describe palpitations (e.g., "flip-flopping," "fluttering," "skipping," "pounding," "racing," or "heart-stopping"), it is usually possible to gain insight into the rhythm disorder by having the patient duplicate the rate and cadence of the palpitation by tapping his or her fingers. This is particularly helpful, since palpitations are often paroxysmal and usually absent at the time of the interview and physical examination. Complaints of "skipped beats" or a "flip-flop sensation" in the chest are usually due to atrial or ventricular extrasystoles. Patients with atrial or ventricular ectopy are often more aware of the postextrasystolic beat, which is associated with an overfilled heart and large stroke volume, than of the premature beat itself. The sensation that the heart has "stopped beating" usually correlates with the compensatory pause following the premature contraction. Fleeting and repetitive palpitations suggest multiple ectopic beats. A gradual onset and cessation of symptoms is typical of sinus tachycardia. If the patient describes the abrupt onset of palpitations and taps out a rapid and regular rhythm, paroxysmal supraventricular tachycardia, atrial flutter, or ventricular tachycardia should be suspected. A rapid but irregular cadence suggests atrial fibrillation or an atrial tachycardia with variable atrioventricular (AV) block. Some patients are perceptive enough to count their pulse during palpitations. Rates of 100 to 140 beats/min suggest sinus tachycardia. Atrial flutter is often associated with a pulse rate of approximately 150 beats/min. A rate exceeding 160 beats/min suggests paroxysmal supraventricular tachycardia or ventricular tachycardia.

B. Precipitating Factors

The patient should be encouraged to describe the circumstances surrounding the onset and termination of palpitations. Specific information should be sought regarding where, when, during what activities, and in whose presence the symptoms become noticeable. The relationship of symptoms to meals, use of caffeine-containing beverages, alcohol intake, smoking, exercise, fatigue, and emotion (particularly anxiety and anger) should be thoroughly explored. A careful drug history is essential, since the use of medications such as antiarrhythmic drugs, diuretics, sympathomimetics, antibiotics, or psychoactive drugs can affect the heart rhythm and precipitate arrhythmias.

Circumstances and other symptoms that provoke arrhythmias will often suggest the diagnosis. A history of palpitation associated with a lump in the throat, dizziness, and tingling in the hands and face suggests sinus tachycardia accompanying an anxiety state with hyperventilation. A history of palpitation during or after strenuous activities may be normal, whereas palpitation during mild exertion suggests the presence of heart failure, anemia, thyrotoxicosis, or poor physical conditioning. When palpitation can be relieved suddenly by stooping, breath-holding, induced gagging, or vomiting, AV nodal reentry or reentrant tachycardia (orthodromic or antidromic) mediated by an accessory pathway is suggested. Palpitation followed by presyncope or syncope suggests either asystole or severe bradycardia following the termination of a tachycardia.

C. Functional and Emotional Consequences

A third purpose of the medical history is to establish the functional and emotional consequences of the arrhythmia, a judgment based largely on the intensity of symptoms (e.g., dizziness, syncope, fatigue, dyspnea, or chest pain) that accompany the palpitations and on the anxiety expressed by the patient concerning a recurrence. This information influences the extent, sequence, and timing of diagnostic tests. For example, a patient in whom palpitation occurs daily and is associated with pulmonary edema and angina will benefit from hospitalization with the anticipation that the heart rhythm during symptoms will be documented within 24 hr. In contrast, initial assessment of a patient with infrequent and mild symptoms would be best served by ambulatory ECG monitoring.

The functional consequences of palpitations must be evaluated in light of the patient's general medical and cardiovascular status. Dizziness and syncope due to arrhythmias are usually caused by extreme bradycardia or tachycardia. In the presence of associated cardiac or cerebral disease, the heart rate required to cause dizziness or syncope is modified. For example, tachycardia will produce syncope at lower heart rates in the presence of severe aortic stenosis. Patients with diffuse cerebrovascular disease may become symptomatic with milder bradycardia. Syncope in otherwise normal young people suggests that the abnormal rhythm is quite dangerous. In patients with coronary artery disease or aortic stenosis, angina may develop during tachyarrhythmias; and in patients with mitral stenosis or ventricular failure, dyspnea or acute pulmonary edema may occur.

Palpitations are often of great psychological significance, since they may be seen as a sign of heart disease. Anxiety may augment the severity of the symptoms. Individual perceptions of arrhythmias are extremely variable; some patients are unaware of the most chaotic arrhythmias, while others are severely incapacitated by palpitations caused by mild rhythm disturbances. In general, palpitations are more likely to be experienced at night and during introspective moments and less likely during activity. Palpitations seem to be more disturbing when they are recent in onset, transient, and episodic. In chronic rhythm disturbances, the patient tends to adapt and become less aware of the abnormal rhythm.

II. PHYSICAL EXAMINATION

The physical examination can provide valuable clues to the diagnosis of cardiac arrhythmia. Although information obtained on physical examination is often redundant, with more extensive and specific information being derived from the standard ECG, the patient may be seen initially in a setting where the recording of an ECG is not possible. The primary sources of information that aid in the diagnosis of arrhythmias are the jugular venous pulse, arterial pulse, and heart sounds (Table 1).

A. Jugular Venous Pulse

The patient should be examined in a quiet room and placed on a bed or examining table having a head section that can be raised or lowered so that the patient's trunk is at a 30–45° elevation from the horizontal. As a rule, atrial activity is best reflected in the right internal jugular venous pulse. During normal sinus rhythm, an a wave precedes the first heart sound and a v wave follows it. The a wave, produced by atrial contraction, is absent during atrial fibrillation. In atrial flutter, rapid and smaller oscillations occurring at a rate of approximately 300/min are typically observed. The venous pulse is particularly valuable in the detection of AV dissociation. When right atrial contraction occurs while the tricuspid valve is closed, a "cannon" a wave will occur in the jugular venous pulse. Cannon a waves may occur regularly or intermittently. When coincident with the arterial pulse, they can result either from supraventricular tachycardia when the PR interval is short or when the P wave follows the QRS or from ventricular tachycardia with 1:1 ventriculoatrial conduction. In supraventricular tachycardia with 2:1 AV block, cannon a waves may occur during every other atrial cycle, coincident with each arterial pulse. Intermittent cannon a waves can be caused by atrial, AV junctional, or ventricular premature depolarizations; the specific etiology can usually be deduced according to the association of these waves with intermittent premature occurrence of the first heart sound and arterial pulse. Regular bradycardia and intermittent cannon a waves are typical of complete AV block. Regular tachycardia and intermittent cannon a waves suggest ventricular tachycardia with AV dissociation.

B. Arterial Pulse

The arterial pulse is often relied on initially to determine the ventricular rate and rhythm. The carotid arterial pulse normally has a single positive wave. An exaggerated carotid pulse may be seen with sinus tachycardia or in patients who are anxious or apprehensive. With complete AV block in adults, the ventricular rate is approximately 40 beats/min, the diastolic pressure is low, and the cardiac stroke volume is increased, thus causing a prominent arterial pulse. For the same reason, 2:1 AV block or sinus bradycardia may also cause an exaggerated arterial pulse. When intermittent premature beats occur, tapping the foot in time with the pulse will usually permit one to distinguish compensatory from noncompensatory pauses—the former pattern suggesting ventricular premature depolarizations and the latter atrial ectopy. Atrial fibrillation produces an irregularly irregular pulse. Under certain circumstances when atrial activation is not transmitted to the ventricles, the peripheral pulses wax and wane in relation to varying time intervals between atrial and ventricular systole. This variation of pulse magnitude occurs most commonly in patients with ventricular tachycardia and in those with AV block or AV dissociation. The pulse is strong when atrial systole precedes ventricular systole by short intervals. When there is a long interval or no preceding atrial contraction, the pulse is weak.

C. Heart Sounds

The most useful heart sounds in the analysis of arrhythmias are S_1 and S_4. S_1 is louder when the PR interval is short, and vice versa. The intensity of S_1 is not particularly useful in the presence of irregular tachycardias, because changes in the cardiac cycle length will also cause the intensity of S_1 to vary. However, in regular tachycardias, marked changes in the intensity of S_1 suggest AV dissociation with intermittent effective atrial contraction. Also, a regular bradycardia with significant variation of S_1 suggests second-degree AV block or complete heart block with AV dissociation. In complete heart block, the relationship of S_4 to S_1 may vary, and more than one S_4 may be heard during a single diastolic phase. Often, auscultation at the apex during the examination of the jugular venous pulse can be very helpful in determining the cause of an arrhythmia. For example, the electrocardiographic (ECG) pattern of regular tachycardia at 150 beats/min and a wide QRS may be seen with paroxysmal supraventricular tachycardia with aberrant conduction, atrial flutter with 2:1 AV block and bundle branch block, or ventricular tachycardia. During supraventricular tachycardias, there will be one a wave per QRS and the amplitude of S_1 will be constant. In atrial flutter, flutter waves may be evident in the jugular venous pulse and S_1 will be constant. If sinus rhythm and AV dissociation exist, ventricular tachycardia will produce occasional cannon a waves and S_1 will vary in amplitude. In circulatory arrest due to ventricular fibrillation, cardiac standstill, or extremely rapid ventricular tachycardia, there is no measurable blood pressure, no arterial pulse, and no audible heart sound. The differential diagnosis between ventricular fibrillation and cardiac asystole cannot be made without an ECG.

III. DOCUMENTATION OF THE HEART RHYTHM
DURING PALPITATION

Optimal management of patients with palpitations requires accurate diagnosis of the cardiac rhythm during symptoms. Specific strategies for selecting the approach to document the heart rhythm during palpitations depend on the frequency, duration, and severity of symptoms.

Table 1 Cardiac Arrhythmias: Physical Examination and Electrocardiographic Characteristics

Arrhythmia	Intensity of S_1	Jugular venous pulse	Ventricular response to carotid sinus massage[a]
Sinus tachycardia	Constant	Normal	Gradual slowing and return to former rate
Sinus bradycardia	Constant	Normal	Gradual slowing and return to former rate
Atrial flutter	Constant; variable if AV block variable	Flutter a waves	Abrupt slowing and return to former rate; atrial flutter remains
Atrial fibrillation	Variable	No a waves	Gradual slowing; gross irregularity remains
AV nodal reentry	Constant, usually decreased	Constant, usually with cannon a waves	Abrupt slowing due to termination of arrhythmia
Orthodromic tachycardia	Constant	Constant, usually with cannon a waves	Abrupt slowing due to termination of arrhythmia
Sinus node reentry	Constant	Normal	Gradual slowing and return to former rate
Intraatrial reentry or automatic atrial tachycardia	Constant; variable if AV block variable	More a waves than v waves	Abrupt slowing and return to former rate; atrial tachycardia remains
Multifocal atrial tachycardia	Variable	Variable relation of a to v waves	No response or gradual slowing with atrial irregularity continuing
Junctional tachycardia	Variable[c]	Intermittent cannon a waves[c]	None
Accelerated idioventricular rhythm	Variable[c]	Intermittent cannon a waves[c]	None
Ventricular tachycardia	Variable[c]	Intermittent cannon a waves[c]	None
Ventricular fibrillation	Absent	Usually absent	None

[a]Lack of a response to carotid sinus massage may occur with any arrhythmia.
[b]Ventricular rate equals atrial rate in absence of AV block.
[c]Constant if atria are captured retrogradely.

66

P waves			QRS complexes		
Rate	Rhythm	Morphology	Rate	Rhythm	Morphology
100–180	Regular	May be peaked	100–180[b]	Regular	Normal
<60	Regular	Normal	<60[b]	Regular	Normal
250–350	Regular	Sawtooth	75–175	Regular in absence of drugs or disease	Normal
400–600	Grossly irregular	Baseline undulation without clear p waves	100–180	Grossly irregular	Normal
120–250	Regular	Inverted	120–250	Regular	Normal
150–250	Regular	Dependent on site of accessory pathway	150–250	Regular	Normal
125–200	Regular	Normal	125–200	Regular[b]	Normal
150–250	Regular	Abnormal	75–200[b]	Regular	Normal
100–150	Grossly irregular	Variable	100–150[b]	Grossly irregular	Normal
60–100[d]	Regular	Normal	70–130	Regular	Normal; may be abnormal but <0.12 sec
60–100[d]	Regular	Normal	50–110	Fairly regular	Abnormal, >0.12 sec
60–100[d]	Regular	Normal	110–250	Regular	Abnormal, >0.12 sec
60–100[d]	Regular	Normal	400–600	Grossly irregular	Baseline undulation; no QRS complexes

[d]Any independent atrial arrhythmia may exist or the atria may be captured retrogradely.
Source: Adapted from Zipes DP Specific arrhythmias: Diagnosis and treatment. In: Braunwald E, ed. Heart Disease: A Textbook for Cardiovascular Medicine. 2d ed. Philadelphia: Saunders, 1984.

A. Electrocardiogram and Rhythm Strip

The cardiac rhythm in patients experiencing palpitations at the time of the interview can usually be determined from analysis of a 12-lead ECG and rhythm strip. For some patients with paroxysmal arrhythmias, the 12-lead ECG is also a satisfactory approach if palpitations last several hours, are not disabling, and the patient has ready access to a medical facility where an ECG can be recorded during symptoms.

B. Ambulatory Electrocardiographic Monitoring

For most patients with paroxysmal palpitations, ambulatory ECG monitoring is the best method to objectively relate specific heart rhythms to patient symptoms. Continuous 24- or 48-hr ECG recordings are the standard. This approach permits analysis of all heartbeats, is indicated for use in patients who experience palpitations at least daily (and preferably several times a day), and provides information on the temporal distribution of arrhythmic events during wake and sleep cycles as well as whether cardiac arrhythmias are associated with antecedent sinus tachycardia, sinus bradycardia, physical exertion, myocardial ischemia, or specific time intervals after the administration of medications.

Advances in ECG signal processing have extended the ability to establish a cause-and-effect relationship between spontaneous cardiac arrhythmias and symptoms in patients with infrequent arrhythmic events that are unlikely to be captured during 24 or even 48 hr of continuous monitoring. Event recorders are now designed for use in patients with infrequent but sustained (at least 3 minutes in duration) palpitations as well as for those with infrequent but fleeting symptoms. Patients with infrequent but sustained palpitations can be provided with ECG event recorders for extended periods of time. When palpitations occur, the patient connects the ECG leads to the monitoring device and activates the recorder. Documentation of the heart rhythm in patients with paroxysmal but fleeting symptoms of palpitations is best accomplished with a continuous-loop ECG recorder. The ECG is monitored continuously but data are stored only when activated by the patient. The memory loop enables documentation of the heart rhythm for up to 60 sec before and 90 sec after patient activation of the recording device, thus maximizing the opportunity to detect brief arrhythmic events.

C. Exercise Testing

Provocative testing is required to relate arrhythmic events to symptoms in patients in whom rigorous attempts with the use of ambulatory ECG monitoring have not produced definitive results. Exercise testing and programmed stimulation (discussed below) are methods used to induce cardiac arrhythmias under controlled conditions. In response to exercise, there is withdrawal of vagal tone and a marked increase in the sympathetic neuroactivity and the level of circulating catecholamines. Sympathetic stimulation plays a major role in the genesis or maintenance of some arrhythmias. Patients with a history of palpitations that are temporally associated with physical or emotional stress are most likely to benefit from exercise testing if ambulatory ECG monitoring has failed to definitively establish a cause-and-effect relationship between spontaneous arrhythmic events and symptoms. Although the number of patients who require excercise stress testing to establish a definitive link between cardiac rhythm and symptoms is small, this approach is particularly useful in patients in whom sinus tachycardia is suspected as the cause of palpitations.

D. Electrophysiological Studies

Invasive electrophysiological studies are used routinely in patients with documented clinical arrhythmias to define mechanisms of arrhythmogenesis, assess the efficacy of antiarrhythmic therapy, and localize and ablate arrhythmogenic tissue. Despite the increasing utilization of these studies in patients with documented arrhythmias, their role in establishing a link between the heart rhythm and symptoms of palpitation is and should remain limited to patients with severe symptoms in whom it is felt unsafe to allow the occurrence of another spontaneous event. Every attempt should be made to establish the relationship between symptoms and underlying cardiac rhythm, using the ECG monitoring techniques described, before proceeding with invasive electrophysiological studies. This caution is necessary because of the low specificity of arrhythmia induction by programmed atrial and ventricular stimulation.

IV. INITIAL ASSESSMENT OF THE HEART RHYTHM

The initial and long-term management of the patient with palpitations caused by a cardiac arrhythmia is dictated by the mechanism of the arrhythmia and its functional and emotional consequences. When initially confronted with the patient having a cardiac arrhythmia, the physician will most likely have to rely on the information contained in the 12-lead ECG to initiate treatment.

A. Analysis of the 12-Lead ECG and Rhythm Strip

In most cases, a systematic analysis of the ECG is sufficient to make a definitive diagnosis. It is best to examine the complete 12-lead ECG in the standard way before analyzing rhythm strips. For rhythm analysis, an ECG lead must be selected that shows distinct P waves and QRS complexes. The mechanism of a cardiac arrhythmia is difficult to determine unless every atrial and ventricular depolarization is identified and used in the analysis. Electrocardiographic calipers are used in examining the rhythm strip. Initial inspection should focus on determining whether the contours and durations of the P waves and QRS complexes are normal. An abnormal P-wave morphology reflects an abnormal atrial depolarization sequence and indicates that the impulse originates outside the sinus node. Absence of the P wave is an important finding and is much more convincing when the tracings from all 12 standard leads are carefully examined. A normal QRS complex virtually eliminates the ventricle as the site of origin for the arrhythmia. If the QRS is widened, it is essential to know whether the QRS morphology is typical of left or right bundle branch block or whether the pattern suggests ventricular preexcitation. A previous ECG is a valuable adjunct to rhythm analysis. In the rhythm strip, each P wave and QRS complex must be identified. The rate and regularity of PP and RR intervals should be ascertained. The typical P-QRS relationships during each of the types of paroxysmal supraventricular tachycardias are summarized in Table 2. One should also establish whether or not the PR interval is constant and whether the number of atrial and ventricular depolarizations is identical. Even when these features are identified, more than one hypothesis may apply.

Ways in which detection of atrial activity may be facilitated are outlined below.

Multiple-Lead Rhythm Strips

Leads aV_F and V_1 recorded at a paper speed of 50 mm/sec are particularly useful for identifying P waves.

Table 2 ECG Diagnosis of Paroxysmal Supraventricular Tachycardia (SVT): P-QRS Relationship

Type	ECG
1. AV node reentry	Retrograde P wave buried in QRS or immediately follows QRS (RP interval <50% RR)
2. AV reentry utilizing a bypass tract (orthodromic SVT)	P wave immediately follows the QRS (RP interval <50% RR)
3. Sinus node reentry	P-wave morphology identical to sinus rhythm, PR related to SVT rate (RP interval >50% RR)
4. Intraatrial reentry	P-wave morphology depends upon site of intraatrial circuit, PR interval related to SVT rate (RP interval >50% RR)
5. Automatic atrial tachycardia	P-wave morphology depends upon site of ectopic focus PR interval related to SVT rate (RP interval >50% RR); first and subsequent P waves have same morphology

Abbreviations: AV = atrioventricular; SVT = supraventricular tachycardia.

70

Adenosine

For patients evaluated in a medical facility, temporary alteration in AV conduction is best achieved with intravenous adenosine (6 to 12 mg).

Carotid Sinus Massage

Vagal maneuvers such as carotid sinus massage often transiently alter AV conduction. External pressure with a gentle massaging motion will stimulate baroreceptors in the carotid sinus, activating a reflex arc that increases the vagal traffic to the heart. The patient should lie supine, with support provided under the shoulders to hyperextend the head and relax the sternocleidomastoid muscle. Electrocardiographic leads should be selected that are most likely to detect P waves when pressure on the carotid sinus causes a pause in rhythm; the use of multiple simultaneous leads increases the likelihood of recording P waves during transient changes in rhythm. The patient's head should be turned to the left for massage of the right carotid sinus. The operator should place the flat portion of the fingertips over the carotid bifurcation near the angle of the jaw. The ECG should be recorded continuously. Initially, only slight downward pressure should be exerted to detect patients with hypersensitive responses. If no response is observed, firm pressure should be applied with a gentle, rotating, massaging motion. Massage should be discontinued after 5 sec. If no response is obtained after several attempts on one side, contralateral massage should be performed. Both carotid sinuses, however, should not be massaged simultaneously. The Valsalva maneuver may be performed in conjunction with carotid sinus massage. The responses of various arrhythmias to carotid sinus massage are listed in Table 1.

Carotid sinus pressure has risks, particularly in older patients. The efferent limb of the baroreceptor reflex may cause peripheral vasodilation and thus lower blood pressure. Stroke following carotid sinus pressure may be due to either cerebral thrombosis or embolism. Carotid sinus massage should be avoided in patients known to have cerebral vascular disease, particularly those with disease in the external carotid system; this condition should be sought by means of history and physical examination when the use of this technique is being considered. Carotid sinus pressure may produce prolonged sinus arrest or high-grade AV block, either of which may cause a dangerous, extended pause in ventricular rhythm. Prolonged sinus arrest after conversion of supraventricular tachyarrhythmias to sinus rhythm is more likely in patients with sinus node dysfunction. If the history suggests sick sinus syndrome and particularly if it includes syncopal episodes, carotid sinus massage should be performed with extreme caution if at all.

Lewis ECG Lead

Special placement of electrodes on the body surface can reveal P waves even when none are discerned in the standard 12-lead ECG. In a method of lead placement attributed to Lewis, the right and left arm leads are positioned in the second and fourth intercostal spaces just to the right of the sternum. Lead I is then recorded, preferably with simultaneous inscription of another lead that displays a well-defined QRS complex.

Esophageal ECG Lead

If a conventional esophageal lead is not available, one can be made by passing an electrode catheter through a nasogastric (NG) tube. The electrode catheter, however, should not extend beyond the distal part of the tube during passage into the esophagus. After the NG tube and catheter are placed approximately 50 cm into the esophagus, the electrode catheter is connected to an exploring (V lead) electrode. The catheter is then extended through the distal end of the NG tube and search is made for electrical activity. If atrial activity is not evident, the NG tube and electrode catheter should be withdrawn in 1-cm increments until P waves and QRS complexes are identified. Having the patient hold his or her breath during midinspiration reduces respiratory interference.

B. Wide QRS Complex Tachycardia

The definitive diagnosis of a wide-QRS-complex tachycardia can be difficult, but correct identification of the underlying etiology is imperative to ensure optimal treatment. There are three etiologies of a wide-complex tachycardia: (a) ventricular tachycardia, (b) supraventricular tachycardia with preexisting or rate-dependent bundle branch block, and (c) supraventricular tachyarrhythmias, including atrial fibrillation, with antegrade conduction through an accessory pathway (Wolff-Parkinson-White syndrome). Historical information is helpful in evaluating a patient with a wide-complex tachycardia. For example, a history of coronary artery disease, prior myocardial infarction, or congestive heart failure favors a diagnosis of ventricular tachycardia. A previously recorded ECG may show bundle branch block during sinus rhythm or ventricular preexcitation. In general, a patient's age is not particularly helpful in evaluating the mechanism of a wide-complex tachycardia. Hemodynamic stability of the tachycardia is also of little diagnostic value.

The ECG is the mainstay for the emergent diagnosis of a wide-complex tachycardia. An irregular rhythm indicates atrial fibrillation with aberrant conduction or conduction via an accessory pathway. A regular rhythm indicates supraventricular tachycardia with aberrant conduction or ventricular tachycardia. Electrocardiographic features that are useful in defining the mechanism of a regular wide-complex tachycardia include the following:

> *AV dissociation.* Although AV dissociation is 100% specific for ventricular tachycardia, it is recognizable in only about 25% of ECGs recorded during ventricular tachycardia.

QRS duration. A QRS duration greater than 140 msec with a right bundle branch block morphology or greater than 160 msec with a left bundle branch block configuration favors ventricular tachycardia. However, if the patient is receiving treatment with antiarrhythmic drugs, the diagnostic power of QRS duration is diminished.

Frontal-plane QRS axis. A frontal-plane QRS axis between -90 and $-180°$, particularly when used in combination with other criteria, is predictive of ventricular tachycardia. The frontal-plane axis, however, is less useful in wide-complex tachycardia having a right bundle branch block QRS morphology.

QRS morphology. Certain QRS morphologies in leads V_1, V_2, and V_6 (Table 3) as well as concordance of the QRS vector in the precordial leads (i.e., predominantly positive or negative deflections in all precordial leads) suggest ventricular tachycardia.

The following stepwise ECG algorithm proposed by Brugada and co-workers has a sensitivity of 98.7% and a specificity of 96.5% for detecting ventricular tachycardia. One proceeds to the next step only if the diagnosis of ventricular tachycardia is not made.

Step 1. Examine the QRS morphology in each precordial lead. Absence of a RS complex in all precordial leads is diagnostic of ventricular tachycardia (100% specificity).

Table 3 Morphological Features of Wide-Complex Tachycardia

Type	Lead V_{1-2}	Lead V_6
RBBB tachycardia		
VT	Monophasic R or biphasic QR or RS pattern	Monophasic R or biphasic QS or QR pattern R/S ratio <1
SVT	Triphasic QRS	Triphasic QRS
LBBB tachycardia		
VT	R wave >30 msec RS (onset of R to nadir of S wave) >60 msec; Notching of the upstroke of S wave	Q wave present (QR or QS pattern)
SVT	If preexisting LBBB is present, morphology is unchanged	Monophasic R wave

Abbreviations: LBBB = left bundle branch block; RBBB = right bundle branch block; SVT = supraventricular tachycardia; VT = ventricular tachycardia.
Source: Adapted from Brugada et al. A new approach to the differential diagnosis of a regular tachycardia with a wide QRS complex. Circulation 1991; 83:1649.

Step 2. Measure the RS interval from the onset of the R wave to the nadir of the S wave. An interval greater than 100 msec is diagnostic of ventricular tachycardia (100% specificity).

Step 3. Examine the ECG for evidence of AV dissociation, which is diagnostic of ventricular tachycardia.

Step 4. Examine the QRS morphology in leads V_1, V_2, and V_6 (Table 3).

Step 5. If the above steps are negative, the cardiac arrhythmia is supraventricular tachycardia with aberrant conduction.

V. INITIAL MANAGEMENT OF SUSTAINED ARRHYTHMIAS

The initial treatment of the patient with a cardiac arrhythmia is dictated by his or her hemodynamic status. Pharmacological and nonpharmacological therapies for each type of cardiac arrhythmia are detailed in Chapters 17 and 18. However, some general principles for the treatment of supraventricular and ventricular tachycardias are summarized in this section.

A. Direct-Current Cardioversion

Cardioversion is the treatment of choice for patients with supraventricular or ventricular tachycardia who are hemodynamically compromised. Cardioversion should be performed using the lowest possible energy to reduce the incidence of complication and the degree of discomfort. A synchronized shock delivered during the QRS complex should be used for all cardioversions except for pulseless ventricular tachycardia, ventricular flutter, and ventricular fibrillation. Initial energy settings should be 25–50 J (joules) for atrial flutter and supraventricular tachycardia, 100–200 joules for atrial fibrillation, 50–200 J (50 J if hemodynamically stable, 200 J if pulseless) for ventricular tachycardia, and 200 J for ventricular fibrillation. Stepwise increases in energy settings should be used if termination of the arrhythmia is not successful.

Elective Cardioversion

Elective cardioversion is indicated if medical therapy fails to restore sinus rhythm. The patient should be fasted for 6 to 8 hr prior to the procedure and serum electrolytes and drug levels (especially digoxin) should be normal. An anticoagulant and antiarrhythmic agent should be administered prior to the procedure in most patients with atrial fibrillation or flutter. A 12-lead ECG should be recorded prior to and following cardioversion. The rhythm should be monitored continuously throughout the procedure. The patient should be supine with the paddles coated with electrode gel and in firm contact with the chest. Two electrode positions are acceptable: (a) a posterior electrode positioned in the left interscapular region, with the anterior electrode over the sternum in the third interspace, or (b) one electrode to the right of the sternum at the level of the second interspace and the other in the left midaxillarly line at the fourth or fifth interspace. Sedation and amnesia should be induced with intravenous diazepam, intravenous midazolam, or a short-acting barbiturate. Personnel skilled in endotracheal intubation should be in attendance. The synchronized artifact should be clearly evident on the monitor. However, if sinus rhythm is achieved only transiently, higher-energy settings are of no value.

The incidence of major complications is small if attention is paid to proper patient selection. If symptomatic bradycardia occurs, 0.5–1.0 mg of atropine should be administered intravenously. A temporary pacemaker may be required occasionally, although the availability of external pacemakers as part of cardioverter-defibrillator systems has decreased the need for transvenous catheters. After sinus rhythm is restored, appropriate antiarrhythmic drugs should be initiated or continued.

Relative Contraindications

A slow ventricular rate during atrial fibrillation (particularly in the absence of medications), marked sinus bradycardia, sinus pulse or sinus arrest, history of the bradycardia-tachycardia syndrome (especially with a history of syncope), and complete AV block are contraindications to cardioversion unless a temporary or permanent pacemaker has been inserted. Automatic tachycardias, including ectopic atrial tachycardias, nonparoxysmal junctional tachycardia, and accelerated idioventricular rhythm are not responsive to direct-current cardioversion. Untreated precipitating factors—including hyperthyroidism, pericarditis, and marked metabolic derangements—make it unlikely that sinus rhythm will be maintained. Whenever possible, precipitating factors should be corrected prior to cardioversion. If hemodynamic compromise is present, immediate cardioversion may be necessary as a temporizing measure.

Therapeutic levels of digoxin do not contraindicate direct-current cardioversion; however, refractory ventricular arrhythmias may develop if toxic levels of digoxin are present. If cardioversion cannot be delayed and high serum levels of digoxin are suspected, lidocaine should be administered and the lowest possible energy setting used.

B. Hemodynamically Stable Supraventricular Tachycardias

The choice of therapy should be guided by the mechanism responsible for the supraventricular tachycardia. The primary goal of therapy is to terminate the tachycardia. If the arrhythmia cannot be terminated, a secondary goal is to slow and regularize the ventricular rate.

75

Vagal Stimulation

The AV node is a critical component of the circuit in supraventricular tachycardias due to AV nodal reentry or reentry utilizing an accessory pathway. Each of these arrhythmias will terminate if conduction block in the AV node is produced, even if for only a single cycle. The sinus node is a critical component in sinus node reentry. Vagal stimulation, including the Valsalva maneuver and carotid sinus massage, alters the electrical properties of the sinus and AV nodes and is likely to terminate these supraventricular tachycardias. Vagal maneuvers generally do not terminate intraatrial reentry or automatic tachycardia but may increase AV block and slow the ventricular rate.

More intense vagal stimulation can be achieved with the diving reflex by placing the patient's forehead, cheeks, and temples into ice water. However, this maneuver can cause ventricular ectopy or asystole and should not be performed in older patients or those with conduction system disease. Vagal stimulation can be augmented by the administration of edrophonium (10 mg over 30 sec following a 1-mg test dose), methoxamine (3–5 mg), phenylephrine (0.1–0.5 mg), or metaraminol (0.5–1.0 mg). The availability of adenosine, however, has essentially eliminated the need to use these drugs in the treatment of supraventricular tachycardias.

Adenosine

Intravenous adenosine (6–12 mg) has become the drug of first choice for terminating supraventricular tachycardia due to sinus or AV nodal reentry or that utilizing an accessory pathway. Due to an extremely short half-life, hemodynamic alterations and side effects abate rapidly.

Verapamil

By increasing AV block, verapamil should be expected to terminate sinus or AV nodal reentry or orthodromic tachycardia utilizing an accessory pathway; verapamil may also slow the ventricular rate during automatic or intraatrial reentrant tachycardias. Administered as an intravenous bolus of 5–10 mg given over 2–3 min, the dose may be repeated every 15–30 min if necessary to a maximum dose of 20 mg. Caution must be exercised in hypotensive patients or those with overt heart failure.

Beta Blockers

Intravenous propranolol or esmolol may terminate supraventricular tachycardia with reentrant circuits involving the sinus or AV nodes or an accessory pathway; it may also slow AV conduction in automatic or intraatrial reentrant tachycardias.

Digoxin

By slowing AV nodal conduction, digoxin may terminate AV nodal reentry or reentry using an accessory pathway. Like verapamil and beta blockers, digoxin may increase AV block and slow the ventricular rate during other forms of supraventricular tachycardia. Digoxin should be given initially in a dose of 0.5 mg intravenously or orally, followed by 0.25 mg every 4–6 hr as needed. The total dose in the first 24 hr, however, should not exceed 1 mg.

Procainamide

Intravenous procainamide (30–50 mg/min over 30 min) will often terminate reentrant and automatic supraventricular tachycardias.

Electrical Cardioversion or Rapid Atrial Pacing

These nonpharmacological approaches can be used if the above methods are unsuccessful. Reentrant forms of supraventricular tachycardia are almost always responsive.

C. Hemodynamically Stable Ventricular Tachycardia

Sustained monomorphic ventricular tachycardia occurs most often in the setting of ischemic heart disease and healed myocardial infarction. If the patient is hemodynamically stable, lidocaine is the drug of first choice to restore sinus rhythm. Initial intravenous therapy should begin with a 1–1.5-mg/kg bolus. At the same time, a continuous infusion of 2–4 mg/min should be started. Additional boluses of 0.5–1.5 mg/kg (to a maximum total dose of 3.0 mg/kg) should be given at 5–10-min intervals to prevent subtherapeutic serum levels as a result of the rapid distribution of lidocaine to the tissue compartment. Maintenance therapy consists of a continuous infusion of 2–4 mg/min.

If lidocaine is not effective, procainamide or bretylium may be administered. Intravenous procainamide should be administered by continuous infusion at a rate up to 50 mg/min until the arrhythmia terminates or a total dose of 17 mg/kg is reached. Following termination of ventricular tachycardia, a maintenance infusion of 1–4 mg/min should be administered. Bretylium should be administered initially as an intravenous bolus of 5–10 mg/kg over 8–10 min, followed by a maintenance infusion of 1–2 mg/kg or repetitive boluses of 5–10 mg/kg every 6–8 hr.

If conversion to sinus rhythm does not occur promptly or the patient's condition deteriorates, direct-current cardioversion is indicated. Occasionally, underdrive or overdrive ventricular pacing may be used to terminate ventricular tachycardia, but it should be performed by experienced personnel.

D. Hemodynamically Stable Wide-Complex Tachycardia

Initial therapy depends on the mechanism of the tachycardia. Supraventricular and ventricular tachycardias should be treated as outlined above. If the diagnosis is uncertain even after a thorough history, physical examination, and interpretation of a 12-lead ECG, therapy should be chosen carefully. A stepwise approach initially utilizing more benign therapy is recommended, thus minimizing risk to the patient. Vagal maneuvers may be diagnostic and therapeutic by terminating a supraventricular tachycardia. As discussed, adenosine is an excellent drug to use in differentiating a supraventricular from a ventricular tachycardia. If vagal maneuvers and adenosine fail to terminate the tachycardia or provide insight into its mechanism, the wide-complex tachycardia should be assumed to be ventricular tachycardia. Lidocaine should be administered. If there is no response, procainamide may be useful. Low-energy cardioversion is very effective in terminating stable wide-complex tachycardias when other means fail.

Verapamil is a potentially dangerous drug to use in the setting of an undiagnosed wide-complex tachycardia and should be avoided. While its AV nodal–blocking capability will terminate some forms of supraventricular tachycardia, it can be catastrophic if it is mistakenly administered to a patient with ventricular tachycardia or a patient with antegrade conduction through an accessory pathway (Wolff-Parkinson-White syndrome). Peripheral vasodilation and decreased contractility may lead to hemodynamic collapse if ventricular tachycardia is treated with verapamil. In the presence of ventricular preexcitation, reflex sympathetic discharge in response to vasodilation can shorten the refractory period of the accessory pathway, resulting in increased pathway conduction and more rapid ventricular rates that can deteriorate to ventricular fibrillation.

SUGGESTED READING

Akhtar M, et al. Wide QRS complex tachycardia: Reappraisal of a common clinical problem. Ann Intern Med 1988; 109:905.

Brugada P, et al. A new approach to the differential diagnosis of a regular tachycardia with a wide QRS complex. Circulation 1991; 83:1649.

El-Sherif N, Samet P. Cardiac Pacing and Electrophysiology. 3d ed. Philadelphia: Saunders, 1991.

Horowitz LN. Current Management of Arrhythmias. Philadelphia: Decker, 1991.

Josephson ME. Clinical Cardiac Electrophysiology: Techniques and Interpretations. 2d ed. Philadelphia: Lea & Febiger, 1992.

5

Syncope and Presyncope

I.	Presentation of the Patient	80
II.	Subsequent Evaluation After Tentative Diagnostic Categorization	85
III.	Situational/Reflexive Syncope	85
IV.	Presumed Cardiac Syncope	90
V.	Diagnostic Yields and Implications	90
	Suggested Reading	92

John D. Fisher, Soo G. Kim, David M. Kaufman, Kevin J. Ferrick, Jay N. Gross, and Ronald Wharton

Syncope is defined as a sudden but transient loss of consciousness and postural tone from which there is spontaneous recovery (barring the effects of secondary injuries). The spontaneous recovery may be partial. Thus, patients with marked bradycardias or tachycardias may regain consciousness as well as movement to some extent, but they remain profoundly impaired while the arrhythmia persists. The onset of syncope may vary from instantaneous to one of brief evolution over several seconds or, rarely, minutes. The same conditions that cause syncope can cause incomplete variations of syncope ranging from light-headedness or "dizziness" to near-syncope or presyncope. The approach to all is similar. Our use of the term "syncope" includes the incomplete variations as well.

Some of these conditions can be associated with cardiac arrest, in which case no spontaneous recovery may occur. When the cause of an initial syncopal episode is unclear, evaluation focuses on possible cardiac arrest as well as more typical cardiac syncope (see below) and is intense. Earlier aggressive and often presumptive therapy such as insertion of an implantable cardioverter-defibrillator (ICD) is common under these circumstances.

I. PRESENTATION OF THE PATIENT

A. Immediate

When a patient arrives in an emergency room or physician's office immediately after a syncopal episode, the evaluating physician has access to fresh data: history, perhaps with witnesses; physical findings; and laboratory results that may be very helpful in making a diagnosis. For example, a very low potassium may indicate an arrhythmia caused by spontaneous or diuretic-induced hypokalemia. An absent or subtherapeutic drug blood level in a patient who is dependent on an antiarrhythmic drug can be virtually diagnostic.

B. Late

In contrast, when a patient first presents days to weeks after an event, the consequent absence of fresh information challenges the physician's diagnostic skills.

C. Initial Data and Tentative Diagnosis

An organized approach to a patient presenting with syncope/near-syncope should result in a tentative assignment to a diagnostic category, often within a few minutes, based on the history, physical examination, and ECG. Diagnostic laboratory results may not be available for some time, but pertinent tests should be ordered promptly. In a patient with a history of syncope caused by tachyarrhythmias that have been suppressed by medications and who presents with recurrent syncope, recurrent palpitations may be described; the electrocardiogram (ECG) may demonstrate abnormalities such as a prolonged QT interval possibly caused by the antiarrhythmic drugs, or the antiarrhythmic drug blood level may be found to be subtherapeutic. Table 1 lists some of the major causes and categories of syncope.

D. History

One should determine whether the patient has had previous episodes of syncope, and if so, their cause. Other questions include the following: What are the circumstances or precipitating factors surrounding the syncopal episode? Were severe coughing spells or straining at the toilet precipitating factors? A variation of this Valsalva maneuver has been seen more than once in truck drivers who pass out when applying the brakes vigorously while approaching toll booths (sometimes with regrettable effects on the toll booth and its attendant).

Table 1 Syncope

Diagnosis to consider based on initial data[a]

Situational/reflexive[b]	Neurological	Non-CV/ nonneurological	Vascular	Cardiac
Noxious stimuli	(Seizures)	Orthostatic	Bruits	Overt bradycardia
needles	(Drop attacks)	blood loss	Asymmetrical pulses	Overt tachycardia
dentists	Migraines syndromes	diuretics	Subclavian steal	ECG:
phlebotomy	orthostatic, plus	drugs	Sudden SOB	WPW
pain (severe)	sphincter	Metabolic	r/o pulmonary emb.	Short PR
fright	impotence	diabetes	Hx: transient ischemic	AV block
Postexertion	tremor	hypoglycemia	attack	BBB
Prolonged standing	rigidity	toxins	cardiovascular	acute MI
esp. if hot, close	Hoarse/tongue or ear pain	Drugs	accident	Long QT
± prior nausea, sweat	glossopharyngeal syncope	antiarrhythmics		etc. abnormal
Sudden position change	Unheralded syncope	illicit		Murmurs
Toilet strain	paroxysmal withdrawal of	ACE inhibitor		Hx: CHF
Cough	sympathetic tone	prazocin		old MI
CSS (+)		insulin		heart surgery
		nitroglycerin		palpitations
		hydralazine		chest pain
		diuretics		congenital heart disease
		Psychological stress,		prior arrhythmia
		Hx		pacer, ICD

[a]History (Hx) physical exam (PE), ECG; send labs hematocrit, electrolytes, glucose, cardiac enzymes, toxicology.

[b]Includes neurocardiogenic syncope (vasovagal syncope, vasoregulatory incompetence, etc.).

Abbreviations: CSS(+) = carotid sinus stimulation; SOB = shortness of breath; r/o = risk of; WPW = Wolff-Parkinson-White syndrome; BBB = bundle branch block; ICD = implantable cardioverter-defibrilator.

Noxious stimuli (see Table 1) usually result in syncope secondary to brady-cardia or hypotension. However, in some instances they may provoke malignant ventricular arrhythmias. If so, a history of syncope associated with any form of excitement is common. A prolonged QT interval may be present, an ECG abnormality associated with torsades de pointes, which is a spiraling polymorphic ventricular tachycardia (VT), usually nonsustained.

Vasoregulatory/vasovagal/neurocardiogenic syncope should be considered in patients who have syncope under conditions such as standing during long services in a crowded and perhaps warm house of worship, while standing in long lines, or after meals.

The "cathedral ceiling syndrome" occurs when a patient extends his or her neck maximally (as in looking at a cathedral ceiling) and has syncope that can be caused by stimulation of the carotid sinus (often related to neckwear) or more typically because of bilateral carotid obstructions that become occlusive when the carotids are stretched by maximal neck extension. Closely related is the "vanity syndrome"—syncope in an older person (who has already had episodes of ataxia) with hyperextension of the neck during a hair-washing session in a beauty salon. Both these types of syncope are attributable to kinking of the basilar arteries. Another variation involves the patient who has syncope upon twisting the neck in one direction or the other—for example, when a driver looks over his or her shoulder to pull out of a tight parking place.

Syncope should be differentiated from drop attacks and epileptic seizures. Drop attacks are usually caused by basilar artery disease and are characterized by sudden loss of postural vascular tone with collapse but without loss of consciousness. Typically, the patient can describe the entire episode accurately.

Witnessed epileptic seizures are often characteristic. Patients may bite their tongues or become incontinent. Many have had previous episodes or give a history of head trauma that can help lead to the diagnosis. Epileptic seizures are usually followed by a postictal period during which the patient may be confused and sleepy for a substantial interval following the event. Todd's paralysis (or paresis) may be present as well.

Situational and cardiac syncope are not usually followed by postictal phenomena unless prolonged, aborted cardiac arrest has occurred. Most patients are typically clear-headed immediately after a syncopal event. There may be retrograde amnesia. Some patients will deny that they have lost consciousness in spite of excellent documentation by witnesses. Occasionally, medical personnel will have the opportunity to witness a syncopal episode associated with asystole documented on an ECG, after which the patient will vehemently deny having lost consciousness. This fact emphasizes the limitations of a history obtained only from the patient. Witnesses to an event can be invaluable.

Patients with a history of heart disease and syncope will often describe palpitations, previous aborted episodes of syncope, or previous documented arrhythmias. The combination of the history and an ECG can then lead to the correct diagnosis.

Neurological causes of syncope besides epilepsy (seizures are not true syncope and are rarely both atonic and aclonic) can include certain types of migraine and a variety of rather rare or unusual syndromes. Two are neurological chronic autonomic insufficiency syndromes that underlie orthostatic hypotension together with intermittent loss of sphincter control, impotence, tremor, and rigidity: a postganglionic benign form and a preganglionic progressive form, both associated with low blood levels of dopamine beta-hydroxylase (the Bradbury-Eggleston and Shy-Drager syndromes). Glossopharyngeal syncope occurs in combination with hoarseness and tongue or ear pain. Unheralded loss of consciousness may occur with the syndrome of paroxysmal withdrawal of sympathetic tone—an unfortunate and untreatable diagnosis of exclusion.

Noncardiovascular-nonneurological causes of syncope may be readily apparent or quite subtle. Major blood loss or metabolic disorders such as diabetes are usually strongly suspected based on the history. With diabetes, severe hypoglycemia or hyperglycemia does not usually produce syncope (sudden but *transient* loss of consciousness and postural tone) because the metabolic abnormality persists after the episode of collapse. True syncope with diabetes is more likely to be caused by orthostatic reflex changes secondary to peripheral neuropathy.

Drug-related syncope should be suspected in anyone taking antiarrhythmic drugs, particularly those in class 1A or class 1C, sotalol, or other drugs known to produce orthostatic changes, especially many antihypertensive and antianginal agents. Illicit drug use, particularly of cocaine, may be denied by the patient but be implicated by toxicology laboratory test results.

Psychological stresses can result in syncopelike conditions. Some psychological stresses can produce typical situational and reflexive syncope that has an organic basis. In other patients, "flight from reality" may be evident, in which the patient appears to have had syncope but is found to have normal vital signs and a normal electroencephalogram (EEG) during episodes.

Pulmonary embolism should be suspected in a patient with a history of peripheral vascular disease, deep vein thrombosis, or prolonged bed rest; occasionally, even without such a history, a patient presents with sudden shortness of breath followed by syncope with continued shortness of breath and other signs of pulmonary embolism after return of consciousness.

Transient ischemic attacks, strokes, and myocardial infarction are not usual causes of syncope. However, they or related conditions can lead to subsequent syncope or seizures.

E. Physical Examination

Irregularities of the pulse; bruits, particularly in the neck; asymmetrical blood pressures in the two arms or in the arms compared with the legs; tachypnea or hyperpnea; cyanosis or extreme pallor; and orthostatic or postural changes in blood pressure can all suggest a specific cause of syncope. The combination of a bruit over the subclavian artery together with syncope with vigorous exercise of the ipsilateral arm suggests a subclavian steal syndrome.

F. Electrocardiogram

Diagnosis is simple if the ECG shows bradycardia caused by second- or third-degree heart block or if it shows tachycardia. Other findings that can be highly suggestive include marked sinus bradycardia, a prolonged QT interval, a short PR interval, especially if it is associated with a delta wave indicative of preexitation and the Wolff-Parkinson-White (WPW) syndrome, bundle branch block, or evidence of an old myocardial infarction, particularly if associated with changes consistent with a ventricular aneurysm and frequent atrial or ventricular premature complexes (VPCs).

Unfortunately, an abnormal ECG can also lead to a diagnostic dead end. The patient with an old infarction, a ventricular aneurysm, and syncope should be suspected of having had an episode of ventricular tachycardia but may have been subject to syncope secondary to vascular and vasoregulatory abnormalities.

The ECG may be normal in patients who have syncope secondary to cardiac arrhythmias. Electrophysiological studies (EPS) may be required to identify those whose syncope is caused by AV node reentry tachycardia or other supraventricular tachycardias (SVT) or by idiopathic ventricular tachycardias (VT), certain abnormalities of sinus node function, or AV block occurring at the infra-Hisian level of the His bundle.

G. Chest X-ray

In patients who have previously been healthy and whose physical examination and ECG are normal, a chest x-ray is of limited value in the initial evaluation of syncope. However, it should be part of an initial screen in patients with characteristics implicating cardiac or pulmonary etiologies.

H. Laboratory Abnormalities

Initial studies should include the following determinations: complete blood count, electrolytes, arterial blood gas values or other estimates of oxygenation, blood glucose, cardiac enzymes (relevant to arrhythmias that may have occurred in conjunction with a symptomatic or silent myocardial infarction), and a toxicology screen. An important and often neglected test is an assay of blood levels of antiarrhythmic drugs for patients taking such medications. Tests such as dopamine beta-hydroxylase, which may be abnormal in some of the neurological orthostatic hypotension syndromes, are usually not part of initial evaluations.

Neurological consultation and extensive neurological workup are usually not indicated. True syncope is only rarely neurological in origin. Only if a general medical evaluation is suggestive of a neurological syndrome should an extensive neurological workup be undertaken early. Low yield and high cost accompany use of routine neurological consultation, EEG, computed tomography, magnetic resonance imaging, and the like, all of which should be reserved for patients in whom there appears to be a likelihood of neurological abnormalities and in whom medical evaluation has failed to identify a nonneurological cause of syncope.

II. SUBSEQUENT EVALUATION AFTER TENTATIVE DIAGNOSTIC CATEGORIZATION

Once the likely cause of syncope has been categorized as tentatively focused, evaluation should be conducted in the most timely, cost-effective, and complete manner possible. Sometimes the cost of multiple tests performed simultaneously is less than the cost of additional hospital delays if the same tests are performed in "a logical sequence." Nevertheless, it is not necessary to perform virtually every test in virtually every patient with syncope.

For the diagnostic categories of neurological syncope, vascular syncope, and nonneurological noncardiovascular syncope, the diagnoses listed in Table 1 can guide subsequent evaluation. For patients with situational/reflexive syncope or cardiac syncope, schemas are presented in Figures 1 and 2.

III. SITUATIONAL/REFLEXIVE SYNCOPE

A. Workups and the Decision Tree

Problems range from trivial to life-threatening. In some instances, simple discharge of the patient to home with advice is appropriate. In others, hospital admission and detailed evaluation are needed. An otherwise normal patient who donates blood, stands up immediately, and has orthostatic hypotension and syncope should be allowed to rest, be given hydration, and sent home. A patient whose initial evaluation is unremarkable and whose syncope was associated with standing for a period of time in a close, warm, stuffy environment can be sent home with advice to avoid such situations insofar as possible, keep the calf muscles moving in the event that the environment is inescapable, and sit down or lie down rather than trying to "fight" impending syncope (see the decision tree in Figure 1).

The question of single compared with multiple episodes of syncope often

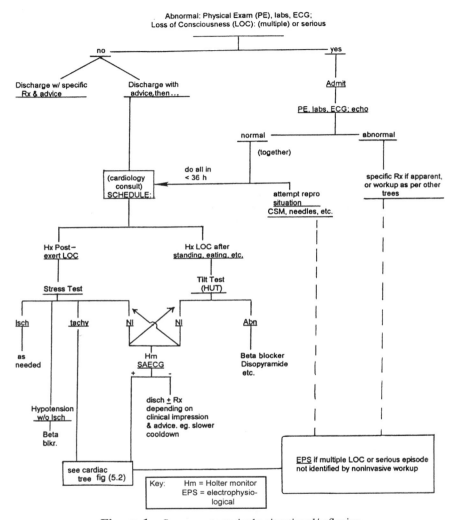

Figure 1   Syncope, tentatively situational/reflexive.

arises but is, in fact, relatively unimportant. Situational syncope may well be recurrent but is not life-threatening. In contrast, syncope secondary to complete heart block or nonsustained but rapid ventricular tachycardia is much more serious. Even a single episode requires a complete evaluation and plan for therapy.

In Figure 1, patients with situational/reflexive syncope are separated into

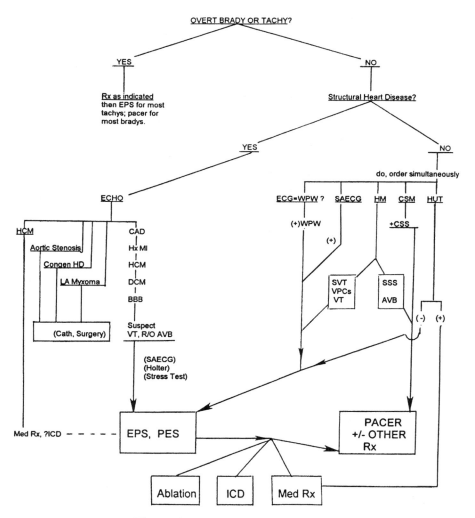

Figure 2   Syncope, tentatively cardiac.

three major diagnostic and therapeutic pathways: (a) those who may be discharged; (b) those who should be admitted because of abnormal findings; and (c) those who should be admitted even though abnormal findings have not yet be identified. Admission is appropriate for a patient with an abnormal physical examination, laboratory studies, or ECG. Abnormalities in patients in the situational/

reflexive category may be less compelling than those in patients in other categories but sufficient to be of concern. An example is a patient with a heart murmur that does not sound like the murmur of aortic stenosis, mild sinus bradycardia, or first-degree AV block with syncope that appears by history to be situational.

Patients should be admitted if they have had multiple episodes of syncope despite avoidance of apparent precipitating factors and adherence to medical advice. Patients who suffer a "serious" syncopal episode should be admitted, including those who have had a virtually instantaneous loss of consciousness and have injured themselves in the process of falling, even if a precipitating factor appears to place the syncope in the situational/reflexive category. Some such patients are ultimately found to have rapid polymorphic nonsustained ventricular tachycardia in response to noxious or exciting stimuli.

In patients with "serious" syncope (Figure 1), an echocardiogram should be obtained to help determine whether structural or functional heart disease is present. If results of all studies are normal, attempts should be made to reproduce the syncope, obtain a cardiology consultation, and schedule tests as outlined in Figure 1.

Carotid sinus massage (CSM) is a diagnostic procedure that can be performed safely in appropriate patients as part of the initial evaluation in an emergency room or elsewhere. Often, hesitancy to perform CSM exists because of the possibility of causing a transient ischemic attack (TIA), stroke, or asystole. However, security is provided by such safeguards as careful auscultation over both carotids with the patient holding his or her breath to exclude bruits; avoidance of CSM in patients with a history of TIAs or strokes; having the patient practice a deep, strong cough and indicating that the initiation of such a cough may be requested immediately (in the event of prolonged asystole); and being prepared and skilled in giving a chest thump, again in the event of prolonged systole. It is extremely unusual for CSM to produce asystole resulting from sinus arrest or complete heart block that persists well beyond the duration of the CSM itself. Induction of SVT, atrial fibrillation, or ventricular tachyarrhythmias is extremely rare. It is, however, always necessary to be prepared for each of these in an emergency room or doctor's office setting.

As indicated in Figure 1, patients with benign situational/reflexive syncopal episodes can often be discharged with specific advice on how to avoid the precipitating circumstances and how to respond to any impending recurrences. Patients whose syncopal episodes were mild, probably situational/reflexive, and whose initial evaluation did not identify abnormalities can be discharged for further evaluation in an outpatient setting.

As indicated in Figure 1, exercise stress testing or a head-up tilt table test (HUT) may be indicated depending on whether the syncope was postexertional or occurred after standing, eating, or another activity. Overlap in syndromes is common. Thus, it may be convenient to perform both tests at the same visit. As indicated in the decision tree in Figure 1, additional evaluation can proceed on the basis of results of the stress test and HUT.

Holter monitoring is "traditional" but has a very low diagnostic yield as an initial test in patients with syncope. It takes 24 hr plus analysis time. Transtelephone event or loop recorders must often be used for longer intervals, but the yield is higher. It is therefore better to proceed with a stress test and HUT if this can be done without delay. As a practical matter, it may be possible to apply the Holter recorder on the night of admission and perform the stress test and HUT the following day. Certainly a negative Holter recording is reassuring, although it is usually not optimally cost-effective. For outpatients, it is more economical to perform a stress test and HUT; of the two, an HUT is more likely to be a positive and therefore more cost-effective. Thus, for outpatients, the sequence of HUT followed by either Holter monitor/even/loop recorder or stress test is preferred.

The objective of a stress test is not only to unearth signs of ischemia but also to elicit changes in rhythm or the QRS complex (appearance of delta waves or intravenous conduction delay) and hypotension occurring during or following the stress test. Rather than recording a rhythm strip every minute or so, it is important to record continuously, so that singular events will not be missed. Cool-down should be abbreviated or matched to the patient's level of activity at the time of syncope to maximize the chances of obtaining a diagnostic finding.

A signal-averaged ECG (SAECG) is a sensitive but not very specific test for inducible ventricular tachycardia in patients with unexplained syncope. Specificity is enhanced in patients who have a history of a myocardial infarction.

The decision tree in Figure 1 entails EPS for patients with multiple episodes of syncope or a serious episode of syncope not identified by a noninvasive workup and those in whom the workup identifies abnormalities consistent with arrhythmias that can be identified by EPS. Identification of multiple causes of syncope is not uncommon. Sometimes there are unsuspected associations. For example, in one study, patients who had SVT with syncope usually had a positive HUT, whereas patients with SVT without syncope had negative HUTs. Accordingly, a positive HUT does not exclude another cause of syncope. Fortunately, beta blockers, the mainstay of therapy for patients with a positive HUT, are also effective for many patients with SVT.

B. Time Frame

Initial evaluation exclusive of obtaining all laboratory results should be accomplished within an hour or so after the patient's presentation. For a patient admitted, it should be possible to schedule and perform all the noninvasive tests within the next 24 to 36 hr. It should be possible to perform an EPS, if indicated, within another 24 hr. Ideally, a diagnostic admission for patients with situational/reflexive syncope should be completed within 2 to 3 days.

IV. PRESUMED CARDIAC SYNCOPE

For patients with overt bradycardia or tachycardia, the cause of syncope is presumptive (Figure 2), and the arrhythmia should be treated immediately. Long-term therapy may be either obvious or may require EPS guidance.

When there is no overt bradycardia or tachycardia, the next question to resolve is whether or not overt structural heart disease is present (organic heart disease, or OHD). In patients without OHD, the ECG should be examined for signs of delta waves indicating the WPW syndrome. Patients with WPW and syncope require therapy; usually radiofrequency (RF) catheter ablation during EPS. For others, CSM should be performed unless contraindicated. If negative, then a SAECG, Holter monitor, HUT, and stress test should be ordered simultaneously. As noted in Figure 2, subsequent diagnostic and therapeutic steps may be needed.

For patients with structural heart disease, an echocardiogram should be performed. Although traditional, echocardiography is rarely of diagnostic and cost-effective value in patients without evidence of OHD reflected by history, physical examination, chest x-ray, and ECG. The echocardiogram can be used to classify patients into two broad categories, those requiring medical or surgical therapy for hemodynamic abnormalities that may cause syncope and those who have abnormalities that often lead to electrophysiological derangements. For the latter, the SAECG, Holter monitor, and stress test may provide useful baseline data, but EPS is usually the major diagnostic modality.

A. Time Frame

Subject to the same constraints and limitations as those applicable to patients with situational/reflexive syncope, noninvasive testing should be completed within 24 to 36 hr after admission. Scheduling and performing EPS may require an additional 24 to 36 hr. Radiofrequency catheter ablation could result in discharge within 24 hr after EPS; implantation of an ICD or open heart surgery would obviously require longer hospitalization.

V. DIAGNOSTIC YIELDS AND IMPLICATIONS

A. General Comments and Principles

The likelihood of identifying a cause for syncope is extremely variable because of differences in patient populations (all patients initially identified as having syncope in an emergency room setting differ from all patients with defined organic heart disease), extent of testing, diagnostic criteria, and many other factors. However, some useful generalities pertain, including the following:

1. Overall, the initial battery of history, physical examination, and basic ECG and laboratory data provide the highest diagnostic yield.
2. A detailed neurological evaluation has a relatively low yield and poor cost-ineffectiveness at initial evaluation.
3. Holter monitoring and long-term event recorders or loop recorders can be helpful but have relatively low diagnostic yields.
4. Head-up tilt is diagnostically effective but positive in many patients in whom syncope is attributable to SVT or VT.
5. Electrophysiological studies are indicated when tachycardia is identified as the cause of syncope.
6. Electrophysiological studies are indicated in patients with syncope whose cause is undetermined after a noninvasive workup when identification of cause is clinically important. Most patients with organic heart disease, particularly that associated with ECG abnormalities, will exhibit a diagnostic abnormality on EPS. In patients who appear to be normal (other than having syncope), EPS will yield diagnostic findings in only 15% (mostly SVT with hypotension followed by lower incidences of VT, sinus node abnormalities, and conduction system disease).
7. "A rose by any other name is still a rose," but diagnostic tests of the same name can differ markedly. Thus, differences in techniques for HUT, exercise stress testing, or thoroughness in EPS can affect the diagnostic yield markedly. Among busy practitioners who limit HUT to 8 min in a frenetic environment, the yield will be lower than with longer tests supplemented by pharmacological stresses.
8. Syncope may be of undetermined origin (SUO). This term has been applied to patients ranging from those who, after superficial evaluation, do not have an identifiable cause of syncope to those whose syncope remains unexplained after a complete noninvasive and invasive (EPS) evaluation. Our preference is for using the term in a fashion analogous to "fever of unknown origin" (FUO)—i.e., to apply it to those whose syncope remains unexplained after thorough noninvasive evaluation. This position is consistent with general usage in the literature.

Early reports of patients with syncope were retrospective and eclectic. Individual series focused on the value of specific diagnostic procedures such as CSM. Electrophysiological testing was widely implemented in the 1980s for the evaluation of syncope. Treatment based on abnormalities identified at EPS generally was associated with elimination or reduction of subsequent syncope. However, many patients with negative EPS and negative noninvasive studies continued to have recurrent syncope. Increased appreciation of the role of the autonomic nervous system and recent emphasis on head-up tilt-table testing have improved diagnostic yields. It is likely that many of the patients of the early 1980s who "passed" noninvasive and EPS testing would have had an abnormal HUT.

Long-term mortality is high in patients when syncope is secondary to a cardiac cause. By contrast, patients with situational/reflexive syncope generally have a benign course, although one punctuated by annoying and rarely disabling recurrences.

SUGGESTED READING

Bass EB, Elson JJ, Rogoros RN, et al. Long-term prognosis of patients undergoing electrophysiologic studies for syncope of unknown origin. Am J Cardiol 1988; 62:1186–1191.

DiMarco JP, Garan H, Harthorne JW, Ruskin JN. Intracardiac electrophysiologic techniques in recurrent syncope of unknown cause. Ann Inter Med 1981; 95:542–548.

Fogel RI, Gest CR, Evans JJ, Prystowsky EN. Are event recorders useful and cost effective in the diagnosis of palpitations, presyncope, and syncope (abstr)? J Am Coll Cardiol 1993; 21:358A.

Gulamhusein S, Naccarelli GV, Ko PT, et al. Value and limitations of clinical electrophysiologic study in assessment of patients with unexplained syncope. Am J Med 1982; 73:700–705.

Kapoor WN. Evaluation and outcome of patients with syncope. Medicine 1990; 69:160–175.

Krol RB, Morady F, Flaker GC, et al. Electrophysiologic testing in patients with unexplained syncope: Clinical and noninvasive predictors of outcome. J Am Coll Cardiol 1987; 10:358–363.

Kushner JA, Kou WH, Kadish AH, Morady F. Natural history of patients with unexplained syncope and a nondiagnostic electrophysiologic study. J Am Coll Cardiol 1989; 14:391–396.

Leitch JW, Klein GJ, Yee R, et al. Syncope associated with supraventricular tachycardia: An expression of tachycardia rate or vasomotor response? Circulation 1992; 85:1064–1071.

Middlekauff HR, Stevenson WG, Saxon LA. Prognosis after syncope: Impact of left ventricular function. Am Heart J 1993; 125:121–127.

Rea RF, Thames MD. Neural control mechanisms and vasovagal syncope. J Cardiovasc Electrophysiol 1993; 4:587–595.

Reiffel JA, Wang P, Bower R, et al. Electrophysiologic testing in patients with recurrent syncope: Are results predicted by prior ambulatory monitoring? Am Heart J 1985; 110:1146–1153.

Rubin AM, Rials SJ, Marinchak RA, Kowey PR. The head-up tilt table test and cardiovascular neurogenic syncope. Am Heart J 1993; 125:476–482.

Sakaguchi S, Shultz JJ, Remole SC, et al. Syncope associated with exercise: A manifestation of neurally mediated syncope. Am J Cardiol 1995; 75:476–481.

Steinbert JS, Prystowsky E, Freedman RA, et al. Use of the signal-averaged electrocardiogram for predicting inducible ventricular tachycardia in patients with unexplained syncope: Relation to clinical variables in a multivariate analysis. J Am Coll Cardiol 1994; 23:99–106.

Teichman SL, Felder SD, Matos JA, et al. The value of electrophysiologic studies in syncope of undetermined origin: Report of 150 cases. Am Heart J 1985; 110:469–479.

Williams RS, Bashore TM. Paroxysmal hypotension associated with sympathetic withdrawal: A new disorder of autonomic vasomotor regulation. Circulation 1980; 62: 901–908.

CARDIAC SIGNS

Evaluation and Treatment of Patients with Signs of Cardiovascular Disease

The astute clinician and, of more importance, the patient are amply rewarded by perceptive clinical observation of often subtle yet remarkably specific signs of cardiac disease. Despite the overwhelming power of modern technologies such as tomographic imaging, electrophysiological mapping, ultrasonic interrogation, and biochemical elucidation of mechanisms of disease, the history and physical examination continue to constitute both cornerstone and lodestone in the evaluation of patients.

Meticulous, focused physical examination can detect signs clarifying the conundrum of shortness of breath such as central cyanosis or methemoglobinemia; a fixed split-second heart sound indicative of an atrial septal defect; physiological variation of heart rate despite no apparent atrial activity indicative of sino-ventricular conduction associated with hyperkalemia; the slatting sail sign of pulmonic stenosis (increased intensity of the midsystolic sound with expiration); dyskinesis of the anterior left ventricular wall indicative of transitory myocardial ischemia underlying an episode of angina; subtle signs of congestive heart failure including unilateral right lower extremity edema, pulsus alternans, a right or left ventricular diastolic gallop (S_3), and loss of high-frequency components of the first heart sound reflecting decreased ventricular contractility; conduction abnormalities manifest by paradoxical splitting of the second heart sound with left bundle branch block; or a pulsatile liver indicative of tricuspid regurgitation; among many others.

Because one sees what one looks for, detection of these and numerous other helpful signs requires a superb knowledge base, vigorous formulation of potential pathophysiology to guide physical examination, and finely honed observational skills. Although the well-used stethoscope does not replace the chest x-ray let alone a CT scan or a pulmonary angiogram, the observer is, in fact, a main determinant of what will be recognized based on what is contemplated. Accordingly, pursuit of signs of cardiac disease is not merely an academic exercise. It is, in fact, the hallmark of epistemology underlying effective differential diagnosis.

6

General Observations

I. Abnormal Pulsations   97
II. Cyanosis/Clubbing/Chest Asymmetry   99

William E. Hopkins

I. ABNORMAL PULSATIONS

It is important to not only recognize the presence of an abnormal pulsation but also to identify it as cardiac, arterial, or venous. Cardiac pulsations are considered in relation to specific disorders such as hypertrophic cardiomyopathy. Here we shall consider abnormal arterial and venous pulsations.

A. Arterial Pulsations

The volume and contour of the arterial pulse are determined by a combination of factors including vascular elasticity, left ventricular stroke volume, and ejection velocity. The carotid pulse provides the most accurate, readily observed representation of the central aortic pulse. The normal carotid pulse rises rapidly to a smooth, rounded peak. Its descending limb is less steep than its ascending limb.

Large, bounding arterial pulses are secondary to an increased pulse pressure and occur in patients with increased stiffness of the vessel wall (aging, atherosclerosis), hyperkinetic states (fever, hyperthyroidism, pregnancy, anemia, exercise), and abnormal runoff of blood (aortic insufficiency, patent ductus arteriosus, arteriovenous malformation). Diminished pulsations are secondary to a decreased pulse pressure and occur in patients with decreased stroke volume. Alternating strong and weak pulsations with a regular rhythm (pulsus alternans) are seen in patients with severe left ventricular dysfunction and detectable by palpation when the difference in magnitude of pulsations exceeds 20 mmHg. Pulsus paradoxus occurs most commonly in patients with pericardial tamponade or obstructive lung disease and is characterized by a perceptible decrease of ≥10 mmHg in the amplitude of the pulse during a normal inspiration. It is often palpable as well as heard by auscultation when the inspiratory decrease is greater than 20 mmHg. A bisferiens pulse is characterized by two systolic peaks. It is seen occasionally in patients with aortic insufficiency or hypertrophic obstructive cardiomyopathy.

Delayed pulses occur when obstruction to flow is present. Obstruction to left ventricular outflow (valvular aortic stenosis, subaortic or supraaortic stenosis) results in a delayed rate of upstroke of the pulse wave (pulsus tardus). Coarctation of the aorta results in bounding carotid and upper-extremity pulses and a delay in the onset of the upstroke of the femoral pulse relative to that of the brachial and radial pulses. Because coarctation of the aorta is often accompanied by a bicuspid aortic valve, either aortic stenosis, aortic regurgitation, or both may be present and can alter the typical arterial pulses otherwise found in patients with coarctation.

Atherosclerotic disease with stenosis, thrombus, embolus, or vasculitis may result in absent or decreased pulses. A proximal subclavian artery stenosis in a patient with a coronary bypass graft of the left internal mammary artery can result in recurrence of angina and should be suspected despite lack of access of the subclavian pulse to physical exam. A bruit may be heard over the vessel, however. Patients with a history of congenital heart disease may have absent or decreased pulses secondary to previous surgery (shunt procedures, coarctation repair), or catheterization in infancy or childhood.

The presence of two pathophysiological abnormalities may alter typical findings in the arterial pulse associated with one of them. For instance, aortic stenosis or a reduced stroke volume may be less apparent in elderly patients because of increased arterial stiffness.

B. Venous Pulsations

The jugular venous pulse reflects right heart dynamics. The normal jugular venous pulse should not be visible more than 3 to 4 cm above the sternal angle (right atrial pressure of 8–9 cmH$_2$O). Elevation of the jugular venous pulse occurs in patients with right atrial hypertension secondary to right ventricular dysfunction, tricuspid valvular disease, pericardial disease from a variety of causes (tamponade, constriction), or myocardial infiltration (restriction). The A-wave amplitude exceeds the V-wave amplitude in normal subjects.

Components of the jugular venous pulse may be abnormal in specific pathophysiological conditions. An elevated A wave occurs in patients with right ventricular hypertension (pulmonary hypertension secondary to primary or secondary pulmonary vascular disease, pulmonary thromboembolism, right ventricular infarction, or pulmonic branch or valve stenosis) or obstruction to right ventricular inflow (tricuspid stenosis or right atrial myxoma). Cannon A waves occur when the right atrium contracts against a closed tricuspid valve in patients with atrioventricular dissociation (heart block, ventricular premature depolarizations, ventricular tachycardia). Patients with atrial fibrillation do not exhibit an A wave. Marked tricuspid regurgitation results in an elevated V wave.

The jugular venous pulse normally falls with inspiration. Elevation of the jugular venous pulse with inspiration (Kussmaul's sign) occurs in patients with pericardial constriction, rarely myocardial restrictive disease, and occasionally after acute right ventricular myocardial infarction.

II. CYANOSIS/CLUBBING/CHEST ASYMMETRY

The following topics are considered in this section: patterns and implications of cyanosis [definition (central versus peripheral), concentration of reduced hemoglobin and the effect of anemia and skin pigmentation, clubbing/hypertrophic osteoarthropathy, differential and reverse cyanosis/clubbing, and methemoglobinemia].

A. Patterns and Implications of Cyanosis

Cyanosis is a blue discoloration of the skin and mucous membranes. Central cyanosis results from decreased arterial oxygen saturation caused by right-to-left shunting of blood or abnormal pulmonary function. Peripheral cyanosis is a result of cutaneous vasoconstriction secondary to reduced cardiac output or exposure to cold. Peripheral cyanosis is seen only in superficial areas such as the skin of the fingers, toes, cheeks, nose, and external parts of the lips. If secondary to cold air or water, it resolves quickly with warming. Arterial oxygen saturation is normal in patients with peripheral cyanosis. Central cyanosis involves the nail beds and the warm mucosa such as the internal part of the lips and cheeks and the tongue.

Cyanosis occurs when the concentration of reduced hemoglobin in cutaneous or mucosal vessels exceeds 3 g/dL. Consequently, cyanosis is less apparent in anemic patients and more apparent in those with erythrocytosis. Central cyanosis is generally not apparent until the arterial oxygen saturation falls below 85% in Caucasians and even lower in subjects with pigmented skin. Central cyanosis in adults with congenital heart disease is almost always associated with clubbing of the fingers and toes (spoon-shaped nails with a loss of the angle at the juncture of the nail and skin and hypertrophy of the soft tissue of the pulp). Severe clubbing is often associated with bony changes in the digits (hypertrophic osteoarthropathy). Hypertrophic osteoarthropathy can also occur in the wrists, elbows, knees, ankles, and long bones of the lower legs and can be chronically painful. Clubbing can also

99

occur in noncyanotic disorders including endocarditis, inflammatory bowel disease, biliary cirrhosis, and carcinoma of the lung.

Differential cyanosis is characterized by cyanosis and clubbing of the toes (and sometimes the fingers of the left hand) and occurs in patients with a nonrestrictive patent ductus arteriosus and Eisenmenger's syndrome. It is a reflection of perfusion of the lower extremities with blood shunted from the pulmonary artery to the aorta. Reverse cyanosis involves clubbing of the fingers only and occurs in patients with a nonrestrictive patent ductus arteriosus, transposition of the great arteries, and Eisenmenger's syndrome.

Methemoglobinemia is a rare cause of cyanosis. In adults, it is generally secondary to exposure to nitrates (infused nitroprusside or inhaled nitric oxide) and is characterized by a normal partial pressure of oxygen in arterial blood but decreased oxygen saturation.

Cherry red "cyanosis" is a hallmark of carbon monoxide poisoning and is characterized by unsaturation disproportionate to P_{O_2} as well.

Chest asymmetry (with left chest prominence) is often seen in adults who had prominent left-to-right shunts in infancy and childhood. Thus, in a cyanotic adult, it may be a clue to the presence of Eisenmenger physiology. It may also be a manifestation of obstruction to cardiac outflow (e.g., congenital aortic stenosis) or other early mechanical derangements such as mitral regurgitation or pulmonic stenosis (right chest prominence).

7

Hypertension

I.	Definitions	101
II.	Essential Compared with Secondary Hypertension	103
III.	Consequences of Elevated Blood Pressure	103
IV.	Management of the Hypertensive Patient	107
V.	Diagnostic Studies for Secondary Hypertension	123
VI.	Adrenal Hypertension	127
VII.	Antihypertensive Therapy	133
VIII.	Hypertensive Emergencies and Urgencies	137
	Suggested Reading	142

Jay M. Sullivan

I. DEFINITIONS

The fifth report of the Joint National Committee on Detection, Evaluation and Treatment of Hypertension (JNC V) has reclassified adult blood pressure levels based on the effect of blood pressure on cardiovascular risk. Normal blood pressure is defined as a systolic blood pressure below 130 mmHg and a diastolic blood pressure under 85 mmHg. High normal pressure lies between 130 and 139 systolic and 85 and 89 diastolic. Stage 1 hypertension includes those with systolic pressure between 140 and 159 and diastolic levels of 90 to 99; stage 2 systolic levels range between 160 and 179 and diastolic levels between 100 and 109; stage 3 systolic levels fall between 180 and 209 and diastolic levels between 110 and 119. Stage 4 applies to individuals with very severe hypertension whose systolic blood pressure exceeds 210 and whose diastolic values are greater than 120. Use of the terms "mild" and "moderate" hypertension is discouraged because of their failure to imply the extent of cardiovascular risk associated with blood pressure levels in this range.

The prevalence of hypertension varies with age, sex, race, education, socio-economic class, and geographic region. In the United States, the prevalence of hypertension rises with age; it is also more common in African Americans than in whites and in males than in females until middle age, at which time the ratio reverses. Data collected in the National Health Examination Survey III of the U.S. Public Health Service on a random sample of the adult U.S. population between the ages of 18 and 79 in 1988–1991 showed that about 20% of adults had diastolic blood pressures higher than 90 mmHg. However, the number of hypertensive adults declined from 58 million in 1976–1980 to 50 million in 1988–1991.

This survey showed that the prevalence of hypertension was roughly twice as great in African Americans as in whites, and when hypertension was found in African Americans, their blood pressure levels were higher than those in whites. As a consequence, hypertensive heart disease, defined as the presence of left ventricular hypertrophy or failure, was present from three to nine times more frequently in subgroups of the African American population than in comparable white subgroups.

Although the JNC V criteria are a convenient "cut point" for epidemiological surveys, they leave unsolved two major clinical problems in dealing with individual subjects. First, an individual's blood pressure varies continually throughout the day, rising with activity, anxiety, discomfort, and even concentration and falling with relaxation or sleep. The severely hypertensive patient might have a consistent elevation of diastolic blood pressure to levels of 115 mmHg or above; but, given this variability, how can we fit an individual into relatively narrow categories of hypertension? First, multiple measurements of blood pressure must be made, in triplicate, on at least three separate days to permit estimation of a patient's representative blood pressure and a decision regarding management. Even transient elevation of blood pressure on casual measurements have been found to be associated with subsequent cardiovascular events.

Next, attention must be paid to the technique of blood pressure measurement. The JNC V report recommends measurement of blood pressure with the patient seated comfortably in a quiet room for 5 min with the forearm supported and the arm muscles relaxed. The upper arm should be exposed and a cuff of suitable size used (i.e., width of 13–15 cm for the adult of average size). The cuff should be inflated while the brachial or radial pulse is palpated until the pulse disappears. A stethoscope should be used for auscultation of the Korotkoff sounds over the brachial artery. Phase IV diastolic pressure is assigned to the level at which the sounds muffle and phase V to that at which sound disappears. Because most studies relating diastolic pressure to risk have used phase V pressures, these should be used to define the need for treatment. Pressures should be obtained in duplicate or triplicate, with readings separated by 2 min and averaged. If readings differ by more than 5 mmHg, additional readings should be obtained.

The second difficulty in the clinical assessment of individual patients is attributable to the fact that hypertension is associated with an increased risk of cardiovascular morbidity and mortality. Insurance actuarial data have shown clearly that increased risk begins at levels of arterial pressure well below 140/90 mmHg. Do all of these individuals in the United States, as well as those elsewhere in the world, require a lifetime of antihypertensive therapy?

II. ESSENTIAL COMPARED WITH SECONDARY HYPERTENSION

Essential hypertension involves blood pressure elevation in patients who do not have a detectable, specific pathophysiological cause responsible for the blood pressure elevation. Secondary hypertension is blood pressure elevation attributable to another specific disease process, such as those listed in Table 1. Discovery of an underlying cause can lead to surgical correction, thus eliminating the need for a lifetime of pharmacological therapy. The timing of a workup to detect secondary hypertension must be determined on an individual basis.

It is estimated that approximately 80% of patients referred to a major medical center with hypertension that is severe or resistant to therapy have essential hypertension, whereas 90 to 95% of patients in a community practice with less blood pressure elevation usually have essential hypertension. Among patients with severe hypertension, the yield of surgically curable forms is relatively high—approximately 10% of the total. Therefore, patients with diastolic pressures above 115 mmHg or those who exhibit evidence of target-organ damage probably should be evaluated for underlying causes of hypertension when they are first diagnosed.

At present, efforts are being directed toward the early detection and treatment of patients with mild blood pressure elevation so as to prevent cardiovascular morbidity. In such patients, the yield of surgically curable secondary forms of hypertension is much lower (Table 2). Thus, it is reasonable to limit the initial evaluation of a patient with mild hypertension to history, physical examination, and a small number of laboratory studies and to pursue a more extensive evaluation of only those patients who fail to respond to antihypertensive therapy.

III. CONSEQUENCES OF ELEVATED BLOOD PRESSURE

In order to adhere to a realistic rationale for treating patients with blood pressure elevation, one must examine those effects of hypertension on the cardiovascular system that lead to the accelerated development of vascular disease. Ever since the development in 1898 of methods for indirect measurement of blood pressure, data acquisition has been extensive. During the subsequent 60 years, patients were, of necessity, followed without effective antihypertensive therapy. It soon became

Table 1   Types of Hypertension

I. Systolic and diastolic hypertension
  A. Primary, essential, or idiopathic
  B. Secondary
    1. Renal
      a. Renal parenchymal disease
        (1) Acute glomerulonephritis
        (2) Chronic nephritis
        (3) Polycystic disease
        (4) Connective tissue diseases
        (5) Diabetic nephropathy
        (6) Hydronephrosis
      b. Renovascular
      c. Renin-producing tumors
      d. Renoprival
      e. Primary sodium retention (Liddle's syndrome, Gordon's syndrome)
    2. Endocrine
      a. Acromegaly
      b. Hypothyroidism
      c. Hypercalcemia
      d. Hyperthyroidism
      e. Adrenal
        (1) Cortical
          (a) Cushing's syndrome
          (b) Primary aldosteronism
          (c) Congenital adrenal hyperplasia
        (2) Medullary: pheochromocytoma
      f. Extraadrenal chromaffin tumor
      g. Carcinoid
      h. Exogenous hormones
        (1) Estrogen
        (2) Glucocorticoids
        (3) Mineralocorticoids: licorice
        (4) Sympathomimetics
        (5) Tyramine-containing foods and MAO inhibitors
    3. Coarctation of the aorta
    4. Pregnancy-induced hypertension
    5. Neurological disorders
      a. Increased intracranial pressure
        (1) Brain tumor
        (2) Encephalitis
        (3) Respiratory acidosis: lung or CNS disease
      b. Quadriplegia
      c. Acute porphyria
      d. Familial dysautonomia

104

Table 1 Continued

      5. Neurological disorders (*continued*)
          e. Lead poisoning
          f. Guillain-Barré syndrome
          g. Sleep apnea
      6. Acute stress, including surgery
          a. Psychogenic hyperventilation
          b. Hypoglycemia
          c. Burns
          d. Pancreatitis
          e. Alcohol withdrawal
          f. Sickle cell crisis
          g. Postresuscitation
          h. Postoperative
      7. Increased intravascular volume
      8. Drugs and other substances
II. Systolic hypertension
    A. Increased cardiac output
      1. Aortic valvular regurgitation
      2. AV fistula, patent ductus
      3. Thyrotoxicosis
      4. Paget's disease of bone
      5. Beriberi
      6. Hyperkinetic circulation
    B. Rigidity of aorta

Source: From Kaplan NM. Systemic hypertension: Mechanisms and diagnosis. In Braunwald E, ed. Heart Disease, A Textbook of Cardiovascular Medicine. 6th ed. Philadelphia: Saunders, 1994.

Table 2 Frequency of Various Diagnoses in Hypertensive Subjects

Diagnosis	Rudnick et al.	Danielson et al.	Sinclair et al.
Essential hypertension	94%	95.3%	92.1%
Chronic renal disease	5%	2.4%	5.6%
Renovascular disease	0.2%	1.0%	0.7%
Coarctation of aorta	0.2%		
Primary aldosteronism		0.1%	0.3%
Cushing's syndrome	0.2%	0.1%	0.1%
Pheochromocytoma		0.2%	0.1%
Oral contraceptive–induced	0.2%	0.8%	1.0%
No. of patients	665	1,000	3,783

Sources: Data from Rudnick KV et al. Can Med Assoc J 1977;117:492. Danielson M, Dammstrom B. Acta Med Scand 1981;209:451. Sinclair AM et al. Arch Intern Med 1987;147:1289.

clear that severely elevated blood pressure was associated with a grave prognosis. Patients with a diastolic blood pressure of 130 mmHg or greater had only brief survival when the elevated pressure was associated with evidence of significant target-organ damage, papilledema, retinal hemorrhages and exudates, congestive heart failure, or diminished renal function. The most frequent symptoms in such patients were visual impairment, headache, gross hematuria, dyspnea, edema, nausea, vomiting, epigastric pain, and malaise. In one series of 105 cases, it was noted that most patients died within 4 months and that only a few patients survived longer than 16 months. In them, the malignant elevated blood pressure was either essential or associated with diseases of the renal parenchyma.

With the development of effective treatment, it soon became apparent that prognosis was improved by the use of antihypertensive agents. The results of several studies showed that antihypertensive therapy lengthened the survival (half-time) of patients with malignant hypertension from approximately 6 months to about 2½ years. Because of progression of underlying renal disease, patients with previous renal damage did not show as great an improvement as those with well-preserved renal function. Patients with impaired renal function (i.e., endogenous creatinine clearance less than 45 mL/min) did not do as well as others with treatment. The prognosis for such patients has been improved by the increased availability of chronic peritoneal or hemodialysis or renal transplantation, both of which substitute for the impaired renal function.

Thus, even partial control of severe hypertension improves prognosis, but those patients with residual blood pressure elevation continue to develop target-organ damage. In 1959, the Build and Blood Pressure Study of the U.S. Society of Actuaries found that blood pressure and longevity were inversely related, starting at levels of around 90/60 mmHg. Observations were confirmed by a similar study in 1979.

In 1954, a total of 5127 residents of Framingham, Massachusetts, began to participate in a long-term study of cardiovascular morbidity and mortality. This investigation was observational, and no therapeutic interventions were initiated. The participants underwent physical and laboratory examination followed by re-evaluations at 2-year intervals. Among the men and women between 30 and 60 years of age who entered the study, 18% of the men and 16% of the women had systolic blood pressures greater than 160 or diastolic pressures greater than 95 mmHg. Of the men, 41% had blood pressure elevations above 140 systolic and 90 mmHg diastolic. Of the women, 48% had pressures within this range. For patients with moderate elevation of blood pressure, the risk of developing congestive heart failure was six times greater than that in subjects with blood pressures less than 140/90. The risk of developing a stroke was three to five times as great and the risk of having a fatal heart attack was two to three times as great. The higher the blood pressure, the shorter the life expectancy. The risk of developing cardiovascular disease was incrementally proportional to the level of blood pressure. These observations applied to women as well as men, were independent of age at the time of initial examination, and held even when other risk factors, such as abnormal lipids, obesity, diabetes, and electrocardiographic (ECG) abnormalities were considered. Deaths in hypertensives were attributable to several cardiovascular disorders, including atherothrombotic brain infarction, coronary heart disease, congestive heart failure, and stroke, both hemorrhagic and nonhemorrhagic. Cerebrovascular accidents were a more prominent cause of death and disability among hypertensive women than among men. In malignant hypertension, death usually occurred from uremia or cerebral hemorrhage, with male and female patients sharing the risk equally. With moderate hypertension, morbidity and mortality from coronary heart disease, hemorrhagic stroke, and thrombotic cerebrovascular accidents constituted the major risks.

IV. MANAGEMENT OF THE HYPERTENSIVE PATIENT

A. Rationale for Treatment

The long-term goal in the treatment of hypertension is to prevent the premature development of cardiovascular disease. The complications of hypertension can be divided into those due solely to elevated blood pressure, including further progression of hypertension, renal failure, hemorrhagic stroke, congestive heart failure, and dissecting aneurysm. Other complications are related to the accelerated atherosclerosis associated with hypertension, including acute myocardial infarction, atherothrombotic cerebral infarction, and intermittent claudication. Even patients with minimal blood pressure elevation are subject to the development of these complications of atherosclerosis.

In the 1950s, it was found that pharmacological reduction of blood pressure prevented the development of necrotic and sclerotic changes in the arterioles of animals with experimental hypertension. Later clinical trials provided evidence that patients with malignant hypertension benefited from therapy. Improved prognosis was limited by the presence of renal damage or underlying renal parenchymal disease. Patients with severely reduced renal function caused by advanced nephrosclerosis did not have a favorable outcome, even with treatment. Although it soon became apparent that patients with accelerated or malignant hypertension benefited from treatment, it was not known whether patients with diastolic blood pressures between 90 and 129 mmHg had anything to gain from the expense and inconvenience of long-term antihypertensive therapy or whether the risks of therapy outweighed the benefits of lowering blood pressure.

A landmark investigation of this problem was the Veterans Administration Cooperative Study of Antihypertensive Agents. Male veterans were hospitalized for an evaluation that excluded those with diastolic blood pressure above 129 mmHg, those with secondary hypertension, and those whose blood pressure dropped beneath 90 mmHg without therapy. Patients who already had evidence of cardiovascular complications were included in the trial. After a placebo lead-in period, the patients were randomized blindly into two groups. One was given placebo and the other hydrochlorothiazide; reserpine and hydralazine were added stepwise as needed to control blood pressure.

It soon became apparent that the patients with the highest blood pressures were developing complications rapidly. As a result, the 143 patients who entered the study with diastolic blood pressures between 115 and 129 mmHg were analyzed after 20 months. Several untreated patients had developed advanced retinopathy, accelerated hypertension, renal failure, dissecting aneurysm, retinopathy with congestive heart failure, stroke, sudden death, or myocardial infarction. In contrast, only one patient in the treated group developed a drug reaction and only one patient suffered a minor stroke. The difference was highly significant, and it was shown that antihypertensive therapy benefited male patients with a diastolic blood pressure between 115 and 129 mmHg.

A subgroup of 380 patients who had entered the study with average, resting diastolic pressures between 90 and 114 mmHg during the initial hospitalization remained. They were followed for as long as 5 years, with an average follow-up of 3.3 years. Terminating morbid events occurred in 35 patients in the control group as opposed to 9 in the treated group; 21 nonterminating cardiovascular events occurred in the control group as opposed to 13 in the treated group, and 20 instances of accelerated hypertension occurred in the control group as opposed to none in the treated group. Fatalities were attributable to seven strokes in the control group and none in the treated group; three myocardial infarctions in the control group and two in the treated group; eight instances of sudden death in the control group as opposed to four in the treated group; and one instance of ruptured arteriosclerotic aneurysm in the treated group. There was a significant reduction of nonfatal strokes and congestive heart failure in the treated group, but the incidence of coronary heart disease did not differ significantly between the two groups.

Based on the data from the subgroup of patients with diastolic blood pressures between 90 and 114 mmHg, it was found that the risk of developing a morbid cardiovascular event during a 5-year period was reduced from 55% in the group receiving a placebo to only 18% in the group on active treatment. The difference between the treated and untreated groups was statistically significant for patients with initial diastolic blood pressures of 105 mmHg or higher. For those patients who entered the trial with lower pressures, the risk of developing a cardiovascular event was not as great and the benefit from antihypertensive therapy was not as marked, although the patients in this subgroup also appeared to benefit from treatment. In no instance did it appear that antihypertensive therapy increased morbidity or mortality, and indeed this study suggests that long-term antihypertensive therapy is relatively benign.

The VA study established that treatment of male patients with a diastolic blood pressure above 105 mmHg conveyed significant benefit to the patient. Women were not studied. Thus, there was no proof that they would benefit equally from therapy. The VA study showed that patients with levels of diastolic blood pressure between 90 and 104 mmHg benefited less from antihypertensive therapy than did their counterparts with higher blood pressures. Thus, in treating patients with mild elevations of blood pressure, it is advisable to weigh the limited benefit of therapy against the greater inconvenience, expense, and risk of side effects from antihypertensive therapy. The risk-benefit ratio in this group did not appear to be as favorable as it was in those individuals who had a persistent diastolic blood pressure above 105 mmHg.

Considering the data from the Build and Blood Pressure Study of 1959, from Framingham, from the VA study, and from other sources, many authorities at the time conservatively recommended that patients with sustained diastolic blood pressures between 90 and 104 mmHg be treated on an individualized basis. A very important factor in reaching a decision to prescribe antihypertensive medications for such patients was the presence or absence of additional cardiovascular risk factors. Because these factors appeared to be additive, a patient with a slight risk imposed by a minor elevation of blood pressure would be thought to have a much greater chance of developing cardiovascular disease if he or she also smoked cigarettes, had diabetes mellitus and/or elevated serum cholesterol, or had a family history of premature cardiovascular disease. In such a case, it will be prudent to attempt to reduce as many risk factors as possible, including mildly elevated blood pressure.

The results of the VA study were extended in an important way by the findings of the Hypertension Detection and Follow-up Program (HDFP), a 5-year, 14-center study involving 10,900 patients that provided the first convincing evidence that mortality in patients with a diastolic blood pressure of 90 to 104 mmHg was reduced by effective antihypertensive therapy.

The participants in HDFP ranged from 30 to 69 years of age and included both men and women. More than 70% of the cohort had diastolic blood pressures between 90 and 104 mmHg. Among patients stratified on the basis of age, sex, race, organ involvement, and prior treatment history and randomized into one of two groups, one group was treated by its usual source of medical care; the other group was given intensive antihypertensive therapy at special centers. Stepped-care therapy was used, consisting of a thiazide diuretic with the addition of reserpine, methyldopa, or, less frequently, propranolol if needed. Hydralazine and then guanethidine were added in sequence if goal blood pressure had not been reached. The therapeutic goal was a lowering of diastolic blood pressure to levels less than 90 mmHg or by 10 mmHg, whichever was lowest. By the end of 5 years, goal had been achieved in 64.9% of the center-care patients and in 43.6% of the referred-care group. The difference was in effectiveness. Although the average starting diastolic blood pressure was about 101 mmHg in both groups, after 5 years blood pressure had fallen to 84.1 mmHg in the center-care group yet to only 89.1 mmHg in the referred-care patients. Mortality from all causes was 17% lower in the center-care group; it was 20% lower in patients whose pretreatment diastolic pressure was 90–104 mmHg. The difference was highly significant ($p<.01$). Similarly, effective treatment lowered deaths from cerebrovascular disease by 45% and death from acute myocardial infarction by 46%.

Metaanalysis of several studies shows that although the reduction of cerebrovascular accidents was as great as predicted from the degree of blood pressure reduction, the decline in coronary events was not as great. It is not clear whether this disparity is attributable to the fact that the trials were not sufficiently long to observe the anticipated reduction or whether adverse metabolic effects of antihypertensive therapy limited the benefit of lower blood pressure.

An Australian trial of therapy in 3427 patients with mild hypertension demonstrated a beneficial effect of treatment of individuals whose pretreatment diastolic blood pressure ranged between 95 and 109 mmHg. In this trial, mortality from cardiovascular disease was reduced by two-thirds over a 4-year period. The trial included a blinded control group treated with placebo, which makes its conclusions particularly convincing. Fully 45% of placebo-treated patients experienced a fall in diastolic pressure to levels beneath 95 mmHg over a 3-year period, suggesting that patients with mild hypertension can be followed for a time while intake of sodium, alcohol, and calories is reduced and levels of exercise increased before a decision is reached regarding the use of antihypertensive drugs.

Thus, blood pressure should be lowered in asymptomatic individuals with diastolic blood pressure between 90 to 95 and 104 mmHg, even if they are free from end-organ damage and even if they are relatively elderly (some of the participants in HDFP were 74 years old at its conclusion). For those individuals with deceptively "mild" hypertension, treatment should begin with weight reduction, salt restriction, and regular exercise, with pharmacological agents added if these measures alone are unsuccessful.

B. Borderline Hypertension

The criteria for entry into the VA study, the HDFP, and the Australian trial included sustained diastolic hypertension. As a result, no firm data exist to prove whether or not therapy of labile or borderline hypertension ultimately benefits the patient, although we do know that borderline hypertension places the patient at risk.

A diagnosis of borderline hypertension creates both diagnostic and therapeutic dilemmas. A patient can have transient elevation of blood pressure to levels above 140/90 mmHg if pain or discomfort is present or if anxiety is prominent. If so, it is necessary to determine how often such elevation of blood pressure occurs. Frequent determinations over a period of 3 to 6 months can help answer the question. Checking the pressure after rest and having a nonphysician or family member check the pressure at home may determine whether the patient's pressure has returned to normal or whether it is fluctuating around a mildly elevated average. Ambulatory blood pressure monitoring can be very useful in these situations.

Data from the Society of Actuaries suggest that even mildly elevated casual blood pressure is associated with increased risk. The group with mild elevation of blood pressure had reduced longevity and was composed of patients with both fixed and labile hypertension. The findings of the Framingham study were based on casual blood pressure determinations and did not separate persons with mild fixed hypertension from those with mild labile hypertension. However, when the Framingham data were analyzed to assess the impact of lability, it was found that for any given average pressure, the degree of variability of the pressure did not affect the risk of cardiovascular events. Thus, it is the average pressure around which repeated readings vary that determines risk.

Borderline hypertension can follow several courses: some affected patients exhibit a return to normal blood pressure levels; some continue to have labile blood pressure elevations, and others develop fixed hypertension. The detection of borderline hypertension demands that the patient continue to be under medical surveillance so that the shortest possible time will elapse between the possible later development of fixed elevation of blood pressure and the initiation of effective antihypertensive therapy. Some advocate the initiation of antihypertensive therapy for most patients with borderline hypertension because of the high likelihood that they will develop fixed hypertension and the probability that early therapy might avoid years of slowly progressive target-organ damage. However, there is as yet no proof that antihypertensive therapy of borderline hypertension increases survival.

Virtually all available antihypertensive agents lower blood pressure in patients with mild, transient elevations. Such patients respond to diuretic therapy. Because hemodynamic studies in some of these patients show a hyperkinetic circulation, they have been treated with beta-adrenergic receptor blocking agents and often respond to very low doses. However, before a decision to treat is made, efforts must be made to evaluate the risk faced by a patient with borderline hypertension, that is, the extent, frequency, and duration of pressure elevation. Hypertensive damage is increased by the presence of other risk factors, and attention must be paid to the use of cigarettes as well as to family history, blood lipid levels, and glucose tolerance. When several risk factors are present, therapeutic intervention is reasonable.

C. Systolic Hypertension

Isolated systolic hypertension (greater than 160 mmHg) is often seen in elderly patients. Ejection of blood from the left ventricle into a rigid aorta causes a wide pulse pressure and an elevated systolic pressure. A few patients with elevated systolic pressure have disorders associated with high cardiac output, such as thyrotoxicosis, anemia, or arteriovenous fistulas. Because systolic hypertension is thought to reflect underlying atherosclerosis, it has often been thought not to be an indication for antihypertensive therapy. However, in the Build and Blood Pressure Study, mortality increased with each increment of systolic pressure at any given level of diastolic pressure and applied to both men and women regardless of age.

Multivariate analysis of the data from Framingham shows that systolic blood pressure correlates with the risk of coronary heart disease even more closely than diastolic or mean pressure, an observation that applies equally to men and women over age 45. However, diastolic pressure seemed to be the strongest determinant of risk in younger men. Data from the Framingham study have shown that isolated systolic pressure in the 140–159 mmHg range (stage I) is associated with an adverse cardiovascular outcome.

Systolic hypertension could reflect the presence of atherosclerosis in the elderly. The possibility exists that systolic hypertension, even though caused by atherosclerosis, may accelerate atherosclerosis, precipitate congestive heart failure, and thus contribute to morbidity and mortality. At present, it is clear that such patients are at increased risk. The Systolic Hypertension in the Elderly Program (SHEP) showed the protective value of lower blood pressure in elderly patients, extending the results of six other trials that included patients older than 60 years and showed that treating diastolic pressures exceeding 90 mmHg improved outcome. SHEP compared treatment with either placebo or low-dose chlorthalidone (with atenolol or reserpine added if necessary) for patients with systolic blood pressure exceeding 160 mmHg but with diastolic pressure less than 90 mmHg. After an average follow-up of 4.5 years, active treatment resulted in 36% fewer strokes and 27% fewer myocardial infarctions. When elderly patients are treated, antihypertensive agents should be started at a low dose and increased gradually, with careful monitoring.

D. Therapeutic Goals

There is no clear dividing line between normal and elevated blood pressure. The lower the naturally occurring blood pressure, the lower the risk of cardiovascular disease. Based on the results of the VA studies and 16 subservient large, randomized clinical trials, the 1994 JNC V report stated that

> The goal of treating patients with hypertension is to prevent morbidity and mortality associated with high blood pressure and to control blood pressure by the least intrusive means possible. This should be accomplished by achieving and maintaining arterial pressure below 140 mm Hg SBP and 90 mm Hg DPB while concurrently controlling other multiple cardiovascular risk factors. Further reduction to levels of 130/85 mm Hg

112

may be pursued with due regard for cardiovascular function, especially in older persons. How far the DBP should be reduced below 85 mm Hg is unclear.

Based on the results of SHEP, isolated systolic hypertension should be lowered to levels between 140 and 160 mmHg.

Reaching an ideal blood pressure must be weighed against the side effects of the drugs required to do so. Persons can have blood pressure reduced to 140/90 on relatively moderate doses of medications and may be entirely free of side effects. Yet, when medications are increased in an attempt to lower the pressure further, patients may be unacceptably sleepy or fatigued and may find that the medications are interfering with their quality of life. Here, the physician must use skill to match medication to patient and judgment in measuring other risk factors to assess how much of a danger the remaining minor elevation of blood pressure poses for the patient. If untoward effects occur that cannot be tolerated or avoided by changing antihypertensive agents, a compromise must be made. Data from the VA study suggest that even partial blood pressure control is beneficial.

Studies showing that reduction of diastolic pressure to levels below 85 mmHg was associated with an increased number of deaths from coronary heart disease led to the development of the "J-curve hypothesis." When arteriosclerosis narrows a blood vessel, flow across the stenosis depends on perfusion pressure. If arterial pressure falls, perfusion of the area distal to the lesion decreases. In the brain, this leads to symptoms of cerebrovascular insufficiency; in the heart, to angina pectoris; in the extremities, to claudication; and in the kidneys, to diminished renal function. In a patient with a history, physical findings, or laboratory tests suggesting the presence of underlying coronary disease, blood pressure must be lowered carefully, with efforts to identify potentially adverse effects of the reduced pressure. It is somewhat reassuring to note that, when treated with antihypertensive agents, the hypertensive survivors of strokes do not exhibit an increased rate of recurrence of stroke.

E. Evaluation of the Patient with Hypertension

History and Physical Examination

In the evaluation of patients with elevated blood pressure, the physician has three major goals: (a) to estimate the severity and rate of progression of the hypertensive process, (b) to assess target-organ damage, and (c) to identify curable forms of hypertension. A complete history and physical examination are essential steps in reaching these goals.

An attempt must be made to date the onset of hypertension. Records should be obtained for confirmation of blood pressure readings. It should be established whether the point of muffling or the point of disappearance of Korotkoff sounds was used to determine the diastolic pressure. The point of muffling tends to overestimate the true diastolic intraarterial pressure. The point of disappearance tends to underestimate the true diastolic pressure and is influenced by arm thickness, length of stethoscope tubing, background noise, and auscultatory skill.

It is important to establish whether the patient, during periods of stress, has had frequent mild, labile elevations that have returned to normal, or whether there is a clear and relentless rise in blood pressure, which may not be greatly elevated at any given time, but has been increasing steadily for years and has now reached a point requiring treatment.

The history should be obtained to identify evidence of target-organ damage. Ordinarily, moderate levels of blood pressure elevation do not cause symptoms until an event occurs that reflects cardiovascular or renal disease.

Symptoms and signs of target-organ involvement vary by organ system. Early cardiac involvement is reflected by increased left ventricular mass on echocardiography—often preceded by diastolic dysfunction—or by left ventricular hypertrophy or strain, evident by ECG. More serious involvement is indicated by clinical ECG or radiological evidence of coronary artery disease, left ventricular systolic dysfunction, or cardiac failure.

Transient ischemic attacks or strokes are often the first manifestation of cardiovascular target-organ damage. Microalbuminuria, proteinuria, or serum creatinine concentrations greater than 1.5 mg/dL indicate renal involvement. Peripheral vascular target-organ damage is manifest by loss of one or more lower-extremity pulses (other than the dorsalis pedis), intermittent claudication, or aneurysm formation. Retinal hemorrhages or exudates, with or without papilledema, indicate hypertensive retinopathy.

Symptoms suggesting secondary hypertension should be elicited. Renal parenchymal disease is the most common secondary cause of hypertension; it is suggested by a history of recurrent urinary tract infections and chronic pyelonephritis, or by episodes of edema, hematuria, and proteinuria in childhood, indicative of acute glomerulonephritis. The most common surgically curable form of secondary hypertension is renal vascular disease, suspected when hypertension appears suddenly before the age of 35 years or after the age of 55, or by hypertension beginning with flank pain or hematuria. Evidence of a source of emboli that might lodge in the renal artery is consistent with a renal cause of hypertension and should be considered if a history of rheumatic fever, heart murmurs (especially the murmur of mitral stenosis), cardiac arrhythmias, or cardiomyopathy is present.

To identify adrenal causes of hypertension, one often searches first for symptoms of pheochromocytoma. These chromaffin cell tumors usually release mixtures of epinephrine and norepinephrine, and the symptoms depend on the relative amount of each catecholamine released. Patients who release norepinephrine show signs of intense alpha-adrenergic stimulation: blanching of the skin, sweating, headache, and reflex slowing of the heart rate. Patients with tumors secreting epinephrine display the signs of beta-adrenergic receptor stimulation: flushing, tachycardia, and at times hypotension. Patients with pheochromocytoma frequently have postural hypotension because of plasma volume depletion. Because an undetected pheochromocytoma can have a fatal outcome, it is essential to keep this diagnostic possibility in mind.

Primary aldosteronism presents with less specific symptoms. The diagnostic hallmark is hypokalemia, which is frequently asymptomatic. When symptoms are present, they consist of episodic muscle weakness, polyuria, polydipsia, nocturia, paresthesia, and tetany.

Cushing's syndrome is usually suspected from the physical examination. The clinical history includes the development of truncal obesity, bone pain, easy bruising, increasing hair growth, and the development of a round, florid face.

Patients with coarctation of the aorta are frequently asymptomatic. When the coarctation is severe, the patient may complain of intermittent claudication or may have headaches because of the elevated blood pressure in the upper part of the body. This diagnosis should be considered in young patients, usually male, with stage I or II hypertension and a "functional" heart murmur.

Patients with hyperparathyroidism may develop hypertension. Points in the history that suggest this diagnosis are depression, constipation, peptic ulcer, and renal calculi.

Space-occupying intracerebral lesions can also present with blood pressure elevation. Most often this consists of systolic hypertension with a wide pulse pressure and a slow pulse rate. The examiner should look for localizing neurological signs and symptoms in evaluating this possibility.

Patients with acute intermittent porphyria may exhibit hypertension during an acute attack. Positive historical features include episodic hypertension, abdominal cramps, and precipitation by drugs such as barbiturates.

It is now well established that the use of oral contraceptive agents can cause hypertension and that the blood pressure elevation so induced may not resolve for as long as 6 months. Other pharmacological agents that can elevate blood pressure are sympathomimetics (e.g., in patients treated with them for asthma, hay fever, and colds), steroids, nonsteroidal antiinflammatory drugs, cyclosporine, erythropoietin, and cocaine or amphetamines.

Knowledge of the patient's family history is important. Although a strict genetic mode of inheritance of hypertension has not yet been elucidated, hypertension appears to be polygenic and blood pressure elevation tends to run in families. The children of two hypertensive parents are especially likely to develop hypertension. Patients often do not know whether their relatives really have hypertension and should be questioned for a family history of premature death or cardiovascular disease.

Examination of the Cardiovascular System

It is essential to measure blood pressure in both arms because atherosclerotic lesions or preductal coarctation of the aorta can result in asymmetrical pressures. This might cause the physician to make a falsely low estimate of the central arterial pressure or miss the fact that atherosclerotic lesions are present. A difference in arm readings of 20 mmHg strongly suggests obstruction. The next step is examination of the neck. The jugular venous pulse is inspected to determine whether the venous pressure is elevated or the pulse contour is abnormal. The carotid arteries must be examined. Thus, the neck is inspected visually for abnormal pulsations and the arteries are palpated and their relative pulse contours assessed. With the hyperkinetic circulation of young patients with labile hypertension, the upstroke of the pulse is brisk. Older patients who might have atherosclerotic lesions somewhere between the aortic valve and the jaw may have a slow upstroke. The presence of carotid or subclavian bruits should be noted. On auscultation of the thorax and lungs, the examiner listens for basilar rales, indicative of congestive heart failure, and for extracardiac bruits, which might point to underlying coarctation of the aorta. In young hypertensive patients, cardiac examination can demonstrate vigorous precordial pulsations and a systolic ejection murmur; together these suggest a hyperkinetic circulation.

The examiner also looks for evidence of hypertensive cardiovascular disease. Inspection of the chest wall and palpation of the cardiac apex can disclose a palpable atrial gallop of S_4, a sign that the ventricle has begun to hypertrophy and that its compliance characteristics have changed; this results in the development of an audible sound as the left atrium forcefully ejects blood into the left ventricle.

Cardiac auscultation can reveal an S_3 gallop that usually indicates cardiac dilatation and failure. However, an S_3 can be a physiological finding in young, athletic subjects with a slow heart rate and a large stroke volume. Systolic ejection murmurs in the older hypertensive suggest calcification of the aortic valve; an apical holosystolic regurgitant murmur suggests dilatation of the left ventricle with mitral valvular insufficiency; and, in severe hypertension, the decrescendo diastolic murmur of aortic insufficiency suggests dilatation of the aorta and aortic valve ring.

Examination of the cardiovascular system extends to the abdomen, where the presence of systolic bruits indicates underlying atherosclerosis of the aorta and bruits occupying both systole and diastole suggest renal artery stenosis. The abdominal aorta should be palpated for evidence of aneurysmic dilitation. Physical examination should include palpation and auscultation of the femoral pulses for evidence of atherosclerosis or coarctation of the aorta. When significant coarctation of the aorta exists, the femoral pulse is diminished, the peak of the pulse is delayed relative to the pulse at the radial artery, and arterial pressure is lower in the legs than in the arms. The popliteal, posterior tibial, and dorsalis pedis pulses should be examined for evidence of peripheral atherosclerosis.

116

Neurological examination should search for focal lesions, either as a cause of the hypertension or as a manifestation of previous intracerebral hemorrhage or infarction.

Retinal Examination

The changes that take place in the optic fundus can be divided into those due to arteriolosclerosis and those due to elevated blood pressure. Retinal exudates can result from other disorders, such as diabetes mellitus, emboli, malignancy, arteritis, hematological malignancies, and primary renal disease. Most of the vessels visualized are true arterioles, at least those beyond one or two disk diameters from the optic disk. The most characteristic hypertensive change is vasoconstriction, but structural changes also take place in the intimal and muscular layers.

Keith and associates described four groups of arteriolar and retinal changes in patients with hypertension—each associated with decreased survival. Patients with group 1 changes, focal or segmental arteriolar narrowing, survived reasonably well. Prognosis was worse in groups 2, 3, and 4. Group 2 changes refer to venous narrowing at the point at which the retinal vein crosses behind a thickened arteriole. Group 3 changes also include retinal hemorrhages and exudates, and group 4 changes include papilledema.

Because hypertension is the most common predisposing factor for the development of arteriolosclerosis, the hypertensive patient might be expected to show the changes of both processes. Arteriolosclerosis can develop also in the absence of hypertension but usually with presence of diabetes mellitus, advanced age, hyperlipidema, or other risk factors. In general, arteriolosclerotic changes correlate roughly with the duration of the blood pressure elevation, and the degree of the hypertensive changes corresponds with the severity of hypertension.

Arteriolosclerosis is a diffuse process that involves thickening of the vessel walls. Involvement of the retinal arteries is reflected by a wide arteriolar light reflex, a silver- or copper-wire appearance, AV crossing changes, and increased arteriolar tortuosity. Healthy young people can also show tortuous arterioles in the absence of underlying arteriolosclerotic disease. Arteriolovenous nicking begins with a mild depression of the vein, followed by obliteration for short distances on either side of the arteriole and later by thickening of the vessel distal to the crossing. AV nicking can occur in the absence of hypertension.

The most striking hypertensive change is retinal hemorrhage, which is associated with severe hypertension and characteristically occurs near the optic disk. The lesions are usually flame-shaped because they occur in the nerve fiber layer and extend between the fibers.

Other forms of hemorrhage can occur in hypertension, but these may be associated with other disease entities. When the hemorrhage is located in the periphery and is solitary and round in shape, it may be a sign of advanced arteriolosclerosis or of arteriolar or venous occlusion. Patients with diabetes mellitus develop capillary aneurysms and may have occluded small vessels, leading to ischemic areas of hemorrhage. Patients with diabetes, stroke, trauma, or leukemia as well as some normal subjects can develop hemorrhages in the deep layer of the retina. Such hemorrhages are usually raised, bright red, and large, with sharp borders.

Two types of retinal exudates can be seen on ophthalmoscopic examination. "Hard" exudates have a sharp margin and are thought to represent the residua of hemorrhages in layers deep to the retinal vessels. These exudates often appear after the initiation of antihypertensive therapy and can persist for a year.

The other common type of retinal exudate is the "cotton wool" or "soft" exudate, which appears suddenly and increases rapidly in size. With the initiation of antihypertensive treatment, the exudates become coarsely granular, develop small red microaneurysms, and gradually disappear. Such exudates are usually located near the optic disk and may represent ischemic infarcts.

The appearance of soft exudates with flame hemorrhages suggests that the hypertensive process is accelerating. These retinal changes can heal completely when the blood pressure is lowered, and the exudates often disappear in several days. Although soft exudates are ordinarily associated with severe hypertension, they can also be seen in lupus erythematosus and dermatomyositis and after occlusion of the central retinal vein. The appearance of soft exudates and striate hemorrhages can be associated with the development of retinal edema, one manifestation of which is a star figure that forms around the macula in hypertensive patients and resolves slowly with antihypertensive therapy.

When soft exudates and striate hemorrhages are accompanied by papilledema, malignant hypertension is present and the patient is commonly threatened by impending renal and cardiac failure. The development of papilledema can be gradual. The patient may develop, in sequence, loss of physiological cupping of the optic disk, blurring of the nasal margins of the disk, distention of the retinal veins, blurring of the temporal margins, and, finally, elevation of the optic disk. With successful antihypertensive therapy, papilledema usually disappears in 2 to 3 months, although some irregularity around the edges of the optic disk may persist for a year. When papilledema appears, brain tumors, cerebral swelling secondary to trauma, intracerebral hemorrhage, pseudotumor cerebri, and lead poisoning should be considered as well.

Controversy remains regarding the role of vasospasm in producing the retinal changes of hypertension. Acute forms of hypertension, such as eclampsia or acute glomerulonephritis, are accompanied by severe retinal arteriolar vasoconstriction. With chronic hypertension, it is difficult to distinguish sclerotic changes from acute vasoconstrictive changes if the vessels do not dilate and constrict during the examination or change acutely in response to therapy. Irregularity of the vessel outline suggests chronic, sclerotic changes.

The development of hemorrhages or exudates signals serious progression of hypertension. This progression from grade 2 to grade 3 retinal changes demands more aggressive management of the elevated blood pressure, often requiring prompt hospitalization.

Laboratory Evaluation

Approximately 50 million Americans have hypertension. Should they all have a costly workup before being treated? In the 10,900 participants of the HDFP, the incidence of secondary hypertension was found to be less than 1%. Thus, an extensive laboratory evaluation to detect secondary causes of hypertension would not have been cost-effective. Procedures such as the intravenous urogram, renal isotope, ultrasound studies, or digital subtraction renal angiograms as well as measurement of plasma or urinary catecholamines or their metabolites and assay of the renin-angiotensin-aldosterone system should be ordered only when specific indications are uncovered by history or physical examination.

However, before the institution of antihypertensive therapy, every patient should undergo a limited number of baseline laboratory studies. The studies recommended by JNC V are listed in Table 3. If the clinical history is suggestive, additional studies should be performed to rule out curable forms of hypertension. Suggested screening and definitive studies for the most common forms of secondary hypertension are given in Table 4. Measurement of urinary microalbumin, echocardiograms, and plasma renin/urinary sodium determinations can be useful in selected cases.

Table 3   Initial Evaluation of the Hypertensive Patient

Medical history
Physical examination
Laboratory studies
1.   To determine severity of vascular disease and possible causes of hypertension
     Complete blood count
     Urinalysis
     Serum creatinine, potassium, calcium
     Electrocardiogram
2.   To assess cardiovascular risk factors and provide baseline for following possible adverse effect of antihypertensive medications
     Total cholesterol
     High-density lipoprotein cholesterol
     Triglycerides
     Fasting plasma glucose
     Serum uric acid

Source: Modified from the 1994 Report of the Joint National Committee on Detection, Evaluation, and Treatment of High Blood Pressure.

Table 4 Screening Tests for Most Common Forms of Secondary Hypertension

Disorder	Primary Screen	Definitive Screen
1. Renal artery stenosis	Captopril renogram, rapid-sequence IVP, transvenous digital subtraction renal angiogram or renal Doppler ultrasound	Renal arteriogram and renal vein renins
2. Renal parenchymal disease	Dipstick urinalysis, serum creatinine	Creatinine clearance, renal ultrasound biopsy when indicated
3. Pheochromocytoma	Urine VMA, metanephrines or catecholamines	Adrenal CT scan, MRI, or arteriograms
4. Primary aldosteronism	Serum potassium	PRA and Aldo after Na^+ restriction, adrenal vein sampling, adrenal CT scan, MRI, or arteriograms
5. Cushing's syndrome	Rapid, overnight dexamethasone suppression test	Longer dexamethasone suppression test, adrenal CT scan, MRI, or arteriograms
6. Coarctation of aorta	Cuff BP in legs	Aortogram

Abbreviations: CT = computed tomography; IVP = intravenous pyelogram; MRI = magnetic resonance imaging; PRA = plasma renin activity; VMA = vanillylmandelic acid.

Cardiovascular Evaluation

Electrocardiogram The electrocardiogram can suggest the presence and define the severity of left ventricular hypertrophy in the following ways: (a) increased voltage, duration, and direction of the main QRS vector; (b) prolonged onset of intrinsicoid deflection in the left precordial leads; (c) leftward and posterior change in director of the initial (0.02-sec) QRS vector; (d) altered repolarization with more anterior and rightward direction of the ST-segment and T-wave vectors; and (e) left atrial abnormality or altered terminal P-wave vector. Some of these abnormalities are directly related to increased left ventricular muscle mass.

Chest X-Ray Routine posteroanterior and lateral chest x-rays are sometime useful in evaluating cardiac size, left ventricular and left atrial enlargement, pulmonary venous congestion, enlargement of the aortic root, tortuosity and calcification of the thoracic aorta, and signs of coarctation of the aorta.

120

Early left ventricular enlargement does not produce significant change in the cardiac silhouette or cardiothoracic ratio. With increasing hypertrophy, there is greater convexity to the left heart border because of enlargement of the left ventricular outflow tract. The lower left heart border enlarges leftward and the apex points downward.

Dilatation, tortuosity, or elongation of the aortic root can result in a widened mediastinal shadow. Uncoiling or tortuosity of the aorta is present in fewer than 3% of persons under 40 years of age; therefore its presence suggests target-organ involvement. In older patients, tortuosity is usually secondary to atherosclerosis.

The chest x-ray suggests coarctation of the aorta when the shadow of the dilated left subclavian artery on the upper mediastinal border, or rib-notching due to dilated intercostal arteries, is seen. The "reversed-three sign" or "E-sign" resulting from aortic dilatation proximal to and distal to the coarctation is another characteristic x-ray finding.

Echocardiography Although ECG criteria of left ventricular hypertrophy (LVH) are associated with a considerable increase in cardiovascular morbidity and mortality, especially if repolarization abnormalities are present, relatively few patients with hypertension exhibit ECG criteria for LVH. In the HDFP, only 5% of the mild to moderately hypertensive participants had LVH evident on the ECG. However, the introduction of echocardiography to the study of hypertensive patients has revealed a much higher frequency of left ventricular involvement. The echocardiogram allows measurement not only of wall thickness but also chamber dimensions, left ventricular mass, and left ventricular wall stress. Devereaux and Reichek compared echocardiographic measurements of left ventricular mass with postmortem measurements in 34 patients and found a correlation coefficient of .96 ($p<.01$) and a sensitivity of 93% with a specificity of 95%. When echocardiography was applied to hypertensive subjects only 3% of whom had ECG evidence of LVH, 48% had increased left ventricular mass or wall thickness demonstrable on the echocardiogram.

Although electrocardiographic evidence of LVH is known to be associated with reduced longevity, increased left ventricular mass detected by echocardiography is associated with increased cardiovascular morbidity or mortality as well. When a muscle is faced with an increased workload, it first undergoes adaptive hypertrophy. If the increased workload is continued and is beyond the capacity of the muscle to adapt, muscle failure results. When blood pressure first rises, the thickness and mass of the left ventricle increase. Thus, the stress per unit of mass is normalized. In order to contract, the left ventricle must develop sufficient tension to overcome the afterload that it faces during shortening. Myocardial wall tension, according to the law of LaPlace, is a direct function of intracavity pressure and ventricular radius and inversely related to wall thickness. Left ventricular mass does not correlate with arterial blood pressure as well as with left ventricular wall stress.

121

An important area of contemporary investigation has been elucidation of the separation of physiological, adaptive hypertrophy from pathological hypertrophy. Data from experimental and clinical studies suggest that the increased left ventricular mass of early adaptive hypertrophy is characterized by preservation of normal diastolic relaxation.

In recent years, attention has been turned to the effect of antihypertensive therapy on LVH and left ventricular function in addition to the effect of pharmacological agents on blood pressure. In the spontaneously hypertensive rat, reversal of hypertrophy occurs upon treatment with methyldopa, captopril, or a combination of reserpine, hydralazine, and hydrochlorothiazide. Treatment with hydralazine alone does not reverse hypertrophy despite control of blood pressure, and treatment with minoxidil alone actually increases hypertrophy. In contrast, ventricular hypertrophy in the rat with renovascular hypertension can be reversed by either unilateral nephrectomy, angiotensin converting enzyme (ACE) inhibition, or calcium channel blockers. These observations suggest that the factors producing hypertrophy—other than increased afterload—differ in different forms of hypertension and that the activity of the adrenergic nervous system may play an important role in the production and reversal of ventricular hypertrophy. Nevertheless, it is now generally agreed that all agents other than direct-acting vasodilators that lower blood pressure effectively also reduce hypertrophy. However, they differ with respect to the rate at which they reduce hypertrophy. The ACE inhibitors and calcium channel blockers have prompt effects. Diuretics or beta blockers act more slowly.

Echocardiographic studies of ventricular function during different phases of the cardiac cycle have provided insights into the pathophysiology of hypertensive heart disease. Unrelieved systemic arterial hypertension results in ventricular hypertrophy, eventually leading to dilation and failure. Accelerated coronary atherosclerosis with myocardial ischemia plays an important role in the genesis of congestive heart failure in the hypertensive patient. Hypertensive patients presenting with pulmonary edema can be separated into two distinct groups by echocardiography: those with dilated ventricles and poor systolic function and those with hypertrophied ventricles with small or normally sized ventricular cavities and well-preserved systolic function, who have impaired diastolic compliance resulting in high ventricular filling pressures. The latter have abnormal diastolic function with a prolonged early diastolic filling period, and reduced peak diastolic dimension increase. Such patients sometimes respond to vasodilator therapy with severe hypotensive reactions.

It is important to distinguish between these two groups of patients because those with dilated ventricles and impaired systolic function often benefit from careful afterload reduction, and those with well-preserved systolic function but high pulmonary capillary wedge pressures because of impaired diastolic function often benefit most from cautious reduction of venous return or even from the use of agents with negative inotropic effects such as verapamil.

122

Renal Evaluation

Routine Urinalysis In the initial evaluation of a patient with newly discovered hypertension, one of the earliest considerations should be the possible presence of undetected renal disease, because chronic parenchymal renal disease is the most common cause of secondary hypertension. Additionally, the intrarenal vasculature and glomerular capillaries are susceptible to hypertensive damage resulting in a loss of function.

The routine urinalysis is useful in assessing these possibilities. A clean-catch midstream specimen is less likely to contain contaminants causing misleading results. The osmolality or specific gravity screens for loss of concentrating ability. Urine should be collected when the patient is relatively dehydrated (e.g., the second voiding after rising). Severe proteinuria and glucosuria can cause elevated specific gravity. The finding of proteinuria should lead to further evaluation. With the semiquantitative methods used in screening examinations, trace amounts may reflect no more than a normal amount of protein. A 1+ designation is abnormal in properly collected specimens and indicates protein concentrations of 10–30 mg/100 mL. Such patients should have quantitative excretion measured.

Microalbuminuria is an early manifestation of hypertensive target-organ damage involving the kidney. Measurement can provide information that is useful in reaching a decision to initiate pharmacological antihypertensive therapy.

Patients with glycosuria should be evaluated for diabetes mellitus, since glomerulosclerosis is associated with renal insufficiency and hypertension.

Microscopic examination of the urine sediment is an important part of the evaluation. A normal urine sediment contains few formed elements—for example, one or two red blood cells, one or two white blood cells, occasional hyaline casts, and a few epithelial cells. Casts indicate parenchymal renal damage if present in an abnormal amount or type. Red blood cell or hemoglobin casts indicate active glomerular injury. Large amounts of white blood cells and bacteria indicate an infection in the urinary tract.

V. DIAGNOSTIC STUDIES FOR SECONDARY HYPERTENSION

A. Renal Parenchymal Disease

Although renal parenchymal disease is the most common cause of secondary hypertension, the manner in which this disorder results in hypertension is not clear. Possibilities include abnormal stimulation of the renin-angiotensin system with inadequate response to the negative feedback signals because of renal damage, inadequate control of sodium and volume homeostasis, and impaired production of renal vasodepressor substances (Table 4).

Although the pathogenesis may differ, the approach to the treatment of patients with renal parenchymal disease is much the same as that of patients with essential hypertension except for a few considerations. Drugs that affect renal function adversely should be used with caution in patients with more mild to moderate reduction of glomerular filtration—that is, those with a serum creatinine above 2.0 mg/100 mL. Thiazide diuretics, chlorthalidone, spironolactone, triamterene, metolazone, angiotensin-converting enzyme inhibitors, and guanethidine all can increase nitrogen retention.

The second consideration regards adjustment of dosage. Loop diuretics such as furosemide are useful in treating patients with severe renal insufficiency, but a larger dose is required as function decreases. Failure to respond to antihypertensive therapy is often attributable to an inadequate dose of diuretic or to excessive sodium intake. The combination of metolazone or thiazide with furosemide results in a potent diuretic regimen that must be used carefully to avoid severe volume depletion. Drugs that are eliminated by renal excretion, such as methyldopa, must be given in lower doses as renal function deteriorates.

B. Renal Function Tests

Costly laboratory tests are not required in the evaluation of patients with hypertension. The serum creatinine is an excellent qualitative measure of glomerular filtration (GFR). When the serum creatinine reaches a value twice that of the mean control level, the GFR is approximately 50%. The endogenous creatinine clearance may be obtained to semiquantify the extent of impairment of glomerular filtration, but it adds little of practical value in patient management when the serum creatinine value is normal.

Quantitative measurement of glomerular filtration and renal plasma flow is possible by measurement of insulin and para-aminohippuric acid (PAH) clearances; this, however, is seldom needed in the evaluation of hypertensive patients.

C. Renovascular Hypertension

In 1914, Volhard postulated that hypertension was caused by stenotic small arteries throughout the renal parenchyma, with systemic arterial hypertension developing as a compensatory mechanism, permitting the circulation to drive blood through the renal "purification system." In 1934, Goldblatt demonstrated that stenosis of a canine renal artery resulted in systemic arterial hypertension and that relief of the stenosis returned blood pressure to control levels. Since then, a number of studies have demonstrated that renal artery stenosis is a cause of hypertension in humans and that correction of the stenosis frequently cures the hypertension.

Renal artery stenosis, probably the most common surgically correctable cause of hypertension in humans, exists in two major forms. The first of these, fibromuscular dysplasia, involves destruction of vascular smooth muscle and fibrous proliferation within the wall of the artery. This condition affects females more often than males by a ratio of about 3 to 1 and often appears in young subjects. The lesions are usually present in the distal two-thirds of the renal artery, although they may also involve other sections.

The second major type of renal artery stenosis is caused by atherosclerosis. It occurs more often in males by a 2 to 1 ratio, is characteristically seen in older age groups, and usually involves the proximal third of the renal artery.

After renal transplantation, stenosis may occur by a different mechanism in which the proliferation of vascular smooth muscle predominates. This condition may be immunologically mediated. The clinical history is rarely of great help in diagnosing renovascular hypertension. However, factors that are consistent with a renovascular etiology are hypertension with a diastolic pressure above 130 mmHg; sudden onset of hypertension with a diastolic pressure above 110 mmHg in patients below 30 or above 55 years of age; accelerated hypertension with hemorrhages, exudates, or papilledema; a history of flank pain, hematuria, or renal trauma; hypertension remaining resistant to pharmacological therapy; and the presence of epigastric of flank bruits throughout systole and diastole. Diastolic are more specific than systolic bruits.

Rapid-sequence intravenous urograms have been thought by many to be the best screening procedures for patients with suspected renal artery stenosis or renal parenchymal disease. However, this test fails to detect about 25% of the cases of renovascular hypertension. An indicator of unilateral stenosis is late appearance of contrast material in the ischemic kidney. Another indication is a difference in renal size. The left kidney is normally 0.5 cm longer than the right. Thus, a difference of 1.5 cm or more when the left kidney is larger or 0.5 cm or more when the right kidney is larger is significant. Because the ischemic kidney reabsorbs filtered water in excess of contrast material, delayed hyperconcentration is another sign of unilateral stenosis, as is scalloping along the course of the ureter secondary to enlargement of collateral ureteric blood vessels.

The radioactive tracer renal scan and renogram or renal Doppler ultrasound provide alternative means of screening. The renogram has an incidence of false-negative results similar to that associated with an intravenous pyelogram (IVP) and does not reveal the anatomic details yielded by intravenous urography, such as hydronephrosis, pyelonephrotic scarring, and reduction in size secondary to glomerulonephritis. A multicenter cooperative study of renovascular hypertension found that about 10% of patients with essential hypertension have abnormal intravenous urograms, whereas 22% of patients with surgically correctable reno-vascular hypertension had normal urograms. Patients with hypertension and ab-normal urograms have about a 50% chance of having surgically correctable reno-vascular hypertension. Digital subtraction intravenous angiography offers the potential to improve detection of significant lesions without the risk of more invasive angiographic procedures, but it often fails to visualize intrarenal vascular stenosis.

In the ischemic kidney, function is maintained via angiotensin II–mediated constriction of the efferent arteriole. A single dose of ACE inhibitor prevents the formation of angiotensin II; therefore renal function fails promptly. This effect can be exploited to amplify differences in uptake of radioactive tracer between the ischemic and normal kidneys, thereby enhancing the diagnostic accuracy of a renal scan measuring scintigraphic images and time-activity curves. Hypertension in most patients with abnormal captopril-augmented renal scans improves after revascularization, making this an excellent non-invasive screening test. A post-captopril scan is done first. If this is abnormal, the scan is repeated without captopril to demonstrate reversible renal function.

Although average peripheral vein renin activity is higher in patients with renovascular hypertension than in those with essential hypertension, there is so much overlap of individual values within the two groups that peripheral renin activity (PRA) is not very useful in screening patients for renovascular hypertension. However, the sensitivity of the test can be enhanced by measuring PRA after the administration of captopril.

When an abnormal intravenous urogram, radioactive renogram, or Doppler ultrasound has been obtained, the next diagnostic step is usually renal arteriography to define the anatomy of any lesion that might be present. In postmortem studies, however, it has been found that about 40% of patients with renal artery stenosis were normotensive during life. Thus, functional assessment of a stenotic lesion is important. The most widely used method is bilateral measurement of renal vein renin activity. Elevated activity on the ischemic side and a renal vein renin ratio of ischemic to uninvolved side of 1.5 or greater correctly predicts results of surgery in about 80% of cases. However, many false-negative results occur. Accuracy is improved somewhat with the use of captopril. When bilateral renal artery stenosis is present, this procedure is less valuable, although it may provide an estimate of which kidney is contributing most importantly to the elevation of blood pressure.

The sensitivity of renal vein renin measurement can be enhanced by sodium depletion. A low-sodium diet plus full doses of oral diuretics for 3 days before measurement of renal vein renin activity improves the predictive value of the test from 35 to 90%. Agents that reduce renin release tend to decrease the sensitivity of the test.

An abnormal intravenous urogram, arterial stenosis demonstrated on arteriography, and a renal vein renin ratio above 1.5 do not automatically indicate that surgical correction is required. Many patients respond to pharmacological therapy with ACE inhibitors, and many are high-risk surgical candidates.

Corrective renovascular surgery in patients with significant extrarenal arteriosclerosis may improve blood pressure but not prolong life. Thus, individual judgment must be applied to each case. It is reasonable to limit renal artery surgery to those patients who fail to respond to pharmacological therapy.

Percutaneous transluminal angioplasty offers a less invasive way—compared with surgery—to relieve renal ischemia. Unfortunately, not all stenotic lesions can be dilated successfully with a balloon-tipped catheter, and many restenose after an initially successful intervention. However, in some patients, periodic redilatation may offer a lower risk of complications and mortality than surgical bypass.

VI. ADRENAL HYPERTENSION

A. Pheochromocytoma

Pheochromocytomas are usually nonmalignant tumors of chromaffin cells of the adrenal medulla or sympathetic ganglia. They occur as isolated lesions, in association with familial neurocutaneous disorders, with thyroid medullary carcinoma, or with hyperparathyroidism.

Pheochromocytomas contain the enzymes needed to metabolize tyrosine to catecholamines. After uptake, tyrosine is hydroxylated to dihydroxyphenyl-alanine (dopa) in a rate-limiting tyrosine hydroxylase–mediated step. Dopa is decarboxylated to dihydroxphenethylamine (dopamine), which in turn is oxidized to norepinephrine in storage granules. In tissues containing phenethanolamine-N-methyltransferase, norepinephrine is methylated to form epinephrine. This enzymatic step usually occurs only in the adrenal medulla.

Symptoms of pheochromocytoma occur as mixtures of catecholamines are released into the circulation. The Valsalva maneuver, exercise, pregnancy, overeating, urination, and ingestion of tyramine-containing foods can precipitate attacks. The most common symptoms are headache, sweating, palpitation, pallor, and nausea. More than 50% of patients with pheochromocytoma have persistent hypertension with spikes; the remainder have intermittent hypertension.

It is not unusual for such patients to be followed for several years before a diagnosis is made. Postural hypotension is found in approximately two-thirds of them.

The cardiovascular effects of catecholamines account for most of the symptoms. Norepinephrine stimulates alpha-adrenergic receptors, causing systolic and diastolic hypertension, reflex bradycardia, and cardiac arrhythmias. Epinephrine stimulates both alpha and beta receptors, causing tachycardia, elevated cardiac output, arrhythmias, and either hypotension or systolic hypertension. Both compounds decrease gastrointestinal motility, inhibit insulin release, and elevate blood sugar, free fatty acids, lactic acid, and basal metabolic rate. Norepinephrine is the major compound produced by most tumors, although predominant production of epinephrine has been reported. Although the two types of tumors cannot usually be separated clinically, it is a reasonable assumption that attacks associated with bradycardia are norepinephrine-mediated, whereas attacks associated with hypotension are epinephrine-mediated.

Management of patients with pheochromocytoma requires confirmation of the diagnosis by biochemical tests and location of the tumor and removal with adequate monitoring after appropriate preparation of the patient.

127

Biochemical tests for urinary catecholamines or their metabolites are the mainstays of diagnosis. Values twice normal or higher are typical. After release of catecholamines, relatively small amounts are excreted unchanged in the urine. Circulating catecholamines are converted to metanephrine and normetanephrine by hepatic catechol O-methyltransferase (COMT). These products are excreted in the urine or metabolized throughout the body by monoamine oxidase to vanillylmandelic acid (VMA). Small amounts of norepinephrine are metabolized to dihydroxymandelic acid within the neuron and converted to VMA by COMT.

Urinary (and plasma) catecholamines are present in only small amounts and are difficult to measure. Elevated values are found in patients taking any catecholamine-containing medication. Measurement of total urinary metanephrine is a reliable procedure in many laboratories, often more reliable than assay of catecholamines. Elevated values occur in patients given monoamine oxidase inhibitors.

Vanillylmandelic acid can be measured by a colorimetric phenolic acid reaction, but results are elevated by ingestion of phenol-containing foods. A more specific spectrophotometric method is not influenced by diet, but values are lowered by monoamine oxidase inhibitors or clofibrate and falsely elevated by nalidixic acid. If urinary levels of one product are elevated, a separate collection should be made and a different product found to be elevated before the diagnosis is considered confirmed. All urine collections should be made in an acid-containing bottle to prevent breakdown of catecholamine metabolites.

Plasma levels of norepinephine and epinephrine are elevated in most patients with pheochromocytoma. However, relying upon measurement of plasma catecholamine as a screening procedure leads to many false-positive results.

The diagnosis of pheochromocytoma should never be made solely on the basis of pharmacological testing. However, provocative tests (e.g., eliciting elevation of blood pressure by administration of histamine, tyramine, or glucagon or inducing a fall in pressure by administration of phentolamine) may be helpful despite many false-positive and false-negative results and some risk.

When the diagnosis of pheochromocytoma has been established, the tumor must be localized. Approximately 80% of pheochromocytomas arise in the adrenals. Another 10–15% arise from intraabdominal sympathetic ganglia or from the organs of Zuckerkandl. Most extraabdominal tumors arise from the thoracic sympathetic chain and can be seen on oblique chest films or with other imaging modalities. Cervical tumors are usually palpable or cause local symptoms.

Intravenous urograms or adrenal tomograms show displacement of the kidney by a suprarenal mass in 50% of cases. Arteriography can localize tumors but may also precipitate acute attacks. Patients should be prepared for study with alpha-adrenergic blocking agents for 1 week before arteriography. Finding one tumor on arteriography does not rule out the presence of others, found in 15–20% of patients. Vena cava catheterization with catecholamine measurement at several sites is sometimes useful in localizing tumors. Computed tomography, magnetic resonance imaging, and scintigraphy with ^{131}I-labeled metaiodobenzylguanidine (MIBG) have been used to locate pheochromocytomas successfully, even in difficult cases.

Preoperative management of the patient with pheochromocytoma requires pharmacological stabilization for 1 or 2 weeks with alpha-adrenergic blockade. Beta-adrenergic blockade is indicated as well when cardiac arrhythmia or serious tachycardia develops but should not be used routinely because of the risk of inducing heart failure in patients who might have occult catecholamine cardiomyopathy. Alpha-methylparatyrosine, an inhibitor of tyrosine hydroxylase, can eliminate many symptoms by interfering with catecholamine biosynthesis and has proved to be useful in the preoperative treatment of patients with pheochromocytoma and in controlling symptoms of those with inoperable or metastatic tumors.

B. Aldosteronism

Aldosterone causes resorption of sodium and secretion of potassium and hydrogen in the distal renal tubule. This leads to the characteristics of primary aldosteronism: hypertension and depletion of body potassium stores. Potassium depletion causes muscle weakness and fatigue and leads to the development of nephropathy, with symptoms of polyuria and nocturia. The hypertension associated with primary hyperaldosteronism is ordinarily mild and well tolerated, although cases of more severe hypertension have been reported. Malignant hypertension secondary to primary aldosteronism is extraordinarily rare.

At present, the most useful screening test for primary aldosteronism is measurement of serum potassium, which is usually less than 3.5 mEq/dL. Because some patients with hyperaldosteronism have mild or borderline hypokalemia, repeat measurements are needed in patients with borderline values. It is necessary to be certain that the patient has not been taking a potassium supplement or restricting dietary sodium. When less sodium is presented to the distal renal tubules, less is exchanged for potassium; thus serum potassium levels remain relatively high.

Many phenomena other than primary aldosteronism result in hypokalemia. The most common is use of diuretic agents. Potassium-wasting renal disease, Cushing's syndrome, juxtaglomerular apparatus, hyperplasia, and aldosteronism secondary to renovascular or renal parenchymal disease are additional possibilities.

Plasma renin activity should be measured under well-defined conditions in patients with unexplained hypokalemia. Patients with primary aldosteronism have retained sodium and water but "escape" before developing edema because of the increased glomerular filtration rate. Because of volume overexpansion, plasma renin levels are usually suppressed. A useful practice is to place patients on a low-sodium diet (10 mEq Na, 100 mEq K) for 4 days and obtain a blood sample for

129

measurement of renin at around noon on the morning of the fourth day, after the patient has been up and about all morning. The combination of upright posture and sodium depletion acts to stimulate renin release, but in patients with primary aldosteronism, because of the volume overexpansion, plasma renin activity remains suppressed.

A patient with suppressed renin activity has either aldosteronism or "low renin" hypertension. Measurement of a high ratio of plasma aldosterone to plasma renin activity, which is normally around 10, suggests primary aldosteronism. Definitive diagnosis of primary aldosteronism requires hospitalization for metabolic studies. The presence of low plasma renin activity despite volume depletion must be confirmed, and elevated plasma or urinary aldosterone that is not suppressed physiologically when the patient is given a salt load must be demonstrated. Once the diagnosis of primary aldosteronism has been made biochemically, tumor should be localized by computed tomography or magnetic resonance imaging, which can detect bilateral enlargement or adenomas as small as 1 cm; by bilateral adrenal venography and sampling of adrenal venous blood for assay of plasma aldosterone levels; or by surgical exploration of both adrenal glands.

Primary aldosteronism, though frequently caused by a single adenoma, can result from at least three other causes. Surgical excision of an adrenal adenoma producing aldosterone ordinarily leads to correction of both hypertension and electrolyte abnormality. Some patients with biochemical evidence of aldosteronism have bilateral nodular hyperplasia of the adrenal cortex. Bilateral adrenalectomy results in correction of electrolyte abnormalities, but the hypertension persists. Although the two groups of patients differ in their responses to changes in salt and fluid balance, distinction between the two before surgery, until recently, required demonstration of a single andenoma by adrenal venography or demonstration of elevated levels of aldosterone in both adrenal veins.

A third group of patients exhibit signs and biochemical manifestations of aldosteronism but respond to the administration of deoxycorticosterone (DOCA) by suppression of urinary aldosterone secretion to normal levels.

A fourth group exhibits glucocorticoid-remediable hyperaldosteronism. The signs, symptoms, and biochemical evidence of aldosteronism are present, but administration of replacement doses of glucocorticoid corrects the blood pressure, suppresses urinary aldosterone secretion, and corrects electrolyte imbalance. This disorder can be diagnosed by measuring urinary excretion of 18-oxo-cortisol or by genetic analysis.

C. Cushing's Syndrome

Patients with excessive cortisol secretion, either from adrenocortical hyperplasia or adrenocortical tumor, frequently develop hypertension. Ordinarily, Cushing's syndrome is apparent on physical examination, with the patient displaying truncal obesity, round face, buffalo hump, purple striae, multiple bruises over thin skin, and bone pain. Diagnosis is supported by positive results of a rapid dexamethasone suppression test, in which the patient is given 1 mg dexamethasone at midnight, which is perceived by the hypothalamus as an elevation of plasma corticosteroids, leading to diminished pituitary adrenocorticotropic hormone (ACTH) release and diminished adrenal secretion of corticosteroids. In normal subjects, measurement of plasma cortisol at 8 A.M. the next morning demonstrates suppression of less than 5 μg/100 mL. Patients with Cushing's syndrome fail to exhibit cortisol suppression and require hospitalization for further evaluation.

D. Adrenal Cortical Enzyme Deficiencies

Congenital disorders exist in which one of the hydroxylase enzymes necessary for the production of corticosteroids is absent or deficient, resulting in diminished serum corticosteroids and elevated pituitary secretion of ACTH. Because steroid synthesis cannot proceed normally through biochemical pathways, the compensatory stimuli result in production of excess amounts of other steroid compounds, including some with salt-retaining properties. The syndrome most frequently seen in adults involves deficiency of 17-hydroxylase, which catalyzes conversion of progesterone to 17-hydroxyprogesterone. Glucocorticoid, estrogen, and androgen production are impaired. Primary amenorrhea, hypertension, and defeminization result. The diagnosis is suspected when urinary excretion of 17-ketosteroids and 17-hydroxysteroids is low or absent, despite hypertension. Dexamethasone, 1 mg daily for 7 to 14 days, should result in correction of the hypertension.

E. Oral Contraceptive Hypertension

In the late 1960s, clinical investigators noted a fall in blood pressure when some hypertensive women discontinued oral contraceptive agents and found that reinstitution of oral contraceptive therapy was followed by a reappearance of the hypertension. Later, prospective studies demonstrated that the administration of oral contraceptives causes a statistically significant rise in systolic blood pressure, by an average of 7 mmHg, and a diastolic pressure rise of 2 mmHg. The incidence of hypertension in users of oral contraceptive agents varies from 1 to 18%, independent of duration of treatment. Blood pressure usually returns to pretreatment levels when contraceptives are discontinued over intervals lasting as long as 6 months.

The pathophysiology of oral contraceptive–induced hypertension is not yet fully understood. The estrogenic component stimulates increased hepatic synthesis renin substrate. As substrate levels rise, plasma renin activity remains constant. Plasma renin concentration would be expected to fall as enzyme release is inhibited. These events occur in both normotensive and hypertensive women and therefore have not been firmly implicated as the cause of hypertension. Other studies have implicated the progestogens.

Patients who are found to develop hypertension must use other means of contraception. If blood pressure is significantly elevated, the patient should be treated with antihypertensive agents for 6 months. The dosage should then be reduced or the drug discontinued to determine whether it is still necessary. If blood pressure elevation is mild, the patient can be observed for a 6-month period before antihypertensive therapy is instituted or workup for other secondary causes of hypertension proceeds.

Certain patients are at greater risk of developing oral contraceptive–induced hypertension, including older women, the obese, and those with a history of hypertension in pregnancies or a family history of hypertension. Such patients can be given oral contraceptives cautiously, under careful medical observation, with blood pressure measured at least every 2 months for the first year and then two or three times a year. Malignant hypertension with irreversible renal failure has rarely been reported secondary to oral contraceptives.

F. Ingestion of Licorice

Licorice contains a salt-retaining compound, glycyrrhizic acid. Ingestion of large amounts of licorice on a daily basis results in sodium retention, potassium excretion, hypertension, and hypokalemia. Because intravascular volume is expanded, plasma renin activity and aldosterone concentrations are low.

G. Hyperparathyroidism

In 40 patients with primary hyperthyroidism studied by Rosenthal and Roy, 13 were found to be hypertensive. Nine patients initially presented with hypertension; of these, seven were discovered to have hyperparathyroidism. The prevalence of primary hyperparathyroidism in hypertensive patients was 7.6%, whereas the frequency ranges between 0.1 and 0.2% in the general population. In 80 patients reported by Madhavan, Frame, and Block, 17.5% were hypertensive, and 50% exhibited reduction of hypertension after parathyroidectomy. This type of hypertension should be considered in patients presenting with a history of depression, recurrent peptic ulcer, bone pain, renal calculus formation, and constipation.

H. Coarctation of the Aorta

Coarctation of the aorta causes hypertension in the upper extremities either by mechanical means or through effects on renal blood flow. Although patients with coarctation of the aorta are ordinarily asymptomatic, certain symptoms—such as pain and coldness of the extremities on exercise, epistaxis, and headache—should suggest this diagnosis. Physical examination shows a decrease, absence, or delayed peak of pulsation in the femoral arteries in comparison with the radial pulse. Measurement of blood pressure with a large cuff in the legs demonstrates a lower pressure than that in the arms. Pulsations may be evident in the intercostal spaces, the axilla, and the interscapular space. A midsystolic murmur is frequently audible anteriorly with radiation to the back. Murmurs may also be heard along the lateral chest wall over dilated collateral vessels.

Coarctation of the aorta is often associated with other congenital cardiac abnormalities, most often a bicuspid aortic valve, patent ductus arteriosus, ventricular septal defect, or valvular aortic stenosis.

Unless contraindications exist, surgical correction should be performed to prevent complications of severe hypertension, rupture of a cerebral aneurysm or of the aorta, left ventricular failure, and bacterial endocarditis.

VII. ANTIHYPERTENSIVE THERAPY

A. Changes in Lifestyle

Early detection and treatment of mild hypertension are essential. Because the risk-benefit ratio for drug treatment cannot be calculated precisely, consideration should be given to nonpharmacological therapy of mild hypertension before hypotensive drugs are prescribed.

B. Obesity

Weight is positively correlated with blood pressure. Weight loss results in reduction of blood pressure, although not invariably. Nevertheless, elimination of obesity is advisable for the control of hyperlipidemias and also to prevent loss of insulin sensitivity.

C. Sodium, Potassium, Calcium, and Magnesium

Populations with high average daily sodium intake are typified by a large fraction of hypertensives. Kempner showed that improvement of severe hypertension by diet required extreme salt restriction—less than 8 mEq sodium daily—a very difficult diet to accomplish even with special salt-free foods. Mild to moderate hypertension improves, however, even when sodium intake is lowered from 150–200 to 50–90 mEq/day. Individual response is variable. It is prudent, however, to advise all hypertensive patients to follow a no-added-salt diet. Blood pressure may be influenced by dietary intake of potassium, calcium, fish oil, and/or magnesium, but proof is lacking.

D. Alcohol

Moderate use of alcohol does not increase blood pressure. However, blood pressure rises as alcohol use increases. Consumption of more than two alcoholic drinks a day increases the risk of hypertension. The caloric implications of alcohol, its adverse effect on the control of type 4 hyperlipidemia, and the dangers of adding the sedative effects of alcohol to those of sympatholytic antihypertensive agents are relevant to any hypertensive patient.

E. Exercise

Strenuous activity and isometric exercise can elevate blood pressure. Thus, it is unwise for hypertensive patients, especially those in the coronary prone age group, to attempt strenuous exercise without initial exercise testing and conditioning. Isometric exercises, such as weight lifting, should be avoided. Regular, moderate isotonic exercise is beneficial. Hypertensive patients on standard antihypertensive regimens are better controlled when they are following a program of regular exercise. For example, Boyer and Kasch observed an average fall in diastolic pressure of 11.8 mmHg in 24 hypertensive men who participated in a walk-jog program.

F. Stress

Hypertension can be provoked by subjecting experimental animals to recurrent stress. Emotional stress elevates blood pressure, even in those whose blood pressure is ordinarily within normal limits. Constant monitoring of blood pressure demonstrates elevation during periods of activity. Major life changes, such as retirement from active professional life, can be followed by reduced hypertension, but regular periods of rest during the day have not proved to be very effective in controlling blood pressure, nor have sedation or administration of tranquilizers. Regular elicitation of the relaxation response for 20 min twice a day has lowered blood pressure in some. However, the therapeutic value of this approach appears to be quite limited. Stress-reduction techniques did not lower blood pressure significantly in the Trial of Hypertension Prevention.

G. Tobacco

Cigarette smoking increases blood pressure transiently, but, on average, smokers have lower blood pressure than nonsmokers. However, cigarette smoking is a strong risk factor for the development of coronary heart disease, which, when combined with hypertension, can be exacerbated. Moderate pipe or cigar smoking does not appear to increase mortality associated with hypertension.

H. Pharmacological Agents

Diverse antihypertensive agents and combinations of agents are available, including thiazide and loop diuretics; agents that block specific components of the sympathetic nervous system; direct-acting vasodilators; ACE inhibitors, which block the renin-angiotensin system; and calcium channel blocking agents. The use of a large dose of a single antihypertensive agent tends to produce more side effects for a given hypotensive effect than does the combined use of smaller doses of several antihypertensive agents with different mechanisms of action. As a result, the concept of "stepped care" has emerged, as recommended by JNC V (Figure 1).

Unless specific indications or contraindications exist, therapy can be initiated with either a thiazide diuretic or a beta blocker, the choice being influenced by the patient's age and race. This recommendation is based on the fact that most major trials that have demonstrated a significant reduction of morbidity and mortality have focused on either thiazides, beta blockers, or both. Similar data are not yet available for ACE inhibitors. Loop diuretics should be reserved for selected patients, such as those with renal failure. If the goal blood pressure has not been reached in 2 to 4 weeks of drug therapy, the next dose should be increased, another drug from a different class should be substituted or added, and, after another few weeks, an additional agent added if necessary.

The art of successful antihypertensive therapy involves the careful matching of medication to patient based on several considerations. For example, selecting beta-blocking agents for patients with angina pectoris or with a history of recent acute myocardial infarction and avoiding them in the treatment of hypertensive patients with asthma, heart failure, or advanced degrees of heart block is essential. The presence of concomitant illness is a major factor influencing the initial choice of a hypertensive agent. Recommended treatment for hypertensive patients with diverse concomitant illnesses is shown in Table 5.

Demographic factors play an important role in the selection of first-step antihypertensive therapy. African Americans tend to be more responsive to diuretics and calcium channel blockers than to beta-blocking agents or to ACE inhibitors. Older patients are more sensitive to all antihypertensive drugs. Those with isolated systolic hypertension can often be controlled with relatively small doses of a thiazide diuretic. Some require the addition of a small dose of beta blocker or other agent.

Quality of life is an important consideration. Several antihypertensive drugs interfere with sexual function. Beta blockers reduce exercise capacity. Centrally acting alpha-adrenergic agents cause fatigue and reduce mental sharpness. Economic considerations are important as well. Many hypertensive patients are elderly, on fixed incomes, and not covered by insurance for prescription costs. The cost of antihypertensive therapy includes costs of periodic laboratory studies and follow-up visits with health-care providers.

Certain physiological measurements sometimes help in the selection of successful antihypertensive therapy. For example, an elevated heart rate may indicate overactivity of the sympathetic nervous system and responsivity to beta blockers. When patients can be kept off antihypertensive medications for 2 to 3 weeks and an accurate 24-hr urine obtained for measurement of sodium excretion, measurement of plasma renin activity can sometimes identify a patient with low

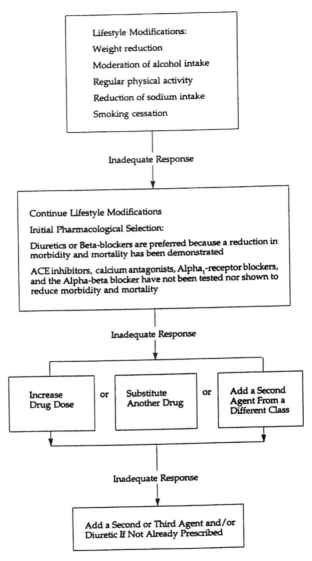

Figure 1 "Stepped-care" treatment algorithm. (Modified from the 1994 Report of the Joint Committee on the Detection, Evaluation and Treatment of Hypertension.)

plasma renin activity who will respond to a diuretic or calcium channel blocker or a patient with high renin who will respond to beta blockers or ACE inhibitors.

In most patients, control of blood pressure can be obtained with a simple program of antihypertensive agents with few side effects. Unless selected on demographic grounds, approximately 50% of patients respond to diuretic or beta-blocker therapy alone. The combination of the two will be effective in 90% of cases. Therefore, unless the hypertension is severe, therapy should be started with diuretics or beta blockers, with additions made as needed.

The pharmacological properties and side effects of the 68 currently available antihypertensive agents are summarized in the report of JNC V.

VIII. HYPERTENSIVE EMERGENCIES AND URGENCIES

In approximately 10% of patients, an accelerated or malignant phase occurs as a complication in almost all types of primary and secondary hypertension. Severe diastolic hypertension, group 3 or group 4 retinopathy, and progressive renal failure are features characterizing this phase. Hypertensive encephalopathy, cerebral hemorrhage, left ventricular failure, and fluid retention are other common findings. Malignant hypertension is associated with a poor prognosis unless it is successfully treated before vascular damage has progressed.

A. Pathophysiology of Malignant Hypertension

The control system for maintaining normal blood pressure involves several negative feedback loops. Physiologically, as blood pressure rises, the stimulus decreases output of one or more forces maintaining pressure. Such negative feedback loops involve the renin-angiotensin-aldosterone system, the atrial natriuretic system, and the sympathetic nervous system, among others. Conversion to a malignant phase occurs when increasing levels of blood pressure and an accelerating rate of vascular damage cause a normal negative feedback loop to become a positive loop. For example, plasma renin activity is usually elevated in patients with malignant hypertension, inappropriately, because the rising pressure should be associated with a declining renin level as a pressure homeostatic mechanism. Because renin levels are high, angiotensin II and aldosterone levels rise and, as a result, sodium and water are retained, effective blood volume increases, and plasma renin levels should fall. However, the high pressure injures the kidney, renin continues to be released despite the increased effective blood volume and blood pressure, and thus a negative feedback loop becomes a positive factor in elevating arterial pressure further.

The malignant phase of hypertension can be reversed by aggressive antihypertensive therapy that arrests progressive vascular damage. Therefore, during

Table 5 Antihypertensive Drug Therapy: Individualization Based on Special Considerations (Guidelines for Selecting Initial Therapy)

Clinical situation	Preferred	Requires special monitoring	Relatively or absolutely contraindicated
Cardiovascular			
Angina pectoris	Beta blockers, calcium antagonists		Direct vasodilators
Bradycardia/heart block, sick sinus syndrome			Beta blockers, labetalol, verapamil, diltiazem
Cardiac failure	Diuretics; ACE inhibitors		Beta blockers, calcium channel antagonists, labetalol
Hypertrophic cardiomyopathy with severe diastolic dysfunction	Beta blockers, diltiazem, verapamil		Diuretics, ACE inhibitors, alpha$_1$ blockers, hydralazine, minoxidil
Hyperdynamic circulation	Beta blockers		Direct vasodilators
Peripheral vascular occlusive disease		Beta blockers	
Post-myocardial infarction	Non-ISA beta blockers		Direct vasodilators
Renal			
Bilateral renal arterial disease or severe stenosis in artery to solitary kidney			ACE inhibitors

138

Condition			
Renal insufficiency			
Early [serum creatinine 130 to 221 μmol/L (1.5 to 2.5 mg/dL)]	Loop diuretics	ACE inhibitors	Potassium-sparing agents, potassium supplements
Advanced [serum creatinine ≥221 μmol/L (2.5 mg/dL)]			Potassium-sparing agents, potassium supplements
Other			
Asthma/COPD			Beta blockers, labetalol
Cyclosporine-associated hypertension	Nifedipine, labetalol	Verapamil,[a] diltiazem,[a] nicardipine[a]	
Depression		Alpha$_2$ antagonists	Reserpine
Diabetes mellitus			
Type I (insulin dependent)		Beta blockers	
Type II		Beta blockers, diuretics	
Dyslipidemia		Diuretics, beta blockers	
Liver disease		Labetalol	Methyldopa
Vascular headache	Beta blockers		
Pregnancy			
Preeclampsia	Methyldopa, hydralazine		Diuretics, ACE inhibitors
Chronic hypertension	Methyldopa		ACE inhibitors

[a]Can increase serum levels of cyclosporine.

Source: From the 1994 Report of the Joint Committee on the Detection, Evaluation and Treatment of Hypertension.

139

the malignant phase of hypertension, reduction of blood pressure is urgent—first to diastolic pressure of 100 to 110 mmHg and subsequently to normotensive levels.

Several hypertensive emergencies require early, expert, and intensive treatment, including subarachnoid hemorrhage, intracerebral hemorrhage, hypertensive encephalopathy, acute left ventricular failure with pulmonary edema secondary to hypertension, aortic dissection, unstable angina, acute myocardial infarction, acute and advancing renal insufficiency, eclampsia, and pheochromocytoma.

Urgent reduction of blood pressure (within 24 hr) is needed for many other conditions, including severe perioperative hypertension and accelerated hypertension without severe symptoms or evidence of worsening target-organ damage. Patients often experience a period of acceleration of hypertension in which the manifestations of vascular damage are not proportionate in all target organs; for example, patients may present with hypertensive encephalopathy in the absence of papilledema, hemorrhages, or exudates. Other patients may present with blurred vision, retinal hemorrhages, and exudates, yet they may have no impairment of consciousness or of renal function. The urgency of lowering blood pressure varies with the specific hypertensive emergency or urgency and the agent to be used. Severely hypertensive patients with subarachnoid hemorrhage or patients with acute left ventricular failure and pulmonary edema secondary to hypertension require more immediate blood pressure reduction than do asymptomatic hypertensive patients with group 3 hypertensive retinopathy and severely elevated diastolic pressure.

The primary objective in the management of hypertensive emergencies is ultimate reduction of diastolic blood pressure to a normal range, with constant attention to maintaining perfusion of vital organs. Patients without preexisting symptoms of vascular insufficiency rarely develop such complications when blood pressure is reduced, although a transient decrease in urine output with a slight rise in serum creatinine is often noted. In the presence of significant coronary or cerebrovascular insufficiency, angina, ECG signs of ischemia, frank myocardial infarction, transient cerebral ischemia, convulsions, and cerebral infarction can occur, primarily as a result of a precipitous drop in arterial pressure. They can usually be avoided by more gradual reduction of pressure and close monitoring of vital-organ function. Persistence is often more important than speed of reduction of pressure.

Parenteral therapy includes agents with a relatively long duration of action, given as a bolus and followed by a variable blood pressure response. Drugs with a short duration of action require constant intravenous infusion and close supervision to effect a controlled and smooth fall of the blood pressure. Gentle diuretic therapy should be employed in most cases to potentiate the effect of other agents and to prevent secondary retention of salt and water, but it should not be used to the extent of inducing intravascular volume depletion, reflex vasoconstriction, and additional renin release and angiotensin II generation. Oral antihypertensive

Table 6 Management of the Hypertensive Crisis: Emergencies and Urgencies[a]

	Dose	Onset	Cautions
Parenteral vasodilators			
Sodium nitroprusside	0.25–10 µg/kg/min as IV infusion Maximal dose for 10 min only	Instantaneous	Nausea, vomiting, muscle twitching; with prolonged use may cause thiocyanate intoxication, methemoglobinemia acidosis, cyanide poisoning; bags, bottles, and delivery sets must be light-resistant.
Nitroglycerin	5–100 µg/min as IV infusion	2–5 min	Headache, tachycardia, vomiting, flushing, methemoglobinemia; requires special delivery system due to drug binding to polyvinylchloride tubing.
Diazoxide	50–150-mg IV bolus, repeated, or 15–30 mg/min by IV infusion	1–2 min	Hypotension, tachycardia, aggravation of angina pectoris, nausea and vomiting, hyperglycemia with repeated injections.
Hydralazine	10–20-mg IV bolus	10 min	Tachycardia, headache, vomiting, aggravation of angina pectoris.
	10–40 mg IM	20–30 min	
Enalaprilat	0.625–1.25 mg every 6 hr IV	15–60 min	Renal failure in patients with bilateral renal artery stenosis, hypotension.
Parenteral adrenergic inhibitors			
Phentolamine	5–15-mg IV bolus	1–2 min	Tachycardia, orthostatic hypotension.
Trimethaphan camsylate	1–4 mg/min as IV infusion	1–5 min	Paresis of bowel and bladder, orthostatic hypotension, blurred vision, dry mouth.
Labetalol	20–80-mg IV bolus every 10 min; 2 mg/min IV infusion	5–10 min	Bronchoconstriction, heart block, orthostatic hypotension.
Methyldopate	250–500-mg IV infusion every 6 hr	30–60 min	Drowsiness.
Oral agents			
Nifedipine (not extended release)	10–20 mg PO, repeat after 30 min	15–30 min	Rapid, uncontrolled reduction in blood pressure may precipitate circulatory collapse in patients with aortic stenosis.
Captopril	25 mg PO, repeat as required	15–30 min	Hypotension, renal failure in bilateral renal artery stenosis.
Clonidine	0.1–0.2 mg PO, repeat every hour as required to a total dose of 0.6 mg	30–60 min	Hypotension, drowsiness, dry mouth.
Labetalol	200–400 mg PO, repeat every 2–3 hr	30 min–2 hr	Bronchoconstriction, heart block, orthostatic hypotension.

[a]Note: It is sometimes appropriate to administer a diuretic agent with any of the above.

Source: From the 1994 Report of the Joint National Committee on the Detection, Evaluation and Treatment of Hypertension.

therapy should be started as soon as possible because its onset of action is relatively slow.

Nine antihypertensive agents are available in the United States for parenteral use in the treatment of hypertensive emergencies and urgencies. Their dosages, onsets of action, and potential adverse effects are summarized in Table 6. Vasodilator drugs are the agents of choice in the treatment of hypertensive emergencies other than those associated with pheochromocytoma, in which alpha-adrenergic receptor blockers are indicated; aortic dissection in which beta-adrenergic receptor blockers are necessary, and perhaps subarachnoid or intracerebral hemorrhage in which vasodilatation may aggravate bleeding. Most hypertensive emergencies are associated with marked elevation of total peripheral resistance. When vasodilators are administered, this declines, facilitating increased cardiac output and organ perfusion. In contrast, agents other than peripheral alpha-receptor blockers that interfere with the activity of the sympathetic nervous system result in a reduction of cardiac output. In the presence of diuretic-induced or intravascular volume depletion resulting from previous diuresis during the development of the crisis, compensatory vasoconstriction can develop, leading to further impairment of organ perfusion. In the absence of target-organ damage or symptoms of hypertensive crisis, severely elevated blood pressure alone does not usually require emergency treatment.

Hypertensive crises with concomitant renal failure present special management problems. Not only patients with malignant hypertension but also those with aortic dissection (because of renal artery obstruction) or acute glomerulonephritis can develop acute renal failure. The retention of salt and water renders such patients less sensitive to antihypertensive agents and can lead to congestive heart failure. Effective hemodialysis can correct these abnormalities and sustain life while fibrinoid necrosis of renal arterioles resolves. Some patients recover sufficiently to be able to live without chronic dialysis.

A few patients with end-stage renal disease become resistant to antihypertensive agents despite removal of salt and water by dialysis. Such patients have extremely high levels of plasma renin activity and become normotensive when the kidneys are removed. Malignant hypertension per se does not preclude successful long-term dialysis and transplantation.

SUGGESTED READING

Applegate WB, Miller ST, Elam JT, et al. Nonpharmacologic intervention to reduce blood pressure in older patients with mild hypertension. Arch Intern Med 1992; 152:1162–1166.

Black HR. Treatment of mild hypertension: The more things change ... JAMA 1993; 270: 757–759.

Collins R, Peto R, MacMahon S, et al. Epidemiology: Blood pressure, stroke, and coronary heart disease. Part 2. Short-term reductions in blood pressure: Overview of randomized drug trials in the epidemiological context. Lancet 1990; 335:827–838.

Cutler JA, MacMahon SW, Furberg CD. Controlled clinical trials of drug treatment for hypertension: A review. Hypertension 1989; 13(suppl I):I-36–I-44.

Dahlof B, Lindholm LH, Hansson L, et al. Morbidity and mortality in the Swedish Trial in Old Patients with Hypertension (STOP-Hypertension). Lancet 1991; 338:1281–1285.

Dzau VJ. Atherosclerosis and hypertension: Mechanisms and interrelationships. J Cardiovasc Pharmacol 1990; 15(suppl 5):S59–S64.

Ferrari P, Rosman J, Weidmann P. Antihypertensive agents, serum lipoproteins and glucose metabolism. Am J Cardiol 1991; 67:26B–35B.

Fletcher AE, Bulpitt CJ. How far should blood pressure be lowered? N Engl J Med 1992; 326:251–254.

Guidelines Subcommittee. 1993 guidelines for the management of mild hypertension: Memorandum from a WHO/ISH meeting. ISH Hypertension News 1993; 3–16.

Joint National Committee on Detection, Evaluation, and Treatment of High Blood Pressure. The fifth report of the Joint National Committee on Detection, Evaluation and Treatment of High Blood Pressure (JNC V). Arch Intern Med 1993; 153:154–183.

Kaplan NM. Clinical Hypertension. 4th ed. Baltimore: Williams & Wilkins, 1994.

Kaplan NM. Non-drug treatment of hypertension. Ann Intern Med 1985; 102:359–373.

Lithell HOL. Effect of antihypertensive drugs on insulin, glucose, and lipid metabolism. Diabetes Care 1991; 14:203–209.

MacMahon S, Peto R, Cutler J, et al. Epidemiology. Blood pressure, stroke, and coronary heart disease: Part 1. Prolonged differences in blood pressure: Prospective observational studies corrected for the regression dilution bias. Lancet 1990; 335:765–774.

Mann SJ, Pickering TG. Detection of renovascular hypertension. State of the Art: 1992. Ann Intern Med 1992; 117:845–853.

Massie BM. Demographic considerations in the selection of antihypertensive therapy. Am J Cardiol 1987; 60:121-I–126-I.

Materson BJ, Preston RA. Angiotensin-converting enzyme inhibitors in hypertension: A dozen years of experience. Arch Intern Med 1994; 154:513–523.

Materson BJ, Reda DJ, Cushman WC, et al. Single-drug therapy for hypertension in men: A comparison of six antihypertensive agents with placebo. N Engl J Med 1993; 328: 914–921.

McCloskey LW, Psaty BM, Koepsell TD, et al. Level of blood pressure and risk of myocardial infarction among treated hypertensive patients. Arch Intern Med 1992; 152:513–520.

McKinney TD. Management of hypertensive crisis. Hosp Prac 1992; 91–109.

Moser M, Hebert P, Hennekens CH. An overview of the meta-analyses of the hypertension treatment trials. Arch Intern Med 1991; 151:1277–1279.

National High Blood Pressure Education Program Working Group. National High Blood Pressure Education Program Working Group report on primary prevention of hypertension. Arch Intern Med 1993; 153:186–208.

Neaton JD, Grimm RH Jr, Prineas RJ, et al. Treatment of mild hypertension study: Final results. JAMA 1993; 270:713–724.

Prisant LM, Carr AA, Bottini PB, et al. Sexual dysfunction with antihypertensive drugs. Arch Intern Med 1994; 154:730–736.

143

Sagie A, Larson MG, Levy D. The natural history of borderline isolated systolic hypertension. N Engl J Med 1993; 329:1912–1917.

Setaro JF, Black HR. Refractory hypertension. N Engl J Med 1992; 327:543–547.

Slataper R, Vicknair N, Sadler R, et al. Comparative effects of different antihypertensive treatments on progression of diabetic renal disease. Arch Intern Med 1993; 153: 973–980.

Stevens VJ, Corrigan SA, Obarzanek E, et al. Weight loss intervention in phase I of the Trials of Hypertension Prevention. Arch Intern Med 1993; 153:849–858.

Sullivan JM. Hypertension and hypertensive heart disease. The International Textbook of Cardiology. New York: Pergamon Press, 1986:543–599.

ter Wee PM, DeMicheli AG, Epstein M. Effects of calcium antagonists on renal hemodynamics and progression of nondiabetic chronic renal disease. Arch Intern Med 1994; 154:1185–1202.

The Systolic Hypertension in the Elderly Program Cooperative Research Group. Implications of the systolic hypertension in the elderly program. Hypertension 1993; 21: 335–343.

The Treatment of Mild Hypertension Research Group. The Treatment of Mild Hypertension Study: A randomized, placebo-controlled trial of a nutritional-hygienic regimen along with various drug monotherapies. Arch Intern Med 1991; 151:1413–1423.

The Trials of Hypertension Prevention Collaborative Research Group. The effects of nonpharmacologic interventions on blood pressure of persons with high normal levels: Results of the Trials of Hypertension Prevention, phase I. JAMA 1992; 267:1213–1220.

Weber MA, Laragh JH. Hypertension: Steps forward and steps backward. The Joint National Committee Fifth Report. Arch Intern Med 1993; 153:149–152.

Weiberger MH. Do no harm: Antihypertensive therapy and the 'J' curve. Arch Intern Med 1992; 152:473–476.

8

Shock

I.	Hemodynamics of Shock	146
II.	Distributive Shock	147
III.	Hypovolemic Shock	148
IV.	Initial Considerations Using Physical Findings	149
V.	Noninvasive Studies	151
VI.	Cardiogenic Shock	152
VII.	Shock Secondary to Cardiac Dysfunction Caused by Mechanical Factors	154
VIII.	Right Ventricular Dysfunction Secondary to Ischemia	156
IX.	Myocardial Rupture	158
X.	Arrhythmias	158

James A. Goldstein and Burton E. Sobel

Cardiovascular collapse underlies inadequate perfusion of vital organs, the *sine qua non* of shock. This syndrome can result from loss of circulating blood volume (e.g., hemorrhage or extracellular fluid and plasma depletion); obstruction to left or right heart output (e.g., aortic stenosis (AS) or coarctation, aortic dissection, and pulmonary emboli or pericardial tamponade); drug toxicity or overdose, or metabolic or endocrine derangements (e.g., uremia, hepatic failure, CO_2 narcosis, hypoxemia, myxedema, adrenal insufficiency, or hyper- or hypocalcemia); anaphylaxis or central nervous system insults (e.g., visceral pain-induced or central hyperthermia); and cardiac failure among other etiologies. Cardiac shock can be mechanical (ruptured papillary muscle or interventricular septum), valvular (aortic stenosis or mitral regurgitation), or myocardiogenic (e.g., associated with acute myocardial infarction). It is the last to which the term cardiogenic shock is generally applied. The nomenclature in this chapter conforms to this usage.

I. HEMODYNAMICS OF SHOCK

Shock is a syndrome predicated on failure of maintenance of adequate perfusion of vital organs. Although the common denominator is a critical reduction of regional blood flow, diverse pathophysiological culprits can be responsible. Shock is generally categorized with respect to the type, mechanism of hemodynamic defects responsible, and underlying etiology. Hemodynamic applications of Ohm's law provide a practical framework for differentiating types of shock and the mechanisms associated with them.

Blood pressure = cardiac output × systemic vascular resistance. Perfusion, the circulatory "bottom line," requires adequate perfusion pressure. At any given driving pressure and cardiac output, systemic vascular resistance determines both systemic output and regional flow distribution. Blood volume is a determinant of both stroke volume (and therefore cardiac output) and systemic vascular resistance.

Shock is usually manifest by systemic arterial hypotension, but the hypotension may be only relative (e.g., in a previously hypertensive patient) or modest (with marked compromise of organ perfusion in the face of high systemic vascular resistance and low cardiac output). Shock can be classified as

1. *hypovolemic*, in which volume loss (attributable to exogenous or endogenous losses of blood, plasma, other fluid or electrolytes, or "third spacing" [ascites, pancreatitis, burns]) results in low cardiac output and hypotension with reflex vasoconstriction but intact cardiac pump function

2. *cardiac*, in which pump failure (secondary to cardiomyopathic processes [myocardiogenic], arrhythmia, or structural lesions including obstruction to outflow or valvular insufficiency) results in diminished stroke volume and low cardiac output with reflex vasoconstriction and volume overload

3. *distributive shock*, related to peripheral vasomotor dysfunction, which can be divided into (a) high or normal peripheral arterial resistance with expanded venous capacitance (attributable to late septic shock, spinal shock, or drug overdose), resulting in high cardiac output but impaired tissue perfusion and microcirculatory pooling; and (b) low resistance due to arteriovenous shunting (attributable to early septic shock, pneumonia, peritonitis, or abscess)

4. *obstructive*, related to extracardiac obstruction of a main channel of blood flow (e.g., venacaval obstruction, cardiac tamponade, or massive pulmonary embolism), which hemodynamically mimics hypovolemic

shock with low cardiac output, hypotension, and vasoconstriction but often with increased blood volume (and pressure) in the central veins attributable to the obstructive lesion (e.g., right heart failure from cardiac tamponade, pulmonary embolism, or obstruction of the superior vena cava).

II. DISTRIBUTIVE SHOCK

Distributive shock is a syndrome of tissue hypoperfusion resulting from perturbations in the distribution of blood flow despite a lack of reduction in total blood volume or cardiac performance, or without obstruction to cardiac output. The derangement may be attributable to diminished systemic arterial resistance and intravascular pooling related to bacteremia (hyperdynamic septic shock), arterial-venous shunting associated with sepsis, or expanded venous capacitance (late phase of septic shock with reflex arterial vasoconstriction, autonomic nervous system blockage, drug overdose, or spinal shock).

The most common cause of distributive shock is septicemia—most frequently with gram-negative bacteremia—a phenomenon occurring in approximately 25–50% of patients with such infections. The pathophysiology is complex and not yet fully delineated. Presumably, components of the bacteria themselves and/or their byproducts (endotoxins) induce peripheral vasomotor dysfunction, including initially selective arterial vasodilatation and venoconstriction. This results in low resistance and peripheral vascular pooling, with an associated increase in cardiac output, unless cardiac function is impaired (as it may be in the elderly), hypotension, and lactic acidosis. The absence of sufficient cardiac filling pressures when combined with an elevated cardiac output help to distinguish distributive shock from low-output states associated with hypovolemia, cardiogenic shock, or intravascular obstruction (e.g., aortic stenosis or coarctation).

As septic shock progresses, cardiac output begins to decrease in association with measurable depression of both right and left ventricular function (RV and LV). The result is further diminution in systemic arterial blood pressure, profound hypoperfusion of vital organs, progressive vascular pooling, and "third spacing" attributable to capillary leak.

A. Evaluation and Management of Septic Shock

In patients with septic shock, quick control of infection is paramount. Regardless—and unfortunately—mortality is high (25–90%). The key to management is (1) recognition that the hemodynamic picture is a manifestation of infection and (2) therapeutic focus on the underlying infection. In patients with hyperdynamic septic shock, hypotension with low filling pressures and high cardiac output is a "red flag" that should stimulate identification of the source of infection (genitourinary, pulmonary, intraabdominal, an inlying catheter or device, or fasciitis).

147

Supportive therapy includes expansion of intravascular volume sufficient to maintain filling pressures consistent with optimal (highest) cardiac output and blood pressure. Because many patients with sepsis develop the acute respiratory distress syndrome, a pathophysiological state in which higher filling pressures exacerbate pulmonary capillary leakage, it is desirable to avoid overexpansion of central blood volume (i.e., keeping patients as "dry" as possible). Careful hemodynamic monitoring with right heart catheterization is essential to guide volume repletion. In young patients with intact cardiac function, the best approach is to maintain low filling pressures and augment cardiac output with the use of agents with positive inotropic effects.

In patients with hypotension but adequate tissue perfusion, vasopressor agents may not be needed. In fact, their use may exact deleterious effects because of vasoconstriction that can compromise tissue perfusion and increase cardiac work by increasing afterload.

In patients with hypotension, hypoperfusion, and impaired cardiac output, pharmacological agents with positive inotropic and vasopressor effects are useful. Dopamine is the initial drug of choice because of its effects on cardiac function and renal perfusion. In patients with hypotension that is unresponsive to high doses of dopamine, addition of dobutamine and/or norepinephrine may be necessary. Despite numerous studies over many years, the efficacy of high doses of glucocorticoids in patients with septic shock continues to be controversial, with results of recent multicenter studies failing to confirm benefit. Several trials with antibodies against endotoxins have been disappointing as well, perhaps because patient selection was not sufficiently focused on candidates for treatment who did indeed harbor susceptible gram-negative organisms.

III. HYPOVOLEMIC SHOCK

Loss of intravascular volume reduces systemic arterial blood pressure because of its effects on both preload (decreased stroke volume) as well as vascular tone. If cardiac pump function is intact, hypovolemia is accompanied by typical responses to neurohormonal compensatory mechanisms including increased heart rate, stimulation of contractility, and reflex vasoconstriction. Loss of less than 20% of blood volume (approximately 1 L in a 70-kg individual) results in postural hypotension and reflex sinus tachycardia. Loss of 20–40% of blood volume (1–2 L) typically results in supine hypotension, brisk reflex tachycardia, and peripheral signs of tissue hypoperfusion, including metabolic acidosis and oliguria. However, if compensatory mechanisms are intact, cerebral perfusion is maintained and patients remain awake and often alert, with good mentation. Loss of 40% or more of blood volume (greater than 2 L) results often in profound circulatory compromise manifest as supine hypotension, tachycardia, peripheral signs of hypoperfusion (cool, clammy, mottled extremities), restlessness or combativeness, and impaired mental status.

A. Clinical Assessment

Diagnosis requires documentation of volume depletion. The history and physical examination should focus on assessment of potential sources of loss of extracellular fluid, plasma, or blood—both exogenous (bleeding, environmental exposure, burns) and endogenous (internal bleeding, diarrhea, vomiting, excessive renal losses). An assiduous search for occult blood loss is essential (e.g., massive GI hemorrhage harbored within the gut, retroperitoneal bleeding, bleeding into the hip or groin following catheterization, and bleeding into intrapleural spaces).

The physical examination will demonstrate features common to many shock states that are nonspecific with respect to hypotension and tachycardia. However, the presence of orthostatic changes is helpful in establishing hypovolemia (although its presence does not absolutely differentiate it from other forms of cardiac and noncardiac shock). Blood volume must be considered from a compartmentalized perspective. That is, a condition of inadequate blood volume in the left ventricle, resulting in a clinical syndrome of low output with intact contractility characteristic of hypovolemic shock, may arise from obstruction to circulatory flow (e.g., ball valve thrombus across the mitral orifice, severe pulmonary embolism, or cardiac tamponade). Therefore, blood volume and correlative pressures should be assessed throughout the "compartments" of the circulation, including the left heart chambers (pulmonary arterial wedge pressure), right heart chambers, and central veins (right atrial and venous pressures). Accordingly, the physical examination should focus on the lung fields and the jugular venous pulse (JVP). Assessment of the JVP should include both the height of the neck vein meniscus as a reflection of mean right atrial pressure and the waveform (A and V waves, X and Y descents), abnormalities of which provide clues to intracardiac pathology. The presence of clear lungs excludes pulmonary edema and heightens the likelihood of hypovolemia as a pathophysiological possibility that can be assessed with volume challenge.

If supine and/or postural hypotension, reflex tachycardia, low central venous pressure (JVP <5 cm mean) and clear lungs are present, volume depletion is likely to be contributing to the hemodynamic abnormalities. However, in patients with hypoperfusion who manifest congested lungs and/or elevated neck vein pressure, total body hypovolemia is effectively excluded.

IV. INITIAL CONSIDERATIONS USING PHYSICAL FINDINGS

The physical examination reflects inadequate tissue perfusion and the circulatory compensatory responses to a low cardiac output. When output is low, the brain is the last organ to be compromised. Thus, in response to hypoperfusion, neurohormonally mediated vasoconstriction shuts off flow to those organs that can best tolerate hypoperfusion (skin, bowel, and skeletal muscle). Accordingly, the initial bedside evaluation starts with careful observation of the patient's general appearance. Signs of impaired mental status reflect the final stages of shock which begin with restlessness, combativeness, and somnolence and lead ultimately to profound depression of cerebral function. (Metabolic and structural derangements unrelated to circulatory compromise must be excluded.)

However, well before the development of signs of cerebral hypoperfusion, important signs of peripheral hypoperfusion may be evident, such as cool, clammy, mottled cyanotic skin, with decreased capillary filling reflecting diminished tissue perfusion and reflex vasoconstriction. Because blood pressure equals cardiac output × systemic vascular resistance, shock can be present despite a normal blood pressure, because shock is the manifestation of severe tissue hypoperfusion—not a particular perfusion *pressure*. Thus, severe hypoperfusion may be present even though blood pressure is still maintained through intense vasoconstriction. Waiting until manifestation of the final stages of shock as frank hypotension results in missed opportunities to diagnose and manage shock before it is most severe and most difficult to treat.

Assessment of heart rate is another critical factor on which to focus in patients with hemodynamic compromise. The presence of reflex sinus tachycardia often signals the beginning of "exhaustion" of compensatory reserve. It is also important to look for both supraventricular and ventricular arrhythmias that may precipitate or exacerbate hemodynamic compromise, as well as chronotropic competence. Evaluation of the respiratory rate provides insight to the extent of pulmonary venous congestion and respiratory compromise.

Assessment of the pulse waveform in the carotid pressure pulse provides insight regarding the contractile state of the left ventricle. Diminished upstroke and reduced amplitude may reflect LV systolic dysfunction (one must exclude carotid disease and aortic stenosis). The carotid pulse may also provide clues to the presence of mechanical complications that may contribute to hemodynamic compromise such as the bounding, collapsing pulses of severe aortic regurgitation, the brisk upstroke with reduced volume of severe mitral regurgitation (MR), and the diminished delayed pulse of aortic stenosis.

The precordial examination reflects the extent of ventricular enlargement, with severe cardiomyopathies attributable to cardiogenic shock typically resulting in a dilated, displaced, and sustained LV impulse. Precordial examination may demonstrate criteria of mechanical complications of acute myocardial infarction (MI), such as a systolic thrill indicative of acute mitral regurgitation or an acquired ventricular septal defect (VSD). The presence of a right ventricular heave indicates RV enlargement that may be related to primary cardiomyopathy or pressure overload from left heart failure, resulting in pulmonary hypertension. Auscultation in patients with severe cardiomyopathy typically reveals a diminished S1 (reflecting decreased LV contractility and elevated filling pressures), an increased S2 associated with passive pulmonary hypertension, an S3 gallop reflecting elevated LV filling pressure, and often a murmur indicating significant mechanical complications (mitral regurgitation, aortic stenosis, VSD). Assessment of the jugular veins provides important information regarding the status of blood volume in general and the presence of right heart failure in particular. Examination of the lungs may indicate the presence of significant pulmonary congestion.

V. NONINVASIVE STUDIES

A. ECG

Careful evaluation of the ECG should include analysis for tachy- and brady-arrhythmias as well as presence of abnormalities suggesting ischemic heart disease or other primary underlying myocardial abnormalities.

B. Chest X-Ray

In patients with shock the chest x-ray is helpful for showing the presence of cardiac enlargement and pulmonary congestion, as well as cardiac chamber dimensions suggesting valvular or congenital heart disease.

C. Echocardiography

Two-dimensional Doppler echocardiographic studies are a critical step in the evaluation of patients with shock. Ultrasound can usually establish whether a shock state is attributable to a cardiac cause, providing data regarding the status of LV size and function, valvular integrity, right heart size and function, pericardial abnormalities, and diseases of the great vessels. In aggregate, these data are usually sufficient to establish the diagnosis and etiologies of cardiac shock (LV systolic dysfunction and mechanical complications).

D. Invasive Assessments

In patients with cardiac shock, invasive evaluation for hemodynamic assessment and determination of coronary anatomy and associated mechanical defects, as well as on-line hemodynamic monitoring during therapy, is essential. Right heart catheterization documents the extent of filling pressure elevation and the severity of reduction of cardiac output and provides on-line monitoring for therapeutic manipulations. Right heart catheterization also helps to detect the presence of important mechanical complications such as acute mitral regurgitation (large V wave in the pulmonary capillary wedge pressure tracing), acute VSD (large V wave in the wedge pressure tracing, oxygen step-up) and RV infarction (dispro-portionate elevation of right heart filling pressures, RV "dip and plateau pattern," and equalization of diastolic filling pressures as in tamponade). Right heart catheterization may be helpful in those patients with noncardiac shock who do not respond to fluid resuscitation alone. Right heart catheterization and on-line monitoring are important in patients with septic shock and respiratory distress syndrome. Improvement may be elicited by maintaining the filling pressures as low as possible, yet consistent with an adequate cardiac output. Left heart catheterization to assess the status of the coronary arteries and further delineate mechanical defects is often crucial.

VI. CARDIOGENIC SHOCK

Cardiogenic shock results from inadequate cardiac output attributable to true "pump failure" (usually depressed LV contractility). It may be associated with other mechanical defects that may in turn cause shock (including aortic stenosis/regurgitation, mitral regurgitation [MR], right ventricular ischemic dysfunction, acute VSD, and myocardial rupture) by limiting stroke volume. Shock can occur because of arrhythmias that profoundly compromise cardiac function primarily and impair myocardial performance secondarily.

A. Primary Pump Failure

Primary depression of LV contractility may be an end result of severe pressure overload (aortic stenosis and systemic hypertension), chronic volume overload (mitral regurgitation, aortic insufficiency, and congenital shunts at the ventricular level) or primary myopathic insults (ischemia, myocarditis, alcohol abuse, cobalt toxicity, and storage diseases, among other disorders). The pathophysiology, natural history, and management of pump failure attributable to pressure or volume overload are distinctly different when primary myopathic processes are present (see Chapter 12, on congestive heart failure). Regardless of the etiology underlying LV pump dysfunction, when the LV ejection fraction is depressed to less than 30%, severe limitations in stroke volume and cardiac output often ensue.

The rapidity of evolution of pump dysfunction influences the extent of hemodynamic compromise as well as its natural history. Thus, massive acute myocardial infarction compromising greater than 40% of LV mass is commonly reflected by severe pump dysfunction and cardiogenic shock. However, it is not uncommon for patients with chronic dilated cardiomyopathies (ischemic and nonischemic) in which the magnitude of pump dysfunction is similar, to be comparatively well compensated. The differences are attributable to factors that include deleterious effects of acute ischemic regional wall motion abnormalities (deleterious effects of regional dyssynergy) on global performance, the time course of evolution of ventricular dilatation and changes in compliance, compensatory hypertrophy and other adaptive remodeling changes, peripheral circulatory adjustments, and other factors.

In patients with severe pump failure, several neurohormonal compensatory mechanisms supervene, including reflex sympathoadrenal activation that may increase LV contractility and heart rate but exacerbate ventricular dilatation because of vasoconstriction and be deleterious to ultimate cardiac viability and performance. The cardiomyopathic ventricle is exquisitely sensitive to increases in afterload, which further limit stroke volume. Thus, reflex vasoconstriction sufficient to maintain systemic arterial blood pressure can reduce output further and perpetuate a cycle of low output and progressive vasoconstriction. This vicious cycle is particularly deleterious when functional mitral regurgitation is present, a common consequence of both ischemic and nonischemic cardiomyopathies. Regurgitation is sensitive to afterload as well. Thus, not only low-output vasoconstriction but also marked increases in pulmonary congestion will occur with a given magnitude of LV pump dysfunction. Increases in preload, contractility, afterload, and heart rate increase oxygen consumption and may result in infarct extension and/or development of ischemia in remote regions supplied by tightly narrowed vessels distant from an initial culprit lesion.

B. Therapeutic Considerations

The mortality associated with cardiogenic shock is 50–70%. The key to therapeutic success is the ability to identify potentially remediable factors before onset of irreversible pump dysfunction. Therefore, identification of ischemic, dysfunctional, but still viable myocardium that may respond to revascularization techniques (thrombolysis, direct angioplasty, surgical revascularization) is crucial. Cardiac catheterization and ventriculography as well as thallium perfusion studies and dobutamine echo are among the procedures designed to determine whether a significant mass of myocardium is still viable. Identification of complicating mechanical lesions (acute mitral regurgitation or a VSD) may provide targets for catheter-based interventions and/or surgery.

The general therapeutic approach to cardiogenic shock involves restoration of circulatory homeostasis, with an initial focus on adequate mean aortic perfusion pressure. Thus, in patients who are hypotensive, initial attempts should be made to ensure optimal blood volume (fluid volume adjusted with reference to lung congestion, jugular venous pulse). In patients whose lungs are relatively clear and neck vein pressure is not elevated, a fluid challenge is appropriate (even patients with dilated cardiomyopathy may be relatively preload deprived such that hemodynamic improvement will occur with a hemodynamically monitored fluid challenge). In patients with obvious volume overload and cardiogenic shock, appropriate diuresis should be initiated. In those who are hypotensive, treatment to restore perfusion pressure should be initiated with parenteral agents with positive inotropic effects. Initially, drugs should be employed that both increase contractility and raise blood pressure through vasoconstriction. Accordingly, agents such as dopamine are most appropriate. If dopamine is not effective, other pressors including norepinephrine may be needed to restore adequate mean aortic perfusion pressure (greater than 60 mmHg). Insertion of an intraaortic balloon pump is often needed not only to restore perfusion pressure but also to simultaneously unload the left ventricle and improve its performance. This intervention is particularly helpful in patients with ongoing ischemia by eliciting hemodynamic improvement as well as improvement of the balance between myocardial oxygen supply and demand. Balloon pumping is helpful also in patients with acute mitral regurgitation or a VSD in whom the unloading effects of the balloon pump will further improve forward output as well as reduce pulmonary congestion.

VII. SHOCK SECONDARY TO CARDIAC DYSFUNCTION CAUSED BY MECHANICAL FACTORS

Mechanical abnormalities rather than primary contractile dysfunction may be a primary cause of or contribute to shock. Such factors include aortic stenosis, mitral regurgitation, acute VSD, ischemic right heart dysfunction, and myocardial free-wall rupture.

A. Aortic Stenosis

Aortic stenosis may be the primary cause of left heart failure (with or without associated "contractile failure"; see discussion in Chapter 12), particularly in the elderly in whom senile degenerative calcific aortic stenosis and concomitant coronary artery disease contribute to LV dysfunction attributable not only to ischemia but also to effects of AS. Because some of the hemodynamic as well as "pump dysfunction" effects of AS may be reversible, and because AS complicates treatment of severe hemodynamic compromise (with respect to aggressive vasodilatation), it is critical to identify aortic valve obstruction in patients with pump dysfunction.

B. Mitral Regurgitation

Acute severe mitral regurgitation can precipitate cardiac shock, exacerbate hemodynamic compromise associated with acute myocardial infarction, and contribute to hemodynamic compromise in patients with primary cardiomyopathic processes.

Acute and severe mitral regurgitation results in profound hemodynamic compromise characterized by pulmonary congestion (often with pulmonary arterial hypertension) and low cardiac output that can lead to shock. Acute mitral regurgitation can be primary (ruptured chordae tendineae, infective endocarditis) or occur as a complication of acute myocardial infarction. In patients with acute MI, it is the mitral valve that most frequently becomes incompetent because of wall motion abnormalities that result in subvalvular tethering and "functional" regurgitation. If so, the mitral incompetence may not be the primary cause of hemodynamic compromise but may exacerbate low output and pulmonary edema in those in whom global LV function is depressed by the primary ischemic insult. Less commonly, acute MI results in a structural defect in the mitral apparatus attributable to frank papillary muscle rupture in which case severe mitral regurgitation that typically precipitates shock occurs even if global ventricular function is depressed only modestly.

Papillary muscle rupture occurs characteristically in the setting of a transmural MI attributable to occlusion of the left circumflex coronary artery (less commonly right coronary artery occlusion), resulting in severe ischemic dysfunction of the posterior-lateral papillary muscles. Patients afflicted typically develop mitral regurgitation 4 to 7 days after infraction, often after a previously stable course. Shock and pulmonary edema develop precipitously as a result of rupture of the papillary muscle caused by necrosis. Whether mitral regurgitation is present with the initial infarction or occurs several days later, the hemodynamic picture is characterized by shock with low cardiac output, reflex vasoconstriction, profound pulmonary edema, and pulmonary hypertension. The mitral regurgitation is manifest by a prominent holosystolic murmur unless cardiac output is profoundly depressed. Although secondary functional MR can be relatively "silent," primary MR is usually manifest by obvious auscultatory findings. Hemodynamic tracings typically reveal a prominent V wave in the wedge pressure trace and often a "rabbit ear" or double-peaked pattern in the pulmonary artery pressure trace, reflecting the retrograde, transmitted V wave. Two-dimensional Doppler ultrasound can easily define the extent and location of the underlying ischemic regional wall motion abnormality, the magnitude of global depression of LV function, the presence of mitral valve tethering, and frank papillary muscle rupture. It can quantify the extent of mitral regurgitation (color flow Doppler).

C. Acute Ventricular Septal Defect (VSD)

Acute rupture of the interventricular septum occurs in approximately 3% of patients with Q wave infarcts that involve the septum. The hemodynamic effects, pathophysiology, natural history, timing of onset, and clinical presentation of a postinfarction VSD are not only similar to but essentially indistinguishable from those seen with acute mitral regurgitation. Acute VSDs occur typically 4 to 7 days after an acute Q wave infarction, at which time necrosis of the interventricular septum leads to rupture and a left-to-right shunt at the ventricular level. Acute VSD is more common with anterior myocardial infarctions in which extensive LV dysfunction is typically present. Thus, global LV function is usually depressed.

However, acute VSDs may complicate anteroposterior septal MIs, in which the presence or absence of associated RV dysfunction secondary to ischemia influences the hemodynamic expression of the acute VSD as well as its natural history and prognosis.

The pathophysiology and clinical manifestations of an acute VSD are similar to those seen with acute mitral regurgitation. Abrupt development of a left-to-right shunt at the ventricular level results in recirculation of blood to the pulmonary bed and subsequently through the left heart chambers. The result is acute left heart volume overload and pulmonary edema. As with acute mitral regurgitation, the shunt further reduces forward output, resulting in a vicious cycle of low output and reflex vasoconstriction. Therefore, patients typically present 4 to 7 days after infarction with shock of abrupt onset and pulmonary edema associated with a pronounced holosystolic murmur.

Postinfarction VSDs and mitral regurgitation are indistinguishable by physical examination, including provocative auscultatory maneuvers. Echocardiography is highly effective not only in detecting a VSD (both two-dimensional imaging and especially color flow Doppler) but also in characterizing the extent of LV systolic dysfunction and the impact of other defects, including mitral regurgitation and RV ischemic dysfunction.

Right heart catheterization provides important clues to and should definitively establish the presence of a postinfarction VSD. Patients affected typically manifest elevated pulmonary capillary wedge pressure with a late V wave evident on the wedge pressure recording resulting from circulatory overload of the left atrium from the left-to-right shunt. Patients with an acute VSD often have falsely elevated values for cardiac output determined by thermodilution, a technique that is predicated on unimpeded passage of a cold bolus injected into the right atrium past the thermistor in the pulmonary artery. The effect of a left-to-right shunt is to "wash out" the cold bolus, thereby leading to a "falsely elevated" estimate of cardiac output.

Patients with acute MI who develop shock and pulmonary edema, a holosystolic murmur, and elevated filling pressures in the presence of a very high cardiac output should be suspected of having a VSD. This diagnosis is generally confirmed by oximetry with demonstration of a significant oxygen saturation set-up in samples drawn from the central and distal ports of a Swan-Ganz catheter.

VIII. RIGHT VENTRICULAR DYSFUNCTION SECONDARY TO ISCHEMIA

Occlusion of the right coronary artery proximal to the RV branches results in RV free-wall dysfunction secondary to ischemia and depressed global RV performance in 50% of patients with Q wave, inferoposterior MI. In approximately 25% of such patients, a unique pattern of hemodynamic compromise develops, characterized by low cardiac output, relatively clear lungs, and disproportionate right heart failure. Despite the fact that virtually all such patients have ischemic involvement of the left ventricle (inferoposterior MI), the pathophysiology of the low output state is distinctly different from that seen in patients with primary LV pump failure. The low output state seen with predominantly RV ischemic involvement is a consequence of reduced LV preload caused by global RV systolic dysfunction, which leads to diminished transpulmonary delivery of LV preload. This limitation of LV filling is exacerbated by effects of acute RV dilatation that shift the interventricular septum from right to left in a reverse-curved orientation that further impairs LV filling through diastolic ventricular interactions. In addition, abrupt dilatation of the ischemic RV can result in sudden elevation of intrapericardial pressure that intensifies diastolic interactions and impairs filling of both the LV and RV. If so, RV systolic performance is determined by LV-septal contractions that generate RV systolic pressure through systolic ventricular interactions mediated by paradoxical septal motion. Thus, the status of global LV function in general, and of septal contraction in particular, is important as a determinant of RV (as well as LV) performance. In fact, patients with acute inferoposterior MI and RV involvement who have had previous anterior-septal LV infarctions are the ones most likely to develop profound and refractory shock because of compromise of both ventricles as well as lack of compensatory LV support for the ischemic right ventricle.

The ischemic, dysfunctional dilated RV is stiff and therefore disproportionately dependent on augmented right atrial transport for optimal filling. Cardiac output becomes dependent on systolic ventricular interactions that contribute to hemodynamic stability. Loss of enhancement of RV function caused by atrioventricular dyssynchrony (e.g., heart block or ventricular pacing) or concomitant right atrial ischemia attributable to proximal right coronary occlusions results in more refractory hemodynamic compromise. The stiff, dilated ischemic right heart has limited stroke volume. Accordingly, maintenance of cardiac output is dependent on both optimal preload and adequate heart rate. For this reason, relative volume depletion (induced by diuretics or venodilators) or inadequate heart rate (frank bradycardia or relative chronotropic incompetence) may exacerbate hemodynamic compromise.

RV dysfunction secondary to ischemia should be suspected in all patients with acute inferoposterior MI even before development of low output. Early recognition may help to prevent precipitation of low-output hypotension by inadvertent administration of vasodilators and diuretics. Right ventricular involvement can be suspected on the basis of clinical criteria (e.g., elevated neck vein pressure). Noninvasive evaluation may demonstrate RV involvement. The right-side chest leads on ECG (ST elevation and loss of R wave in $V_{3-4}R$) are sensitive criteria for the presence of RV involvement but not its severity. Two-dimensional echocardiograph effectively delineates the presence and extent of RV dilatation, RV free-wall motion abnormalities, and the magnitude of depression of global RV systolic function. Invasive hemodynamic evaluation reveals characteristic patterns consisting of disproportionate elevation of right heart filling pressures and low cardiac output despite intact global LV contractility. The RA waveform may indicate augmented RA contraction (increased A wave amplitude— the W pattern) or ischemic RA dysfunction (diminished A wave amplitude—the M pattern), RV pressure "dip and plateau" (actually, the plateau is the abnormality), and equalized left and right heart diastolic filling pressures.

IX. MYOCARDIAL RUPTURE

Frank rupture of the ventricular wall occurs in approximately 1% of patients with Q wave myocardial infarction. Pathogenesis and timing of events are similar to those associated with necrotic rupture of a papillary muscle (leading to acute MR) or ventricular septum (leading to acute VSD). The vulnerability of inflamed zones of infarction is greatest 4 to 7 days after onset of a Q wave infarction. Factors that can increase the propensity for this catastrophic complication include advanced age and possibly thrombolysis.

Frank rupture of the ventricular free wall results typically in abrupt and profound hemodynamic compromise that may present initially as shock but more typically as abrupt electromechanical dissociation. The onset of deterioration may be heralded by recurrent chest pain but more frequently occurs without warning. Rupture may be "contained" and localized by the pericardium, evident clinically by recurrent chest pain with ultrasound evidence of an assymmetric pericardial effusion or "pseudoaneurysm." The detection of perforations before development of hemodynamic collapse is crucial. Survival of patients who develop electromechanical dissociation is dismal. However, in patients with contained rupture or frank rupture with shock but with no electromechanical dissociation, surgical intervention may be life saving.

X. ARRHYTHMIAS

Bradyarrhythmias and tachyarrhythmias commonly complicate acute myocardial infarction and may precipitate or exacerbate hemodynamic compromise. Hence rhythm status must be characterized, monitored, and rendered optimal. Tachyarrhythmias contribute to hemodynamic compromise by increasing myocardial oxygen demands, thus further exacerbating myocardial dysfunction. The increased heart rate shortens the diastolic filling period, thereby compromising ventricular filling and further impairing cardiac performance. Both supraventricular and ventricular tachyarrhythmias result in loss of atrioventricular synchrony and therefore loss of an effective atrial transport mechanism needed for optimal ventricular filling. Because ischemic ventricles (both LV and RV) are more critically dependent on atrial booster pump function for optimal filling and performance, loss of this important enhancer of cardiac filling may contribute to hemodynamic compromise, especially in patients with disporportionately stiff ventricles, whether because of ischemia or hypertrophy. Bradyarrhythmias can contribute to hemodynamic compromise not only by limiting rate and therefore cardiac output—particularly in ventricles with limited preload that are disproportionately dependent on chronotropic competence to maintain cardiac output—but also through loss of atrioventricular synchrony. Therapeutic ventricular pacing may induce pathologic rhythms if atrioventricular synchrony has not been restored.

Because ischemic dysfunctional ventricles are stiff, they generally cannot maintain a high stroke volume. Thus, cardiac output is disproportionately dependent on heart rate. Accordingly, it is essential that rhythm be viewed in relationship to cardiac output, and attention paid to the "optimal" rate for any given set of conditions. If, for example, heart rate is 70 beats/min when normal sinus rhythm prevails, normal cardiac output and blood pressure may be anticipated in a physiologically normal subject. However, in a patient with severe pump failure and low output, a physiologically appropriate rhythm would be reflex sinus tachycardia. Accordingly, the presence of a heart rate in the 60–90 range would be inappropriate and a reflection of "chronotropic incompetence." It would be wise to institute pharmacological measures or pacing designed to increase heart rate.

9

Suspicions of Cardiovascular Disease Raised by Results of "Routine" Diagnostic Tests

I.	Findings Seen on the Chest X-ray	161
II.	Electrocardiographic Findings	162
III.	Abnormal Results of "Routine" Laboratory Tests	164
IV.	Echocardiography	164

Allan S. Jaffe

Abnormalities detected by routine diagnostic tests may occur as isolated or associated phenomena. They should be considered with respect to each other and to the patient's history and overall status.

I. FINDINGS SEEN ON THE CHEST X-RAY

1. Occult congestive heart failure is suggested by cardiomegaly, pulmonary vascular redistribution, and pleural effusions, which are generally greater on the right side. The presence of cardiomegaly is the most compelling feature suggestive of heart failure.
2. Aortic dissection is suggested by a widened mediastinum and an aortic shadow lateral to a region of calcification within the aortic wall. The absence of such findings does not exclude a dissection that is suspected on other grounds.
3. Septal defects and coarctation as well as other forms of congenital heart

disease may be implied by findings evident on the chest film as well. A right-sided "mirror image" aortic arch may suggest tetralogy of Fallot and rib notching may suggest aortic coarctation. Specific chamber enlargement (see below) and shunt vasculature (dilated proximal pulmonary arteries and plethoric distal pulmonary vessels) are among the most obvious signs of septal defects encountered.

4. Pulmonary hypertension is suggested by accentuated narrowing of the pulmonary arterial vessels in the peripheral lung fields with apparent tapering of the vessels and an appearance of oligemia.

5. Right ventricular enlargement (for example, that seen with atrial and some ventricular septal defects, pulmonary hypertension, or right heart failure) may be evident. Enlargement of the right ventricle is usually most evident on a lateral chest x-ray in which the retrosternal space is occupied by the enlarged chamber.

6. Left ventricular enlargement suggests coronary disease, hypertension, or congestive heart failure attributable to another cause. When it is present, the left ventricular apex tends to "sit on" the left hemidiaphragm and impinge on what is normally a clear space between the spine and the posterior aspect of the heart evident on the lateral chest x-ray.

7. Left atrial enlargement may be suggestive of mitral valvular disease and/or atrial hypertension with elevated left ventricular end-diastolic pressure. The left heart border may be straightened and the left main stem bronchus may be splayed upward.

8. Pulmonary vascular shunts including small arteriovenous malformations (AVMs) may be evident. Occasionally, large regions of the lung are involved. Thus, extensive pulmonary arteriovenous shunting with collapse of even a whole lobe can occur as in the scimitar syndrome, in which a curvilinear area of lung collapses (usually on the right in association with anomalous pulmonary venous return).

9. Straightening of the left heart border may indicate corrected transposition of the great vessels in appropriate patients.

10. Poststenotic dilatation of the pulmonary artery suggests pulmonary stenosis.

11. Loss of definition of the aortic, pulmonary, and left atrial appendage shadows may be indicative of a pericardial effusion.

II. ELECTROCARDIOGRAPHIC FINDINGS

1. The electrocardiogram (ECG) is neither sensitive nor specific for the detection of left ventricular hypertrophy (LVH). The earliest change as LV mass begins to increase is usually left atrial enlargement, best diagnosed by the presence of a negative deflection in the P-wave in lead V^1, with an area at least equivalent to that of the positive deflection and occupying 1 mm^2 or more on the electrocardiographic paper. Subsequently, increased QRS voltage may

develop. Criteria based on R-wave amplitude in leads I and aV_L are highly specific in the absence of left axis deviation, but they are not sensitive. Other criteria, based on voltage in the precordial leads and ST/T-wave changes tend to yield underestimates of the incidence of LVH.

2. Conduction defects may be a manifestation of underlying structural heart disease, including sclerodegenerative changes of the conduction system itself (Lev's and Lengre's diseases).

   a. Left bundle branch block is usually a manifestation of primary or secondary sclerodegenerative disease, hypertension, infiltrative processes, coronary disease, or other entities that cause left ventricular dysfunction.

   b. Right bundle branch block can be a manifestation of sclerodegenerative disease, but, more often than left bundle branch block, it is a manifestation of an acute ischemic event. Because of the abruptness with which right bundle branch block can occur, its prognostic significance in the setting of acute MI is more adverse than that of left bundle branch block. When either abnormality occurs in an acute setting, especially in association with first-degree AV block, pacing should be implemented prophylactically to prevent progression to complete heart block.

3. Results of longitudinal studies indicate that the presence of frequent runs as well as multifocal and/or multiform ventricular premature complexes (VPCs) is a marker of increased cardiovascular risk. Frequent VPCs may presage sustained ventricular arrhythmias. Nevertheless, aggressive pharmacological treatment to suppress VPCs does not decrease mortality. Indeed, in the absence of sustained ventricular arrhythmias or symptoms associated with hemodynamic impairment caused by ventricular arrhythmias, treatment of VPCs per se is not indicated.

4. ST-segment abnormalities have a more adverse prognostic significance than T-wave abnormalities alone, although either can be nonspecific. ST-segment depression that is planar or downsloping is more likely to be a manifestation of ischemic heart disease than are other patterns. Deep, symmetrical T-wave inversion in leads V_1 through V_3 can occur with a variety of conditions, including stroke and cerebral vascular disease, but it may be a marker of severe left anterior descending coronary artery disease.

5. Abnormal Q waves should lead to the consideration of remote myocardial injury, including infarction. However, contusion, muscular dystrophy, and other types of injury can result in similar findings. Patterns called pseudo-infarction, resembling the ST-segment depression that occurs with acute myocardial infarction, can occur in patients with hypertrophy.

6. Criteria of right ventricular hypertrophy (RVH), including large terminal R waves in lead V_1 or V_2 and/or right axis deviation, should lead to the consideration of entities such as atrial septal defect, pulmonic stenosis, chronic recurrent pulmonary emboli, primary pulmonary hypertension, tricuspid regurgitation, and mitral stenosis. Such ECG findings are not specific

163

for RVH; for example, tall, thin subjects can manifest a rightward axis and other ECG signs compatible with RVH.

7. If a narrow QRS complex is present, indicative of a junctional rhythm, and the patient is otherwise well, the rhythm is generally benign regardless of the severity of heart block unless the signs are a reflection of digitalis toxicity or other toxicity. Wide-complex escape rhythms are unstable and are an indication for pacing when heart block is persistent or of high degree.

III. ABNORMAL RESULTS OF "ROUTINE" LABORATORY TESTS

1. Elevated total and/or MB creatine kinase (CK) can occur with skeletal muscle myopathy, acute or chronic; hypothyroidism, because of reduced clearance of the enzyme; renal failure; pulmonary embolism, especially if associated with right ventricular infarction; and diabetes, especially with ketoacidosis. Because MB CK is expressed in skeletal muscle, although minimally, elevations of MB CK can be seen with crush injury or rhabdomyolysis. Artifacts can account for unexpected reports of increased MB CK, especially when complexes with other serum proteins contribute. Generally, MB CK elevations in patients with skeletal muscle injury persist rather than rise and fall in a temporal pattern (12 to 36 hr), typical of that seen with acute myocardial infarction. Percentage criteria based on the relationship of MB to total CK improve specificity for the diagnosis of cardiac damage, but at the price of decreased sensitivity.

2. Elevations of serum cholesterol in acutely ill patients should lead to later characterization of potential lipid abnormalities for which preventive measures would be indicated. Lowering of elevated serum cholesterol is effective, as judged from results in secondary prevention trials. It is likely to be beneficial in primary prevention as well.

3. Increases in acute phase reactants including C-reactive protein and other nonspecific markers of inflammation (e.g., elevated whole blood cell count or erythrocyte sedimentation rate) may reflect subtle acute or smoldering disorders affecting the heart. Thus, patients with cardiovascular symptoms with such findings are more likely to harbor a serious cardiovascular process than is the case in those without them.

IV. ECHOCARDIOGRAPHY

A variety of findings may be obtained serendipitously, leading to the detection of the following:

1. Cardiac tumors or masses, which are generally benign. The most common is atrial myxoma, often with attachment to the atrial septum. Most

tumors require resection. Vegetations are generally confined to valve leaflets.

2. Ventricular thrombi are common in the left ventricles of patients with ischemic heart disease. If the clot is laminated, it is generally of less risk than if it is protruding into the cavity and appears friable. For high-risk thrombi, anticoagulation is indicated. Fibrinolytic agents have been used to dissolve thrombi, but definitive studies of their efficacy and safety are not yet available.

3. Atrial clots are rarely seen on transthoracic echocardiograms but relatively often in transesophageal studies. They are generally a manifestation of atrial pathology. Formation of thrombi (e.g., after electrical cardioversion) can lead to the appearance of "smoke" on transthoracic or transesophogeal echocardiograms in the region of the left atrial appendage.

4. Pericardial effusions are common in patients with heart failure and acute infarction and not of pathophysiological significance in the absence of signs or symptoms indicative of compression of the right ventricular or atrium.

5. Aortic root disease can often be identified with good echocardiographic views of the aortic root that can localize dissection and dilatation. Transesophageal echocardiography can often identify the site of origin of a dissection.

6. Diverse phenomena—including mitral valve prolapse and clinically trivial tricuspid or pulmonary regurgitation—are commonly recognized. Additional evaluation is not required unless symptoms or signs clearly mandate otherwise. Even when mitral valve prolapse is detected, it is not clear that it is responsible for neuropsychiatric symptoms. If it is present, prophylaxis for thromboembolic phenomena can generally be accomplished with antiplatelet agents alone unless overt thrombi are present, in which case anticoagulants should be implemented. Prophylaxis for endocarditis is indicated only if mitral regurgitation or a pressure gradient is present.

III

CARDIAC TREATMENT

Management of
Specific Cardiac Problems

Effective cardiac treatment is predicated on definitive diagnosis, principles derived from the underlying pathophysiology, and a focus on proximate cause of
signs and symptoms. As in all branches of medicine, "fashions" in treatment
change, sometimes diametrically, as a result of acquisition of new knowledge. For
example, the treatment of heart failure, which relied until recently on use of agents
with positive inotropic effects and diuretics, now focuses on afterload reduction to
diminish cardiac work and enhance perfusion. This modality increases life expectancy in addition to ameliorating symptoms. Another example is the previous old
saw that patients with Eisenmenger's syndrome should be treated with digitalis,
diuretics, and phlebotomy. Modern approaches are predicated on the recognition
that signs and symptoms can be best ameliorated by augmentation of systemic
cardiac output. Thus, vasodilators in patients with ventricular dysfunction or
valvular regurgitation (to decrease peripheral arteriolar resistance and increase
output) are useful despite their potential to increase the volume of right-to-left
shunting. Their use elevates mixed venous blood oxygen saturation secondary to
the increased systemic output, resulting in less desaturation caused by the shunt
despite its increased magnitude. Recent information demonstrating a less steep
rise in blood viscosity with increasing hematocrit under conditions simulating
those in the microcirculation (low shear) underlies another paradigm shift in the
treatment of patients with Eisenmenger's syndrome. Phlebotomy is now generally
avoided despite the presence of an elevated hematocrit. Diuretics are recognized

167

as being potentially deleterious because of their propensity to diminish plasma volume, augmenting hematocrit without increasing red cell mass, and thereby compromising microcirculatory hemodynamics. In fact, it appears that the single most powerful determinant of well being of patients with this syndrome is "red cell cardiac output," that is, the capacity to deliver oxygen to viscera and the periphery supplied by the systemic arterial circulation. Thus, a high hematocrit reflecting increased red cell mass rather than contraction of plasma volume is beneficial.

Equally striking paradigm shifts have occurred in the management of patients with arrhythmia. In the recent past, primary reliance was placed upon drugs; but adverse clinical outcomes despite apparently favorable effects on suppression of ventricular ectopy and even episodes of ventricular tachycardia have led to increasing use of radiofrequency catheter ablation procedures for ventricular as well as supraventricular tachyarrhythmias, implantation of devices including "smart" pacemakers to abort spontaneously occurring tachycardias, and anti-fibrillatory devices for patients at high risk of ventricular fibrillation and cardiac arrest. Pacemakers have virtually completely replaced drug therapy in the management of patients with bradycardia attributed to conduction system disease and heart block.

The treatment of acute myocardial infarction, previously focusing on reduction of myocardial oxygen requirements, analgesia, oxygenation, and suppression of deleterious arrhythmias, now focuses largely on revascularization induced pharmacologically with fibrinolytic agents or mechanically with new devices and conventional balloon angioplasty, and sometimes on early surgery. Increasing recognition is being given to the need to prevent progression of the underlying coronary disease or the enhancement of its regression with lipid-lowering measures.

In each of these therapeutic challenges, paradigm shifts have accompanied increased elucidation of fundamental pathophysiology. The same can be said for many other aspects of cardiology in which treatment has reduced not only morbidity but also mortality. On the horizon, somatic gene therapy, the use of small molecules to modulate gene expression, the marriage of interventional cardiology with local delivery of agents that modify the evolution of vascular lesions, correction of biochemical defects responsible for heart failure including that seen in mitochondrial myopathies and other definitively elucidated conditions are likely to advance therapeutics even more effectively. The clinician is in the privileged position of applying these modalities to patients in whom the specific diagnosis and elucidation of pathophysiology continue to provide the foundation for effective management and intervention. In this part, medical management is considered in the context of specific diagnostic entities and treatment predicated on pathophysiology.

Management of Patients with Chest Pain of Cardiac Origin

I.	Stable Angina Pectoris	169
II.	Pharmacological Management of Stable Angina	171
III.	Pharmacological Management of Patients with Unstable Cardiac Pain (Unstable Angina or Non-Q-Wave Infarction)	176
IV.	Selection of Patients for Angiography	180
V.	Patients Requiring Revascularization	181
VI.	Specific Management Issues	182
VII.	Management of Patients with Angina	184
VIII.	Unstable Angina	186
IX.	Management of the Patient with Inoperable Coronary Disease and Frequent Unstable Symptoms	187

Allen J. Solomon and Bernard J. Gersh

I. STABLE ANGINA PECTORIS

After the diagnosis of angina pectoris has been established, it is essential to tailor treatment to the patient's stability of signs and symptoms or lack thereof. A patient is considered to have stable angina if the frequency, severity, and duration of chest pain remains unchanged over time. Chest pain that is new, occurs at rest, or exhibits a changing pattern is considered indicative of an unstable coronary syndrome including variant angina, non-Q-wave myocardial infarction, or post-infarction angina.

Therapy of stable angina consists of pharmacological and nonpharmacological interventions. Its goals are to relieve symptoms, prevent myocardial infarction and associated morbidity, and decrease mortality. Nonpharmacological therapy consists of several lifestyle modifications. Pharmacological therapy is directed at risk factors for coronary artery disease, precipitating factors, improving the balance between myocardial oxygen supply and demand, and inhibiting platelet aggregation.

Initial treatment requires cessation of cigarette smoking. This must be discontinued because smoking leads to progression of atherosclerosis and induces deleterious acute coronary hemodynamic effects, including coronary vasoconstriction. It predisposes to atherosclerotic plaque instability and rupture. Dietary modifications are essential. Hyperlipidemia should be treated by a reduction in saturated fat and cholesterol intake, a decrease in total calories to achieve ideal body weight, and increased consumption of fruits, vegetables, and fiber. Dietary control is crucial to the management of hypertension and diabetes mellitus as well. An exercise program is helpful in resolving hypercholesterolemia, hypertension, and obesity as well as improving exercise performance and a sense of well-being.

Pharmacological therapy is two-tiered. One tier is aimed at the risk factors indicative of and potentially underlying the coronary artery disease itself. Thus, management of hypercholesterolemia, hypertension, and diabetes mellitus is essential. In women, the use of estrogens has been associated with a reduction in progression of overt coronary heart disease and cardiovascular mortality.

The second tier is directed at increasing the ratio of myocardial oxygen supply to demand and inhibition of platelet aggregation. An important adjunct to both pharmacological and nonpharmacological therapy is the treatment of conditions known to precipitate or exacerbate angina pectoris, such as anemia, hyperthyroidism, infection, arrhythmias, and valvular heart disease.

The prognosis of patients with stable angina is dependent upon the severity of ischemia, quality of left ventricular function, and electrophysiological stability. In patients with mild stable angina and normal left ventricular function randomized to initial medical therapy in the Coronary Artery Surgery Study (CASS), the 10-year survival rate was 86%, which was not different from that in the surgical cohort. Thus, patients with stable angina should be treated medically with a goal of reducing or eliminating angina and ischemia and preventing myocardial infarction.

The initial approach to patients with stable angina should include aggressive risk-factor modification, regular exercise, use of prophylactic nitroglycerin, avoidance of cold weather, and avoidance of exercising after meals. Aspirin should be initiated and nitroglycerin used as needed to control symptoms.

A second step, if needed on the basis of symptoms or results of electrocardiographic monitoring or stress testing, involves the initiation of a long-acting nitrate, with a nitrate-free interval, and a beta blocker or calcium channel antagonist. A beta blocker is ideal for patients with silent ischemia or a high sympathoadrenal tone (reflected by a relatively high resting heart rate). A calcium channel antagonist is best suited for patients with obstructive pulmonary disease, peripheral vascular disease, insulin-dependent diabetes mellitus, or angina with a strong vasospastic component.

A third step, if needed based on refractoriness to the above, is the combination of a beta blocker with a calcium channel antagonist. If verapamil or diltiazem is chosen, the patient should be monitored closely for bradycardia or heart block, especially if he or she is an elderly subject and has preexisting conduction system disease. Accordingly, a dihydropyridine calcium channel antagonist is often helpful instead for use in combination therapy. Pharmacological treatment comprises the use of four classes of drugs: nitrates, calcium channel antagonists, beta blockers, and antiplatelet agents.

II. PHARMACOLOGICAL MANAGEMENT OF STABLE ANGINA

A. Nitrates

The therapy of chronic stable angina frequently begins with nitrates (Table 1). Nitrates are safe, effective, and inexpensive. They are available in a variety of preparations, including sublingual, buccal, oral, topical (ointment or patch), and intravenous forms. They are used to treat symptoms associated with stable angina, silent ischemia, or both. They can and should be used prophylactically, before activities that often precipitate chest pain otherwise. The prophylactic use of nitrates tends to be underemphasized but should be taught to all patients, since it

Table 1 Nitrates

Drug	Route of administration	Daily dosage (mg)	Frequency of administration
NTG[a]	Sublingual	0.3–0.4	prn
NTG	Aerosol	0.4	prn
NTG	Buccal	1–3	prn
Pentaerythritol tetranitrate	Oral	30–120	tid
Isosorbide dinitrate	Oral	30–120	tid
Isosorbide mononitrate	Oral	40	bid
NTG ointment	Topical	½–2″	tid
NTG patch	Topical	0.2–0.4/hr	Off at night
NTG	Intravenous	10–200 μg/min	Continuous

[a]NTG = nitroglycerin.

171

markedly reduces the frequency of symptoms and improves quality of life. Although nitrates improve symptoms and lessen ischemia, they do not retard the progression of atherosclerosis or reduce mortality.

Nitrates increase myocardial oxygen supply and decrease demand. Myocardial oxygen supply is increased by the dilatation of epicardial coronary arteries, relief of coronary artery vasospasm, and dilatation of collateral coronary vessels, all of which result in an increase in blood flow to the subendocardium, the most vulnerable region of the heart because of its distance from the coronary perfusion head and the high wall stress to which it is subjected. Myocardial oxygen demand is reduced by the vasodilatory actions of nitrates on venous capacitance vessels, resulting in a decrease in ventricular preload and a subsequent decrease in myocardial wall stress. Peripheral arterial vasodilatation may contribute by reducing ventricular afterload.

If nitrates are given continuously, tolerance develops rapidly. Thus, patients will experience less antianginal effects. Tolerance results in part from depletion of sulfhydryl groups required for the production of nitric oxide [endothelial derived relaxation factor (EDRF)], derived from the organic nitrates and thought to account for their pharmacological actions. It can be prevented by including an 8- to 12-hr nitrate-free interval in the dosing schedule. For example, topical nitrates can be removed at bedtime or the nighttime dose of an oral preparation can be withheld. However, if symptoms are typically nocturnal, the nitrate-free interval can be shifted to daytime. Pharmacological approaches to nitrate tolerance, such as administration of *N*-acetylcysteine and captopril, rich in sulfhydryl groups, are currently being studied.

Adverse reactions are common, especially in the elderly, but rarely serious. Most commonly, patient develop headache, flushing, tachycardia, or hypotension. Hypotension is usually a sign of insufficient preload, as is seen with relative or absolute hypovolemia. Nitrate tablets must be kept in airtight containers and stored in the cold to avoid loss of potency.

For treatment of episodes of chest pain, the usual initial choice is sublingual nitroglycerin. A 0.3- to 0.4-mg tablet should be taken immediately at the onset of pain or prophylactically. If there is no response, doses can be repeated in 5-min intervals up to a total of three. The onset of action is 1–3 min, with a duration of 10–15 min. Initial therapy can be via tablets, spray, or buccal preparations. If no relief is achieved after three doses and after 15 min, the patient should be seen by a physician or in an emergency facility immediately because of the likelihood that infarction is impending or evolving.

Long-term therapy utilizes oral preparations or transdermal delivery systems. Both are effective in eliminating or reducing episodes of angina and increasing exercise tolerance. The oral preparations generally have an onset of action of 15–60 min and act for 2–6 hr. Transdermal systems have an onset of action of 30–60 min and continue to deliver drug for as long as the patch is in place beyond the

8- to 12-hr nitrate-free interval that should be initiated. To avoid skin irritation, the site of placement of patches should be varied.

B. Calcium Channel Antagonists

The calcium channel antagonists are heterogenous drugs that block the influx of calcium ions into myocytes and vascular smooth muscle cells, resulting in increased coronary blood flow and decreased myocardial oxygen demand (decreased contractility and afterload). They are effective in the treatment of hypertension, supraventricular tachyarrhythmias, left ventricular diastolic dysfunction, vasospastic (Prinzmetal's) angina, and stable cardiac chest pain syndromes. Calcium channel antagonists are especially useful when beta blockers are relatively or absolutely contraindicated, as in patients with asthma, chronic obstructive lung disease, peripheral vascular disease, or insulin-dependent diabetes mellitus. When coronary vasospasm is predominant, as in cold-induced angina, calcium channel antagonists are often superior to beta blockers. Results of the INTACT and other studies suggest that calcium channel antagonists may reduce progression of coronary artery disease, although this point remains controversial.

Calcium channel antagonists are classified as papaverine derivatives (verapamil), benzodiazaepine derivatives (diltiazem), dihydropyridines (nifedipine, isradipine, felodipine, amlodipine, nicardipine, and nimodipine) and mixed calcium, sodium, and potassium blockers (bepridil). Each type exhibits unique features (Table 2). Verapamil, at one end of the spectrum, causes the greatest effect of slowing of conduction within the AV and SA nodes and depression of myocardial contractility, as well as the least extent of peripheral vasodilation. At the other end of the spectrum are the dihydropyridines. They cause the most marked peripheral vasodilation and the least reduction of cardiac conduction velocity. The effects of diltiazem are intermediate.

Nifedipine, amlodipine, nicardipine, diltiazem, verapamil, and bepridil are approved in the United States for the treatment of stable angina pectoris. They decrease the frequency and severity of episodes of angina and increase exercise tolerance. They are well suited for use in hypertensive patients with angina pectoris. Diltiazem and verapamil are especially useful in patients with left ventricular diastolic dysfunction or supraventricular tachyarrhythmias as well as angina.

Calcium channel antagonists are relatively well tolerated, but many adverse effects, some of which may be serious, have been reported The most common are attributable to vasodilatation and include headache, flushing, palpitations, dizziness, and peripheral edema. Adverse effects are less frequent with the use of long-acting preparations. Rarely, a coronary artery steal phenomenon can result in an exacerbation of angina. Both verapamil and diltiazem can cause bradycardia and heart block, especially when used in combination with a beta blocker. Verapamil is

Table 2 Calcium Channel Antagonists[a]

Drug	Heart rate	Cardiac condition	Myocardial contractility	Peripheral vasodilation	Daily dosage (mg)	Frequency of administration
Verapamil	↓	↓	↓↓	↑	240–360	tid
SR					120–480	qd
Diltiazem	↓	↓	↓	↑	90–270	tid
CD					120–300	qd
Nifedipine	↑	—	↓	↑↑	30–120	tid
XL					30–120	qd
Nicardipine	↑	—	—	↑↑	30–60	tid
SR					30–60	qd
Amlodipine	↑	—	↓	↑↑	5–10	qd
Bepridil	↓	↓	V	—	200–400	qd

[a]Approved in United States for the treatment of angina.

Key: ↑ = increase

↓ = decrease

— = no change

V = variable.

the most likely calcium channel antagonist to exacerbate congestive heart failure. All of these agents, however, may do so, particularly when used in conjunction with beta blockers. The dihydropyridines generally do not depress cardiac function in vivo because of the induction of increased sympathoadrenal tone secondary to vasodilatation and relative hypotension.

The most common adverse effect of verapamil is constipation. Bepridil should be reserved for patients who have failed to respond to other antianginal drugs because of an incidence of induction of life-threatening ventricular tachyarrhythmias, including torsades de points and agranulocytosis.

Calcium channel antagonists can cause profound hypotension in patients with aortic stenosis. They can exacerbate hyperglycemia in diabetics by antagonizing insulin release. Withdrawal of calcium channel antagonists may lead to rebound. Thus, discontinuation should be gradual.

C. Beta Blockers

Beta blockers compete with endogenous catecholamines for beta adrenoreceptors in the heart and peripheral vasculature. This results in a reduction in myocardial oxygen demand primarily because of the decreasing heart rate and blood pressure (especially with exercise) and decreased myocardial contractility. Oxygen supply may be increased by a shift in the oxygen-hemoglobin curve to the right with increased oxygen delivery to the tissues and by a shift in coronary blood flow to the subendocardium because of decreased left ventricular wall stress secondary to decreased contractility.

Beta blockers are classified according to their pharmacological properties (Table 3). Metoprolol, atenolol, acebutolol, bisoprolol, betaxolol, and esmolol are cardioselective. They block only β_1 receptors when given in low doses and are advantageous in patients with bronchospasm, diabetes mellitus, or peripheral vascular disease. Pindolol, oxprenolol, labetalol, acebutolol, carteolol, and penbutolol have intrinsic sympathomimetic activity with partial agonist activity and less slowing of the resting heart rate. Beta blockers are used in the treatment of many cardiovascular disorders in addition to angina pectoris, including hypertension, supraventricular and ventricular arrhythmias, acute myocardial infarction, aortic dissection, hypertrophic cardiomyopathy, the long-QT syndrome, and congestive heart failure. They are more effective than calcium channel antagonists in the treatment of silent ischemia. Beta blockers should be titrated to reduce resting heart rate to 50–60 beats/min and limit the increase to less than 110 beats/min with exercise. Dosing schedules for approved beta blockers are shown in Table 3. Discontinuation should be gradual, over 5 to 10 days, to avoid rebound angina or hypertension.

Beta blockers are safe and generally well tolerated. Most of their adverse effects are a consequence of their therapeutic and pharmacological properties. These effects include bradycardia, heart block, hypotension, congestive heart failure, hypoglycemia, bronchospasm, claudication, lethargy, cold extremities, sleep disturbances, and impotence. Contraindications to their use include symptomatic bradycardia, advanced heart block, peripheral vascular disease (relative), severe diabetes mellitus, or bronchospasm. They may be helpful in patients with dilated cardiomyopathy (by reducing myocardial injury) but must be used judicially and at low doses initially in this setting. In general, beta blockers should be avoided in patients with uncontrolled heart failure.

Table 3 Beta Blockers[a]

Drug	CS	ISA	Route of elimination	Daily dosage (mg)	Frequency of administration
Propranolol	—	—	Hepatic	40–240	qd–qid
Nadolol	—	—	Renal	20–240	qd
Metoprolol	+	—	Hepatic	50–200	qd–bid
Atenolol	+	—	Renal	25–100	qd

[a]Approved in United States for the treatment of angina.
Abbreviations: CS = cardioselective; ISA = intrinsic sympathomimetic activity.

175

D. Antiplatelet Agents

Aspirin selectively acetylates an enzyme-mediating synthesis of platelet prostaglandins and thromboxanes, resulting in irreversible loss of cyclooxygenase activity. Consequently, the formation of thromboxane A_2, a very potent vasoconstrictor and activator of platelets, is blocked. Because platelets contribute to the pathogenesis of acute ischemic syndromes, aspirin plays an important role in the treatment of both coronary and peripheral arterial disease.

Aspirin is valuable in therapy of unstable angina, other acute coronary syndromes, and stable angina as well as in secondary and possibly primary prevention of coronary, cerebrovascular, and peripheral vascular disease. Treatment with aspirin acutely reduces mortality in patients with unstable angina pectoris or myocardial infarction. Long-term use decreases late mortality, nonfatal myocardial infarction, and stroke (secondary prophylaxis) in patients who have sustained acute myocardial infarction, episodes of unstable angina pectoris, transient ischemic attacks, and stroke. It helps to maintain patency in patients with peripheral arterial grafts and reduces thromboembolic episodes in patients with nonvalvular atrial fibrillation and those with prosthetic heart valves, in whom it is used as an adjunct to warfarin.

The utility of aspirin in the primary prevention of occlusive coronary disease is somewhat controversial. Because the event rate in healthy subjects is low, it is difficult to prove consistent benefit. However, in patients with overt coronary disease manifest by chronic stable angina but no myocardial infarction, the risk of a first myocardial infarction is reduced. For example, in the Swedish Angina Pectoris Aspirin Trial, patients with chronic stable angina treated with 75 mg of aspirin daily exhibited a reduction in the combined incidence of a first myocardial infarction and sudden death by 34%.

Thus, all patients with chronic stable angina who do not have contraindications should be given aspirin with a loading dose of 160–300 mg followed by 75–100 mg daily as maintenance. Adverse effects are usually minor, primarily dose-related gastrointestinal toxicity, bleeding, and rare renal insufficiency. Gastrointestinal tract toxicity is exacerbated by alcohol intake.

III. PHARMACOLOGICAL MANAGEMENT OF PATIENTS WITH UNSTABLE CARDIAC PAIN (UNSTABLE ANGINA OR NON-Q-WAVE INFARCTION)

A. Nitrates

Nitrate therapy plays a pivotal role in the treatment of unstable and stable cardiac chest pain syndromes. Initial therapy is with sublingual nitroglycerin. However, unlike the case with stable cardiac chest pain, intravenous therapy is the key to

176

successful treatment of unstable cardiac chest pain. It provides rapid onset and certain absorption and is initiated at a low dose (e.g., 10 μg/min with increases in 10 μg/min increments every 5 min to a maximum dose of 200 μg/min titrated in the individual patient, with relief of pain as the endpoint. Doses should be reduced if adverse effects such as hypotension develop. Despite the development of some tolerance, intravenous nitroglycerin can be continued for several days, although it may be necessary to increase the rate of infusion after 24 hr to maintain efficacy.

B. Calcium Channel Antagonists

All of the calcium channel antagonists used in the treatment of stable cardiac chest pain are effective in controlling unstable cardiac pain (Table 2). They are particularly useful when coronary artery vasospasm is playing a predominant role or when beta blockers are contraindicated. Although, like nitrates and beta blockers, they clearly decrease angina, they have not been shown to decrease mortality or progression to myocardial infarction. Thus, calcium channel antagonists should be reserved as third-line therapy, behind nitrates and beta blockers, in patient with ongoing or recurrent chest pain. These agents (especially the papaverine- and benzodiazepine-based drugs) should be avoided in patients with pulmonary edema or left ventricular dysfunction. Dihydropyridines such as nifedipine should be used only in combination with a beta blocker, because reflex tachycardia encountered otherwise may increase the incidence of myocardial infarction.

C. Beta Blockers

As is the case with stable cardiac chest pain, beta blockers are effective for most patients with unstable angina (Table 3), with the same precautions and contraindications. These agents are especially useful in patients with a high level of sympathoadrenal tone, reflected by relative tachycardia and sometimes hypertension. However, beta blockers should probably be avoided in patients with known primary vasospastic angina because of the risk of relative increases in unopposed alpha-adrenergic tone. They can be combined with nitrates or calcium channel antagonists. Beta blockers can complement nitrates by preventing reflex tachycardia and the sympathetically mediated increase in contractility and myocardial oxygen demand that may occur with nitrates alone. Combination with calcium channel antagonists is effective also, but the addition of diltiazem or verapamil to a beta blocker regimen can precipitate excessive bradycardia, heart block, or hypotension.

For high-risk patients, intravenous beta blockade should be initiated. Metroprolol, given in 5-mg increments every 5 min to a total dose of 15 mg, can be followed in 1 to 2 hr by 25–50 mg orally every 6 hr. Propranolol can be given in an initial dose of 0.5–1.0 mg followed in 1–2 hr by 20–80 mg orally every 6–8 hr. Atenolol can be given in an initial dose of 5–10 mg, followed by 100 mg orally.

A metaanalysis of results with beta blockers compared with placebo in unstable angina demonstrated a 13% reduction in the risk of progression to myocardial infarction. Although a mortality benefit has not been shown in unstable angina, randomized trials in acute myocardial infarction and stable angina with silent ischemia have shown a mortality benefit for beta blockers. Thus, these agents are indicated in the treatment of unstable chest pain syndromes.

D. Antiplatelet Agents

Although conventional antianginal therapy with nitrates, beta blockers, and calcium channel antagonists is effective in controlling pain, the primary pathophysiological substrate is not necessarily affected. Because platelet activation plays an integral role in the pathogenesis of unstable chest pain syndromes, treatment with aspirin is appropriate. In four major trials in patients with unstable angina, aspirin has been shown to decrease mortality and the incidence of nonfatal myocardial infarction in the doses ranging from 75–1300 mg/day. Adverse effects occurred more commonly with higher doses. When 1300 mg (325 mg qid) were used, 44% of patients reported gastrointestinal adverse effects. Higher doses can decrease vasodilatory prostacyclin release from the arterial endothelium. Thus, low-dose aspirin (80–324 mg/day) is the optimal approach for maintenance treatment of patients with unstable chest pain.

In patients intolerant of aspirin, ticlopidine is a reasonable alternative. Ticlopidine has a slower onset of action (several days) because it is active only on megakaryocytes rather than mature platelets. It inhibits platelet aggregation mediated through adenosine diphosphate (ADP). Ticlopidine has been shown to decrease cardiovascular mortality and the incidence of nonfatal myocardial infarction in patients with unstable angina pectoris. The recommended daily dose is 250 mg twice daily. The most common adverse effects are gastrointestinal or dermatological; however, severe neutropenia or agranulocytosis occurs in approximately 1% of patients treated.

The potential benefit of initial treatment with aspirin in combination with heparin (see below) has not yet been firmly established. The combination is clearly more effective than aspirin alone but may not be superior to heparin alone. However, the risk of major bleeding with the combination is increased. Other antiplatelet agents, including sulfinpyrazone and dipyridamole, are not effective in the treatment of unstable angina. Agents that block platelet fibrinogen receptors (specifically the glycoprotein IIb/IIIa receptor) are currently under active investigation and offer a promising approach.

E. Anticoagulation and Thrombolysis

Several large studies have confirmed the value of heparin in the initial treatment of patients with unstable chest pain syndromes. Heparin affects the underlying pathophysiological substrate because of its antithrombin and consequently indirect as well as direct antiplatelet effects. The benefits of heparin in reducing mortality and the incidence of nonfatal myocardial infarction as well as relief of refractory angina in patients with unstable angina are well documented.

All patients with unstable cardiac chest pain who do not have contraindications should be treated for 2 to 5 days with full-dose continuous intravenous heparin. A conventional regimen entails an initial bolus of 80 U/kg body weight (to saturate endothelial cell heparin binding sites) followed by a maintenance infusion targeted to induce a partial thromboplastin time of 55–85 sec. Heparin withdrawal has been associated with recurrent chest pain, which may be ameliorated by coadministration of aspirin or by giving heparin subcutaneously for several days before discontinuing therapy completely. Most adverse effects are related to bleeding and are usually minor.

Although platelet aggregation and thrombosis are integral components of the pathophysiology of unstable angina, thrombolytic agents have not been shown to be useful, even though they do result in a reduction in the extent of thrombosis visualized angiographically. Paradoxically, a trend toward an increased incidence of recurrent infarction in patients with unstable cardiac pain who have been treated with thrombolytic agents has been observed, in striking contrast to results in patients with Q-wave myocardial infarction. Thus, thrombolytic agents are at least relatively contraindicated at present in patients with unstable angina. Failure may be related to factors including the modest thrombus burden, plaque size or nature, and thrombus composition (platelet-rich opposed to erythrocyte-rich).

Novel antithrombin and antiplatelet drugs are currently being investigated for use in unstable chest pain syndromes. Hirudin and hirulog are direct-acting inhibitors of thrombin, in contrast to heparin, which acts in concert with cofactors, including antithrombin III. Because these new drugs require no cofactors, they are more active against fibrin-bound thrombin associated with intracoronary thrombi. Antiplatelet agents including chimeric Fab antibody fragments against the glycoprotein IIb/IIIa receptor are particularly promising, but a potential for serious bleeding exists.

F. Support of the Circulation with Devices Such as the Intraaortic Balloon Pump

When unstable cardiac chest pain does not respond to medical management, circulatory support is often helpful. It results in an increase in diastolic blood pressure, which can increase coronary blood flow, and a decrease in systolic blood pressure, which results in reduced myocardial oxygen demands. Relief of the cardiac chest pain is common. The support can act as a bridge to more definitive therapy, specifically revascularization. The most common complications are vascular and occur in about 10% of patients. Intraaortic balloon pumps (IABPs) are contraindicated in patients with severe peripheral vascular disease, aortic insufficiency, or aortic aneurysms.

Definitive revascularization is predicated on elucidation of coronary angiographic anatomy.

IV. SELECTION OF PATIENTS FOR ANGIOGRAPHY

A. Stable Angina

The objectives of coronary angiography are definition of prognosis and selection of medical treatment or revascularization, either percutaneous or surgical. In patients with stable cardiac chest pain, coronary angiography is indicated when symptoms are refractory to maximal medical therapy. Coronary angiography should be considered when severe ischemia is demonstrated with exercise or pharmacological stress testing. The presence of left ventricular dysfunction and clinical evidence of multivessel coronary artery disease are indications for coronary angiography as well. In patients with multiple admissions for chest pain of unknown etiology and no objective evidence of coronary artery disease, coronary angiography is helpful in delineating or excluding important pathology.

Patients with normal left ventricular function but with symptoms of angina who are not candidates for revascularization should be given a trial of medical therapy guided by adequacy of symptom relief and improvement evident by successful completion of exercise or pharmacological stress tests. If failure is encountered or angina is refractory, revascularization should be considered.

B. Unstable Angina

Angiography will demonstrate normal coronary anatomy or minimal coronary artery obstructive disease in 10–20% of patients, in which case subsequent treatment is targeted toward variant angina, syndrome X, or a noncardiac source of chest pain. Most patients with unstable chest pain syndromes will exhibit major obstructive coronary arterial lesions. Left main coronary artery disease will be present in 5–10%, three-vessel disease in 15–25%, two-vessel disease in 25–30%, and single-vessel disease in 30–40%. Compared with patients with stable cardiac chest pain, those with unstable chest pain generally harbor more severe coronary artery disease with longer, more eccentric, more irregular, and frequently thrombus-rich coronary artery lesions. Angiography may delineate a "culprit lesion" undergoing dynamic change and responsible for the instability of symptoms leading to the study.

Indications for coronary angiography in patients with unstable angina are dependent on the group into which the patient has been stratified (low-, intermediate-, or high-risk). Coronary angiography is indicated in all high-risk patients. Patients with a previous revascularization procedure, those with depressed left ventricular function, and those who have been stratified initially into low- or intermediate-risk groups but in whom a subsequent exercise or pharmacological stress test is markedly positive should be studied as well.

Variant (Prinzmetal's) Angina

Coronary artery vasospasm can lead to chest pain at rest, often in a circadian pattern, associated with ST-segment elevation and usually with nonobstructive atherosclerosis, as well as spasm occurring at the site of modest coronary narrowing. Deranged vascular smooth muscle contractility, endothelial vasodilator function, and autonomic regulation may contribute. The diagnosis hinges upon the demonstration of reversible ST-segment elevation associated with episodes of pain or the demonstration of focal coronary artery vasospasm in the catheterization laboratory in response to intracoronary infusion of ergonovine maleate or acetylcholine. Coronary artery vasospasm can rarely lead to myocardial infarction, heart block, or ventricular tachyarrhythmias. Prognosis depends on the severity of the spasm, the extent of underlying obstructive coronary artery disease, and left ventricular function.

Initial therapy usually comprises administration of nitrates and calcium channel antagonists. Sublingual nitroglycerin is often effective for individual episodes. Long-term administration of calcium channel antagonists (all are effective) is helpful. Calcium channel antagonists act directly on vascular smooth muscle to inhibit coronary artery vasospasm. This results in reduction of symptoms in more than 50% of patients and a reduction in the risk of myocardial infarction. Cyproheptadine may be useful as well. Theoretically, beta blockers may worsen vasospasm by blocking $beta_2$ receptors and tipping the balance toward relatively unopposed alpha-adrenergically mediated increased coronary vasomotor tone. Because atherosclerosis is usually present, aspirin should be included in the medical regimen. Coronary artery bypass graft surgery with plexectomy may be necessary in the rare, medically refractory patient.

V. PATIENTS REQUIRING REVASCULARIZATION

Although the indications for coronary angiography differ for patients with stable compared with unstable cardiac chest pain, once coronary anatomy and left ventricular function have been defined, treatment decisions are similar. Its objectives are to improve symptoms, increase exercise capacity, and decrease subsequent morbidity and mortality.

A. Percutaneous Transluminal Coronary Angioplasty

The initial use of percutaneous transluminal coronary angioplasty (PTCA) in patients with single-vessel coronary artery disease has been expanded to increas-

181

ing numbers of patients with multivessel disease. In comparison with coronary artery bypass graft (CABG) surgery, PTCA is associated with a shorter hospital stay and lower initial costs. Long-term costs, however, are similar because of an increased need for subsequent revascularization procedures of the initially targeted lesion and for repeat coronary angiography in patients treated with PTCA rather than CABG, especially in those with multivessel disease. Initial complications of PTCA include abrupt coronary closure (thrombotic) (3–5%), myocardial infarction (2–5%), and death (approximately 1%). The Achilles' heel of angioplasty continues to be restenosis. It occurs in 30–50% of patients. In comparison with coronary artery bypass graft surgery, a lower rate of complete revascularization following PTCA has been well documented in patients with multivessel coronary artery disease. Its impact on long-term outcome is presently under intense investigation.

B.   Coronary Artery Bypass Graft Surgery

Coronary artery bypass graft surgery is indicated for any patient with a left main coronary artery stenosis greater than or equal to 50% diameter reduction. It is indicated as well in patients with three-vessel coronary artery disease (with stenoses $\geq$ 70%) and severe two-vessel disease with high-grade proximal left anterior descending coronary artery stenosis ($\geq$ 95%) and depressed left ventricular systolic function (e.g., ejection fraction $\leq$ 50%).

In comparison with medical therapy, long-term control of angina and increased quality of life can be expected with CABG. Perioperative mortality is generally 1–2%. In comparison with PTCA, long-term morbidity and mortality are similar. Although PTCA requires a shorter initial hospital stay and lower initial costs, it leads to a greater number of subsequent, repeat revascularization procedures. Therefore its long-term costs are equivalent.

VI.   SPECIFIC MANAGEMENT ISSUES

A.   "Syndrome X"

Patients with syndrome X (cardiac chest pain with angiographically normal coronary arteries) experience chest pain consistent with myocardial ischemia, angiographically normal epicardial coronary arteries, and no other identifiable cause of chest pain. Many show ECG changes typical of ischemia during stress testing. The incidence is greater in female subjects. The prevalence of depression and panic disorders is increased among these patients. Frequently, right ventricular stimulation or intracoronary adenosine may reproduce the symptoms. The mechanisms responsible are unknown but may include endothelial dysfunction in the coronary microvasculature, inadequate vasodilator reserve, or locally deranged metabolism.

Treatment is targeted toward relief of symptoms. Long-term prognosis is generally excellent. Nitrates and calcium channel antagonists are often helpful but unlikely to abolish symptoms completely. Antidepressants such as imipramine may reduce the frequency of chest pain by approximately 50% at a dose of 25 mg qhs for 1 week and 50 mg qhs subsequently. Clonidine has been thought to be effective in some patients as well.

B. High-Risk ECG Subsets of Patients with Unstable Angina

Diffuse ST-segment depression with pain and deep anterior T-wave inversions is common in patients with three-vessel coronary artery disease and proximal left anterior descending coronary artery disease, respectively. Patients in these high-risk subsets should be treated with aggressive medical therapy. If this is not successful within 1 hr, angiography should be performed with consideration of prompt revascularization.

C. Unstable Angina and Poor Left Ventricular Function

Initial therapy should comprise aggressive medical management including anti-anginal agents and control of congestive heart failure with diuretics and afterload-reducing agents. Avoidance of drugs that can further depress left ventricular function—such as beta blockers, verapamil, and diltiazem—should be considered. If a calcium channel antagonist is used, a dihydropyridine such as amlodipine should be the first choice. Coronary angiography should be initiated relatively early, because many patients will require prompt revascularization.

D. Unstable Angina and Hypertension or Anemia

In patients with unstable angina and poorly controlled hypertension, therapy should be directed at both. Beta blockers, nitrates, or calcium channel antagonists should be titrated until chest pain resolves and blood pressure normalizes. Additional antihypertensive agents such as angiotensin converting enzyme (ACE) inhibitors, clonidine, labetalol, or sodium nitroprusside may be helpful. Maintenance of normotension will decrease myocardial oxygen demands. However, special efforts must be directed toward avoiding excessive decreases in diastolic blood pressure that could compromise coronary artery perfusion pressure and flow.

When anemia contributes to unstable angina, the impairment in myocardial oxygen supply can limit the effectiveness of conventional antianginal therapy. Transfusions of packed red blood cells to a hematocrit equal to or greater than 30% is helpful. Diuretics to reduce pulmonary congestion may be necessary before transfusion.

E. Non-Q-Wave Myocardial Infarction

In contrast to Q-wave myocardial infarctions, total coronary occlusion of an infarct-related vessel is infrequent. Coronary angiography usually demonstrates high-grade coronary artery stenosis in the infarct-related artery. In-hospital mortality is lower than that seen with Q-wave myocardial infarction; however, the subsequent incidence of recurrent ischemia and reinfarction is higher, leading to a similar or perhaps slightly worse overall long-term prognosis. Accordingly, management of a non-Q-wave myocardial infarction should be aggressive. It is quite similar to the treatment of unstable angina pectoris. Because recurrent ischemia is common, most patients will require coronary angiography and subsequent revascularization. Diltiazem may be particularly useful following non-Q-wave myocardial infarctions in patients with normal left ventricular function.

Thus, all patients with unstable cardiac chest pain and ongoing ischemia should be admitted to a coronary care unit. Initial therapy should consist of aspirin, heparin, nitroglycerin, and beta blockers. If the chest pain does not resolve, calcium channel antagonists should be added. Aggressive medical management can control the presenting episode of ischemia in most patients. However, cardiac catheterization and coronary angiography should be performed in patients who cannot be stabilized with medical therapy and those who manifest recurrent unstable angina as well as in those with previous revascularization procedures, depressed left ventricular function, or markedly positive exercise or pharmacological stress tests to identify the need for revascularization and guide selection of a specific modality.

VII. MANAGEMENT OF PATIENTS WITH ANGINA

Management of patients with stable and unstable angina is considered in Chapters 1 and 11. General principles are discussed in Chapter 11. When angina is associated with other disorders, specific management issues arise that are considered here.

A. Angina and Hypertension

The objectives of treatment in patients with stable angina and hypertension are to eliminate the angina and control the blood pressure. In many patients, standard antianginal therapy with beta blockers, calcium channel antagonists, and nitrates will achieve both. However, other patients will require additional antihypertensive therapy because control of blood pressure decreases myocardial oxygen demands. In patients with angina, hypertension, and depressed left ventricular function, ACE inhibitors are particularly useful. Excessive decreases in diastolic blood pressure must be avoided to prevent compromise of coronary perfusion pressure. Lipid levels should be monitored in patients given beta blockers because of the occasional nontrivial depression of high-density lipoprotein (HDL) and elevation of low-density lipoprotein (LDL) cholesterol that may be induced.

B. Angina and Diabetes Mellitus

The management of diabetic patients focuses on three major issues. First, silent ischemia is common and must be recognized. Elimination of ischemia, as opposed to pain, is the optimal endpoint. Second, beta blockers must be used judiciously because they can mask the features of hypoglycemia. When necessary, a cardio-selective agent such as metoprolol or atenolol should be chosen. Third, hyper-glycemia must be controlled, because diabetes is a powerful risk factor for progression of atherosclerosis.

C. Angina and Poor Left Ventricular Function

Agents that depress left ventricular systolic function—such as beta blockers, verapamil, and diltiazem—should not be used as first-line agents. For initial therapy, nitrates and a dihydropyridine calcium channel antagonist are preferred. Combined angina and left ventricular dysfunction identifies a patient with a poor long-term prognosis on medical therapy alone. Long-term outcome can be im-proved substantially by coronary revascularization. Such patients should be treated with an ACE inhibitor or a combination of hydralazine and nitrates.

D. Angina and Lung Disease

In patients with severe chronic obstructive pulmonary disease or asthma, beta blockers should be avoided or used only with extreme caution. Patients with mild bronchospastic airway disease may tolerate low doses of a cardioselective beta blocker. Nevertheless, calcium channel antagonists and long-acting nitrates are generally the agents of choice.

E. Angina and Valve Disease

Aortic Stenosis

When aortic stenosis is moderate to severe, any decrease in preload or afterload can be disastrous. Accordingly, all antianginal agents must be started at low doses and titrated gradually. The treatment of angina combined with aortic stenosis requires complete assessment of the severity of both the coronary artery disease and the valvular stenosis with a view towards aortic valve replacement, coronary artery bypass graft surgery, or both.

Aortic Regurgitation

To prevent progressive ventricular dilatation, afterload reduction must be part of medical management. To achieve this, ACE inhibitors, dihydropyridine calcium channel antagonists, and hydralazine are useful. Again, the severity of coronary artery disease and valvular regurgitation must be quantified with an eye toward surgery.

F. Atypical Stable Angina

When coronary artery vasospasm is implicated in the pathogenesis of angina, calcium channel antagonists should be the first-line therapy. Each of the agents is effective. Nitrates are the second choice.

G. Additional Tests

Exercise and pharmacological stress testing are useful to make a diagnosis, assess therapy, and define prognosis, and monitor the results of revascularization. Results enable the clinician to titrate medical therapy, especially in patients with silent ischemia.

Coronary angiography is indicated in high-risk patients and those who fail to respond to maximal medical therapy. It will define the presence and severity of obstructive (and often vasospastic) coronary artery disease. The information obtained is critical in determining whether revascularization is necessary, and if so, whether percutaneous or surgical revascularization is likely to be most beneficial.

VIII. UNSTABLE ANGINA

A. Surgery

Coronary artery bypass graft surgery is indicated for any patient with left main coronary artery stenosis equal to or greater than 50% and those with three-vessel coronary artery disease or severe two-vessel coronary artery disease with depressed left ventricular systolic function. Bypass surgery improves long-term control of angina compared with medical therapy.

The objectives of long-term management in patients who have undergone surgery are to maintain graft patency and prevent the progression of coronary atherosclerosis in grafts and native vessels. Control of risk factors for coronary artery disease is pivotal. Cigarette smoking must be discontinued, blood pressure should be normalized, hyperlipidemia should be controlled with LDL cholesterol reduced to less than 100 mg/dL by diet and when necessary, lipid-lowering drugs. In older women, hormone replacement therapy alone or in combination with other lipid-lowering agents may be used. With these measures, progression of obstructive atherosclerotic lesions and particularly the clinical manifestations of unstable plaques is retarded or actual regression of obstruction is induced. Long-term management requires aspirin as well, to decrease the early and late likelihood of graft occlusion and thereby possibly reduce graft atherosclerosis. Aspirin should be continued indefinitely in view of its long-term effects on native coronary arteries as well as on bypass grafts.

A. Percutaneous Transluminal Coronary Angioplasty

Medical stabilization is preferred before coronary angioplasty to reduce the likelihood of abrupt closure, myocardial infarction, the need for emergency surgery, and death. In medically refractory patients, angioplasty is frequently the revascularization procedure of choice. Often, a "culprit" lesion can be dilated as either definitive treatment or as a bridge to subsequent surgical revascularization. In patients with single, double or triple vessel coronary artery disease, PTCA can be performed. With the exception of patients with left main disease or severe two- or three-vessel disease with left ventricular dysfunction, PTCA and CABG result in generally similar long-term mortality and cost.

The objectives of long-term management are the prevention of restenosis and progression of coronary atherosclerosis. Aggressive risk-factor modification is essential, just as with surgery. Antiplatelet agents play an important role as well. Major trials have shown clearly that pretreatment with aspirin alone or aspirin plus dipyridamole or ticlopidine significantly decreases the incidence of acute closure, periprocedural myocardial infarction, and the need for emergency CABG. Aspirin should be used in long-term management after PTCA. To date, no agent has been found that reduces restenosis. Investigational approaches include the use of omega-3 fatty acids, blockers of receptors in smooth muscle cells, inhibitors of cytokines and growth factors, thrombin inhibitors, and monoclonal antibodies directed against platelet surface membrane receptors. Novel devices such as stents are currently being explored in the hope of decreasing the incidence of restenosis.

IX. MANAGEMENT OF THE PATIENT WITH INOPERABLE CORONARY DISEASE AND FREQUENT UNSTABLE SYMPTOMS

In patients with inoperable coronary artery disease, maximal medical therapy is required. This consists of antiplatelet therapy and triple antianginal therapy (nitrates, beta blockers, and calcium channel antagonists). In addition, aggressive risk-factor modification is critical. If symptoms persist, coronary angioplasty of the culprit lesion is often helpful. Consideration of cardiac transplantation may be required if other measures are impractical or fail.

11

Management of Patients with Acute Myocardial Infarction

I.	General Principles	189
II.	Diagnosis of Acute Myocardial Infarction	190
III.	Initial Management of Patients with Acute Myocardial Infarction	195
IV.	Pulmonary Artery Catheterization and Management of Hemodynamic Subsets	206
V.	Management of Bradyarrhythmias and Conduction Abnormalities in Patients with Myocardial Infarction	211
VI.	Management of Tachyarrhythmias and Ventricular Arrhythmias in Patients with Myocardial Infarction	213
VII.	Rehabilitation and Secondary Prevention After Myocardial Infarction	216
	Suggested Reading	218

Paul R. Eisenberg

I. GENERAL PRINCIPLES

Optimal management of patients with acute myocardial infarction requires, in part, recognition of subsets at higher risk for recurrent infarction, hemodynamic deterioration, or death. The most common cause of death from acute myocardial infarction is ventricular fibrillation (VF) occurring within the first 2 hr after the onset of symptoms. Prompt recognition of symptoms indicative of acute infarction and activation of the emergency medical system are the most effective means for preventing early death from myocardial infarction. Early management should emphasize rapid diagnosis, immediate reversal of VF should it occur, and rapid institution of recanalization of thrombotically occluded culprit coronary arteries (see Section III). Unfortunately, only 30–40% of patients with acute myocardial infarction are candidates for reperfusion with fibrinolytic drugs. Most of those who arrive at the hospital too late for optimal intervention are in cardiogenic shock or have concomitant conditions that render their prognosis poor.

The extent of left ventricular dysfunction and the adequacy of restoration of perfusion to jeopardized myocardium are important predictors of long-term morbidity and mortality. Accordingly, initial management of patients with suspected myocardial infarction should focus on induction of sustained coronary patency to the infarct region whenever possible and initiation of treatment to optimize left ventricular function (and hence effective perfusion of myocardium). To accomplish these treatment objectives, initial clinical evaluation should include characterization of myocardial function with noninvasive tests and, in higher-risk patients, early invasive procedures with right and left heart catheterization and coronary angiography.

II. DIAGNOSIS OF ACUTE MYOCARDIAL INFARCTION

Acute myocardial infarction should be considered in patients who present with either prolonged chest discomfort, new electrocardiographic (ECG) changes consistent with ischemia or myocardial injury, or increased concentrations of plasma enzyme markers of myocardial necrosis. Typically, at least two of these criteria will be present.

A. Characteristic Symptoms

Symptoms are similar to those associated with unstable angina but are more prolonged or severe. Often symptoms of shorter duration and/or lesser severity precede those of the index, acute infarct. Chest discomfort in patients with acute infarction is often associated with dyspnea, diaphoresis, nausea, or vomiting. Less frequently, palpitations, presyncope, or syncope occur. In elderly patients, those with diabetes, or patients with multiple medical problems, chest discomfort may be minimal, atypical, or absent. Dyspnea, diaphoresis, or nausea often predominates. In such patients the onset of atypical symptoms should prompt immediate evaluation, including the ECG. In patients in an intensive care unit (ICU) because of multiple medical problems or the need for postoperative care, myocardial infarction may be manifest only by signs such as unexplained tachycardia, worsening congestive heart failure, or the appearance of ventricular arrhythmias.

B. Electrocardiographic Findings Associated with Acute Infarction

A good-quality 12-lead ECG should be obtained immediately in patients who present with prolonged chest discomfort or other symptoms suggestive of acute infarction. Many initial treatment decisions are based on the recognition of specific ECG abnormalities.

ST-Segment Elevation

ST-segment elevation equal to or greater than 1 mm in two or more contiguous leads is consistent with acute myocardial injury and should prompt immediate evaluation of the patient for treatment with either thrombolytic agents or primary angioplasty (see Chapter 1, Section XV). In patients with ST segments abnormal at baseline due to left ventricular hypertrophy, early repolarization changes, or bundle branch block, recognition of ST-segment elevation attributable to acute myocardial infarction may be difficult. Immediate echocardiography may be useful in defining a wall motion abnormality indicative of infarction. Alternatively, coronary angiography and primary angioplasty may be preferable if they can be performed immediately. However, angioplasty entails a substantial risk of late restenosis (40%) and the need for multiple subsequent invasive procedures. If no contraindications militate against treatment with fibrinolytic agents, they should be instituted promptly when symptoms and ECG findings are suggestive of an acute myocardial infarction.

ST-Segment Depression

Patients who present with symptoms of acute infarction and ST-segment depression on the initial ECG are generally not considered to be candidates for recanalization because total occlusion of a coronary artery is often absent. However, coronary artery thrombosis may be present. Thus, aspirin and anticoagulants are needed. The exception is patients with ST-segment depression in precordial leads (i.e., V_1 through V_3) reflecting true posterior wall infarction, which should be managed more aggressively.

T-Wave Changes

Peaked T waves (i.e., "hyperacute" T waves), even with minimal or absent ST-segment elevation, may be seen in some patients with acute infarction. Serial ECGs, particularly if symptoms do not resolve with sublingual nitroglycerin, often show rapid progression of ECG changes to ST-segment elevation and should prompt treatment with fibrinolytic agents or coronary angioplasty.

New T-wave inversion with or without ST-segment depression is common in patients with unstable angina or non-Q-wave infarction. Such patients often

191

have an unstable thrombotic coronary artery or partially occlusive lesion and should be treated with aspirin and anticoagulants. Deep, symmetrical T-wave inversion in leads V_1 through V_6 suggests a high-grade left main or left anterior descending lesion and warrants aggressive stabilization of the patient with close monitoring and medical therapy.

Q Waves

Evolution of new Q waves (> 0.4 sec) occurs rapidly in the patient who presents with acute infarction and ST-segment elevation. Their presence should not preclude treatment with fibrinolytic agents or primary angioplasty within 24 hr of the onset of symptoms. However, extensive evolution of Q waves, particularly in patients who present more than 6 hr after the onset of symptoms of acute infarction, suggests that the extent of myocardial injury is already such that salvage will be minimal. Q waves develop infrequently in patients with myocardial infarction who present with ST-segment depression or T-wave changes alone. Patients with non-Q-wave myocardial infarction typically have subtotal coronary artery occlusion associated with acute thrombosis and a high risk of recurrent infarction associated with total coronary occlusion.

C.   Cardiac-Specific Enzymes and Proteins

Myocardial infarction results in release into plasma of intracellular macromolecules, including enzymes and structural proteins. Diagnosis of acute myocardial infarction is based on measuring abnormally elevated plasma levels of these "cardiac" enzymes, e.g., aspartate immunotransferase (AST or SGOT), creatine kinase (CK), or lactate dehydrogenase (LDH). Increased concentrations may occur with noncardiac muscle injury or other noncardiac pathological processes; however, increases in the concentration of the MB isoenzyme of creatine kinase (MB-CK) and the LDH_1 isoenzyme are relatively specific criteria of myocardial injury. Assays of myoglobin, cardiac-specific troponin I or T, and cardiac-specific myosin light chains have been developed to exhibit high specificity for the diagnosis of myocardial necrosis. Increases in plasma concentrations of macromolecules may not be detectable for 4 to as many as 12 hr after the onset of symptoms. Accordingly, although plasma assays are essential in confirming the diagnosis of myocardial infarction, they are of little value in the early exclusion of the diagnosis and therefore not pivotal in the immediate management of patients with suspected myocardial infarction.

Creatine Kinase

Both the MB and MM isoenzymes of creatine kinase (CK) are expressed in myocardium. The percentage of the MB isoenzyme in noncardiac skeletal muscle is very low (generally $< 1\%$). Therefore, increases in plasma MB-CK are usually due to myocardial necrosis. Increases in MB-CK into an abnormal range usually occur within 4–6 hr after the onset of symptoms and peak in 12–20 hr. The time to peak is abbreviated in patients in whom myocardial reperfusion is induced. Levels of MB-CK generally return to the normal range within 36–72 hr.

Increases in plasma MB-CK may result from causes other than acute infarction. In such instances, the characteristic temporal sequence of the rise and fall associated with acute myocardial infarction may not be observed (Table 1). The magnitude of increase in MB-CK is directly related to the extent of myocardial necrosis; therefore, the peak value is useful in defining the extent of infarction. Stuttering or late increases in MB-CK after an initial rise associated with acute infarction is generally indicative of recurrent infarction, which may be asymptomatic.

Isoforms of MB-CK and MM-CK can be measured in plasma and are of value in early diagnosis. Intracellular MM- and MB-CK contain lysine residues at the carboxyl terminus of each of the subunits of the enzyme (M subunit or B subunit), which are cleaved by a carboxypeptidase in plasma over time. Increased relative concentrations of the intracellular form compared with cleaved isoforms in plasma can be detected as early as 1 hr after the onset of symptoms of infarction.

Lactate Dehydrogenase (LDH)

The concentration of the LDH_1 isoenzyme is increased relative to that of the other four isoenzymes of LDH in myocardium. A ratio in plasma of $LDH_1:LDH_2$ greater than 1 is consistent with an acute myocardial infarction and can be detected typically in samples obtained 12–24 hr after the onset of symptoms. Increased concentrations of LDH reach a peak within 24–48 hr after myocardial infarction, but—in contrast to creatine kinase—persist for up to 10 to 14 days (because of slower clearance in continued elaboration from red blood cells involved in the inflammatory exudate in myocardium). Increases in the $LDH_1:LDH_2$ ratio are relatively insensitive and nonspecific criteria of acute myocardial infarction because other processes—such as hemolysis, acute renal failure, megaloblastic anemia, and neoplasms—can induce elevation of LDH_1.

Troponin

Troponin is a structural protein in the contractile apparatus of myocardium and striated muscle that consists of three polypeptide subunits called troponin I (inhibitory), troponin C (catalytic), and troponin T (tropomyosin). With myocardial necrosis, each is released into blood, troponin I and T within 2–4 hr, with elevations persisting for up to 14 days. Thus, increased plasma troponin I and T can be detected long after CK has returned to normal. Troponin T increases with unstable angina, perhaps because of occult myocardial cell death in minute regions. In patients with elevated CK from noncardiac sources, troponin I and T may be more specific for myocardial injury than MB-CK. Elevations of troponin I

Table 1   Causes of Increases in MB-CK Besides Myocardial
Infarction

I.   Increased MB-CK and increased troponin and/or $LDH_1 > LDH_2$
    a.   Myocarditis
    b.   Pericarditis
    c.   Myocardial contusion
    d.   Cardiac surgery
    e.   Repetitive cardiac defibrillation
II. Increased MB-CK and normal troponin
    Low percentage MB-CK relative to total CK
    a.   Extensive muscle trauma
    b.   Rhabdomyolysis
    High percentage MB-CK relative to total CK
    a.   Polymyositis
    b.   Muscular dystrophy
    c.   Other skeletal muscle myopathies
    d.   Chronic renal insufficiency (probably secondary to myopathy)
    e.   Vigorous athletic training (e.g., marathon runners)
    f.   Nonmuscle sources of MB-CK (e.g., neoplasm)
    g.   Delayed clearance of CK (e.g., hypothyroidism)

may be more specific than those of troponin T. Increases in troponin in patients with unstable angina without CK-MB isoenzyme elevations on admission are indicative of high risk for recurrent ischemic events.

Clinical Use of Assays of Cardiac Enzymes and Other Macromolecular Markers

Blood samples should be obtained for measurement of CK and MB-CK from patients with suspected myocardial infarction on admission and at 12 and 24 hr after admission. In patients in whom MB-CK levels are within normal limits but plasma LDH is elevated on admission, LDH isoenzymes should be assayed. If the $LDH_1:LDH_2$ ratio is below 1.0 on admission but infarction is suspected clinically, the assay should be repeated. Elevated troponin I or T in patients with normal plasma MB-CK is highly suggestive of a recent myocardial infarction (perhaps within the past few days).

D.   Noninvasive Cardiac Imaging in Patients with Suspected Myocardial Infarction

Radionuclide procedures and two-dimensional echocardiography are of considerable value in initial evaluation when ECG findings are not diagnostic. However, the lack of availability of noninvasive cardiac imaging should not prohibit prompt implementation of measures to initiate reperfusion.

194

Two-Dimensional Echocardiography

Echocardiography is the modality of choice for imaging the ascending aorta, pericardium, cardiac chambers, and valves. With the use of Doppler and color-flow Doppler techniques, valvular regurgitant and stenotic lesions can be defined rapidly, as can complications of infarction such as ventricular septal rupture. When the ECG is nondiagnostic, a posterior wall motion abnormality can identify infarction in a patient with anterior ST-segment depression. However, echocardiography cannot visualize all segmental wall motion abnormalities. Furthermore, wall motion abnormalities are neither specific nor sensitive criteria of acute myocardial infarction. Nevertheless, echocardiography should be performed as soon as possible in patients with cardiogenic shock so as to exclude potentially treatable mechanical causes such as cardiac rupture, ventricular septal rupture, or papillary muscle rupture and acute and severe mitral regurgitation. Trans-esophageal echocardiography is indicated for patients in whom acute aortic dissection is suspected or those in shock in whom adequate transthoracic images cannot be obtained.

Technetium 99m Pyrophosphate

Uptake of ^{99m}Tc-pyrophosphate is increased in infarcted myocardium. However, imaging does not become positive for infarction until 2 to 5 days after the acute event. Accordingly, this scintigraphic criterion is not useful in initial evaluations unless detection of relatively temporally remote infarction is a major consideration.

Sestamibi Scintigraphy

Myocardial uptake of sestamibi parallels perfusion and is decreased in regions of ischemia or infarction. However, sensitivity is not sufficient to exclude infarction. Thus, imaging is not essential in the initial evaluation of patients with suspected myocardial infarction.

III. INITIAL MANAGEMENT OF PATIENTS WITH ACUTE MYOCARDIAL INFARCTION

A. General Measures

Admission and Monitoring

Admission to an intensive care unit and continuous ECG monitoring are essential. Twelve-lead ECGs should be obtained on admission, on recurrence of symptoms, and at least daily.

Oxygenation

Hypoxemia is common and may exacerbate ischemia. Oxygen should be given by nasal cannula (2 to 4 L/min) and oxygenation monitored with a transcutaneous

195

sensor or by measurement of arterial blood gases (arterial puncture should be deferred for at least 12 hr in patients who will be or have been treated with thrombolytic agents). Higher concentrations of oxygen in the inspired gas should be provided to patients with pulmonary edema (face mask with inspired oxygen concentration of 40–60%). Those who have been intubated to manage severe respiratory dysfunction should be maintained on a ventilator set to provide full assisted support of ventilation (i.e., "assist control" mode) at a rate sufficient to attenuate respiratory efforts by the patient that would otherwise increase the work of breathing. In patients with pulmonary edema, modest amounts of positive end-expiratory pressure (e.g., < 10 cm H_2O) are indicated to increase pulmonary residual volume, optimize oxygenation, and modestly decrease left ventricular preload.

Activity

Patients with suspected myocardial infarction should be at complete bed rest for 24 hr. If necessary, sedation should be provided with low doses of a benzodiazepine or other anxiolytic agent (see Table 5, Chapter 30).

Diet

During the first 24 hr, food intake by mouth should be limited or avoided, particularly in patients who are hemodynamically unstable or in whom invasive procedures may have to be performed. After this, clear liquids are appropriate in high-risk patients. In others, a 1200- to 1800-calorie, low-sodium, low-cholesterol diet can be provided, with dietary restrictions as indicated for other medical problems (e.g., diabetes). Decaffeinated beverages are preferred to caffeinated ones. Stool softeners or mild laxatives should be prescribed to avoid constipation and straining.

B. Risk Stratification

The prognosis of patients with acute myocardial infarction is dependent on the extent to which the patency of the infarct-related artery can be promptly restored and sustained and on the extent of left ventricular dysfunction. Short-term prognosis is determined also by the presence or absence of complications such as acute valvular regurgitation, ventricular septal rupture, or life-threatening ventricular arrhythmias. Initial management should focus on detection and management of significant left ventricular dysfunction, complications of infarction, and induction and maintenance of patency of the infarct-related artery.

Prompt myocardial reperfusion induced with either thrombolytic agents or by primary angioplasty is essential. In patients who, on ECG, present with ST-segment depression or non-Q-wave myocardial infarction, the challenge is not only to restore infarct artery patency but also to prevent subtotal thrombotic coronary artery occlusive lesions from progressing to total occlusion. Initial management entails aspirin and prompt anticoagulation with intravenous heparin. Anticoagulant therapy should be monitored closely. Such patients are often candidates for mechanical interventions such as angioplasty, atherectomy, or coronary artery bypass grafts (CABG), depending on clinical stability, coronary angiographic anatomy, and left ventricular function.

The extent of left ventricular dysfunction is a primary descriptor for short- and long-term morbidity and mortality. Initial evaluation should detect left or right ventricular dysfunction. Prompt institution of therapy to optimize ventricular function is necessary. Angiotensin-converting enzyme (ACE) inhibitors should be used early in the management of most patients with myocardial infarction, particularly when moderate to extensive left ventricular dysfunction is present. Long-term treatment with ACE inhibitors and other afterload-reducing agents reduces morbidity and mortality by favorably influencing ventricular remodeling after infarction.

In 10–20% of patients, acute myocardial infarction is secondary to factors that markedly alter the balance between myocardial oxygen delivery and demand resulting in subendocardial necrosis. Examples include infarction precipitated by severe anemia, aortic regurgitation, marked hypertension, or aortic stenosis. A non-Q-wave myocardial infarction asociated with ST segment depression on the initial ECG is often present. Immediate management should focus on relieving the derangements that induce the infarction (e.g., transfusion, support of blood pressure). Subsequent management of left ventricular dysfunction is similar to that in patients in whom infarction is attributable to unstable coronary atherosclerotic lesions.

Clinical Criteria Useful for Risk Stratification

Low-risk subgroups are characterized by normal blood pressure and heart rate, lack of signs of pulmonary congestion, and a relatively unremarkable cardiac examination (Killip class I). When such patients are treated promptly to induce reperfusion, prognosis is excellent. In-hospital mortality is below 5%. Even in the absence of prompt reperfusion, prognosis is excellent if the extent of infarction is modest (modest elevation of peak MB-CK and limited extent of infarction on the ECG) and the infarction is an initial one.

Pulmonary congestion or an S_3 gallop (Killip class II) suggests more extensive left ventricular dysfunction and is associated typically with more extensive infarction. When early coronary reperfusion is inducible, prognosis is excellent and similar to that in Killip class I patients. Patients in whom coronary reperfusion is induced only late and those in whom it is not inducible are at higher risk for complications and have a greater in-hospital and 1-year mortality.

High-risk patients are characterized by evidence of extensive left ventricular dysfunction, often manifest by severe pulmonary edema (Killip class III) or hypotension and shock (Killip class IV). Morbidity and mortality are extremely high, particularly with shock (80%). All high-risk patients should be evaluated promptly, and whenever possible echocardiographically, to define the extent of left or right ventricular dysfunction and exclude or identify and treat mechanical complications such as acute mitral regurgitation or ventricular septal rupture. Prognosis is improved when prompt reperfusion can be induced with fibrinolytic agents or by primary angioplasty. The latter is preferable in patients in shock when appropriate facilities are immediately available. Initial support with intravenous vasopressors, agents with positive inotropic effects, or circulatory support with intraaortic balloon counterpulsation or left ventricular assist devices is useful in stabilizing such patients and permitting immediate primary angioplasty when necessary. The long-term prognosis is extremely poor in patients with extensive left ventricular dysfunction in whom infarct-related arterial patency cannot be restored.

Right ventricular infarction in patients with inferior wall infarction is an important reversible cause of cardiogenic shock. Systemic hypotension associated with clear lung fields on chest x-ray and elevated jugular venous pressure is characteristic. Electrocardiographic criteria such as ST-segment elevation in the right-sided precordial leads, particularly V_{4R}, may be helpful in confirming the diagnosis.

Estimation of Infarct Size

Morbidity and mortality after acute myocardial infarction are related closely to the extent of infarction (i.e., infarct size). The peak elevation in MB-CK is a semi-quantitative measure of the extent of infarction. Similarly, the number of ECG leads in which ST segment elevation is present as well as the extent of loss of R-wave amplitude after infarction are useful in estimating the extent of infarction, particularly in patients with anterior or lateral wall infarcts. However, enzyme and ECG criteria are less useful in patients in whom reperfusion is implemented. In general, such criteria provide only a semiquantitative measure of the extent of infarction.

Noninvasive cardiac imaging with Doppler/two-dimensional echocardiography or radionuclide ventriculography (RVG) are the most readily available noninvasive modalities for assessment of the extent of left ventricular dysfunction following acute myocardial infarction. Doppler echocardiography has the advantage of defining cardiac structural and valvular abnormalities as well.

Left-Heart Catheterization and Coronary Angiography

Cardiac catheterization and angiography are of value in the early evaluation of patients with suspected myocardial infarction, particularly those with cardiogenic shock, a history of coronary bypass surgery, known multivessel coronary artery disease, previous myocardial infarction, or cardiac disease that may be complicated by acute infarction (e.g., aortic stenosis). In those with contraindications to thrombolytic agents, immediate angiography and primary angioplasty should be considered.

C. Management Contingent on Risk Stratification

Low-Risk Patients

Patients at low risk for complications of myocardial infarction include those with relatively small, completed initial infarcts and those with minimal or only modest left ventricular dysfunction in a setting in which early reperfusion has been induced or subtotal thrombotic coronary obstruction is present. Patients who have been treated with thrombolytic therapy or primary angioplasty as well as those with non-Q-wave infarction require specific management to prevent progression of coronary artery thrombosis and recurrent infarction. Thus, aspirin and anticoagulants should be administered immediately. Patients with small, completed infarctions and preserved left ventricular function can often be managed less aggressively and discharged from the hospital within 5–7 days.

Patients with Small Completed Initial Myocardial Infarcts   Total occlusion of a coronary artery supplying a small area of myocardium is usually the culprit, and a left ventricular ejection fraction of greater than 40% is usually present after infarction. The ECG often exhibits Q waves. However, particularly with infarction involving the circumflex artery distribution, Q waves may not evolve. Peak elevations of MB isoenzymes usually do not exceed 100 IU/L. In some instances, differentiation of such patients from those with non-Q-wave infarction due to a subtotal thrombotic obstruction may be difficult. Management should include the following:

Aspirin.   Aspirin, 180 to 320 mg PO daily, should be continued long term for secondary prevention. Enteric-coated aspirin is often best tolerated.

Beta Blockers.   Beta blockers have been shown to reduce long-term mortality, sudden death, and rates of reinfarction (see Table 1, Chapter 30). In patients with well-preserved left ventricular function, the long-term benefit of beta-blocker therapy is less well established. Nonetheless, it is reasonable to continue treatment for at least 2 years in patients without contraindications.

ACE Inhibitors.   Initiation of treatment with ACE inhibitors within 24 hr of the onset of acute myocardial infarction and continuation for 6 weeks modestly improves survival, independently, in part, of improvement in left ventricular function and remodeling. The initial dose of an ACE inhibitor should be half of the maintenance dose or less (see Table 1, Chapter 30). Subsequent doses should be titrated to maintain systolic blood pressure above 100 mmHg. The value of longer-term treatment (more than 6 to 8 weeks), with ACE inhibitors in patients with normal or only minimal left ventricular dysfunction has not been established.

Patients with Small Infarcts Who Have Not Been Treated to Induce Coronary Recanalization

No Recurrent Ischemia. Patients without recurrent ischemia should undergo noninvasive testing for long-term risk stratification. Symptom-limited, submaximal exercise stress testing can be performed safely within 5 to 7 days after infarction and provides critical information regarding the likelihood of severe coronary artery disease and the potential for recurrent ischemia or infarction. When the ECG is normal, a treadmill or bicycle exercise ECG test can differentiate high- from low-risk patients. High risk is typified by ST-segment depression of 0.2 mV or more with exercise, particularly if present in leads outside the infarct zone; poor exercise capacity; chest discomfort; ventricular arrhythmias; or hypotension during the test. Patients who can complete the exercise protocol without evidence of ischemia are at low risk for cardiac events over the next year.

In patients with ST-segment abnormalities at baseline or left bundle branch block on the ECG, imaging of the myocardium during the exercise test with thallium, radionuclide ventriculography, or echocardiography is of value. In patients unable to exercise, pharmacological stress testing with dipyridamole or adenosine, thallium imaging, or dobutamine echocardiography appear to be safe and potentially useful for risk stratification.

Patients with strongly positive exercise tests or other clinical criteria of high risk of significant three-vessel coronary, left main, or proximal left anterior descending artery disease should be evaluated by coronary angiography.

Postinfarction Ischemia. Patients with postinfarction ischemia, even that following small infarcts, are at risk for recurrent infarction. Many may have unstable subtotal thrombotic coronary occlusion. Recurrent ischemia associated with ECG changes in a region distinct from that involved with the initial infarction suggests three-vessel disease.

Ischemia occurring at rest after an acute infarction is more typically indicative of unstable coronary disease than is that associated with exercise. Patients with recurrent symptoms should be evaluated by ECG at the time of chest discomfort. Blood samples should be obtained for assay of cardiac enzymes. When unstable coronary disease is suspected clinically, anticoagulation with heparin should be either reinstituted or optimized when necessary. Aggressive medical therapy—including titration of the dose of beta blocker to yield a heart rate of 55 to 60 beats/min, sublingual or intravenous nitrates to resolve acute symptoms, and calcium-channel blockers—is indicated if symptoms persist. Most patients with postinfarction angina will require coronary arteriography, and some will need angioplasty.

Patients with Mild Left Ventricular Dysfunction After Early Myocardial Reperfusion Patients with initially successful early reperfusion have an excellent short- and long-term prognosis. The main concern is maintenance of patency of the infarct-related artery long term. Aspirin and anticoagulants, in addition to beta-blocking agents and ACE inhibitors, are useful.

Aspirin.   Aspirin should be administered at a dose of 180–325 mg daily, starting at the time of initiation of fibrinolytic agents or before primary angioplasty, and should be continued indefinitely.

Anticoagulants.   Intravenous heparin should be administered to all patients treated with tissue plasminogen activator and the dose should be titrated to maintain the activated partial thromboplastin time (aPTT) at approximately 2.5 times normal control, usually in a range of 60–85 sec. Doses of heparin associated with excessive prolongation of the aPTT may contribute to intracranial bleeding and should be avoided (see Table 10, Chapter 30). If coronary angiography is planned, heparin should be continued until the procedure is performed or for at least 3 days. The benefits of intravenous compared with high-dose subcutaneous heparin (12,500 U SC, q 12 hr) in patients treated with intravenous streptokinase or urokinase are not as well defined. However, optimal anticoagulation is more easily achieved with intravenous administration of heparin and is preferred in institutions where aPTTs can rapidly be performed. Long-term anticoagulation with warfarin does not improve long-term infarct-related arterial patency compared with aspirin in patients who have been treated with fibrinolytic agents and should not be used in low-risk patients.

Beta Blockers.   In patients treated with fibrinolytic agents, immediate intravenous administration of beta blockers followed by oral administration decreases the incidence of nonfatal infarction and serious ventricular arrhythmias in hospital. It is reasonable to treat patients without contraindications with beta blockers for up to 2 years. However, many elderly patients will experience subtle, often unrecognized depression requiring cessation or dose reduction by an astute physician alert to this possibility.

ACE Inhibitors.   ACE inhibitors appear to enhance recovery early after myocardial reperfusion and should be started within the first 24 hr of the onset of infarction (see above).

Patients with Initially Successful Reperfusion and Minimal Left Ventricular Dysfunction   Recurrent ischemia after coronary thrombolysis, particularly in association with recurrent ST-segment elevation, should be evaluated with urgent coronary angiography to determine whether reocclusion is threatened or has occurred. It is often seen in patients being given suboptimal doses of anticoagulants. Unfortunately, heparin has only limited efficacy in the treatment of high-grade unstable coronary thrombotic lesions. Accordingly, angioplasty may be necessary. Newer anticoagulants—such as the direct-acting antithrombin hirudin—are promising for more effective prevention of reocclusion.

Patients with recurrent chest discomfort at rest after thrombolysis but no ECG signs of reocclusion should be evaluated with coronary angiography to determine the severity of the residual infarct-related coronary lesion and the presence of coronary disease in other vessels. Ideally, angiography should be delayed for several days to permit maximal resolution of the initial coronary thrombosis.

Results of the second Thrombolysis in Myocardial Infarction (TIMI-2) study do not support the routine use of angiography and infarct-related artery angioplasty in low-risk patients without recurrent ischemia after thrombolysis. To reduce the likelihood of unnecessary coronary revascularization in patients with minimal left ventricular dysfunction, noninvasive tests are useful in identifying those who should undergo angiography. In low-risk patients with normal stress tests, morbidity and mortality with conservative medical management appear to be similar to those in patients in whom catheterization is performed and more aggressive treatment is pursued.

Risk stratification in patients who have undergone primary angioplasty is not yet optimal. Because the extent of coronary disease is known, revascularization is often applied to lesions other than those associated with the acute infarction. Whether this approach improves survival remains to be seen.

Patients with Mild Pulmonary Edema and Minimally Decreased Left Ventricular Function The prognosis of these patients is similar to that in those without signs or symptoms of pulmonary congestion, particularly when early reperfusion has been accomplished. In addition to the management outlined above, diuretics and low-dose nitrates are useful. When renal function is normal, furosemide, 10 to 20 mg IV, is effective in inducing diuresis, decreasing lung water, and reducing (virtually immediately) pulmonary venous pressure through pulmonary venous dilatation. Excessive diuresis should be avoided because most patients are not volume overloaded. ACE inhibitors may be particularly beneficial. Beta-blocking agents should be used as well if other contraindications are absent.

High-Risk Patients

Patients with extensive infarction and moderate to severe left ventricular dysfunction are at risk of short- and long-term morbidity and mortality. Significant left ventricular dysfunction may be manifest only by subtle signs such as tachycardia or oliguria. Alternatively, pulmonary edema and shock may supervene. Markedly elevated MB isoenzymes, ECG indications of extensive infarction, and severe left ventricular dysfunction demonstrable by two-dimensional echocardiography help to identify those at high risk.

Patients with Moderate to Severe Left Ventricular Dysfunction Without Pulmonary Edema Patients with moderate to severe left ventricular dysfunction (left ventricular ejection fraction < 40%) are a high-risk subgroup whose long-term morbidity and mortality is improved by treatment with afterload-reducing agents, particularly ACE inhibitors. Their benefit appears to reflect favorable effects on left ventricular remodeling. Long-term patency of the coronary artery favorably influences outcome. Accordingly, aggressive anticoagulation with aspirin and anticoagulants is indicated in patients in whom early reperfusion has been induced. Revascularization in patients without initial recanalization may improve ultimate left ventricular function and long-term survival as well, though the favorable effect is by no means certain.

Aspirin. At a dosage of 180 to 325 mg PO daily, aspirin should be started on admission and continued long-term in all such patients except those treated with long-term warfarin.

Beta Blockers. These agents are indicated even in patients with left ventricular dysfunction; however, the dose should be titrated slowly over several days or longer when the condition is severe. Beta blockers should not be used in patients with marked first-degree AV block (PR interval > 0.24 sec), new bundle branch block, second- or third-degree AV block, or reactive airway disease (e.g., a history of asthma or wheezing on examination). In patients with pulmonary edema or uncompensated left ventricular failure, beta blockers should be deferred until left ventricular function has been optimized with diuretics and afterload-reducing agents. Beta blockers should not be used in patients with hypotension or shock.

ACE Inhibitors. Early initiation of treatment with ACE inhibitors improves early survival in high-risk patients. Long-term treatment appears to provide additional benefits. Thus, these drugs should be started within 24 hr except when systolic blood presure is below 100 mmHg. Initial doses should be half or less of maintenance doses (see appendix table for doses of ACE inhibitors). Subsequent doses should be adjusted to maintain systolic blood pressure above 100 mmHg. Pulmonary artery catheterization is indicated in most patients with severe left ventricular dysfunction and borderline blood pressure to delineate left ventricular filling pressure and cardiac index before these agents are initiated.

Nitrates. Intravenous nitroglycerin may enhance left ventricular remodeling in patients with moderate to severe left ventricular dysfunction, even though improved survival has not been demonstrable. Intravenous nitroglycerin is useful in high-risk patients for treatment of recurrent ischemia, congestive heart failure, and mild hypertension. It should be initiated as an infusion of 10 μg/min with increases of 10 μg/min as needed to a maximum of 200 μg/min. Blood pressure should be monitored closely and dose adjusted to avoid a reduction in systolic blood pressure greater than 10–15%. Hypotension is due to low preload. In patients with inferior wall myocardial infarction complicated by right ventricular dysfunction, intravenous nitrates should be used cautiously and preferably only after volume expansion sufficient to provide adequate left ventricular filling pressure (18–22 mmHg).

Anticoagulants. Intravenous heparin should be administered to most high-risk patients with acute myocardial infarction, even those who have not been treated with fibrinolytic agents or by angioplasty. It can prevent deep venous thrombosis as well as mural thrombus and preserve coronary patency. Intravenous heparin is preferred to the subcutaneous form. Although high-dose subcutaneous

203

heparin has been used, it can result in both under- and overanticoagulation. More consistent therapeutic anticoagulation can be obtained with intravenous heparin. Patients with extensive anterior infarction and apical dyskinesis or documented mural thrombus should be treated with warfarin for 3 to 6 months, with dose adjusted to maintain the international normalized ratio (INR) between 2 and 3. Heparin can be discontinued in other patients when they become fully ambulatory.

Patients with Pulmonary Congestion or Pulmonary Edema   In patients with acute myocardial infarction, increases in lung water are common, ranging from mild pulmonary congestion to severe pulmonary edema and respiratory failure. Initial management should be based on assessment of the extent of left ventricular dysfunction. Patients with minimal left ventricular dysfunction and mild pulmonary edema are at low risk for complications of infarction. High-risk subgroups are those in which pulmonary edema and moderate to severe left ventricular dysfunction are present.

Mild Pulmonary Edema and Mild to Severe Left Ventricular Dysfunction. Diuretics should be used cautiously in patients with moderate to severe left ventricular dysfunction after acute myocardial infarction because such patients often require high filling pressures to maintain optimal cardiac output (see Section IV.E.1). Intravenous nitroglycerin is often useful. However, titration requires monitoring of cardiac pressure via a pulmonary artery catheter. The ACE inhibitors are of particular value and should be continued long term. Digoxin may be useful long term but should be avoided in the acute setting. In patients with systolic blood pressure below 100 mmHg, oliguria, or failure to improve with initial therapy, pulmonary artery catheterization is indicated to guide further management.

Moderate to Severe Pulmonary Edema with Moderate to Severe Left Ventricular Dysfunction.   In these patients, more aggressive management is required, because hypoxemia and the increased work of breathing associated with pulmonary edema may give rise to myocardial ischemia, arrhythmias, and respiratory failure. Patients should be given oxygen by face mask or intubated if respiratory distress ensues. Pulmonary artery catheterization is indicated to guide early management, which often includes nitrates, diuretics, and ACE inhibitors. In patients who are intubated, mechanical ventilation should provide fully assisted support for breathing (i.e., "assist control" mode), and low levels of positive end-expiratory pressure (i.e., < 10 mm H_2O) are indicated.

Mechanical cardiac complications such as acute mitral regurgitation or, less frequently, ventricular septal rupture always should be considered. Two-dimensional echocardiography with Doppler can usually define their presence, but mitral regurgitation may be intermittent because of papillary muscle dysfunction and may be revealed only by the intermittent appearance of V waves in the pulmonary artery occlusive pressure tracing, often in association with exacerbation of symptoms. Patients with severe pulmonary edema and severe mitral regurgitation or ventricular septal rupture will usually require intra-aortic balloon counterpulsation in addition to aggressive afterload reduction with nitroprusside.

Pulmonary Edema with Hypotension/Cardiogenic Shock. In these patients, prognosis is poor. Initial evaluation should always include two-dimensional and Doppler echocardiography to exclude mechanical complications such as acute mitral regurgitation or ventricular septal rupture. Early coronary angiography and primary angioplasty may be of value in patients who present within 24 hr of the onset of infarction. If moderate to severe respiratory distress or shock is present, intubation and mechanical ventilation should be instituted promptly to improve oxygenation and decrease the work of breathing. Pulmonary artery characterization is indicated to monitor cardiac pressures and the response to treatment, including support of blood pressure with agents with positive inotropic effects, such as dobutamine, and afterload reduction. Intra-aortic balloon counterpulsation can be supportive for those with reversible mechanical complications of infarction and those who benefit from urgent coronary revascularization with improvement of left ventricular function.

Patients with Hypotension or Cardiogenic Shock Without Pulmonary Edema Immediate intervention is required in these patients to prevent myocardial and vital organ hypoperfusion, which exacerbates ischemia and shock. Hypotension or shock may be caused by right or left ventricular dysfunction. Clinical criteria may be helpful in determining its cause, but often additional invasive and noninvasive evaluations will be necessary. The first objective is to increase blood pressure (volume expansion if tolerated) and intravenously administer vasopressors and cardiotonics. In patients without pulmonary edema, initial treatment should include a fluid challenge with 500 mL to 1 L of normal saline infused rapidly over 15 to 30 min.

1. Extensive left ventricular dysfunction may be present in any patient with hypotension who presents with anterior wall or extensive posterolateral wall myocardial infarction or infarction in the setting of previous ischemic left ventricular dysfunction or severe aortic stenosis. Initially, pulmonary edema may be absent. Hypotension results from decreased stroke volume, which may be improved by volume challenge in some patients. More often, it is indicative of myocardiogenic shock and will not respond to volume expansion. Intravenous dopamine at doses of 5 to 20 μg/kg/min can support blood pressure. With severe hypotension, intravenous norepinephrine, starting at a dose of 0.5 μg/min and titrated to maintain blood pressure, may be necessary. However, its use may entail unavoidable deleterious effects on jeopardized myocardium. In patients who present within 24 hr after the onset of infarction, emergency primary angioplasty may improve prognosis. Two-dimensional echocardiography with Doppler should be performed to identify or evaluate for left ventricular free wall rupture (which may be subacute), pericardial tamponade, acute mitral regurgitation, and ventricular septal rupture. The latter two complications are invariably accompanied by

pulmonary edema. Intra-aortic balloon counterpulsation is indicated in patients with cardiogenic shock caused by extensive left ventricular dysfunction and those with a mechanical complication if a reversible process is thought to be present as well.

    2. Right ventricular dysfunction should be considered as a cause of cardiogenic shock in patients with acute inferior wall myocardial infarction. If it is present, aggressive volume expansion (e.g., 2 to 5 L of normal saline) is often necessary to increase blood pressure. Intravenous vasopressors should be used to maintain systolic blood pressure above 90 mmHg if the response to initial fluid is inadequate. Early pulmonary artery catheterization is particularly important to avoid overadministration of fluids and to guide further management with intravenous agents such as dobutamine (see Section IV.E.5).

High-grade atrioventricular conduction block often complicates extensive right ventricular infarction (e.g., third-degree AV block). The consequent loss of atrial systole exacerbates right ventricular systolic dysfunction. Temporary atrioventricular pacing may improve cardiac output. Acute atrial fibrillation complicating right ventricular infarction and shock should be cardioverted promptly as well.

    3. Massive pulmonary embolism is a cause of severe right ventricular dysfunction and cardiogenic shock, which can mimic shock caused by inferior and right ventricular myocardial infarction. If this diagnosis is suspected and can be confirmed by ventilation perfusion scintigraphy or pulmonary angiography, thrombolysis is indicated to improve right ventricular function. Initial management should include volume expansion and administration of vasopressors and agents with positive inotropic effects.

    4. Pericardial tamponade may mimic cardiogenic shock. Two-dimensional echocardiography is the modality of choice for diagnosis of pericardial tamponade and should be used to guide emergency pericardiocentesis, which is often life-saving.

    5. Acute aortic dissection may mimic acute myocardial infarction and cardiogenic shock. Proximal ascending aortic dissection can be complicated by acute aortic insufficiency and pericardial tamponade. When it is suspected, transesophageal echocardiography or aortography should be performed immediately. In affected patients in shock, emergency surgical repair of the aortic dissection is the only alternative, but it entails high mortality.

IV. PULMONARY ARTERY CATHETERIZATION AND MANAGEMENT OF HEMODYNAMIC SUBSETS

A. Common Indications

Listed below are common indications for bedside pulmonary artery catheterization with a balloon-tipped catheter in patients with acute myocardial infarction:

- Pulmonary edema with moderate to severe left ventricular dysfunction
- Moderate to severe left ventricular dysfunction with persistent tachycardia and/or borderline hypotension
- Cardiogenic shock and/or hypotension in patients with myocardial infarction unresponsive to initial volume expansion
- Infarction complicated by significant mitral regurgitation, ventricular septal rupture, or potentially hemodynamically significant pericardial infusion
- Oliguria in patients with moderate to severe left ventricular dysfunction unresponsive to volume expansion
- Unexplained severe cyanosis, persistent hypoxemia, or acidosis
- Monitoring of parenterally administered vasoactive agents in high-risk patients requiring aggressive treatment

Systemic blood pressure should be monitored with an intra-arterial radial or femoral catheter in patients with marked hypotension requiring parenteral vasopressor agents. When the blood pressure can be auscultated, it should be measured frequently either with a noninvasive automatic device or manually. All patients with complicated high-risk myocardial infarction should have their urine output monitored closely; this often requires an indwelling catheter.

B. Bedside Pulmonary Artery Catheterization with Balloon-Tipped Catheter

Devices required should be inserted under sterile conditions by individuals trained in their use and in interpretation of hemodynamic waveforms. After insertion, catheters should be maintained patent and sterile by trained personnel. Catheters should be left in place generally for no more than 72 hr and almost never for longer than 96 hr. Careful adherence to sterile insertion, dressings, and limited duration of catheterization reduces the potential for episodes of catheter-related sepsis, which should not occur more than 3–5% of the time. Hemodynamic measurements should be obtained by staff trained to appropriately calibrate and establish a 0 mmHg reference point (typically at the midaxillary line) before acquiring data. Pressures should be measured at end-expiration and recorded. Appropriate catheter position should be confirmed by x-ray immediately after each procedure is performed. Waveforms should be reviewed and validated before results are used to guide patient management.

C. Measurements Obtained by Pulmonary Artery Catheterization

Balloon-tipped pulmonary artery catheters permit measurement of hemodynamic variables and cardiac output by thermodilution. Special catheters are available that permit measurement of continuous pulmonary artery blood oxygen saturation and right ventricular ejection fraction as well. At the time of insertion of the catheter, mixed venous blood can be obtained from the right atrium, right ventricle, and pulmonary artery to determine whether a step up in oxygen saturation is present, indicative of a left-to-right shunt. Such a shunt in a patient with acute myocardial infarction is usually caused by ventricular septal rupture. The following measurements and calculations should be considered:

Right atrial pressure (RAP). Both a and v waves should be present and mean right atrial pressure should be recorded.

Right ventricular pressure (RVP). Increased right ventricular end-diastolic pressure suggests right ventricular dysfunction.

Pulmonary artery pressure (PAP). The PAP should be monitored continuously. Pulmonary artery end-diastolic pressure is similar to the pulmonary artery occlusive pressure in patients without underlying pulmonary vascular disease.

Pulmonary artery occlusive pressure (PAOP). The PAOP is obtained by inflating the balloon at the tip of the catheter. Its waveform should exhibit a and v waves similar to those observed in the right atrial pressure recording but delayed relative to the QRS complex on a simultaneously recorded ECG tracing. The pre-a-wave pressure is the best reflection of left atrial pressure. Large v waves in the PAOP tracing are suggestive of mitral regurgitation.

Pulmonary artery or mixed venous blood oxygen tension. This measurement is of value in patients with significant left ventricular dysfunction to characterize arterial-venous oxygen differences and calculate cardiac output by the Fick principle. Continuous monitoring may be useful in patients with severe left ventricular dysfunction or combined respiratory and cardiac failure.

Cardiac output (CO). The CO should be measured by thermodilution in most patients. Cardiac index [cardiac output/body surface area (CI)] is usually the best reflection of adequacy of CO. Results may be inaccurate in patients with severe tricuspid or mitral regurgitation, marked intracardiac shunts, and/or markedly decreased cardiac output (CI < 1.5 L/min/m^2). If so, CO should be measured by the Fick principle.

Systemic vascular resistance (SVR) and systemic vascular resistance index (SVRI). These measurements are important variables [SVR = (mean arterial pressure − RAP)/CO × 80]. An adequate response to afterload reduction should result in decreased SVR (normal range is 900 to 1350 dynes/sec/cm^{-5}).

Stroke volume (SV) and stroke volume index (SVI). The SV and SVI are calculated by dividing cardiac output by heart rate and are useful in patients treated with agents with positive inotropic effects to determine whether CO improves secondary to an increase in stroke volume, heart rate, or both.

D. Guidelines in Interpreting Hemodynamic Measurements

It is important to establish baseline measurements and follow trends rather than rely on a single measurement. Sudden changes should prompt review of potential misinterpretation attributable to artifact. Hemodynamic data should be considered in the context of blood pressure, pulse, and urine output. Valid changes should correlate with changes noted in the physical examination and symptoms. Patients should not be managed based only on target values for a single hemodynamic variable.

E. Hemodynamic Subsets Characterized by Pulmonary Artery Catheterizations

1. *Decreased left ventricular filling pressures (PAOP < 15–18 mmHg).* In patients with hypotension decreased cardiac index (< 2.5 L/min/m^2), oliguria or persistent sinus tachycardia suggests relative volume depletion. A rapid infusion of 1 L of normal saline may be beneficial. If left ventricular compliance is decreased (e.g., with anterior wall infarction), optimal left ventricular end-diastolic volume usually requires PAOP of 15–18 mmHg or more. Effective volume expansion should increase with PAOP and stroke volume. To avoid development of pulmonary edema, fluid administration should be restricted when PAOP exceeds 18–22 mmHg.

2. *Elevated left ventricular filling pressures (PAOP > 18 mmHg) with a normal cardiac index (> 2.5 L/min/m^2).* This indicates volume overload or decreased left ventricular compliance. Intravenous nitroglycerin or topical nitrates can decrease left ventricular filling pressure if total-body fluid overload is present; diuretics should also be used. This hemodynamic pattern is often seen in patients with marked systemic hypertension and left ventricular hypertrophy. Management of elevated systemic blood pressure and modest diuresis are often beneficial.

3. *Elevated left ventricular filling pressure (PAOP > 18 mmHg), decreased cardiac index (< 2.5 L/min/m^2), and systolic atrial blood pressure > 100 mmHg.* These indicate moderate to severe left ventricular dysfunction. Afterload reduction is the treatment of choice as long as systolic blood pressure exceeds 100 mmHg. In patients with acute myocardial infarction, nitroglycerin is the preferred agent. In addition to decreasing left ventricular filling pressures and afterload, it may improve blood flow to ischemic myocardium. Early oral administration of ACE inhibitors is indicated in hemodynamically stable patients.

Intravenous nitroprusside is a potent vasodilator and can improve hemodynamics in patients with moderate to severe left ventricular dysfunction. However, in patients with acute myocardial infarction, blood flow to ischemic regions may be decreased (i.e., coronary steal). Intravenous nitroprusside is nonetheless the drug of choice to control persistent, marked hypertension.

Most patients with moderate to severe left ventricular dysfunction will respond to initial therapy with nitrates, ACE inhibitors, and modest diuresis. However, if systemic blood pressure drops below 100 mmHg or the cardiac index does not increase, an agent with positive inotropic effects, typically dobutamine or amrinone, should be added.

4. *Elevated left ventricular filling pressures (PAOP > 18 mmHg), decreased cardiac index (< 2.5 L/min/m²), and systolic arterial blood pressure < 100 mmHg* indicate severe left ventricular dysfunction, and — in patients with organ hypoperfusion (e.g., oliguria, confusion) — shock. If systolic blood pressure is between 90 and 100 mmHg, support with dobutamine is usually indicated. Cautious administration of ACE inhibitors will often improve cardiac function without further decreasing blood pressure. If systolic blood pressure is below 90 mmHg or if cardiogenic shock is present, intravenous vasopressors should be used to increase the systolic blood pressure to at least 90 mmHg. Dopamine is preferred, but in patients with severe hypotension, norepinephrine may be necessary. In patients with treatable mechanical complications of infarction such as severe mitral regurgitation or ventricular septal rupture or in those who are candidates for heart transplantation, intra-aortic balloon counterpulsation can provide stabilization to "buy time" until a definitive procedure can be performed.

5. *Right ventricular myocardial infarction.* This diagnosis is usually suggested by clinical signs and confirmed by finding a decreased cardiac index (< 2.5 L/min/m²) with elevated right atrial pressure (> 10 mmHg) and relatively low or normal PAOP (8–12 mmHg). Right atrial pressure may not be elevated until after intravenous fluids have been administered. If systolic blood pressure is 90–100 mm Hg and the cardiac index is depressed, fluids should be administered until PAOP is 15–18 mm Hg. If the cardiac index remains depressed or hypotension is severe, dobutamine should be administered. Patients with both extensive right ventricular and right atrial infarction may be particularly difficult to manage. Complicating atrial arrhythmias or AV conduction block can cause atrial-ventricular dysynchrony. In that case, AV sequential pacing may be helpful.

F. Recognition and Management of Complications of Invasive Procedures

All invasive vascular procedures can cause bleeding— minor or life-threatening. The risk depends in part on the adequacy of hemostasis. Patients treated with fibrinolytic agents are at the highest risk. Even treatment with aspirin alone increases risk modestly. Percutaneous venous or arterial puncture carries the highest risk of minor bleeding complications. Cutdowns carry less risk. In patients treated with fibrinolytic agents, even apparently uncomplicated internal jugular or subclavian vein catheterization can result in serious or life-threatening bleeding (e.g., hemothorax, hemopericardium). Although femoral vein catheterization is often performed when hemostasis is impaired, severe retroperitoneal bleeding may result. All patients who have undergone invasive vascular procedures should be monitored closely to detect and reverse potential complications.

A thorough physical examination before and after the procedure is essential. A chest x-ray should be obtained after placement of central venous lines, transvenous pacemakers, or pulmonary artery catheters. Invasive vascular procedures should not cause more than minor local discomfort. Complaints of lower back or groin pain after placement of a femoral venous or arterial catheter suggest extravascular bleeding. Sudden shortness of breath or chest discomfort after placement of a jugular or subclavian vein catheter usually indicates hemothorax, pneumothorax, or hemomediastinum. Complications are particularly frequent in patients who have undergone invasive arterial procedures after treatment with fibrinolytic agents. Catheterization site hematomas, retroperitoneal bleeding, pseudoaneurysms, and arteriovenous fistulas may occur. In patients with minor bleeding around arterial catheter sheaths, placement of a larger sheath may sometimes be of value.

Management varies depending on the specific complication. All patients with serious bleeding should be transfused immediately to yield a hematocrit of approximately 30%. Whenever possible, anticoagulants should be discontinued, and, if necessary, fresh-frozen plasma administered. Patients with moderate to severe left ventricular dysfunction with or without pulmonary edema may require placement of a pulmonary artery catheter to monitor the response to aggressive infusion of blood and/or plasma. Platelet transfusions may be needed in patients who develop thrombocytopenia. Often, surgical exploration can be avoided if the underlying bleeding diathesis is corrected. However, it may be necessary; if so, it should not be delayed.

V. MANAGEMENT OF BRADYARRHYTHMIAS AND CONDUCTION ABNORMALITIES IN PATIENTS WITH MYOCARDIAL INFARCTION

A. Bradyarrhythmias and Atrioventricular Conduction Abnormalities

These occur frequently. Management depends on diversity and adverse consequences, usually hypotension and additional conduction abnormalities. Temporary transvenous pacing can stabilize patients with severe bradyarrhythmias or conduction abnormalities and is justified prophylactically in those at high risk of progression to third-degree heart block.

Asymptomatic bradycardias and atrioventricular conduction abnormalities include sinus bradycardia and first-, second-, and third-degree atrioventricular blocks, which frequently occur without accompanying symptoms or hypotension. In asymptomatic patients, temporary transvenous pacing is indicated only if the risk of progression to complete heart block is high.

In patients with inferior wall myocardial infarction, atrioventricular conduction blocks are particularly frequent at the time of presentation and often resolve with reperfusion. Transient high-grade second- and third-degree atrioventricular blocks require close monitoring but not necessarily insertion of a pacemaker. However, third-degree block and bradycardia can be exacerbated in patients with inferior wall infarction when reperfusion is induced, particularly with primary angioplasty. Prophylactic transvenous pacing is indicated in those with persistent third-degree atrioventricular block and those thought to be at particularly high risk for exacerbation.

In patients with anterior wall myocardial infarction, new second- and third-degree atrioventricular conduction blocks are suggestive of extensive infarction and associated with a poor prognosis. Even in asymptomatic patients, a temporary transvenous pacemaker should be inserted when Mobitz type II second-degree atrioventricular block or third-degree atrioventricular block is present or when Mobitz type I atrioventricular block is accompanied by intraventricular conduction block (QRS > 0.12 sec). Patients with these manifestations are likely to have involvement of the conduction system below the atrioventricular node and are at high risk for progression to complete heart block.

New conduction block is usually indicative of extensive myocardial damage and is associated with a high risk of progression to complete heart block and death. Placement of a temporary transvenous pacemaker should be considered in asymptomatic patients who present with right bundle branch block with either left anterior or posterior fascicular block of new or indeterminate age or new left bundle branch block, particularly in the setting of an anterior infarction. Preexisting left bundle branch block generally does not require a prophylactic temporary transvenous pacer. However, if marked first-degree AV block and anterior infarction are present or pulmonary artery catheterization is planned, temporary pacing is usually indicated.

Sinus bradycardia and junctional rhythm (impaired AV conduction) occur frequently in patients with acute inferior infarction and may give rise to hypotension (in part because of lack of well-timed atrial transport function). Symptomatic patients should be treated initially with intravenous atropine at a dose of 0.5 mg, which can be repeated to a maximum of 2 mg. In patients who are unresponsive to atropine (with both correction of the bradycardia and the hypotension), temporary transcutaneous external pacing can be instituted to improve hemodynamics until a transvenous pacemaker can be inserted. The most common error is administration of an insufficient amount of atropine or failure to recognize that a given heart rate is indicative of relative bradycardia in the setting of hypotension. Most symptomatic atrioventricular blocks are high-grade Mobitz I or Mobitz II second-degree block or third-degree block. Some patients with inferior wall myocardial infarction and second-degree AV block will respond to atropine alone and require no further treatment. For most of the remainder, temporary transvenous ventricular pacing is sufficient. In patients with right ventricular infarction or those with extensive left ventricular infarction, temporary atrioventricular pacing may be needed to improve cardiac output to a greater extent than that induced by ventricular pacing alone.

Indications for Permanent Pacing After Myocardial Infarction

Persistent high-grade second- or third-degree atrioventricular block after infarction should be supported with permanent pacing if infarction has been extensive. Permanent pacemaker insertion should be delayed for at least 5 to 7 days because many conduction disturbances will revert spontaneously by then. Placement of a permanent pacemaker is indicated in patients with bundle branch block and transient atrioventricular block and in selected patients with high-grade second-degree AV block if conduction system disease below the level of the atrioventricular node is present.

VI. MANAGEMENT OF TACHYARRHYTHMIAS AND VENTRICULAR ARRHYTHMIAS IN PATIENTS WITH MYOCARDIAL INFARCTION

A. Life-Threatening Ventricular Arrhythmias

Ventricular fibrillation and sustained ventricular tachycardia occur frequently within the first 24 to 48 hr after onset of infarction and are the most common cause of early death. Immediate treatment is discussed in Chapter 19, dealing with advanced cardiac life support. Patients who have been successfully resuscitated should be treated with intravenous lidocaine by infusion of 2–4 mg/min for 24–48 hr after admission. Doses should be reduced in patients who are more than 70 years of age, are lean, and have severe congestive heart failure as well as hepatic or renal dysfunction, neurological disease, or shock. Blood levels should be monitored in high-risk patients who are treated for more than 24 hr.

Recurrent ventricular fibrillation or sustained ventricular tachycardia may reflect extensive left or right infarction and be difficult to manage.

Bretylium is used to prevent recurrent ventricular fibrillation or tachycardia unresponsive to lidocaine. After a loading dose of 5 mg/kg over 8 to 10 min, repeated once, a continuous infusion of 1 to 2 mg/min can be given. Long-term infusions may induce hypotension; therefore close monitoring is required.

Procainamide is used when ventricular arrhythmias are refractory to lidocaine. A loading dose of 17 mg/kg should be administered at a rate not exceeding 30 mg/min, followed by a 1- to 4-mg/min maintenance infusion. Hypotension, prolongation of the QT interval, and QRS widening may occur. The infusion should be stopped if hypotension or QRS widening greater than 50% occurs.

Ventricular tachycardia refractory to drugs may be suppressed by overdrive atrioventricular or ventricular pacing when the coupling interval between the sinus beat and the onset of the tachycardia is sufficiently long.

Patients with recurrent ventricular fibrillation or sustained ventricular tachycardia, particularly occurring 48 hr or more after the onset of infarction, are at high risk of subsequent sudden death and should be studied electrophysiologically to define optimal long-term treatment (see Chapter 17, on electrophysiology).

B. Electromechanical Dissociation, or Pulseless Electrical Activity

Electromechanical dissociation or pulseless electrical activity in patients with suspected acute myocardial infarction is an ominous condition presaging an extremely high mortality. It is often caused by cardiac rupture or extensive irreversible left ventricular injury and dysfunction. Rupture occurs typically within the first week after acute infarction and is often preceded by persistent chest pain refractory to medical therapy.

Pulseless electrical activity may occur with conditions other than acute myocardial infarction, including tension pneumothorax, cardiac tamponade, massive pulmonary embolism, severe hypoxia, and severe hypotension due to shock. Many of these can accompany or complicate infarction. Treatment is reversal of the underlying condition whenever possible. Patients may respond to aggressive volume expansion, epinephrine 1 mg IV repeated every 3 to 5 min, vasopressors, or, rarely, atropine, 1 mg IV, for treatment of severe bradycardias.

C. Symptomatic but Non-Life-Threatening Arrhythmias

Nonsustained ventricular tachycardia, particularly when episodes are prolonged, may be associated with hypotension, ischemic chest pain, or worsening of heart failure. Recurrent symptomatic ventricular tachycardia after myocardial infarction can increase the risk of sudden death. Patients affected should undergo electrophysiological evaluation to define long-term therapy. Intravenous lidocaine, at a loading dose of 1 to 1.5 mg/kg followed by 0.75 to 1.5 mg/kg for 5 to 10 min if needed, is usually effective as initial treatment. A continuous infusion of

2–4 mg/min should follow. In patients who do not respond to lidocaine, procainamide should be given in a loading dose of 17 mg/kg at a rate less than or equal to 30 mg/min. Bretylium is a third-line choice for the treatment of recurrent symptomatic ventricular tachycardia. Unfortunately, prolonged infusions can induce hypotension. In patients unresponsive to lidocaine or procainamide, bretylium can be administered at an initial dose of 5 mg/kg over 8 to 10 min, followed by a second 5-mg/kg loading dose and a subsequent continuous infusion of 1 to 2 mg/min.

Patients given doses of these agents should be monitored closely for widening of the QRS, prolongation of the QT interval, or hypotension. Overdrive atrioventricular pacing may help in patients whose arrhythmias are refractory to drugs (see Chapter 16).

Supraventricular tachycardias such as sinus tachycardia, paroxysmal supraventricular tachycardia, atrial fibrillation, and atrial flutter are common and are often associated with exacerbation of myocardial ischemia, congestive heart failure, or hypotension. The first step in their initial management is exclusion of sinus tachycardia. If tachycardia is present, it is often indicative of severe left ventricular dysfunction requiring evaluation with cardiac imaging and pulmonary artery catheterization (see Section IV). Unstable patients with supraventricular tachycardia that is not sinus tachycardia should be treated by cardioversion immediately. In patients who are clinically stable, intravenous adenosine is the drug of choice for terminating atrioventricular nodal reentry tachycardias, and it may help to define the nature of the tachycardia. It should be given as 6 mg IV via rapidly pushed bolus over 3 to 5 sec followed by a 20-ml flush of the intravenous line with saline or 5% dextrose in water. A second dose of 12 mg should be administered, if needed, to revert the arrhythmia to sinus rhythm, in the same manner. In stable patients with recurrent supraventricular tachycardia or supraventricular tachycardia refractory to adenosine, other drugs such as diltiazem, verapamil, propranolol, or digoxin can be used (see Chapter 16 on the management of supraventricular tachycardias).

Atrial fibrillation or flutter may occur secondary to acute myocardial infarction or to factors such as hypoxia, pulmonary embolism, or thyrotoxicosis in patients who present with suspected myocardial infarction. A rapid ventricular response in patients with infarction may exacerbate cardiac ischemia and worsen ventricular function because of loss of the atrial contribution to ventricular filling. Accordingly, patients who are either symptomatic or who manifest signs of hemodynamic compromise should be sedated and the rhythm cardioverted electrically beginning with energy of 100 J to a maximum of 300 J. If electrical cardioversion is unsuccessful, a loading dose of intravenous procainamide can be administered and electrical cardioversion attempted again. In patients with possible digitalis toxicity, electrical cardioversion is contraindicated because of the risk of inducing ventricular arrhythmias mediated by the Wedensky effect. Rapid atrial overdrive pacing may be of help.

Atrial fibrillation or atrial flutter that does not compromise hemodynamics can be managed with intravenous diltiazem, beta blockers, or digoxin to control the rate of the ventricular response. These rhythms are often transient and may convert to normal sinus rhythm without specific antiarrhythmic therapy. All patients who have new-onset atrial fibrillation in the setting of acute myocardial infarction should be anticoagulated with heparin.

D. Asymptomatic Arrhythmias

Accelerated idioventricular rhythm (AIVR) often occurs at the time of reperfusion in patients with acute myocardial infarction treated with fibrinolytic agents. The AIVR is a wide-QRS-complex rhythm typically at a rate of 60 to 100 beats/min; it is usually not responsible for hemodynamic compromise and is benign. Rarely, AIVR persists or results in hypotension because of loss of the atrial filling function. Then either atropine— to accelerate sinus rate and overdrive and suppress the AIVR—or overdrive atrioventricular or ventricular pacing is necessary.

Nonsustained ventricular tachycardia does not require treatment in patients with acute myocardial infarction, even though it is a sign of risk for sudden death. Patients affected should be evaluated electrophysiologically.

Premature ventricular contractions (PVCs) occur frequently in patients with acute myocardial infarction and should not be treated when they are isolated or unassociated with precipitation of sustained or symptomatic ventricular tachycardia or VF. In patients who require suppression of PVCs, lidocaine, procainamide, and, rarely, bretylium may be needed, as outlined in Chapter 16.

VII. REHABILITATION AND SECONDARY PREVENTION AFTER MYOCARDIAL INFARCTION

A. Activity

The level and progression of physical activity after acute infarction is dependent, in large part, on whether the patient is at low or high risk of complications. Low-risk patients initially should be kept at bed rest but encouraged to sit up and dangle their feet over the side of the bed during the first 24 hours. Subsequently, they should be encouraged to provide their own personal hygiene and use a beside commode, undertake limited walking on the third day, and gradually increase activity over the next few days while being monitored by telemetry. They can usually be discharged within a week—some (successful reperfusion and minimal left ventricular dysfunction) have been discharged as early as 3 days after admission.

High-risk patients generally require hospitalization for 7 to 10 days or more if late coronary revascularization becomes necessary. During the first 3 days, high-risk patients on vasodilators should be evaluated to detect and obviate orthostatic changes in blood pressure. Use of a bedside commode should be deferred until intravenous vasodilators have been discontinued. Subsequently, patients should walk slowly with blood pressure and pulse monitored to detect orthostatic changes. Close monitoring by telemetry is needed while progressive ambulation is implemented over days 5 to 7. Discharge within 10 days is anticipated unless the course is complicated by refractory left ventricular dysfunction, recurrent arrhythmias, or the need for late coronary revascularization.

B. Counseling

Counseling should begin during hospitalization to the reduce risk of subsequent cardiac events. Smoking cessation programs provided by the hospital or the American Heart Association should be encouraged. Control of hypercholesterolemia, hypertension, or diabetes should be emphasized. Dietary restrictions should be reviewed with the patient before discharge. Postdischarge counseling is essential for reinforcement.

After discharge, activity at home should be increased gradually. Walking should be encouraged and increased daily at home, outside in warm weather, or in an indoor walking program facility. Heavy lifting, driving, stair climbing, and sexual activity should be avoided until inducible ischemia has been excluded by appropriate monitoring. A supervised exercise rehabilitation program may be of considerable assistance.

C. Risk Stratification After Myocardial Infarction

Low-risk patients (defined in Section III) should undergo submaximal exercise testing 6 to 10 days after infarction. Those with inducible ischemia should undergo coronary angiography. High-risk patients should undergo either early submaximal stress testing (i.e., 6 to 10 days) or symptom-limited exercise testing 2 to 3 weeks after infarction. Those who have undergone coronary angiography but not coronary bypass surgery should be evaluated by symptom-limited exercise testing after hospital discharge. Patients with inducible ischemia are at high risk for subsequent cardiac events and should be evaluated by coronary angiography for possible revascularization.

D. Secondary Prevention

Management of Risk Factors

See Chapter 27, "Preventive Cardiology."

Medical Therapy

Long-term treatment with aspirin, beta-blocking agents, and ACE inhibitors decreases morbidity and mortality after myocardial infarction and should be implemented.

217

SUGGESTED READING

Anonymous. ACC/AHA guidelines for the clinical application of echocardiography: A report of the American College of Cardiology/American Heart Association Task Force on Assessment of Diagnostic and Therapeutic Cardiovascular Procedures (Subcommittee to Develop Guidelines for the Clinical Application of Echocardiography). J Am Coll Cardiol 1990; 16:1505–1528.

Anonymous. ACC/AHA guidelines for cardiac catheterization and cardiac catheterization laboratories: American College of Cardiology/American Heart Association Ad Hoc Task Force on Cardiac Catheterization. J Am Coll Cardiol 1991; 18:1149–1182.

Anonymous. Guidelines and indications for coronary artery bypass graft surgery: A report of the American College of Cardiology/American Heart Association Task Force on Assessment of Diagnostic and Therapeutic Cardiovascular Procedures (Subcommittee on Coronary Artery Bypass Graft Surgery). J Am Coll Cardiol 1991; 17:543–589.

Anonymous. Guidelines for percutaneous transluminal coronary angioplasty: A report of the American College of Cardiology/American Heart Association Task Force on Assessment of Diagnostic and Therapeutic Cardiovascular Procedures (Committee on Percutaneous Transluminal Coronary Angioplasty). J Am Coll Cardiol 1993; 22: 2033–2054.

Cummins RD, ed. Textbook of Advanced Cardiac Life Support. Dallas: American Heart Association, 1994.

Dreifus LS, Fisch C, et al. Guidelines for implantation of cardiac pacemakers and antiarrhythmia devices: A report of the American College of Cardiology/American Heart Association Task Force on Assessment of Diagnostic and Therapeutic Cardiovascular Procedures (Committee on Pacemaker Implantation). J Am Coll Cardiol 1991;18: 1–13.

Gruppo Italiano per lo Studio della Sopravvivenza nell'Infarto Miocardico. GISSI-3: effects of lisinopril and transdermal glyceryl trinitrate singly and together on 6-week mortality and ventricular function after acute myocardial infarction. Lancet 1994; 343:1115–1122.

Gunnar RM, Passamani ER, et al. Guidelines for the early management of patients with acute myocardial infarction: A report of the American College of Cardiology/American Heart Association Task Force on Assessment of Diagnostic and Therapeutic Cardiovascular Procedures (Subcommittee to Develop Guidelines for the Early Management of Patients with Acute Myocardial Infarction). J Am Coll Cardiol 1990; 16:240–292.

Lavie CJ, Gersh BJ. Mechanical and electrical complications of acute myocardial infarction. Mayo Clin Proc 1990; 65:709–730.

Moss AJ, Benhorn J. Prognosis and management after a first myocardial infarction. N Engl J Med 1990; 322:743–753.

Pfeffer MA, Braunwald E, et al. Effect of captopril on mortality and morbidity in patients with left ventricular dysfunction after myocardial infarction. Results of the survival and ventricular enlargement trial. The SAVE Investigators [see comments]. N Engl J Med 1992; 327:669–677.

Simoons ML. Myocardial infarction: ACE inhibitors for all? For ever? Lancet 1994; 344:279–281.

Swedberg K, Held P, et al. Effects of the early administration of enalapril on mortality in patients with acute myocardial infarction: Results of the Cooperative New Scandinavian Enalapril Survival Study II (CONSENSUS II) [see comments]. N Engl J Med 1992; 327:678–684.

Topol EJ, Holms DR, et al. Coronary angiography after thrombolytic therapy for acute myocardial infarction. Ann Intern Med 1991; 114:877–885.

12

Management of Patients with Congestive Heart Failure

I.	Definition of Terms	221
II.	Predominantly Diastolic Dysfunction	223
III.	Left Ventricular Systolic Dysfunction	225
IV.	Pathophysiology of Congestive Heart Failure Related	
	to Left Ventricular Systolic Dysfunction	225
V.	Clinical Presentations	227
VI.	Evaluations	227
VII.	Treatment of Congestive Heart Failure	229

James A. Goldstein

I. DEFINITION OF TERMS

"Congestive heart failure" (CHF) is a term applied to diverse clinical presentations of syndromes with diverse etiology, pathogenesis, prognosis, and requirements for treatment. It conjures an image of a dilated, poorly pumping left ventricle in which impaired systolic function is manifest by depressed ejection fraction and cardiac output. These result in "forward failure" characterized by fatigue and reduced exercise tolerance and later by low output and sometimes cardiogenic shock. Associated diastolic dysfunction leads to "backward failure," resulting in exertional dyspnea early and pulmonary edema in its most severe form. When a result of a myocardial insult (secondary to ischemia, myocarditis, or alcohol abuse, among other phenomena), the extent of left ventricular (LV) systolic dysfunction determines not only the magnitude of hemodynamic impairment and severity of symptoms but the gravity of prognosis as well.

Numerous conditions can result in similar symptoms (fatigue, dyspnea, leg swelling) and signs (hypoperfusion, rales, elevated venous pressures, peripheral edema) of CHF in the presence of normal LV systolic function, and some may be independent of any LV pathology whatsoever. For example, patients with primary LV diastolic dysfunction (attributable to hypertrophy or an infiltrative cardiomyopathy) may present with exertional dyspnea or frank pulmonary edema despite normal LV function or hypercontractility. Clearly, treatment and prognosis differ from those for CHF caused primarily by depression of LV systolic function.

Mitral valve disease (both regurgitation and stenosis) can result not only in pulmonary congestion but also in right heart failure precipitated by postcapillary pulmonary hypertension. Such a presentation is often termed CHF, but the left ventricle may, in fact, be entirely normal.

The term "CHF" is applied liberally to syndromes in patients who present with symptoms related to predominant right heart failure, characterized by elevated jugular venous pressure, peripheral edema, hepatomegaly, and ascites alone or in combination. Although such clinical findings, reflecting increased central venous pressures, are typically attributable to right heart pathology, they may be stigmata of extracardiac venous obstructions (e.g., the superior vena caval syndrome). Furthermore, even when they are indicative of elevated right heart filling pressures, they may reflect pericardial disease (constriction or tamponade), tricuspid valve abnormalities (incompetence or obstruction), left-to-right atrial shunt with an atrial septal defect (ASD), a right ventricular cardiomyopathic processes (restrictive or dilated), or pulmonary arterial hypertension (resulting from primary lung disease, pulmonary valvular disease, pulmonary vascular disease, pulmonary thromboembolism, or pulmonary venous hypertension attributable to left heart disease).

Accordingly, the term "CHF" can be misleading, as exemplified by the patient with acute exacerbation of chronic obstructive lung disease who presents with intense dyspnea (related to intrinsic lung disease) with secondary pulmonary hypertension ("cor pulmonale"), resulting in symptoms and signs of right heart failure. Such a constellation of findings is often termed CHF; in fact, it represents pure right heart failure without left heart involvement, requiring evaluation and management and associated with a prognosis totally different from those in patients with CHF related to severe depression of LV systolic function. It is imperative that patients who present with symptoms and signs consistent with CHF be differentiated according to the pathophysiological mechanisms and etiologies responsible for hemodynamic derangements. Specific considerations include (a) determining whether the clinical presentation reflects derangements of the left heart, right heart, or both; (b) whether the underlying pathophysiological derangement is attributable to myocardium, valves, or pericardium; (c) determining whether "myocardial failure" is diastolic, systolic, or both; and (d) whether pathophysiological-hemodynamic derangements result in diastolic "backward" failure, systolic "forward" failure, or both.

II. PREDOMINANTLY DIASTOLIC DYSFUNCTION

Predominantly diastolic dysfunction results in backward failure. Left heart diastolic dysfunction results in pulmonary venous congestion, leading to dyspnea and pulmonary edema (with potential complications of secondary "postcapillary" pulmonary hypertension and right heart failure), whereas right-sided diastolic dysfunction results in systemic venous congestion. Severe diastolic limitations on either side of the heart may occur with myocardial abnormalities accompanying hypertrophy (both primary and that from pressure overload), ischemia, and infiltrative and fibrotic processes; valvular stenotic obstruction of the semilunar valves (aortic or pulmonary) or obstruction of the atrioventricular (AV) valves (tricuspid and mitral); or pericardial abnormalities (constriction or tamponade). Most clinical presentations include evidence that the ventricles are stiff and that preload is relatively modest. However, volume overload resulting from regurgitant lesions of the semilunar or AV valves as well as shunts at the ductal, atrial, or ventricular level can lead to ventricular dilatation with manifestations of diastolic dysfunction in a volume-overloaded chamber with still intact contractility.

Appreciation of the compliance characteristics and diastolic performance of the cardiac chambers is critical to an understanding of the pathophysiology of predominantly diastolic dysfunction. Cardiac chambers (both atria and ventricles) operate on diastolic pressure-volume filling curves that characterize their compliance. Stiff, noncompliant chambers (hypertrophic ventricles or those with infiltrations such as amyloid) require high filling pressures for myofibrillar stretch in accommodating a given diastolic volume. However, the diastolic properties of a given chamber are influenced by factors besides intrinsic stiffness of the chamber volume. One is the diastolic filling period, which, when reduced, exacerbates diastolic dysfunction because of the inward preload required (i.e., end-diastolic pressure) to maintain ventricular filling. Accordingly, increased heart rate, which shortens the diastolic filling period, can exacerbate or precipitate diastolic hemodynamic abnormalities.

Chamber compliance can be altered extrinsically by pericardial compression or restraint (tamponade or constriction), or through chamber interactions in diastole, through which the compliance and filling of one chamber (atrium or ventricle) is altered by pressure and/or volume overload of its contralateral neighbor, mediated by a shared septum. Such adverse interactions are intensified by the presence of the normal pericardium, which tightly, functionally links the cardiac chambers. When the ventricle is stiff, the atrial contribution (mediated by atrial contraction) to ventricular filling becomes critical not only with regard to main-

223

taining optimum preload and ventricular output but particularly with respect to delivering the preload at a mean atrial pressure sufficiently low to preclude signs and symptoms of backward failure. The importance of the atrial "booster pump" transport function is underscored by the potentially profound, deleterious effects of its loss (associated with supraventricular tachycardias, AV block, or primary atrial contractile dysfunction related to ischemia), which can precipitate both backward failure and a low forward output when ventricular compliance is low.

A. Evaluation of Predominantly Diastolic Dysfunction

In patients who present with symptoms and/or signs of backward left or right heart failure, differentiation of their origins with respect to myocardium, valves, or pericardium is essential. For those with myocardial derangements, delineation of the status of ventricular systolic performance is critical to differentiate primary diastolic from secondary diastolic abnormalities (e.g., those associated with primary systolic dysfunction). Although pertinent aspects of the history and physical examination can help in the evaluation of patients with "backward" failure and in establishing underlying etiology, two-dimensional ultrasound is the most effective, widely applicable, and accurate noninvasive method with which to distinguish myocardial, valvular, and pericardial abnormalities and to assess ventricular systolic function. Echocardiography provides data delineating abnormal wall thickening and thickness, valvular obstruction or regurgitation, chamber enlargement, and pericardial effusion, constriction, or thickening. Doppler echocardiography provides data relevant to ventricular compliance with respect to filling and flow patterns across the AV valves—data particularly relevant to hemodynamically significant diastolic abnormalities. Invasive hemodynamic assessment may be helpful and necessary in some patients to define the presence and patterns of hemodynamic abnormalities, relate perturbations to symptoms, delineate etiological and pathophysiological factors (e.g., demonstrate constrictive or restrictive physiology), and monitor therapy. Invasive studies, including endomyocardial biopsy, may be helpful in establishing etiology (e.g., restrictive cardiomyopathies related to infiltrative processes such as sarcoid or amyloid.

B. Management of Primary Diastolic Dysfunction

The therapy of diastolic heart failure is determined predominantly by the nature of the underlying pathophysiological abnormality and etiology and the severity of impairment. Thus, therapy targeted toward derangements in the pericardium and pericardial space (tamponade and constriction) or valves (obstructions and leaks) can be definitive. In patients with primary myocardial disease, some specific etiologies lend themselves to specific interventions (e.g., antihypertensive therapy for patients with hypertension and hypertrophy, ventricular pacing for those with hypertrophic obstructive cardiomyopathy, and pharmacological interventions for those with ischemic heart disease with predominant diastolic abnormalities). However, for most patients with primary ventricular diastolic dysfunction and some with pericardial and valvular disease in whom direct interventions are either unwarranted or unsuccessful, nonspecific therapy designed to "unload" the stiff chambers (diuretics and venodilators) may be helpful. Caution must be employed because the optimum filling pattern may be very narrow, and even moderate diuresis or venodilatation may result in suboptimal filling and subsequent low output. In patients with hypertrophic hearts, agents that depress contractility (beta blockers, calcium channel blockers with negative inotropic effects, disopyramide, and amiodarone) may be beneficial. Beta blockers may be particularly helpful not only because they reduce contractility but also because the blunting heart rate at rest and with exertion thereby increasing diastolic filling time and potentially improving diastolic performance. In patients with symptomatically severe and functionally limiting predominant diastolic dysfunction refractory to other interventions, cardiac transplantation may be required.

III. LEFT VENTRICULAR SYSTOLIC DYSFUNCTION

The availability of effective technology and pharmacological agents has altered the natural history of congestive heart failure (CHF) resulting from severe left ventricular systolic dysfunction. In the past, CHF in the western world was most frequently a result of rheumatic heart disease, untreated hypertension, and ischemia. Over the past 10 to 20 years, the incidence of rheumatic heart disease has declined, and hypertension has been detected earlier and treated more effectively. Concomitantly, therapeutic advances have increased the survival of patients with ischemic heart disease, including those with impaired ventricular performance. Earlier recognition and more aggressive treatment of acute and chronic manifestations of ischemic heart disease have facilitated detection of left ventricular dysfunction at early stages.

Ischemia is now the most common etiological culprit in patients with CHF. Affected patients frequently present at an advance age with many associated cardiovascular problems, such as coronary disease, aortic stenosis, and arrhythmias as well as concomitant dysfunction in other organ systems including kidney, liver, and brain, all of which influence the pathophysiology, natural history, and management of CHF.

IV. PATHOPHYSIOLOGY OF CONGESTIVE HEART FAILURE RELATED TO LEFT VENTRICULAR SYSTOLIC DYSFUNCTION

Cardiovascular hemodynamics can be viewed as an analogy to Ohm's law, with blood flow determined by the pressure difference (voltage) driving flow across the

225

organ vascular bed divided by the vascular resistance within the bed (resistance). Cardiac output, determined by the stroke volume generated by the left ventricle with each beat and heart rate, underlies perfusion, but the system is pressure-dependent. Thus, circulatory homeostatic mechanisms sustain blood pressure, thereby maintaining perfusion. Blood pressure sensors (baroreceptors) are present in vessels within or supplying organs that are particularly vulnerable to hyperperfusion, such as the brain and the kidney. Thus, reduced blood pressure elicits a coordinated neurohormonal response that tends to sustain the vital organs. The initial response, mediated by baroreceptors, leads to reflex stimulation and activation of the sympathetic nervous system, which increases blood pressure by inducing systemic arterial vasoconstriction and augmenting cardiac output through stimulation of heart rate and myocardial contractility. In response to hypoperfusion, the juxtaglomerular apparatus of the kidney secretes renin, which stimulates the hepatic conversion of angiotensinogen to angiotensin I and which is, in turn, then converted by angiotensin converting enzyme (ACE, most particularly in the lung) to the potent arterial vasoconstrictor angiotensin II. Angiotensin II tends to increase blood pressure through intense vasoconstriction (venular and arteriolar) and through release of aldosterone from the adrenal gland, which expands blood volume through renal salt and water retention, thus further increasing blood pressure and cardiac output.

Neurohormonal activation reflects not only the severity of depressed left ventricular function and deranged hemodynamics but may also perpetuate the pathophysiology. Although neurohormonal activation plays a crucial role in maintaining cardiovascular homeostasis under conditions of low output, it may, in patients with CHF, may have deleterious as well as compensatory effects. Hypoperfusion, from an evolutionary perspective, is due to to loss of blood volume, attributable to dehydration or hemorrhage; in this case, survival would depend on neurohormonal activation until volume could be restored. When CHF is present, neurohormonal activation may have deleterious hemodynamic effects. Specifically, because the depressed left ventricle is sensitive to increased impedance (afterload) to ejection, stroke volume may decline. Neurohormonally mediated systemic vasoconstriction will then decrease LV stroke volume, resulting in a vicious cycle of low output and further reflex vasoconstriction. Depressed LV ejection leads to LV dilatation. Stimulation of the renin-angiotensin-aldosterone system through right atrial stretch axis further expands blood volume, leading to increased LV preload, which exacerbates backward failure. In addition, sympatho-adrenal stimulation leads to tachycardia and stimulation of contractility which, in combination with increased LV loading, results in increased myocardial oxygen requirements, thus compounding LV dysfunction associated with ischemia.

The abnormal loading conditions typical of CHF can lead to further deterioration in LV function through adverse "remodeling," where, by progressive dilatation, myofibrillar stress and dysfunction occur. Remodeling appears to be particularly prevalent in patients suffering substantial myocardial infarction (especially anterior), who, even if initially stable hemodynamically, are prone to develop progressive LV dysfunction. Although they may not manifest CHF initially, progressive deterioration of LV function often occurs over time. Mechanisms that may contribute to progressive LV dysfunction include recurrent ischemia and infarction, stunned or hibernating myocardium—in which viability hangs in a balance between oxygen supply and demand, and "remodeling" related to the chronically increased LV preload and afterload. Presumably, normal regions of the heart that are contracting well at the time of an acute infarct may undergo functional deterioration over time because of the mechanical stresses imposed by abnormal loading related in part to neurohormonal activation.

V. CLINICAL PRESENTATIONS

Congestive heart failure related to LV systolic dysfunction may present in an insidious manner or as acute hemodynamic compromise. Chronic complaints include fatigue and diminished exercise tolerance resulting from low cardiac output as well as breathlessness [dyspnea on exertion, paroxysmal nocturnal dyspnea (PND), or orthopnea], all of which reflect pulmonary venous congestion. When ventricular dysfunction results in chronic elevation of left atrial pressure (> 25 mmHg), pulmonary hypertension results, which may lead to right heart failure manifest by peripheral edema, ascites, anorexia, and weight loss. Left ventricular systolic dysfunction may present in a more acute fashion, either as an end stage of insidious progression culminating in a decompensated state or a precipitous decline precipitated by decompensating factors [acute myocardial ischemia, arrhythmias, infection, pulmonary embolus, metabolic abnormalities, drugs, increased afterload (hypertension), renal failure, transitory hyper- or hypotension, and noncompliance with diet or therapy].

VI. EVALUATION

Evaluation and management of heart failure requires (a) determination of the pattern of pathophysiological abnormalities, (b) definition of the underlying etiology, (c) identification and treatment of remediable factors, (d) assessment of functional and hemodynamic status, (d) initiation of therapy, and (e) monitoring the response to therapeutic interventions.

A. Etiological Considerations

Initial evaluation of patients with CHF should focus on differentiating primary myocardial abnormalities from valvular or pericardial disease. In patients with CHF related to impaired LV systolic performance, it is critical to differentiate "contractile failure," which results from disorders that primarily depress the contractile apparatus (ischemia, myocarditis, alcohol and other toxins, metabolic diseases, and neuromuscular defects) from "pump failure," in which LV systolic performance is depressed because of pressure overload (aortic stenosis, severe hypertension) or volume overload [aortic regurgitation, mitral regurgitation shunts secondary to a nonrestrictive ventricular septal defect (VSD) or patent ductus arteriosus (PDA)]. This differentiation has implications with regard to identification of potentially remediable conditions and specific management because primary pressure and volume overload conditions can impair LV systolic performance yet not induce depression of the contractile apparatus. Thus, "pump failure" does not necessarily imply "contractile failure." When the pressure or volume overload is relieved, the pump failure may resolve. This is particularly true in patients with severe aortic stenosis and CHF, in whom valve replacement may result in dramatic improvement in LV performance.

Numerous entities may depress the contractile apparatus, resulting in LV systolic dysfunction with resulting volume overload secondary to the depressed ejection fraction. The most common cause is ischemic heart disease. Others are inflammatory myocarditis [viral, autoimmune associated with systemic lupus erythematosus (SLE), and rheumatoid arthritis], toxins (alcohol and drugs), endocrine abnormalities (thyrotoxicosis, myxedema, pheochromocytoma, carcinoid), nutritional disease (hypocalcemia, beriberi, kwashiorkor), neuromuscular disorders (muscular dystrophy, myotonic dystrophy, Friedreich's ataxia), and metabolic diseases (glycogen storage disease, hemochromatosis, Wilson's disease, sarcoid, amyloidosis).

The initial evaluation should include an assiduous search to exclude remediable lesions (aortic stenosis and ischemic, stunned, or hibernating myocardium) as well as reversible alterations in the metabolic milieu that may have precipitated heart failure (thyroid disorders, hypocalcemia, anemia, hypoxia, and sepsis). It is of paramount importance to exclude arrhythmias as a precipitating factor leading to hemodynamic decompensation inpatients with LV systolic dysfunction. Both bradyarrhythmias and tachyarrhythmias can precipitate hemodynamic compromise because of loss of atrial transport, which contributes up to 40% of cardiac output when the ventricle is stiff; impaired ventricular filling secondary to shortened diastole (particularly important when it occurs in association with loss of atrial contractile contributions to LV filling); increased myocardial oxygen consumption secondary to increased heart rate; and impaired coronary blood flow attributable to increased heart rate, diminished diastolic filling, and hypotension.

Noninvasive evaluation with echocardiography helps to exclude treatable valve lesions, provides critical information regarding LV size and function, and delineates mechanical factors associated with severe cardiomyopathy such as function, AV valvular regurgitation, secondary pulmonary hypertension, and right heart failure. Ultimately, invasive evaluation including coronary angiography should be performed to define potential coronary artery disease as well as the presence and severity of associated valve lesions by hemodynamic assessment. In patients with ischemic cardiomyopathy, myocardial viability studies are essential to determine whether extensive hibernating or stunned myocardium amenable to revascularization is present. Accordingly, even in patients with long-standing ischemic cardiomyopathy, initial evaluation by thallium perfusion scintigraphy (with delayed rest imaging or reinjection images), positron emission tomography, or stress echocardiography (with exercise, dipyridamole, or dobutamine) may be helpful. In patients with relatively recent onset of CHF (within 3 to 6 months), endomyocardial biopsy should be considered if previous tests have not established the etiology of an apparent dilated cardiomyopathy. Endomyocardial biopsy is essential in patients in whom the clinical presentation suggests the possibility of viral myocarditis, systemic autoimmune disorders (including SLE, rheumatoid arthritis, or periarteritis nodosa), or a systemic "infiltrative disease" (such as amyloidosis, sarcoidosis, or hemochromatosis).

VII. TREATMENT OF CONGESTIVE HEART FAILURE

A. Goals of Therapy

Because therapeutic interventions entail potential risk, therapy should be tailored to specific pathophysiological derangements and focused on specific short- and long-term objectives, including (a) improvement of symptoms, (b) increasing exercise tolerance, (c) improving LV function and hemodynamics, (d) preventing of further LV damage, and (e) increasing longevity. In patients with severe, decompensated CHF, the primary goal is to improve hemodynamics, reduce symptoms, and improve exercise tolerance. By contrast, in patients with mild CHF with comparatively well-preserved LV function, prevention of further deterioration in LV function is paramount. However, in all patients with LV systolic dysfunction and CHF, reducing the very high mortality associated with this condition is the ultimate objective.

The most effective immediate treatment for severe congestive heart failure is to improve LV contractility and minimize further LV damage. Thus, patients with severe coronary artery disease and ongoing ischemia should be considered for revascularization [percutaneous transluminal coronary angioplasty (PTCA) or coronary artery bypass grafting (CABG)]. Aortic valve replacement may improve LV function when aortic stenosis is severe; reversal of metabolic derangements may improve it when the derangements are major contributing factors to CHF; immunosuppressive agents may be beneficial in patients with active myocarditis (although proof is lacking); and corticosteroids may improve ventricular performance when it is depressed by inflammatory processes such as those seen with lupus.

General therapy for CHF should be tailored to the pattern and magnitude of clinical and hemodynamic derangements. Thus, it should focus on the pathophysiological components of the cycle of low-output reflex vasoconstriction, elevated blood volume and preload, increased heart rate, and generalized neurohormonal activation. When diastolic dysfunction leads to pulmonary congestion manifest as dyspnea, reduction of preload is helpful. Diuretics are a cornerstone of therapy by virtue of their ability to reduce total blood volume and decrease cardiac preload specifically. They are particularly useful in patients with manifest systemic and/or pulmonary venous congestion. However, their use entail risks, including (a) deterioration of renal function and further exaggeration of neurohormonal stimulation when reduction in blood volume and hypovolemia are excessive and (b) metabolic derangements, including hypokalemia, that may contribute to arrhythmogenesis. Deleterious reductions in preload can be exaggerated by concomitant administration of other agents with venodilating effects, such as nitrates and ACE inhibitors.

Systolic dysfunction leads to low output with reflex vasoconstriction and perpetuates low output and progressive ventricular dilatation. Reduction of systemic resistance, arterial vasodilators such as parenteral nitroprusside, oral ACE inhibitors, and hydralazine can improve cardiac output and exercise tolerance. By enhancing output, these agents attenuate neurohormonal activation, thereby ameliorating the vicious cycle of low-output vasoconstriction. Venodilators not only reduce preload—and therefore filling pressures—but also intramyocardial wall tension. Thus, cardiac performance may improve. The advent of potent and well-tolerated vasodilators has improved clinical and hemodynamic status and survival as well.

Vasodilators can be categorized in terms of their sites and mechanisms of vasodilating action. Drugs that exert predominantly venodilating effects are exemplified by the nonparentally administered nitrates (oral, patch, and paste). The exert moderate venodilating effects and lesser effects on systemic arteries. The mechanism responsible involves vascular smooth muscle relaxation mediated by increased cyclic guanosine monophosphate (GMP).

Nitrates increase venous capacitance and thereby reduce systemic and pulmonary venous pressure and ventricular filling pressure. However, they do not increase cardiac output. When combined with arterial vasodilators, long-term nitrate therapy improves exercise tolerance and increases longevity.

Parenteral administration of nitroglycerin leads to more striking arterial dilation. Nitroprusside is a balanced vasodilator with relatively equivalent venodilating and arterial dilating effects. Both agents reduce preload and improve output.

The most common side effect of nitrate therapy is headache, which usually subsides within several days. Excessive dosage may lead to hypotension because of decreased ventricular filling, particularly when diuretics and arterial vasodilators are employed concomitantly. If concentrations of nitrate are maintained, tolerance can limit efficacy. This limitation can be overcome, at least in part, by a daily nitrate-free interval of 8–12 hr.

Angiotensin converting enzyme inhibitors (see below) exert potent venodilating as well as arterial dilating effects.

B. Arterial Dilators

Hydralazine, which directly relaxes vascular smooth muscle, is the prototype arterial vasodilator. When administered to patients with severe congestive heart failure, hydralazine decreases systemic vascular resistance, with a resultant increase in forward cardiac output, usually with little or no effect on arterial pressure and heart rate. However, pulmonary capillary pressure and left ventricular filling pressure are usually unaltered. Given in combination with a nitrate, hydralazine improves hemodynamics and exercise tolerance and lowers mortality. However, at the dosages of the hydralazine-nitrate combination that are necessary, 15–20% of patients develop side effects necessitating discontinuation.

Angiotensin converting enzyme inhibitors are the most effective agents in patients with LV systolic dysfunction and CHF, which results in stimulation of the renin-angiotensin-aldosterone system, intensifying vasoconstriction, impeding ejection from a depressed LV, promoting further left ventricular damage, and contributing to mortality. Angiotensin converting enzyme (ACE) inhibitors exert balanced venodilating effects (which reduce preload) as well as causing arteriolar dilatation, which reduces afterload. The combined effect increases cardiac output and reduces filling pressures. Angiotensin converting enzyme inhibition improves symptoms and exercise tolerance and lowers mortality. Administration of ACE inhibitors early after infarction in patients with moderate LV dysfunction may, by altering abnormal loading conditions and attenuating neurohormonal activation, diminish ventricular remodeling and deterioration in LV function and hemodynamics.

The side effects of ACE inhibitors include hypotension, skin rash, cough, and, in very high doses or when other disorders are present, proteinuria and neutropenia. As with all vasodilating drugs, hypotension can lead to deterioration of renal function in patients with severe heart failure. The ACE inhibitors may be particularly likely to precipitate renal dysfunction in patients with end-stage heart failure, in whom activation of the renin-angiotensin system is responsible for maintaining blood pressure and efferent arteriolar resistance and hence renal perfusion when cardiac output is depressed. Hyponatremia, associated with pre-existent renal hypoperfusion, may help to identify patients at greatest risk for developing renal failure after administration of ACE inhibitors; such a development is particularly likely if concurrent diuretic doses are not reduced.

Calcium channel blockers exert a potent dilating effect by blocking the entry of calcium into vascular smooth muscle. Since calcium mediates the contraction of vascular smooth muscle, these drugs result in vascular smooth muscle relaxation, thereby decreasing systemic vascular resistance and increasing cardiac output. However, by interfering with calcium entry into myocardial cells as well, some calcium blockers depress myocardial contractility. Among available calcium channel blockers, verapamil has the most potent negative inotropic effect and is absolutely contraindicated in patients with severe CHF. Diltiazem may exert deleterious side effects as well.

Some patients with severe ischemic cardiomyopathy and recurrent ischemia tolerate and possibly benefit from calcium blockers that affect primarily vascular smooth muscle (e.g., nicardipine and amlodipine).

The primary underlying problem in severe cardiomyopathy is depressed LV contractility; accordingly, therapy with agents having positive inotropic effects has been utilized. Before the advent of vasodilators, digitalis was considered a cornerstone of therapy, as were diuretics. It improves symptoms and exercise tolerance in patients with severe CHF and is helpful for rate control when CHF is complicated by supraventricular arrhythmias such as atrial fibrillation. Parenteral agents (e.g., dopamine, dobutamine, or amrinone) are indispensable in stabilizing patients with severe decompensated or refractory failure. Parenteral support of contractility is essential in patients with severe low output manifest by hypotension and pulmonary edema and often helpful when CHF leads to renal insufficiency and liver and bowel congestion. Although patients with these manifestations may improve with bed rest and intravenous diuretics administered concomitantly with oral vasodilators, diuretics, and digitalis, recovery is more rapid and more complete when initial support includes parenteral agents with positive inotropic effects. Such parenteral support may facilitate optimal titration of vasodilating drugs, particularly ACE inhibitors, since absorption can be impaired by bowel congestion secondary to right heart failure and dosage can be limited by renal failure and/or hypotension. Parenteral agents are particularly important in patients with decompensated CHF and renal failure, in whom they may avoid the need for discontinuation of ACE inhibitors.

Although most patients with decompensated CHF who require stabilization with parenteral agents can be successfully weaned and sent home on a regimen of oral vasodilators, diuretics, and digitalis, some will remain dependent on cardiotonic drugs despite maximal medical therapy guided by invasive hemodynamic monitoring. Such patients should be considered for cardiac transplantation. Whether or not transplantation is an option, some such patients can be rendered reasonably functional and discharged home with the use of a chronic dobutamine infusion program. However, long-term results with such an approach, whether with dobutamine or with other oral agents such as beta blockers and phosphodiesterase inhibitors, have been disappointing. Sustained hemodynamic functional benefit is limited and, of even greater concern, mortality may be increased, perhaps through a proarrhythmic effect.

Although beta blockers had been thought to be absolutely contraindicated in patients with CHF, it is now clear that chronic beta-blocker therapy may improve LV function, hemodynamics, and symptoms in some patients with dilated cardiomyopathy. The failing heart is chronically exposed to intense sympathetic stimulation and high catecholamine levels that downregulate the number and affinity of myocardial beta-adrenergic receptors. Beta blockade is thought to restore responsiveness of the myocardium to endogenous adrenergic stimulation and thereby improve ventricular performance. There is no definitive means by which to predict which specific patients will benefit from this intervention. Improvement occurs slowly over several months. The agents must be titrated cautiously and judiciously. Patients with tachycardia at rest or with mild exertion may be the best candidates.

13

Management of Patients with Pulmonary Vascular Diseases

I.   Primary Pulmonary Hypertension   235
II. Secondary Pulmonary Hypertension   237

Stuart Rich

I. PRIMARY PULMONARY HYPERTENSION

The treatment of primary pulmonary hypertension has improved markedly over the past decade. Goals are to reduce symptoms, stabilize the disease process, and improve survival.

A. Digoxin

The value of digoxin is unproven in patients with pulmonary hypertension. However, its use is based on a rationale similar to that in patients with left ventricular failure. Besides providing support of cardiac contractility in patients with right ventricular failure, digoxin may elicit beneficial effects by restoring baroreceptor function and reducing sympathetic activation.

B. Diuretics

Diuretics can be extremely helpful in stabilizing and improving the symptoms of patients with pulmonary hypertension associated with right ventricular failure. Because the extent of edema and/or ascites is variable, diuretics should be prescribed whenever elevated central venous pressure is documented by bedside examination or catheterization studies. Patients with overt right ventricular failure require diuretic therapy, often with high doses of loop diuretics, occasionally in combination with thiazide diuretics, to promote a prompt diuresis. Hypotension is generally not a problem if right atrial filling pressure remains elevated. Diuretics often relieve dyspnea that may be related to increased lung water developing in patients with pulmonary hypertension.

C. Vasodilators

Vasodilators may exert very beneficial effects in some patients with pulmonary hypertension, although they may be dangerous and can result in deterioration. It is advisable to first test pulmonary vasodilator reserve with a potent short-acting vasodilator such as intravenous adenosine or inhaled nitric oxide. Failure to respond to these agents appears to predict failure to respond to the oral vasodilators. Their short half-lives permit incremental dosage with little systemic effect, thus defining maximal pulmonary vasodilator reserve. In addition, the short half-life provides a good margin of safety should an untoward response occur.

Among the available oral vasodilators, calcium channel blockers have had the most consistent record of producing substantial reductions in pulmonary artery pressure and pulmonary vascular resistance. Because the dose that will be effective is highly variable from patient to patient, these agents must be titrated until a maximum physiologically effective dose can be ascertained. Calcium channel blockers, however, possess negative inotropic effects and can induce overt right heart failure and cardiovascular collapse. Therefore, initiation of calcium channel blockers to treat patients with pulmonary hypertension requires consultation and often invasive monitoring. Calcium channel blockers have not been particularly effective in patients with secondary forms of pulmonary hypertension. Their administration in this setting is often associated with adverse effects.

D. Anticoagulants

Anticoagulants appear to improve survival in patients with primary pulmonary hypertension and are indicated in all patients, irrespective of the severity of the disease. They should not, however, be expected to improve patients' symptoms immediately. Warfarin should be adjusted to reduce an international normalized ratio (INR) of two to three times control so as to provide effective anticoagulation without an undue risk of bleeding.

E. Prostacyclin

Prostacyclin is effective in reducing symptoms and improving survival in patients with primary pulmonary hypertension refractory to conventional treatment. It can be given only intravenously. Thus, the patient must have permanent venous access (e.g., via a Hickman catheter) so that the drug can be given on a daily basis. A constant infusion pump system is required. Although prostacyclin is considered to be primarily a bridge to lung transplantation, some patients may have such a favorable response that the need for lung transplantation, at least immediately, is reduced. Associated risks of catheter-based infection and thrombosis are significant; these complications must be prevented or, if they occur, managed aggressively.

II. SECONDARY PULMONARY HYPERTENSION

Treatment of secondary pulmonary hypertension has similar objectives but is even more difficult. Among the most difficult patients to treat are those patients with underlying collagen vascular disease. Although vasculitis is presumed to affect the lung, there is little distinction histologically between patients with this form of pulmonary hypertension and those with primary pulmonary hypertension. However, patients with collagen vascular disease appear to be far less responsive to vasodilators, perhaps because of the chronicity of the disease process. Attempts have been made to initiate or intensify anti-inflammatory and immunosuppressive therapy in these patients, but to date, no documentation of any consistent effectiveness of this strategy exists. Most affected patients are not candidates for organ transplantation because of the systemic nature of this disease.

Patients whose pulmonary hypertension results from chronic obstructive pulmonary disease (COPD) are best managed with diuretics and chronic nasal oxygen therapy. Vasodilators have not been effective in this group and may be associated with worsening gas exchange and exacerbation of right heart failure. In the subset of patients with COPD and cor pulmonale, the only therapy that improves hemodynamics and prolongs survival is long-term administration of oxygen.

Some patients with pulmonary hypertension have underlying interstitial lung disease. As in patients with COPD, vasodilators are not effective and may induce worsening gas exchange by dilating pulmonary vessels in areas of poor ventilation, creating intrapulmonary right-to-left shunting. Treatment should be directed against the underlying cause of the lung disease.

14

Management of Patients with Valvular Heart Disease

I.	General Considerations	239
II.	Lesions Affecting the Aortic Valve	241
III.	Aortic Regurgitation	248
IV.	Mitral Valve Disease	251
V.	Mitral Regurgitation	255
VI.	Tricuspid and Pulmonary Valve Disease	258
VII.	Tricuspid Stenosis	260
VIII.	Pulmonary Regurgitation	261
IX.	Pulmonary Stenosis	263
X.	Mechanical and Surgical Interventions Required in the Management of Patients with Valvular Heart Disease	264
	Suggested Reading	265

Burton E. Sobel, Matthew W. Watkins, and James A. Goldstein

I. GENERAL CONSIDERATIONS

Although most clinicians immediately think of heart murmurs when they contemplate valvular heart disease, other manifestations are of considerably more importance in the detection of its presence, assessment of its severity, and implementation of management in the context of its prognosis. Thus, for example, a loud first heart sound is often a signpost of the presence of mitral stenosis; left ventricular hypertrophy is often a critical criterion reflecting severity of aortic stenosis or regurgitation as well as mitral regurgitation; and the intensity of murmurs may decline markedly when cardiac output falls in association with high-grade valvular lesions.

Major decisions confronting the clinician caring for patients with valvular heart disease include the need to determine and implement, if necessary, prophylaxis for endocarditis (see Chapter 28). Wisdom is necessary in differentiating, for example, a patient with the click-murmur syndrome (mitral valve prolapse) who has mitral regurgitation manifest by a murmur and who is therefore a good candidate for antibiotic prophylaxis from one with a click only and no regurgitation despite prolapse documented objectively by echocardiography or another modality.

Among the most difficult aspects of assessment and management of patients with valvular heart disease are those related to combined lesions. Textbook descriptions of entities such as aortic stenosis or mitral regurgitation are usually couched in terms of the pathophysiology of a single lesion, diagnostic criteria, manifestations and functional consequences, and strategies for management. Such an approach, although invaluable from a pedagogical point of view, skirts the difficult clinical issue of assessment of the functional significance of a given lesion when multiple lesions are present. Thus, repair of mitral stenosis in the face of moderate aortic stenosis can lead to an exacerbation of the functional consequences of the aortic valve lesion when ventricular filling is freed from the constraint of the stenotic mitral valve. Alternatively, when the left ventricle is unloaded, mitral regurgitation may exacerbate the limitation in forward cardiac output resulting from otherwise moderate aortic stenosis. Thus, although we shall present management considerations in terms of specific individual valvular lesions, the astute clinician will always keep in mind the importance of considering the lesion in a given patient in the context of other lesions that may be present concomitantly.

Among the most critical decisions that must be made in the care of patients with valvular heart disease are those related to the necessity for and timing of surgical repair or replacement of valves and, in some instances, valvuloplasty. In general, a decision to intervene surgically is based on the severity of physiological impairment experienced by the patient. Patients who are asymptomatic and can tolerate high levels of exercise and other physical activity [New York Heart Association (NYHA) class I] generally do not require valve repair or replacement. Those who experience symptoms at less than normal levels of activity (NYHA class III) generally do. Surgical risk is least in patients whose physiological compromise is minimal; accordingly, the "golden moment for intervening" is often the hypothetical moment present while the patient can still perform normal levels of activity without becoming symptomatic (class II) but is about to deteriorate to a class III status. Unfortunately, identification of such a "golden moment" is at best difficult, even when regular follow-up is meticulous and noninvasive testing is used to enhance recognition of a change in functional status.

Another principle underlying the decision to undertake valve repair or replacement relates to the performance of specifically affected chambers of the heart. Thus, for example, a patient with aortic insufficiency who begins to manifest progressive ventricular dilatation and hypertrophy is a good candidate for valve replacement, whereas a patient with regurgitation without chamber enlargement can usually be managed successfully medically. Assessment of the physiological response to exercise is often helpful in unmasking functional impairment. The pivotal requirement is meticulous follow-up and serial assessment of left ventricular chamber dimensions, the magnitude of regurgitation, and the functional consequences of its presence.

II. LESIONS AFFECTING THE AORTIC VALVE

The aortic valve comprises three semilunar cusps in the aortic root juxtaposed to the sinuses of Valsalva. The cusps or leaflets are not separated from the wall of the aorta by fibrous tissue, in contrast to the case with the mitral valve annulus; as a result, the aortic root is susceptible to dilatation.

A. Causes of Aortic Stenosis

Several congenital abnormalities—including the presence of a unicuspid valve (presenting with severe obstruction in infancy); a bicuspid valve, seen in as many as 2% of the population; and other, rare malformations—may result in "fixed" aortic stenosis. Conditions such as hypertrophic cardiomyopathy result in dynamic obstruction to left ventricular outflow, simulating, to some extent, aortic stenosis. Subaortic stenosis and supravalvular aortic stenosis can also occur in the presence of an anatomically normal aortic valve.

Bicuspid valves predispose to aortic stenosis relatively late in life as a result of turbulence and long-standing trauma to the leaflets, with degenerative changes including fibrosis and calcification contributing to obstruction to left ventricular outflow in patients in the range of 50 years of age. In a substantial subset, earlier onset with a gradient, left ventricular hypertrophy, and functional impairment can occur—even in childhood or in the teenage years. Detection of a bicuspid valve is of particular importance because of the need to protect patients with degenerative changes from infective endocarditis.

Acquired aortic stenosis can be the result of rheumatic heart disease. If so, mitral valve disease is virtually always present as well. Degenerative calcific aortic stenosis (aortic stenosis of the elderly) is the most common form of acquired aortic stenosis in the United States, with functional consequences generally evident in patients in the seventh and eighth decades of life. Its incidence is increased in patients with hyperlipidemia or diabetes.

All forms of acquired and congenital aortic stenosis can be associated with aortic regurgitation. Although one hemodynamic lesion generally predominates (a highly stenotic valve will often not permit large volumes of regurgitant flow), functionally "mixed" lesions are seen in as many as 50% of patients.

Other causes of acquired aortic stenosis include collagen vascular diseases such as rheumatoid arthritis and lupus erythematosus (the latter with lesions typically on the mitral valve), infective endocarditis including mycotic endocarditis, and marantic endocarditis associated with an imbalance between thrombosis and fibrinolysis.

B. Functional Consequences of Aortic Stenosis

Obstruction to left ventricular outflow is compensated by generation of higher left ventricular systolic pressures and prolongation of left ventricular ejection time, which, in combination, maintain stroke volume initially at normal levels with the patient at rest. The increased left ventricular wall tension is a stimulus for concentric left ventricular hypertrophy. The hypertrophied left ventricle becomes less compliant and highly dependent on adequate left ventricular filling and preload. This is the reason why patients with aortic stenosis who develop atrial fibrillation deteriorate hemodynamically regardless of heart rate when the atrial transport function is accordingly lost. The stiff left ventricle gives rise to diastolic dysfunction and pulmonary vascular congestion, particularly when diastolic filling time is limited by tachycardia. As the disorder progresses, stroke volume declines disproportionately to acceleration of heart rate, and cardiac output falls not only with exertion but also at rest. Fatigue and presyncope or syncope are attributable to a relatively or absolutely fixed cardiac output because of the limitaton to preload, fixed obstruction, and exercise-induced vasodilataton.

The increased myocardial oxygen requirements associated with increased wall stress predispose some patients with aortic stenosis to myocardial ischemia. Thus, consequences of coronary artery disease that would be well tolerated in a patient without valvular dysfunction are manifest, including angina pectoris and myocardial infarction. For this reason, the presence of aortic stenosis should be considered in any patient with coronary artery disease, and the presence of coronary artery disease should be considered in any patient with aortic stenosis. Treatment of either one alone when both are present is inadequate. Conversely, the high afterload caused by the stenosis can cause systolic dysfunction (pump dysfunction) in the absence of impaired contractility.

C. Mixed Aortic Stenosis and Aortic Regurgitation

Hemodynamically important aortic regurgitation is particularly prominent in association with bicuspid valves and with aortic stenosis caused by rheumatic heart disease. However, any stenotic valve that becomes infected can become severely regurgitant. The functional consequences of stenosis are magnified substantially when concomitant regurgitation is present because of the left ventricular volume overload that results, coupled with the limitation of effective forward cardiac output. The presence of regurgitation leads to underestimation of cardiac output with indicator dilution techniques that measure effective forward output only. Consequently, estimates of aortic valve area will be erroneous, with overestimation of the severity of valvular stenosis. For this reason, stroke volume is best calculated on the basis of imaging (left ventriculography, echocardiography, or other, tomographic methods).

A. Signs and Symptoms

Shortness of breath resulting in part from increased pulmonary vascular pressure, fatigue (often a reflection of limited augmentation of cardiac output with exertion), angina pectoris, limitation of exercise capacity, and syncope are salient features in patients with aortic stenosis. Syncope is generally the result of increased left ventricular pressure with resultant effects on left ventricular chamber baroreceptors. It results from the consequent failure of occurrence of reflex changes in response to vasodilatation accompanying exercise or assumption of a sitting or standing posture, among other stimuli. Vasoconstriction that would otherwise occur, mediated by carotid sinus baroreceptor sensing of decreased arterial pressure, does not occur because the brainstem is "misinformed" by the ventricular baroreceptors and therefore senses erroneously that arterial pressure is high. A failure of mediation of reflex vasoconstriction results.

Syncope can, of course, be a manifestation of arrhythmia as well. Administration of vasodilator agents or diuretics and extracellular volume contraction from any cause, as well as progression of the decline in left ventricular ejection fraction, predispose to syncope. The appearance of any symptom in a patient with aortic stenosis presages rapid deterioration, morbidity, and increased mortality. In general, when angina pectoris is the presenting symptom, life expectancy is in the range of 5 years. When syncope is the initial symptom, life expectancy is generally 3 years or less. The most ominous presenting symptoms are those indicative of congestive heart failure and left ventricular systolic functional impairment, in which case life expectancy is as little as 2 years. Rarely, the presenting event is sudden cardiac death, presumably attributable to a malignant ventricular arrhythmia occurring in an asymptomatic patient. For this reason, screening programs for competitive athletics in schools should focus on the detection of occult aortic stenosis, among other conditions.

Sudden exacerbation of previously consistent symptoms often reflects the onset of atrial fibrillation, with the loss of atrial transport compromising cardiac output; tachycardia of any cause, with consequent diminution of left ventricular filling time and left ventricular preload; the occurrence or progression of aortic regurgitation as a result of hemodynamic stresses and further degeneration of the aortic valve or superimposition of infective endocarditis; or myocardial infarction, reflecting increased myocardial oxygen requirements resulting from aortic stenosis coupled with underlying coronary artery disease.

Systemic embolization can, of course, occur as a result of thrombus formed on and released from a diseased aortic valve. Thus, cerebral vascular accident, myocardial infarction, bowel ischemia or infarction, and other complications may ensue.

B. Physical Findings

The carotid arterial pulse (and peripheral pulses in general) exhibits a slow rate of rise and low amplitude with a delayed peak when aortic stenosis is severe. A palpable shudder (thrill) may be present. Left ventricular enlargement is often evident, with a sustained apical impulse, an often palpable fourth heart sound (unless atrial fibrillation is present), and a systolic thrill over the precordium. The intensity of the aortic component of the second heart sound is frequently diminished when calcification is present. The second heart sound may be split paradoxically if left ventricular dysfunction is severe or simply as a result of prolongation of ejection time. In congenital aortic stenosis, an aortic ejection sound is common. With acquired aortic stenosis, ejection systolic murmurs are typical and best heard along the left sternal border with the intensity increasing, the time to peak intensity increasing, and the presence of a palpable thrill over the precordium and often over the carotid arteries indicative of severe obstruction. As cardiac output declines with progressive impairment of left ventricular function, these signs may paradoxically diminish. When the aortic systolic ejection murmur does not exhibit the characteristic crescendo-decrescendo pattern and when it radiates to the axilla, it may be confused with the holosystolic murmur of mitral regurgitation (Gallavardin's phenomenon). In aortic stenosis of the elderly, the murmur is much less obviously of ejection quality compared with the case in other forms of aortic stenosis because of the absence of jet lesions through a single narrow orifice. In hypertrophic obstructive cardiomyopathy, the systolic murmur may mimic that of aortic stenosis despite being associated with a bisferious carotid pulse and a characteristic increase with the Valsalva maneuver, in contrast to the decrease seen with valvular aortic stenosis during the straining phase as cardiac output declines.

The aortic stenosis murmur is usually distinguished readily from that of mitral regurgitation, which increases with handgrip exercise as a result of increased peripheral vascular resistance, in contrast to the case with aortic stenosis, in which the murmur changes little or not at all and decreases with administration of amyl nitrite (a diagnostic maneuver now used only rarely) because of systemic arterial vasodilatation. This is in contrast to the case with an aortic stenosis murmur that increases. In contrast to the murmur of mitral regurgitation, beats with long RR intervals increase and those with short RR intervals decrease the intensity of the aortic stenosis murmur.

The severity of aortic stenosis can be assessed at the bedside. Delayed occurrence of the aortic component of the second heart sound (A_2)—with consequently narrow or paradoxical splitting or an absent A_2 (with calcific aortic stenosis), a palpable thrill, late peaking of the murmur, and a sustained apex impulse—suggests severe aortic stenosis. Delayed upstroke of the arterial pulse is typical when aortic stenosis is severe, particularly in young subjects, but the sign may be absent in elderly subjects because of decreased arterial compliance and consequent augmentation of pressure wave transit and intensity.

C. Laboratory Findings

Electrocardiographic (ECG) manifestations of aortic stenosis include left atrial enlargement manifest by negative or biphasic P waves in the right precordial leads, left ventricular hypertrophy manifested by voltage, and often ST- and T-wave criteria. The chest x-ray may demonstrate left ventricular enlargement, pulmonary vascular congestion (especially in the upper lobes—so-called pulmonary vascular redistribution), calcification of the aortic valve, and occasionally poststenotic aortic dilatation. Valvular morphology can be delineated by two-dimensional echocardiography, as can valve motion, valve area, concomitant changes in the aortic root, left ventricular and left atrial cavity dimensions, the presence of regional wall motion abnormalities that may be indicative of coronary artery disease, systolic ventricular function, and the possible presence of associated mitral and other valve lesions. Doppler echocardiography permits estimation of the pressure gradient across the stenotic aortic valve and, with concomitant application of the continuity equation (see below), estimates of aortic valve area. It is helpful in detecting and defining the severity of associated aortic regurgitation and other valve lesions as well as left ventricular compliance, reflected in the transmitral flow profile.

Cardiac catheterization defines transvalvular pressure gradients and valve area, left ventricular function and dimensions, the presence and severity of obstructive coronary artery disease, aortic regurgitation (with aortography), and the presence and severity of left atrial, pulmonary arterial, and pulmonary capillary wedge pressure elevations. Ventriculography is useful in defining not only cardiac output and stroke volume but also wall stress.

The advent of two-dimensional and Doppler echocardiography has profoundly affected the management of patients with valvular heart disease. Both facilitate early noninvasive diagnosis, anatomic characterization, quantitative assessment of transvalvular pressure gradients and stenotic valvular orifice areas, and semiquantitative assessments of the severity of regurgitation. In the case of aortic stenosis, optimal echocardiographic information can differentiate etiologies, define maximal instantaneous transvalvular pressure gradients by application of the modified Bernoulli equation [Δ pressure (mmHg) = $4 \times v^2$ (with v = velocity in m/sec)], and determine aortic valve area by application of the continuity equation that relates mean laminar flow velocity through a conduit to the conduit's cross-sectional area. Although serial assessment of severity of aortic stenosis is enhanced, several limitations of continuous-wave Doppler data acquisition are relevant. The modified Bernoulli equation derives pressure gradients from peak flow velocities, estimates of which are critically dependent on the angle of the continuous-wave Doppler being parallel to blood flow. Thus, suboptimal imaging can lead to underestimation of the transvalvular pressure gradients, especially in the presence of prosthetic valves. Conversely, small high-velocity jets associated with normal prosthetic valve function can lead to overestimation of true pressure gradients across a prosthetic valve.

The continuity equation permits estimation of valve orifice area independent of measurements of cardiac output (velocity $\times$ area through one valve = velocity $\times$ area through a valve related to the first valve by continuity of flow, with each velocity corrected by division by the cosine of the intercept angle). However, its accuracy for this purpose is dependent on accurate measurements of left ventricular outflow tract diameter. In the continuity equation, valve area is a function of the outflow tract diameter squared. Thus, a small underestimation of diameter leads to a marked overestimation of the severity of the aortic stenosis. Accordingly, echocardiographic assessments tend to overestimate transvalvular gradients with mild stenosis and to underestimate transvalvular gradients with severe stenosis.

The direct measurement of transvalvular pressure gradients and application of the Gorlin formula [valve area = flow/(44.5 $\times$ a hydraulic constant specific for the type of valve multiplied by the square root of the pressure gradient)] to estimate valve orifice area at cardiac catheterization is independent of limitations related to outflow tract morphology, acoustic windows, acoustic reverberations and shadowing seen with echo with prosthetic valves, and the angle of Doppler beam interrogation. However, the hydraulic constants used in the Gorlin formula are not, in fact, constant in the setting of low cardiac output or under conditions seen with extremes of heart rate. In addition, significant concomitant valvular regurgitation can lead to an underestimation of true transvalvular flow and thus an overestimation of the severity of valvular stenosis.

In the case of regurgitant valvular lesions, both echocardiography and cardiac catheterization provide only semiquantitative assessments of severity. Color Doppler mapping of an increased velocity indicative of regurgitant flow cannot be correlated directly with regurgitant volume because of the load-dependence of the velocity envelopes. The changes in contractility and loading conditions associated with left ventricular angiography limit quantitative assessment of valvular regurgitation in the catheterization laboratory. An even more fundamental factor limiting both techniques is the lack of available criteria by which the appropriate timing of surgical intervention can be determined in terms of the measured severity of valvular aortic and/or mitral regurgitation.

Thus, echocardiography has been relied upon increasingly for the early diagnosis, morphological characterization, and serial evaluation of patients with valvular heart disease. With some important caveats, high-quality echocardiography is often sufficient. Cardiac catheterization may be required for early diagnosis and management when concomitant coronary artery disease is suspected, complex mixed valvular lesions are present, or a prosthetic valve is dysfunctional. In the case of isolated valvular disease, cardiac catheterization is frequently used in a confirmatory fashion at the time of consideration of surgical intervention and to delineate the presence and severity of associated coronary artery disease.

D. Management

Effective management of patients with aortic stenosis requires delineation of etiology; quantification of the severity and rate of progression of functional consequences of aortic stenosis, including left ventricular hypertrophy and left ventricular systolic function; delineation of the potential presence of concomitant disorders, including coronary artery disease; and results of monitoring, with assessment of functional class, physical findings, and results of noninvasive tests to define patients who are candidates for valve repair or replacement. Once symptoms have appeared, medical management is relatively ineffective. When systolic dysfunction is prominent, cardiotonic agents including digitalis glycosides may be helpful. When diastolic dysfunction is prominent, diuretics may be helpful despite the risk they entail of exacerbating syncope. Very judicious use of vasodilators is helpful in some patients, but all such agents entail a risk of precipitating or exacerbating episodes of syncope. In patients with advanced disease, parenteral administration of agents with positive inotropic effects is relatively ineffective, and circulatory support with an intraaortic balloon pump may be necessary as a bridge to valve replacement or repair. However, significant aortic regurgitation interdicts use of an intraaortic balloon pump, which would overload the left ventricle in diastole.

For patients with mild aortic stenosis, generally associated with an aortic valve area of equal to or greater than 0.75 cm^2 and a pressure gradient of less than or equal to 50 mmHg, no specific therapy is generally required. Follow-up should occur at a frequency of at least 6-month intervals and should include annual echocardiography. Sudden death is rare when aortic stenosis is asymptomatic. Even when it is severe, with a valve area less than 0.75 cm^2 and a gradient exceeding 50 mmHg, mechanical interventions can be deferred if the patient truly belongs in functional class I and left ventricular systolic function is normal despite the presence of left ventricular hypertrophy. However, follow-up should be more frequent and valve replacement should be undertaken when symptoms develop or if the presence of a concomitant disorder, particularly coronary artery disease, is documented. Strenuous exercise, including that employed in stress testing, should be avoided when valve area is equal to or less than 0.75 cm^2.

For patients with symptomatic aortic stenosis or a critical valve area (0.5 cm^2), valve replacement or repair should be undertaken.

E. Definitive Measures

Treatment of severe aortic stenosis generally requires valve replacement. Even when left ventricular function is severely compromised, results of surgery are often good. Nevertheless, left ventricular systolic functional impairment is the strongest descriptor of surgical mortality, which can be as high as 25% when left ventricular ejection fraction is severely depressed.

A recently developed alternative to surgery is balloon valvuloplasty, a procedure that is sometimes effective for prolonged intervals in patients with congenital unicuspid or bicuspid valves. Unfortunately, however, in acquired aortic stenosis, valvuloplasty generally does not provide acceptable long-term restoration of function despite an initial reduction of the pressure gradient and increase in valve area of approximately 50%. Generally, within 6 months, 50% of the benefit dissipates. Nevertheless, in some patients, particularly those of very advanced age with limited life expectancy, valvuloplasty can offer considerable symptomatic relief. In others, it may provide a bridge to surgery.

III. AORTIC REGURGITATION

In addition to occurring as part of the combined lesion of aortic regurgitation and aortic stenosis, aortic regurgitation may exist as an independent entity. It is caused by either aortic root dilatation or aortic valvular disease. Root dilatation is seen with connective tissue disorders such as Marfan's syndrome, ankylosing spondylitides including rheumatoid arthritis and Reiter's syndrome, syphilis, aortic dissection (often secondary to cystic medial necrosis, traumatic injury, or hypertension), and long-standing hypertension per se.

Regurgitation caused by aortic valve disease can occur with congenital disorders including a bicuspid aortic valve, a membranous ventricular septal defect (VSD) with inadequate support of the leaflets and aortic valve prolapse potentiated by a Venturi effect associated with the VSD, or myxomatous valves (often called floppy valves) seen alone or as a manifestation of a connective tissue disorder such as Marfan's syndrome. Acquired aortic regurgitation can result from rheumatic heart disease, infective endocarditis, and valvulitis associated with collagen vascular disorders including peripheral rheumatoid arthritis and lupus erythematosus. Rarely, trauma can cause aortic valvular regurgitation because of leaflet avulsion or rupture.

A. Acute Versus Chronic Aortic Regurgitation

The classic manifestations of aortic regurgitation (wide pulse pressure, bounding pulses, pistol-shot sounds over the femoral artery, left ventricular dilatation, and hypertrophy, among others) are typical of chronic aortic regurgitation with well-maintained left ventricular contractility and a gradual left ventricular compensatory response to this slowly progressing regurgitation. Acute aortic regurgitation is associated with diminished forward output and shock, peripheral vasoconstriction, a narrow pulse pressure, lack of cardiac dilatation, and often pulmonary edema, all of which reflect the immediate lack of compensatory response of the left ventricle to the sudden imposition of regurgitation. Thus, the physiology can resemble that of constrictive pericardial disease with equalization of left ventricular and right ventricular filling pressures. Acute aortic regurgitation is often associated with premature closure of the mitral valve, evident by the occurrence of the first heart sound before the QRS complex is inscribed on the ECG. It virtually always requires prompt invasive diagnostic evaluation (catheterization if coronary disease is potentially present or transesophageal echocardiography, which may be adequate otherwise), circulatory support, and surgery.

Acute aortic regurgitation is caused most often by proximal aortic dissection, infective endocarditis, or trauma. It frequently presents as cardiovascular collapse, shock, and pulmonary edema and constitutes a genuine cardiac emergency. In contrast to the case with chronic aortic insufficiency, peripheral signs of aortic insufficiency are absent.

B. Functional Manifestations

Chronic aortic regurgitation leads to left ventricular dilatation and is associated with maintenance of effective forward stroke volume at the expense of an overall large increase in total cardiac output. Massive cardiomegaly may occur. A wide pulse pressure associated with systolic hypertension and diminished peripheral vascular resistance is typical. Because of the high shear forces associated with the high overall cardiac output, aortic root dilatation may progress regardless of the initial etiology.

With chronic aortic insufficiency, left ventricular compliance is generally well maintained. Accordingly, regurgitation can be well tolerated for years in some patients even with exertion. As the cardiac compensatory mechanisms begin to fail, left ventricular systolic function declines, often associated with eccentric hypertrophy. In very advanced disease, pulmonary congestion may predominate. Prominent symptoms include those related to bounding pulses, chest pain—often suggestive of but atypical for angina pectoris, and exercise intolerance, dyspnea, and signs of initially left and ultimately biventricular heart failure with very advanced disease. Salient signs in chronic aortic regurgitation include systolic pressure greater than 140 mmHg with popliteal artery systolic pressure often as much as 60 mmHg greater than brachial arterial pressure (Hill's sign); diminished diastolic arterial pressure; water hammer pulses (Corrigan's sign); pistol-shot sounds over the femoral artery (Traube's sign); a two-component murmur over the femoral artery (Duroziez's sign); visible capillary pulsations in the nail beds with partial compression of the fingertips (Quincke's sign); lateral displacement of the left ventricular impulse, which is sustained and hyperdynamic; an audible and palpable third heart sound; and often a diastolic decrescendo murmur and thrill heard and felt best at the left upper sternal border. This diastolic murmur must be differentiated from Graham Steell's pulmonary insufficiency murmur seen with mitral stenosis and pulmonary hypertension and often associated with an accentuated pulmonic component of the second heart sound.

With acute aortic regurgitation, the signs typical of chronic regurgitation are absent but the diastolic murmur is present, although sometimes abbreviated because of the very high left ventricular end-diastolic pressure. Because abbreviation of the diastolic murmur accompanies diastolic dysfunction of the left ventricle, the duration of the murmur with chronic aortic regurgitation is not a reliable sign of severity. A fourth heart sound is often heard in patients with either acute or chronic aortic regurgitation but has little diagnostic utility because of its frequent occurrence with hypertension of any cause and its nonspecificity.

A sometimes useful differentiating feature of aortic regurgitation caused by root dilatation as opposed to aortic valvular disease per se is the greater intensity of the diastolic murmur on the right side of the sternum, as opposed to the left, in the interspace in which the murmur is loudest when root dilatation is its cause. When aortic regurgitation is severe, it may be associated with an Austin-Flint murmur (hydraulic mitral stenosis) attributable to the partial closure of the mitral valve as the left ventricular filling caused by aortic regurgitation in diastole occurs and/or fluttering of the anterior mitral valve leaflet caused by the regurgitant jet impinging on the juxtaposed aortic wall. In contrast to the case with mitral stenosis, an opening snap is absent and the first heart sound is generally soft (as a result of premature closure of the mitral valve).

In both acute and chronic aortic regurgitation, the relatively or absolutely increased forward flow across the aortic valve frequently results in a systolic ejection murmur that may not be indicative of obstruction but results simply from turbulence associated with ejection of a high volume of blood.

C. Laboratory Results

Left ventricular hypertrophy (with a volume overload pattern in QRS changes on the ECG) with left atrial enlargement is often seen with chronic aortic regurgitation. In fact, among all valve lesions, aortic regurgitation results in the most massive left ventricular hypertrophy (LVH). The chest x-ray demonstrates left ventricular enlargement. Echocardiography is of particular value in the detection of manifestations of chronic aortic regurgitation and their severity, including elevated left ventricular diastolic volume, maintenance of a normal or high left ventricular ejection fraction until the disorder has become severe, and the presence of aortic root dilatation either as the primary cause of the regurgitation or as a consequence of its progression. Stress echocardiography is useful to determine whether the physiological response to exercise is intact. The echocardiogram is particularly useful in the diagnosis of acute aortic regurgitation in which left ventricular and diastolic volume may be modestly or markedly increased in the absence of left ventricular hypertrophy and in association with premature closure of the mitral valve. In both chronic and acute aortic regurgitation, echocardiography can define the architecture of the aortic valve, the presence or absence of vegetations, and the status of the aortic root. If proximal dissection is present, its entry site can often be identified as well. Definitive diagnosis of dissection requires aortography or alternative imaging modalities including nuclear magnetic resonance (NMR), computed tomography (CT) with contrast, or transesophageal biplane echocardiography.

D. Management

Medical management of patients with aortic regurgitation is appropriate despite severe long-standing disease as long as left ventricular ejection fraction has not decreased. Because mortality increases markedly as left ventricular ejection fraction declines, regular follow-up is essential. Aortic valve replacement improves symptoms in virtually all patients, even those with left ventricular dysfunction pre-operatively, in whom impaired function usually persists. Medical management for patients who are decompensated because of left ventricular dysfunction should focus on the use of vasodilator agents to reduce ventricular afterload. Digitalis glycosides and diuretics may be helpful as well.

The same considerations pertinent to detection and assessment of the severity of concomitant disorders, particularly coronary artery disease as those noted with respect to surgical treatment of aortic stenosis, apply to surgical treatment of aortic regurgitation.

IV. MITRAL VALVE DISEASE

The mitral valve can be stenotic as a result of congenital anomalies or acquired insults, including rheumatic heart disease, valvulitis secondary to collagen vascular diseases such as lupus erythematosus, infiltrative processes including deposition of amyloid, mucopolysaccharides in children with hereditable metabolic disease, and excess calcium, as in elderly patients with degenerative calcific disease of the annulus. Conditions simulating mitral stenosis include obstruction of the orifice by thrombus, tumor, or a membrane (as in cor triatriatum) or extrinsic compression secondary to constrictive pericarditis. A rare cause of true mitral valve stenosis is pulmonary carcinoid syndrome, presumably attributable to the flooding of the mitral valve with noxious mediators released by the tumor and reaching the valve via the pulmonary veins.

A. Functional Consequences of Mitral Stenosis

Hemodynamic derangements are not usually evident unless the mitral valve area is reduced from its normal 4 to 6 cm^2 to less than 2 cm^2. In patients with acute rheumatic fever who develop rheumatic heart disease, the evolution of mitral stenosis to an extent that markedly impairs function occurs slowly. Consequently, symptoms often do not appear for 5 to 20 years or more after the initial insult. When the mitral valve area is reduced progressively by any process, left atrial pressure rises, leading ultimately to pulmonary venous and subsequently pulmonary arterial hypertension. With prolonged elevation of pulmonary arteriolar pressures, the pulmonary vascular bed undergoes structural modification, leading to increased pulmonary vascular resistance. The elevated left atrial pressure leads to left atrial dilatation, predisposing to thrombosis in the atrial appendage and in the atrial cavity and to atrial arrhythmias including atrial fibrillation.

Salient symptoms include dyspnea on exertion, orthopnea, and paroxysmal nocturnal dyspnea; marked limitation of exercise tolerance; fatigue; and ultimately right heart failure secondary to the increased pulmonary vascular resistance. Because of the dependence of left heart output on the atrial transport function, the occurrence of atrial fibrillation often heralds exacerbation of symptoms and functional deterioration. It may also precipitate acute pulmonary edema, as may any process that increases cardiac oxygen demands, such as a febrile illness that reduces oxygen supply because of tachycardia and abbreviation of the diastolic filling period.

Signs of mitral stenosis and left atrial enlargement can include hemoptysis and hoarseness because of the impingement of the dilated left atrium on the recurrent laryngeal nerve (Ortner's syndrome). All of the signs of right heart failure—including hepatomegaly, edema, ascites, and sometimes anasarca—coupled with systemic venous hypertension are typical of very advanced disease. Signs and symptoms associated with systemic thromboemboli (originating from left atrial thrombi) or pulmonary thromboemboli (developing because of stasis in the pulmonary vascular bed) may be initial manifestation of mitral stenosis. Risk of endocarditis is high regardless of the nature of mitral stenosis; accordingly, antibiotic prophylaxis is essential.

Prominent physical findings are those related to low cardiac output, including flushed cheeks (mitral fascies). The intensity and contour of peripheral arterial pulses are consistent with a low stroke volume. The a wave may be exaggerated in the jugular venous pulse because of right ventricular hypertrophy and elevated right ventricular and atrial pressures. If the v wave is prominent, tricuspid regurgitation (either secondary to the hemodynamic consequences of mitral stenosis or, less commonly, to primary tricuspid valvular disease in patients with rheumatic heart disease) is likely. The constraint on left ventricular inflow is reflected by a quiet precordium. A right ventricular heave is often present when pulmonary hypertension is marked. A palpable thrill over the apex impulse may accompany the diastolic murmur of mitral stenosis.

Early in the course of mitral stenosis, the first heart sound is accentuated. When the valve becomes calcified, this finding disappears. Similar considerations apply to the opening snap, which is present when the leaflets are supple. The interval between the aortic second sound and the opening snap is a good index of the severity of mitral stenosis. It decreases as left atrial pressure rises. In addition, a loud pulmonary component of the second heart sound becomes evident as pulmonary hypertension progresses.

The classic murmur of mitral stenosis is a low-pitched diastolic rumble beginning with an opening snap and often exhibiting presystolic accentuation. Its detection can be elusive because it is often localized to the apex and sometimes heard only when the patient is in the left lateral recumbent position or subject to a physiological stress such as exercise.

B. Laboratory Findings

The ECG demonstrates left atrial enlargement without left ventricular enlargement unless mitral regurgitation or another cause is present. Right ventricular hypertrophy and right atrial enlargement are evident in patients with pulmonary hypertension. The chest x-ray demonstrates left atrial enlargement, pulmonary venous congestion, right ventricular enlargement when pulmonary hypertension is present, a dilated proximal pulmonary artery, and often Kerley B lines and pulmonary vascular congestion with upper-lobe vascular redistribution. In addition, a miliary pattern may be evident as a result of deposition of hemosiderin in fixed pulmonary macrophages.

Echocardiography demonstrates the anatomic characteristics of the stenotic mitral valve and consequences of its dysfunction, including pulmonary hypertension, left atrial enlargement, and right heart failure. Valvulitis in other sites in patients with rheumatic heart disease may be evident. Two-dimensional Doppler echocardiography can delineate the limited mobility, doming, and restriction of excursion with calcification in valve leaflets; decreased orifice area; enlarged left atrium and right heart chambers; the magnitude of the pressure gradient across the mitral valve; and a prolonged pressure half-time, i.e., the interval required for decline of the pressure gradient between the left atrium and left ventricle to 50% of its maximum.

High-quality ultrasonic interrogation of the heart (transthoracic or transesophogeal echocardiography) permits assessment of mitral stenosis without the need for catheterization in most patients. However, when a mixed lesion is present (mitral regurgitation and mitral stenosis), the status of the coronary vascular tree is uncertain, or the clinical picture is complex, cardiac catheterization remains the definitive means for assessment in patients who are potential candidates for valve repair or replacement.

C. Management

Because of the risks of endocarditis, thromboembolism, and catastrophic complications of both, definitive interventions are appropriate for patients with mitral stenosis that is sufficiently severe to induce symptoms regardless of the calculated valve area. Intervention is not appropriate if the symptoms are a consequence of tachycardia with resultant decreased time for left ventricular filling in diastole. Critical mitral stenosis (with a valve area of < 1.0 cm^2) requires definitive intervention whether or not symptoms are present. In patients with mild mitral stenosis and no symptoms, exercise testing should be used to define the functional significance of the lesion and repeated at yearly intervals for the same purpose. Arrhythmias such as atrial fibrillation can be managed conventionally with beta-adrenergic blocking agents or digitalis glycosides, among other agents and options. If minimal symptoms are present, such as dyspnea only with severe exertion, beta blockers (to slow heart rate and provide a prolonged interval for ventricular filling) may be helpful. When and if signs of left heart failure occur in patients who cannot be treated definitively, diuretics may be helpful.

Definitive therapy may entail balloon valvuloplasty or surgical commissurotomy. Valvuloplasty generally increases mitral valve area by 50–100% and is associated with a mortality of less than 1% (albeit with 5% risk of embolism) and a 5-year survival in excess of 95%. Mitral regurgitation or excessive mitral valve calcification or subvalvular fibrosis sufficiently severe to require mitral valve replacement occurs in at least 2% of patients.

Open surgical commissurotomy was the procedure of choice before the development of prosthetic valves. When anatomic and structural criteria are favorable, results are excellent, with survival of 95% or more in the first 5 years. An alternative when left atrial thrombus is demonstrably absent and anatomy is demonstrably favorable is closed commissurotomy. With both procedures, restenosis occurs in 50% of patients within 10 years. Occasionally, mitral regurgitation is encountered during follow-up.

Both valvuloplasty and commissurotomy are inappropriate when mitral regurgitation is present because of the severity of the deformity of the valve responsible. Its presence and other factors—including episodes of thromboemboli, atrial fibrillation, massive left atrial enlargement, or endocarditis at any time—are contraindications to commissurotomy and valvuloplasty, as is the presence of aortic valve disease. Under these conditions, mitral valve replacement or surgical repair are the procedures of choice. Relative contraindications include heavy calcification and subvalvular disease.

V. MITRAL REGURGITATION

In addition to deformity of the mitral valve itself, papillary muscle dysfunction or rupture and chordal rupture can underlie mitral regurgitation. Mitral regurgitation can be a result of the following:

dilatation of the mitral annulus

floppy mitral valve leaflets on a congenital basis (myxomatous degeneration)

inflammatory processes affecting the valve leaflets, including rheumatic heart disease

collagen vascular diseases

infection, destruction, or dysfunction of the mitral valve supporting apparatus including the chordae tendineae and the papillary muscles as a result of inflammatory disorders such as rheumatic heart disease or ischemia secondary to coronary artery disease

the click/murmur mitral valve prolapse syndrome that may be familial (Barlow's syndrome)

myxomatous degeneration

disorders affecting ventricular or atrial function in view of the contributions of each to mitral valve closure and competence.

Degenerative, infiltrative, and inflammatory processes—including diverse entities such as scleroderma, Takayasu or giant cell arteritis, Marfan's or Ehler's-Danlos syndromes, degenerative calcification of the mitral annulus, and leaflet perforation or deformity secondary to infective endocarditis—must be considered. Mitral valve incompetence can occur with hypertrophic cardiomyopathy because of malposition of the papillary muscles and may be seen with eccentric left ventricular hypertrophy regardless of its etiology.

A. Functional Manifestations

Because the elevated left atrial pressure associated with mitral regurgitation is relieved by decompression accompanying left ventricular filling with each cardiac cycle, mitral regurgitation is generally better tolerated than mitral stenosis. For the same reason, the left atrial enlargement does not predispose to atrial fibrillation and other arrhythmias to the same extent that it does in patients with mitral stenosis. The severity of mitral regurgitation can be reduced dramatically by reduction of left ventricular afterload with vasodilators or mechanical interventions when concomitant disorders such as aortic stenosis are present. Because of the potentiation of mitral annular dilatation, mitral regurgitation is self-perpetuating.

Salient symptoms include dyspnea and related signs of left heart failure, fatigue, and other signs and symptoms of pulmonary hypertension, hemoptysis, and hoarseness, as in mitral stenosis. Thromboemboli are less common than with mitral stenosis but still a prominent risk.

Physical findings are those associated with the underlying disorder (e.g., arachnodactyly in patients with Marfan's syndrome) and those reflective of the hemodynamic derangements attributable to the mitral regurgitation. Peripheral arterial pulses are brisk, with a rapid upstroke. The precordium is hyperdynamic, with a left ventricular heave and a laterally displaced and sustained point of maximal impulse. A systolic thrill may be palpable, as may left atrial systolic expansion reflected by a left parasternal impulse. Pulmonary hypertension gives rise to an intense pulmonary component of the second heart sound with narrow splitting and a right ventricular heave with or without signs of tricuspid regurgitation.

The first heart sound is generally of diminished intensity and followed immediately by a holosystolic murmur at the apex. When mitral regurgitation is severe, a diastolic rumble is audible, often because of the overall increase in transmitral flow in diastole. The mitral regurgitant murmur can be confused with that of a ventricular septal defect, especially when it is accompanied by a thrill, but oximetry can readily differentiate the two conditions. It can be confused also with a tricuspid insufficiency murmur, generally heard best to the right of the sternum.

When mitral valve prolapse is responsible for mitral regurgitation, an early systolic click is present along with the murmur. The click occurs earlier when left ventricular dimensions are reduced (e.g., as a result of the patient's assumption of an upright posture or with administration of amyl nitrite). Conversely, the click moves further into systole when left ventricular dimensions are augmented (e.g., by handgrip). In contrast to the case with a split first heart sound that varies with respiration, the interval between the first heart sound and the click remains quite constant independent of respiration.

B. Laboratory Findings

The ECG often demonstrates left atrial enlargement accompanied by left ventricular enlargement and right ventricular hypertrophy when pulmonary hypertension is present. Echochardiography is useful in delineating anatomic features indicative of specific etiologies and of the severity of regurgitation (often best assessed with color Doppler echocardiography). As in the case of aortic regurgitation, the severity of the insult is reflected primarily by the response of specific chambers affected. Thus, left ventricular hypertrophy and marked left atrial dilatation are hallmarks of severe mitral regurgitation. A recent promising approach to quantifying transvalvular regurgitation per se echocardiographically is predicated on isovelocity spherical envelopes (actually isovolume transport calculations).

Echocardiography is particularly useful in differentiating mitral regurgitation secondary to severe left ventricular dysfunction, such as that caused by ischemia (in which case regional wall motion abnormalities are likely to be present) or cardiomyopathy from primary mitral regurgitation. Thus, for example, a dilated annulus in a patient with dilated cardiomyopathy may certainly give rise to secondary mitral regurgitation associated with poor left ventricular systolic performance, in contrast to the case in a patient with rheumatic mitral regurgitation in which left ventricular ejection fraction may be elevated.

Cardiac catheterization is useful in defining the severity of mitral regurgitation in terms of the magnitude of elevation of pulmonary capillary wedge pressure and amplitude of the v wave in the left atrial pressure recording, the status of left ventricular function—particularly left ventricular end-diastolic pressure and volume, the presence and severity of pulmonary hypertension, the extent to which pulmonary hypertension is attributable to increased pulmonary vascular resistance as opposed to elevated left atrial pressure, and the presence of associated manifestations including regional wall motion abnormalities indicative of coronary artery disease.

C. Management

Asymptomatic patients with mild mitral regurgitation require no specific therapy. The use of ACE inhibitors and other vasodilating agents is reasonable to reduce ventricular remodeling. Patients who are symptomatic and in whom left ventricular ejection fraction is not depressed are candidates for surgery if mitral regurgitation leads to symptoms and objective signs of elevated pulmonary capillary wedge pressure at rest or with mild exertion. Mitral valve replacement generally ameliorates symptoms but is less beneficial when left ventricular enlargement is extensive preoperatively and particularly when left ventricular systolic function is impaired. When the anatomy is favorable (as in patients with myxomatous valves), mitral valve repair is preferable to mitral valve replacement. Mitral repair is relatively contraindicated when ejection fraction is equal to or less than 25%. However, it is desirable even with chordal disease and prosthetic valves to preserve ejection fraction and diminish left ventricular remodeling. If left ventricular dilatation is severe or associated with early systolic dysfunction, surgery is generally indicated even in an asymptomatic patient. When compromise of systolic function is severe in a patient who has become symptomatic, the patient may no longer be able to tolerate surgery.

When mitral regurgitation is acute (usually as a result of acute myocardial infarction and papillary muscle rupture or endocarditis), vasodilators and circulatory support with an intra-aortic balloon pump can "buy" the time needed to improve the outcome of surgery by allowing healing in an infarct zone or an initial response to antibiotics. However, if left heart failure is refractory, mitral regurgitation is secondary to an acute ischemic insult, or the regurgitation is life-threatening, surgery should not be delayed.

VI. TRICUSPID AND PULMONARY VALVE DISEASE

Tricuspid regurgitation can result from dilatation of the tricuspid annulus secondary to right ventricular pressure or volume overload. It is commonly seen in association with pulmonary hypertension from any cause, including primary pulmonary hypertension, chronic recurrent pulmonary embolic disease, cor pulmonale as a result of chronic pulmonary disease, increased pulmonary arteriolar resistance secondary to mitral stenosis, protracted and severe left heart failure with elevated pulmonary capillary wedge pressure, rare congenital anomalies such as cor triatriatum, pulmonary venous obstruction, and an Eisenmenger reaction in association with a nonrestrictive ventricular septal defect or an atrial septal defect with protracted pulmonary hypertension and the evolution of obstructive pulmonary vascular disease late in life. Processes affecting the tricuspid valve structurally cause primary tricuspid regurgitation and include rheumatic heart disease, infectious endocarditis, inflammatory disorders and vasculitis, ischemic insults resulting in right ventricular infarction or infarction of papillary muscles supporting the tricuspid valve, tumors including myxoma (more commonly seen in the left heart), and traumatic injury. Even when right ventricular ischemic injury does not affect the supporting apparatus of the tricuspid valve, right ventricular infarction associated with increased pressure and dilatation of the chamber induces tricuspid regurgitation because of dilatation of the annulus. Infective endocarditis is a particularly important consideration. When it involves the right heart, the tricuspid valve is more often the site (95% of the time) than is the pulmonary valve. Chemical and drug abuse, particularly intravenous drug use, induces endocarditis on anatomically normal valves all too often. With this cause, the tricuspid valve is frequently involved, usually with concomitant aortic and mitral endocarditis. In less than 50% of instances, the tricuspid valve is the only valve involved.

Fortunately, right heart endocarditis is better tolerated than left heart endocarditis, in part because systemic venous congestion is relatively well tolerated and less life-threatening. Furthermore, forward cardiac output can be well maintained even when right atrial pressure is markedly elevated. Accordingly, treatment with antibiotics can often be continued sufficiently long and with sufficient intensity to produce a genuine cure of infective endocarditis involving the tricuspid valve, whereas surgical intervention is more often necessary with left heart endocarditis.

Rare causes of tricuspid regurgitation include the carcinoid syndrome, with mediators reaching the right atrial endocardium through the systemic venous circulation. Carcinoid heart disease is usually associated with metastatic carcinoid tumors involving the liver. Endocardial fibrosis frequently results in tricuspid regurgitation and more rarely tricuspid stenosis or a mixed lesion. The pulmonary artery may be involved as well. When carcinoid tumors are present in the lung, analogous morphological changes occur in the left heart and can produce mitral valve disease.

A. Functional Manifestations

Chronic tricuspid regurgitation is often well tolerated because of the compliance of the right heart and pericardium. Acute tricuspid regurgitation is less well tolerated because of insufficient time available during which the right ventricle and pericardium can accommodate to increased pressures. When tricuspid regurgitation is secondary to right ventricular pressure and volume overload, it initiates a vicious cycle of self-propagation with exacerbation of right ventricular dilatation and right heart failure. When tricuspid regurgitation is severe, left ventricular filling is compromised because of diminished pulmonary blood flow and the impingement of the interventricular septum on left ventricular volume as a result of reversed curvature of the interventricular septum or increased diastolic ventricular interaction. Atrial fibrillation is, of course, frequently associated with right ventricular dilatation secondary to tricuspid regurgitation.

Salient signs and symptoms associated with tricuspid regurgitation are those of profound right heart failure including elevated venous pressure, edema or anasarca, hepatojugular reflex, hepatomegaly, bowel edema with malabsorption or a protein-wasting enteropathy, ascites, abdominal pain, anorexia, fatigue, and shortness of breath. The elevated right heart pressures result in a prominent v wave in the jugular venous pulse, hepatojugular reflux, a right ventricular heave and occasional systolic thrill, and a right-sided third heart sound. The murmur of tricuspid regurgitation is holosystolic, particularly when it is secondary to right ventricular pressure overload. It increases with inspiration (Carvallo's sign) and may be associated with a diastolic rumble because of very high antegrade flow over the tricuspid valve when the tricuspid regurgitation is severe. Physical findings of pulmonary hypertension, including an accentuated second component of the second heart sound with close splitting, may implicate pulmonary hypertension as the cause of the tricuspid regurgitation.

B. Laboratory Findings

In addition to the right atrial enlargement evident electrocardiographically, signs of right ventricular hypertrophy implicate pulmonary hypertension as the cause of tricuspid regurgitation. Doppler echocardiography can quantify the extent of pulmonary hypertension, thereby helping to define treatment options. The chest x-ray is useful in the same fashion in delineating right ventricular enlargement and a potential cause of pulmonary hypertension, such as mitral stenosis or pulmonary vascular disease. The echocardiogram is particularly useful in differentiating primary organic tricuspid regurgitation from secondary tricuspid regurgitation with an intact valve structure associated with severe right ventricular dilatation and often diminished systolic function. When tricuspid regurgitation is severe, the interatrial septal curvature is often reversed in association with profound enlargement of the right atrium. Systolic flow reversal in the superior vena cava and in the inferior vena cava is demonstrable by Doppler echocardiography, as is the extent to which the tricuspid regurgitant jet enters the right atrial cavity. Hepatic venous pulsations can often be detected as well.

When pulmonary stenosis is not present, pulmonary arterial pressure can be calculated on the basis of velocity of the tricuspid regurgitant jet and the magnitude of right atrial or jugular venous pressure.

C. Management

Because right heart lesions are generally better tolerated than left heart lesions, treatment of tricuspid regurgitation should focus on the underlying condition (e.g., bacteriological cure of infective endocarditis, correction of left heart valve lesions, relief of pulmonary hypertension, and unloading of the right ventricle to obviate its performing on the descending limb of the Franck-Starling curve, as it does when dilatation is excessive). Medical management incorporates the use of diuretics and vasodilators, particularly those with prominent effects on the systemic venous system. When right heart failure dominates transitory support with agents with positive inotropic effects may be helpful.

Surgical intervention is required only rarely for primary tricuspid regurgitation, because right ventricular performance often can be well maintained despite its presence. However, when symptoms are severe or refractory, repair of the tricuspid valve, annuloplasty, or tricuspid valve replacement are reasonable options.

VII. TRICUSPID STENOSIS

In addition to processes responsible for organic tricuspid regurgitation, all of which can result in a mixed lesion or tricuspid stenosis, congenital abnormalities including tricuspid atresia (the most extreme form of tricuspid stenosis), primary cardiac tumors, or metastases and thrombi can produce tricuspid stenosis. Manifestations include signs of chronic right heart failure with jugular venous pressure elevation and edema but a blunted "y" descent in contrast with the brisk descent seen with tricuspid regurgitation. The presentation may mimic that of cirrhosis or constrictive pericarditis. Just as with mitral stenosis, the first heart sound may be intensified (the tricuspid component being the second component of a split first heart sound) and an opening snap (right-sided) may be present. The murmur of tricuspid stenosis is heard best at the lower left or right sternal border and is often accentuated in middiastole, increasing with inspiration because of increased right heart filling accompanying the negative intrathoracic pressure.

A.   Laboratory Findings

The ECG demonstrates right atrial enlargement, and the chest x-ray is usually essentially normal when tricuspid stenosis is the sole cardiac lesion. In most instances, tricuspid stenosis is associated with aortic and mitral valve disease, manifestations of which are evident on the ECG and chest x-ray. Structural abnormalities of the tricuspid valve accounting for stenosis are often demonstrable by echocardiography, particularly transesophageal echocardiography. Thus, thickening and calcification of the leaflets or abnormalities of the chordae tendineae may be seen with partial occlusion of the valve orifice and doming of the valve. Doppler echocardiography can quantify the severity of the stenosis based on measurement of transtricuspid flow velocity. When stenosis is severe, right ventricular chamber dimensions are diminished unless concomitant left heart valve disease is present.

An important form of tricuspid valve disease (usually tricuspid regurgitation) is Ebstein's abnormality—namely ventricularization (malpositioning) of the tricuspid valve. Major manifestations include tricuspid regurgitation, cyanosis (if an atrial or ventricular septal defect is present), tachyarrhythmia with or without a preexcitation syndrome (Wolff-Parkinson-White), and audible sounds associated with chattering of the tricuspid valve heard on auscultation. An interesting variant is left-sided Ebstein's, seen in association with other anomalies including transposition of the great vessels.

B.   Management

In addition to a focus of treatment on the underlying condition, conventional medical management of right heart failure with diuretics and vasodilators is indicated. Effective right ventricular filling may, however, require maintenance of high right atrial pressure. When left heart valve repair or replacement is being undertaken, concomitant open valvulotomy may be employed to ameliorate tricuspid stenosis. If tricuspid valve replacement is required (only rarely), a bioprosthetic valve is the appropriate choice.

VIII.   PULMONARY REGURGITATION

The etiology is usually pulmonary hypertension secondary to left heart disease, pulmonary vascular disease, and pulmonary thromboembolic disease. When pulmonary regurgitation occurs in the absence of elevated distal pulmonary arterial pressure, the cause is typically structural. Outflow tract or valve abnormalities on a congenital basis, connective tissue disorders, infective endocarditis, and rarely the carcinoid syndrome or rheumatic heart disease may be responsible. The most common cause of organic pulmonary regurgitation is unfortunately infective endocarditis in drug abusers, in whom the implicated organism is most frequently the gonococcus.

A. Functional Manifestations

Severe pulmonary regurgitation overloads right ventricular volume, a generally well-tolerated derangement in the absence of pulmonary hypertension. When pulmonary hypertension is present, the volume overload is complicated by pressure overload, with consequent right ventricular dilatation and ultimately systolic dysfunction. Massive right ventricular dilatation can impair left ventricular filling through adverse diastolic interactions, thereby inducing signs of secondary left heart failure.

When pulmonary regurgitation is acute, right ventricular volume overload is not well tolerated and may lead to severe symptomatic right heart failure manifest by markedly elevated jugular venous pressure, edema, hepatomegaly, bowel congestion, and ascites.

The murmur of pulmonary regurgitation is generally decrescendo and heard best in the second left intercostal space. When the regurgitation is severe, it may be associated with a diastolic thrill. If the second heart sound's pulmonic component is accentuated, the regurgitation is likely to be secondary to pulmonary hypertension. If it is inaudible, destruction of the pulmonary valve is implicated.

In patients with mitral stenosis secondary to rheumatic heart disease, secondary pulmonary regurgitation is common as a result of the pulmonary hypertension accompanying high left atrial pressure. Under these circumstances, a decrescendo diastolic murmur of pulmonary regurgitation is often heard (the Graham-Steell murmur). The duration of the murmur of pulmonary regurgitation is a reflection of the interval required for equalization of pressures retrograde from the pulmonary artery to the right ventricle in diastole.

B. Laboratory Findings

The ECG and chest x-ray are useful in detecting the potential presence of pulmonary hypertension. Echocardiography (particularly transesophageal echocardiography) may be helpful in determining the presence or absence of structural abnormalities of the pulmonary valve and the severity of the pulmonary regurgitation and consequent right ventricular chamber dimensions and pump functions. The severity of pulmonary regurgitation can be quantified in a fashion similar to that used for aortic regurgitation by Doppler echocardiography based on the Bernoulli equation and the peak flow velocity across the pulmonary valve. Pulmonary, mitral, and aortic regurgitation are very dependent on loading conditions and therefore problematic with respect to the definition of the volume of regurgitation as a reflection of valve lesion severity. Cardiac catheterization is helpful in defining the presence and severity of pulmonary vascular resistance changes in patients with pulmonary hypertension and the response of pulmonary vascular resistance to oxygen and vasodilators.

C. Management

Medical management focuses on treatment of the underlying disease process and right heart failure with diuretics and vasodilators. When pulmonary hypertension is the cause of pulmonary regurgitation, high right heart filling pressures are necessary to sustain cardiac output; accordingly, diuretics and vasodilators must be used cautiously. Pulmonary valve replacement is rarely necessary. An exception is the need for cure of pharmacologically refractory infective endocarditis.

IX. PULMONARY STENOSIS

Pulmonary outflow tract obstruction occurs secondary to right ventricular hypertrophy in the presence of pulmonary hypertension under diverse circumstances including, for example, those prevailing in patients with tetralogy of Fallot. Most valvular pulmonary stenosis is congenital. It is often associated with other complex congenital abnormalities. Acquired pulmonary stenosis attributable to the pulmonary valve per se is rare but sometimes seen in patients with carcinoid tumors that have metastasized to the liver or as a result of infective endocarditis. Pulmonary stenosis can be mimicked by proximal pulmonary emboli and extrinsic pulmonary artery compression by tumor.

A. Functional Manifestations

The effects of obstruction to right ventricular outflow on the right heart resemble those of left ventricular outflow tract obstruction on the left heart. The hemodynamic derangements induce fatigue and signs and symptoms of right heart failure. Thus, elevation of the jugular venous pressure, right ventricular enlargement with a heave detectable on physical examination, accentuation of the pulmonic component of the second heart sound sometimes associated with a systolic ejection click (paradoxically decreasing with inspiration, the so called slatting-sail sign), wide splitting of the second heart sound because of delayed pulmonic closure as a result of the pulmonary stenosis, and a systolic ejection murmur peaking late when the stenosis is severe are typical. When right ventricular failure ensues, signs of secondary tricuspid regurgitation may dominate.

B. Laboratory Findings

Right ventricular enlargement is evident on the ECG, often with right atrial enlargement. The chest x-ray demonstrates chamber enlargement and often post-stenotic dilatation of the main, left, or right pulmonary artery with oligemic lungs. The echocardiogram is particularly useful for delineating structural abnormalities of the pulmonic valve, the magnitude of chamber enlargement, and the status of right ventricular systolic performance. Cardiac catheterization is particularly useful in delineating specific causes of pulmonary hypertension, such as pulmonary embolic disease, that can simulate pulmonary stenosis.

C. Management

Congenital pulmonic stenosis is generally treated by balloon valvuloplasty when the gradient across the valve exceeds 50 mmHg. Among all balloon targets of valvuloplasty, the success rate is highest and recurrence rate lowest for correction of pulmonic stenosis. Surgery is employed when the pulmonic stenosis is associated with other complex lesions. Surgical intervention is rarely needed in the treatment of patients with acquired pulmonary stenosis.

X. MECHANICAL AND SURGICAL INTERVENTIONS REQUIRED IN THE MANAGEMENT OF PATIENTS WITH VALVULAR HEART DISEASE

The ultimate decision regarding the selection of a mechanical intervention for treatment of a particular patient should, of course, rest with the interventional cardiologist or surgeon who is responsible. Relevant considerations are legion.

Valve replacement is a palliative rather than a curative procedure. Accordingly, the choice of valve to be used must depend on numerous considerations, including the age of the patient, the presence or absence of pregnancy, estimated life expectancy, ability to adhere to a regimen of prolonged anticoagulation, risk factors for infective endocarditis, activities of daily living, and the presence or absence of concomitant illnesses, among others. Any prosthetic valve is a potential nidus for infective endocarditis, hemolysis, and valve failure. Mechanical valves include high-impedance and low-impedance varieties and generally require long-term anticoagulation. Advantages include proven endurance and widespread utilization over many years. Bioprosthetic valves are fabricated with diverse materials (e.g., pericardium, heterologous or autologous tissue valves, heterografts, or orthotopic or isotopic homografts, among others). Compared with mechanical valves, their advantages include tolerance without the need for long-term anticoagulation (although it is still desirable for bioprosthetic valves in the mitral position) and the avoidance of stenosis associated with structural components of mechanical valves. Disadvantages compared with mechanical valves include valve failure over 1–20 years attributable to degenerative changes in the prostheses. Both stenosis and regurgitation may result beginning within 5 years after implantation with an incidence of 20–50% in 10 and 70% in 15 years. Homografts may be less prone, however, to degeneration.

In planning for an appropriate prosthetic valve, the risks of reoperation, should it become necessary, are relevant. Despite remarkable advances in cardiac surgery, repeat operations are confounded by adhesions and difficulty in acquiring adequate access, increased incidence and severity of perioperative complications, and excess mortality.

Prosthetic valves are of most value in the treatment of left heart lesions. Isolated tricuspid valve replacement is almost never an optimal choice. Nevertheless, technical considerations markedly favor bioprosthetic over mechanical valves when placement is to be in the tricuspid position and to a lesser extent in the mitral position. Recent success with bioprosthetic valves or homografts in the aortic position has been impressive.

When complications potentially attributable to the previous insertion of a mechanical or bioprosthetic valve are suspected, rigorous evaluation—including two-dimensional echocardiography, Doppler echocardiography, and often transesophageal echocardiography—is helpful. Cardiac catheterization can overcome uncertainties in estimates of concomitant stenosis and regurgitation echocardiographically with prosthetic valves obviating the confounding impact on Doppler-based estimates of small high-velocity transvalvular jets. Both procedures are helpful in elucidating the presence or absence of structural derangements and the need for further interventions. When mechanical valves are impaired functionally by thrombosis, thrombolytic agents are often helpful, despite some attendant risk. An alternative is surgery.

SUGGESTED READING

Abrams J, ed. Essentials of Cardiac Physical Diagnosis. Philadelphia: Lea & Febiger, 1987.
Braunwald E. Valvular heart disease. In: Braunwald E, ed. Heart Disease: A Textbook of Cardiovascular Medicine. Philadelphia, Saunders, 1992: 1007–1077.
Perloff JK, ed. The Clinical Recognition of Congenital Heart Disease. Philadelphia, Saunders, 1987.

15

Management of Patients with Pericardial Disease

I.	Anatomy and Pathophysiology	267
II.	Physiological Properties of the Normal Pericardium	268
III.	Pericardial Functions	269
IV.	Pathophysiology	269
V.	Primary Diseases of the Pericardium	270
VI.	Evaluation	271
VII.	Differential Diagnosis	272
VIII.	Management	273
IX.	Cardiac Tamponade	274
X.	Noninvasive Diagnostic Procedures	276
XI.	Cardiac Catheterization	276
XII.	Hemodynamic Assessment of Pericardial Effusions: Clinical Algorithms	277
XIII.	Management	277
XIV.	Constrictive Pericarditis	281

James A. Goldstein

I. ANATOMY AND PATHOPHYSIOLOGY

The pericardium is a bilayered, flask-shaped sack consisting of an inner visceral layer made up of a thin elastic membrane of mesothelial cells and a thick, stiff, outer parietal layer consisting predominantly of collagen and elastic fibers. It envelops the cardiac chambers but does not directly attach to them at any point. Instead, it reflects up and around the great vessels (forming the arterial and venous mesocardia), creating two major serosal tunnels (the transverse and oblique sinuses) between the great vessels and the adjacent veins (systemic and pulmonary) as they enter their respective atria. It is noteworthy that the left atrium is not entirely an "intrapericardial" structure. The pericardium has important ligamentous attachments to surrounding thoracic structures (including the sternum and diaphragm) that provide structural support for the heart within the thoracic cage and thereby limit excessive cardiac motion, particularly with changes in body position.

II. PHYSIOLOGICAL PROPERTIES OF THE NORMAL PERICARDIUM

An appreciation of the physiology of the venous circulations, the effects of intrathoracic pressure (ITP) and respiratory motion on cardiovascular physiology, and the dynamics of right and left heart interactions is critical to understanding pericardial physiology and pathophysiology. The interventricular septum (IVS) is predominantly an architectural and mechanical component of the left ventricle (LV). However, even under physiological conditions, septal contraction contributes to right ventricular (RV) performance through systolic ventricular interactions. When the RV free wall is dysfunctional, such interactions mediate critically important compensatory mechanisms maintaining global RV function. Hemodynamically important diastolic ventricular interactions also occur. Pressure or volume overload of one ventricle results in decreased compliance and filling of the contralateral ventricle through diastolic ventricular interactions medicated by the thick IVS; these interactions are enhanced in the presence of the pericardium. Similar interactions occur between the atria across the thinner intraatrial septum.

Under physiological conditions, venous return to both atria is biphasic, with a systolic peak determined by atrial relaxation [corresponding to the "X" descent of the right atrial (RA) and jugular venous pressure (JVP) waveforms] and a diastolic peak determined by tricuspid valve (TV) resistance and RV compliance (corresponding to the "Y" descent of the RA and JVP waveforms). Systemic venous return is augmented with inspiration, as the inspiratory decrease in ITP reduces intrapericardial pressure (IPP), thereby enhancing the caval:RA gradient and augmenting venous return flow by 50–60%, which increases right heart filling and output. In contrast, left heart filling, stroke volume, and aortic systolic pressure decrease with inspiration (up to 10–12 mmHg), a phenomenon termed (normal) pulsus paradoxus or paradoxical pulse. The mechanisms responsible for this normal inspiratory oscillation in aortic pressure include ventricular competition for intrapericardial volume related to leftward septal displacement induced by augmented right heart filling, increased LV "afterload" imposed by the differential effects of decreased ITP on the heart relative to the extra thoracic great vessels, and inspiratory delay of augmented RV output through the lungs.

268

III. PERICARDIAL FUNCTIONS

Although an intact pericardium is not critical to maintenance of cardiovascular function (as evidenced by the innocent effects of incision and subsequent lack of pericardial closure after surgery), potentially important subsidiary functions have been attributed to the pericardium. These include (a) limitation of intrathoracic cardiac motion; (b) balancing right and left ventricular output of through diastolic and systolic interactions; (c) buffering of positional changes in chamber filling and therefore output; (d) suction filling; (e) limitation of acute dilatation; (f) lubricant effects that minimize friction between cardiac chambers and surrounding structures; and (g) lymphatic/immunological functions, mediated in part through anatomic barriers that help prevent spread of infection from contiguous structures, especially the lung. The pericardium behaves initially as a stiff, noncompliant shell with pressure-volume characteristics analogous to those of the ventricles when increments in intrapericardial volume are sudden. The result is elevation of IPP. The normal pericardium has a small capacitance reserve (150–250 mL) whereby initial increments in intrapericardial volume result in trivial increases in IPP. However, once this capacitance has been exceeded, further increases in intrapericardial volume result in steep increments in IPP.

IV. PATHOPHYSIOLOGY

Elevated IPP is the major mechanism by which the pericardium exerts adverse hemodynamic effects, not only by limiting chamber filling and therefore forward output (systolic limitations) but also through adverse diastolic effects whereby external pressures dictate that whatever filling can be achieved must occur at elevated pressures, resulting in backward (diastolic) failure. Elevation of IPP may result from primary disease of the pericardium itself, either secondary to accumulation of fluid within the pericardium (effusion resulting in tamponade) or increased stiffness of the pericardial layers (constrictive pericarditis). However, IPP may be increased in conditions in which the pericardial layers and space themselves are normal. The elevated IPP results from acute chamber dilatation within the noncompliant pericardial shell, with the pericardium acting as an "innocent bystander." Furthermore, the pericardium cannot differentiate between increments in intrapericardial volume resulting from fluid accumulation within the pericardial sack (effusion) as opposed to acute chamber dilatation (e.g., acute LV dilatation secondary to mitral regurgitation or acute RV dilatation secondary to RV infarction). Regardless of whether increments in intrapericardial volume result from effusion or acute chamber dilatation, the magnitude of IPP elevation will be influenced by several common factors, the most important of which are the extent of intrapericardial volume "overload" and the rapidity with which it develops. Given time, the pericardium can stretch, exhibit increased compliance, and therefore accommodate increased intrapericardial volume at lower IPP. However, even with chronic intrapericardial volume overload, a point is reached at which the pericardium elicits a steep segment of the pressure-volume curve, at which time even small additional increments in intrapericardial volume result in sharp increases in IPP, with severe and often precipitous hemodynamic consequences.

V. PRIMARY DISEASES OF THE PERICARDIUM

A. Acute Pericarditis

The most common affliction of the pericardium is acute pericarditis, in which inflammation of the pericardial surfaces results in a syndrome characterized by chest pain, pericardial friction rub, and serial electrocardiographic (ECG) abnormalities. Acute pericarditis is most often idiopathic, with specific identifiable etiologies most frequently resulting from acute viral (most common are Coxsackie and echo) and nonviral (tuberculosis, bacterial, and fungal) infections. Important noninfectious entities include acute myocardial infarction (MI), delayed postinfarction Dressler's syndrome (also postsurgical pericardiotomy delayed pericarditis syndromes), uremia, neoplastic involvement, radiation, systemic inflammatory states [systemic lupus erythematosus, rheumatoid arthritis, other connective tissue diseases, forms of vasculitis, drugs (e.g., hydralazine), aortic dissection, trauma (blunt, penetrating, and—most commonly in this era—that following cardiac surgery)]. Acute pericarditis is characterized pathologically by inflammation with fibrinous exudate that may involve not only the pericardial layers themselves but also the epicardial surface of the myocardium. Accumulation of pericardial fluid (effusion) is common and occasionally hemodynamically significant. Specific underlying disease entities may distort the characteristic pathophysiological changes (e.g., neoplastic involvement or irradiation) by directly altering pericardial stiffness.

Acute pericarditis may be clinically silent but is most often heralded by pleuritic-type chest pain. Although pericardial pain may vary in quality and location, it is typically localized to the retrosternal and left precordial regions, with radiation to the shoulder and neck. The pain is often exacerbated by coughing or deep inspiration. However, in contrast to pure pleuritic pain, pericardial pain is often aggravated when the patient lies supine or swallows and alleviated when the patient sits up and leans forward. Acute pericarditis may be manifest by dyspnea resulting from an unconscious alteration to a shallower pattern of respiration in avoidance of pericardial pain. Dyspnea may more ominously signal the presence of a hemodynamically significant pericardial effusion and cardiac tamponade.

The physical examination is influenced by the underlying etiological disease entity and the presence or absence of a hemodynamically significant pericardial effusion. Patients are typically febrile and may appear "systemically ill." The pathognomonic clinical feature of acute pericarditis is a scratchy, leathery, high-pitched pericardial friction rub with multiple components all related to the cardiac cycle. Such rubs may be evanescent. Their presence, pitch, quality, and number of components may vary, and they may be heard even in the presence of significant pericardial effusion. Pericardial friction rubs must be differentiated from pleural rubs (the latter typically more lateralized in the chest and varying with respiration rather than cardiac motion) and mediastinal (Hamman's) crunch (a harsh, cracking, substernal auscultatory phenomenon caused by mediastinal air). A single-component rub must be differentiated from a harsh cardiac murmur (aortic stenosis, hypertrophic obstructive cardiomyopathy, and mitral or tricuspid regurgitation). Assessment of the presence and hemodynamic significance of associated pericardial effusions is critical.

The major complications of acute pericarditis result from the inflammation and underlying disease. The major acute complication of pericarditis is cardiac tamponade (see below). Over time, pericarditis may smolder and result in fibro-calcific changes (particularly in the parietal layer), leading to constrictive pericarditis (see below). Factors that influence the development of pericardial constriction have not been fully delineated. However, constriction is more common when the antecedent acute pericarditis is related to trauma with hemopericardium, tuberculosis, or after mediastinal irradiation. Acute pericarditis is occasionally associated with arrhythmias, most commonly innocent PACs and/or PVCs and less commonly supraventricular tachycardias. It is almost invariably accompanied by sinus tachycardia.

VI. EVALUATION

Noninvasive studies are usually sufficient for assessment of acute pericarditis. The ECG is sensitive (acute abnormalities evident in over 90% of cases) but non-specific. Demonstration of characteristic ECG abnormalities, in particular their serial "evolution" over time, is helpful in establishing the presence of acute pericarditis and differentiating it from acute myocardial ischemia. The classic ECG changes of pericarditis evolve sequentially and include: (a) ST-segment elevation with upright T waves and depressed PR segment; (b) isoelectric ST segments with flat or inverted T waves and depressed PR segment; (c) isoelectric ST segments, inverted T waves and isoelectric PR segment; and (d) normalization. The first accompanies the acute onset of chest pain; the second and third evolve over several days, and the fourth may not occur for weeks or months. With the exception of sometimes showing diffuse low voltage, however, the ECG is not helpful in detecting associated pericardiac effusions.

The plain chest film is not helpful in detecting pericardial inflammation itself but may provide useful information regarding the presence or absence of a significant effusion (evident as cardiomegaly with a "water bottle–shaped" heart), and abnormalities associated with specific underlying disease entities (e.g., pulmonary infections, cancer, acute MI resulting in heart failure). Echocardiography may be unrevealing in simple, uncomplicated acute pericarditis but is a critical test to establish the presence and define the hemodynamic significance of pericardial effusions, detect abnormalities of the pericardial layers themselves, and delineate underlying cardiac abnormalities such as regional wall motion abnormalities associated with acute MI. Blood tests are not usually helpful but may slow elevations of cardiac enzymes (positive MB creatine kinase) resulting from epicardial inflammation associated with primary acute pericarditis. The differentiation from acute myocardial infarction, with which the echocardiogram will often show regional wall motion abnormalities, and secondary pericarditis is critical.

VII. DIFFERENTIAL DIAGNOSIS

Establishing the etiology of acute pericarditis is of paramount importance, most particularly with respect to the therapeutic implications of underlying disorders such as acute myocardial infarction, treatable infections (tuberculosis, bacterial pericarditis), and aortic dissection. The most important entities to identify promptly include the following.

A. Acute Myocardial Infarction

Acute pericarditis may mimic or be caused by acute MI. Acute transmural myocardial infarction (particularly anterior) may induce acute pericarditis because of inflammation contiguous to transmural necrosis. Acute pericarditis developing weeks or months after acute MI (Dressler's syndrome) is presumed to be of autoimmune origin; a similar syndrome; and postpericardiotomy pericarditis, may occur early or late after open-heart surgery. In patients presenting with acute chest pain and nonspecific ECG changes in which initial differentiation of primary acute pericarditis from acute myocardial ischemia or infarction may be difficult, noninvasive testing by two-dimensional echocardiography to identify wall motion abnormalities and subsequent evaluation of serial ECGs and cardiac enzymes can establish the correct diagnosis. Identification of acute pericarditis associated with acute MI may have implications with regard to anticoagulation and the use of thrombolytic agents. Although not absolutely precluded, fibrinolytic drugs must be used with caution and awareness of the risk of induction of pericardial effusion.

B. Infectious Pericarditis

Treatable infections resulting in pericarditis include tuberculosis and purulent pericarditis (caused by bacterial, rickettsial, and other pathogens). Consideration

272

of unusual infections (e.g., fungal or retroviral) in susceptible individuals should stimulate consideration of testing appropriate for specific entities. However, even in immunocompromised hosts, pericardial infection is rarely primary. Therefore assiduous investigations to identify regional or systemic infection is essential. Pericarditis may complicate infective endocarditis (penetrating contiguous myocardial abscess, ruptured aortic abscess or eroding septic coronary arterial embolus), at which stage primary infection of the heart is usually obvious from echocardiograms. "Idiopathic" acute pericarditis most often results from viral infections (e.g., Coxsackie and echo B), which can be identified retrospectively with acute and convalescent serological testing.

C. Neoplastic Pericarditis

Both solid-organ and hemopoietic tumors metastasize to the heart, a common manifestation of which is acute pericarditis. Insidious or abrupt effusion may be the presenting problem. Initial screening of patients with acute pericarditis for tumor (e.g., lung, breast, lymphoma, melanoma, and leukemia) with physical examination, chest x-ray, and blood studies is sufficient unless an otherwise unexplained bloody effusion is identified, which should stimulate a search for occult malignancy.

D. Miscellaneous

Identification of systemic inflammatory states and metabolic disorders that may result in acute pericarditis is important, particularly such entities as connective tissue disease, drug-induced vasculitides, uremia, and myxedema.

VIII. MANAGEMENT

Once appropriate steps have been taken to establish the underlying etiology of pericarditis, therapy should be targeted not only at the underlying condition but also at the pericardial inflammation itself. In general, acute pericarditis should be initially evaluated and managed in-hospital, so that underlying associated acute myocardial infarction, treatable infections, or other potentially life-threatening conditions as well as the presence, development, and progress of pericardial effusions and arrhythmias can be recognized and managed appropriately. Patients should be put at bed rest until pain and systemic inflammation (fever) have abated. Telemetry is appropriate for the first 24 hr. Pericardial pain typically responds to nonsteroidal anti-inflammatory drugs (aspirin 650 mg q 6–8 hr or indomethacin 25–50 mg q 6 hr); analgesics (meperidine hydrochloride or morphine) should be administered as needed. For severe or refractory pericardial pain, oral or intravenous corticosteroids may be necessary. The patient should be examined on a daily basis to ascertain potential development of hemodynamically important pericardial effusion. In the vast majority of patients, conservative measures will suffice and thereby can be tapered over 3 to 7 days.

Acute viral pericarditis may occasionally be recrudescent, with episodes over several months, which may predispose to development of constrictive pericarditis. Such recurrences should be managed with reinstitution of anti-inflammatory drugs, initially nonsteroids but including short courses of corticosteroids in more recalcitrant cases.

Pericardial effusions associated with idiopathic or acute viral pericarditis usually abate over several weeks or months. Therefore, if the echocardiogram demonstrates a small effusion and the initial course is uncomplicated, follow-up with serial chest x-ray and clinical examination is usually sufficient. In patients with initially more substantial effusions, an echocardiogram should be repeated several weeks after an uncomplicated course or earlier hemodynamic abnormalities are present. When effusions persist or increase despite optimal therapy or a pyogenic process or neoplastic source is suspected, diagnostic and potentially therapeutic pericardiocentesis is indicated.

IX. CARDIAC TAMPONADE

Cardiac tamponade is a life-threatening hemodynamic condition resulting from a pericardial effusion that increases IPP sufficiently to externally compress and restrict filling of cardiac chambers and constrain cardiac output, inducing backward failure. The most common causes include effusions secondary to neoplasm, cardiac surgery, catheter- or pacemaker-induced myocardial perforation of the right atrium or ventricle, idiopathic pericarditis, acute myocardial infarction with cardiac rupture, and uremia. Hemodynamic consequences reflect the volume of the effusion, rapidity of its accumulation, compliance of the pericardium and myocardium, cardiac compensatory mechanisms (contractility and heart rate), and total blood volume. For any given magnitude of effusion, the interval over which it accumulates is a critical determinant of hemodynamic impairment. Thus, acutely developing effusions of even 300 to 400 mL (e.g., related to pacemaker-induced chamber perforation) can abruptly elevate intrapericardial pressure and induce tamponade. However, given time, the pericardium can stretch and exhibit compliance. Accordingly, slow accumulation of fluid (even in amounts greater than 1 L, associated with neoplasms) may be tolerated with little or no hemodynamic compromise. At some point, however, even chronic effusions can accumulate sufficiently to encroach on the limits of pericardial compliance. Then, even small increments in intrapericardial volume sharply increase IPP and compromise hemodynamics.

Once IPP exceeds 8 to 10 mmHg, cardiac filling is compromised. Hemodynamically significant effusions compress the cardiac chambers throughout diastole, limiting chamber filling and cardiac output. Although chamber volumes are markedly decreased (evident by echocardiography as diminished chamber volumes with chamber compression), filling pressures are markedly increased, reflecting not only the actual transmural distending pressure within the ventricle but also the external resistance of the pericardium. Increased contractility and, most importantly, sinus tachycardia, which can signal the presence of a hemodynamically important effusion and herald hemodynamic collapse, are compensatory mechanisms. Hemodynamically important pericardial effusions increase pulsus paradoxus (inspiratory decrease in aortic systolic pressure $\geqslant$ 15 mmHg) by rendering RV filling more dependent on inspiratory increases in systemic venous return and compromising LV filling when RV filling is relatively augmented.

A. Clinical Presentations

Hemodynamically significant cardiac effusions may induce dyspnea, mimic predominant right heart failure, and present with hypotension, unexplained sinus tachycardia, easy fatigability, or asymptomatic cardiomegaly. With tamponade, a constellation of these manifestations may be present. The most severe form presents a severe right heart failure with clear lungs and low cardiac output. Jugular venous pressure (JVP) is elevated and the waveform abnormal, as is arterial blood pressure. The sine qua non of cardiac tamponade is elevation of JVP pressure. Elevated IPP greater than 10 mmHg will be evident as increased JVP with a sharp X descent (reflecting systolic intrapericardial depressurization coincident with ventricular emptying), but a blunted Y descent (reflecting pandiastolic resistance to RV filling because of the resonant interplay of increasing ventricular volume in a confined space with external pressure transmitted to the atria and ventricle by the effusion). The waveforms are best delineated by timing the most visually dramatic collapse of the JVP to the carotid upstroke. Collapse that occurs coincident with the carotid upstroke is the systolic X descent. That following the carotid peak is the diastolic Y descent. In patients in sinus rhythm who are breathing spontaneously, pathological pulsus paradoxus is evident, best measured by initially determining peak systolic pressure over several beats, then inflating the blood pressure cuff to this level during quiet held expiration, and then slowly deflating the cuff with held full inspiration and defining the systolic drop. Profound tamponade may result in palpable paradox, evident by marked diminution of disappearance of the brachial pulse with inspiration. Activation of cardiac compensatory mechanisms maintaining cardiac output and blood pressure becomes clinically evident with evolving tamponade, most notably sinus tachycardia and peripheral vasoconstriction. When these compensatory mechanisms can no longer sustain cardiac output, low output and hypotension develop rapidly. Although cardiac tamponade elevates filling pressures, cardiac volumes are reduced. Thus, the precordium is quiet. Despite the fact that left and right heart filling pressures are elevated and equalized, the amount of fluid in the pulmonary veins is modest. Accordingly, the lungs are typically clear despite sometimes profound dyspnea.

X. NONINVASIVE DIAGNOSTIC PROCEDURES

The chest x-ray typically shows cardiomegaly, often with a "water bottle shape." Lung fields are characteristically oligemic. The ECG may show diffuse low voltage and nonspecific ST-T changes. In patients with severe hemodynamic compromise, electrical alternans, which is ominous, may appear. Two-dimensional echocardiography can detect pericardial effusions, assess its hemodynamic significance, and guide therapeutic pericardiocentesis. It is essential to assess not only the volume of the effusion itself but also its effects on the cardiac chambers. Accordingly, echocardiographic documentation of reduced chamber volume associated with compression of the inferior vena cava or RA reflects severe embarrassment. Free wall compression of the RV is indicative of even greater compromise.

XI. CARDIAC CATHETERIZATION

Elevated and equalized diastolic filling pressures in the RA, RV, pulmonary artery capillary wedge position, and LV are typical of tamponade. Characteristic waveform alterations in the RA with a prominent A wave reflecting augmented RA contraction into a stiff, noncompliant RV and pericardium, a steep X descent reflecting both accelerated atrial relaxation and systolic intrapericardial depressurization, and a blunted Y descent indicative of pandiastolic resistance to RV filling are likely.

Equalized diastolic filling pressure is not specific. It may also be seen in constrictive pericarditis, restrictive cardiomyopathy, RV infarction, and with conditions of sudden chamber dilatation in the left heart (e.g., acute and severe mitral regurgitation). Conversely, preexisting pathological conditions may preclude equalization of filling pressures, particularly those associated with intrinsic cardiac disease. Diastolic pressure may be increased and unrelated to pericardial abnormalities.

Severe effusions typically result in low stroke volume and cardiac output, despite neurohormonally mediated reflex sinus tachycardia and elevation of systemic vascular resistance. Before the wide availability of two-dimensional echocardiography, invasive hemodynamic evaluation was essential in assessing the hemodynamic significance of pericardial effusions. However, ultrasonography has preempted the need for invasive hemodynamic assessment in most patients. In compromised patients in whom echocardiography is definitive, invasive studies before pericardiocentesis are unnecessary. Their performance may waste precious time in the case of a life-threatening tamponade. However, when the hemodynamic significance of large effusions is not clear from physical examination and

276

results of noninvasive studies or when combined effusive and constrictive or restrictive physiology is suspected, invasive hemodynamic assessments are often needed.

XII. HEMODYNAMIC ASSESSMENT OF PERICARDIAL EFFUSIONS: CLINICAL ALGORITHMS

Cardiac tamponade is a potentially life-threatening emergency that responds dramatically to properly performed and optimally timed pericardial damage and decompensation. The most critical initial step in management is establishing the magnitude of hemodynamic compromise. Hemodynamic assessment may be necessary in "asymptomatic" patients, in whom an effusion is initially identified incidentally in noninvasive studies (i.e., chest x-ray or echocardiography), and in patients presenting with primary hemodynamic abnormalities consistent with a diagnosis of cardiac tamponade. Regardless of the circumstances, the hemodynamic impact of effusions can be categorized as (a) hemodynamically important effusion: effusion present by ultrasound (may be large), but without chamber compression. The JVP is less than 5 to 7 mmHg; blood pressure, heart rate, and respiratory rate are normal; clinical stigmata of impaired perfusion are absent as is dyspnea; (b) hemodynamically important but compensated effusion: echocardiography shows prominent effusion with mild compression of the inferior vena cava, RA, and/or RV free wall; JVP is elevated. Pathological pulsus paradoxus may be present, but neither hypotension nor tachycardia are seen. Perfusion is not compromised and dyspnea is absent; (c) hemodynamically severe effusion with compensatory mechanisms maximally activated: prominent effusion is seen on ultrasound with chamber collapse; JVP is elevated with a sharp X but blunted Y descent, pathological paradoxical pulse is prominent, but there is no hypotension and perfusion is adequate. The patient is often tachypneic, and resting tachycardia is present; and (d) hemodynamically severe effusion, decompensated: ultrasound shows prominent effusion with chamber collapse. The heart may be swinging in pericardium, giving rise to electrical alternans affecting all components of the ECG waveform (P, ORS, and T waves). The JVP is markedly elevated, pathological pulsus paradoxus is severe, sinus tachycardia is pronounced, tachypnea is marked, hypotension is striking, and compromise of perfusion is evident clinically. Of note, modest effusions that accumulate rapidly may produce such profound hemodynamic effects.

XIII. MANAGEMENT

Regardless of the underlying cause of a hemodynamically significant effusion, echocardiographically-guided pericardiocentesis is the initial drainage procedure of choice. Pericardiocentesis provides prompt relief of hemodynamic compromise and may be lifesaving.

Echocardiographic monitoring increases the safety, success and efficacy of pericardiocentesis. Surgical intervention is now rarely required. Under optimal conditions, echocardiographically guided pericardiocentesis is best performed in a procedure room equipped with electrocardiographic and hemodynamic monitoring. Fluoroscopic monitoring is not necessary. Pericardiocentesis can be performed either at the bedside or in a cardiac care unit as well. In profoundly compromised patients, pericardiocentesis should be performed "on site" (emergency room, regular ward); in those with impending or manifest cardiovascular "collapse" (systolic blood pressure < 70 mmHg with signs of cerebral hypoperfusion), done blindly if necessary even without echocardiographic monitoring. The following is a practical procedure protocol suitable for use in most urgent circumstances.

Under controlled conditions, pericardiocentesis should be performed with the patient lying at an angle of approximately 45–90° (depending on patient comfort), with ECG and digital blood pressure monitoring. The patient should be gowned with a cap and a mask to enhance sterility, and the patient's head should be turned away from the operator. Patients with even mild hemodynamic compromise should be given a volume challenge while being closely monitored. Those with hypotension or hypoperfusion should be given dopamine to support cardiac output. While the subxiphisternal area is being prepared, an echocardiographic assistant should establish an optimal apical four-chamber monitoring view. The skin over the xiphisternum should be rendered sterile and infiltrated with 1–2% lidocaine. A small superficial incision should be made with a #11 scalpel blade. The pericardiocentesis needle is attached to an anesthetic-filled syringe and the syringe is advanced on a path under the xiphisternum toward the tip of the left scapula under constant echocardiographic imaging with constant aspiration and with anesthetic infiltrated intermittently as necessary for patient comfort. Resistance is typically encountered through the first several centimeters of soft tissue. However, a "give" or "release" indicates penetration of the needle through the diaphragm, following which the needle is slowly but steadily directed forward with constant aspiration and monitoring of the apical four-chamber view for evidence of entrance into the pericardial sac (indicated by the emergence of a bright, echogenic density in the area of the apex or RV free wall). Should aspiration of fluid be noted at any time while the needle is being advanced, the syringe should be aspirated to its full volume and the fluid "banked" immediately for microbiological, chemical, and cytological analyses. Whether the fluid is serous, serosanguinous, or frankly bloody, a syringe filled with agitated saline should be attached to the needle as soon as free aspiration is noted, the syringe plunger aspirated slightly to assure a fluid-fluid interface, and the agitated saline injected rapidly under echocardiographic monitoring to define optimal positioning of the needle tip within the pericardium, as indicated by the appearance of bright swirling echogenic contrast bubbles ("popcorn" echodense appearance) within the pericardial sac. Contrast bubbles within the cardiac chambers indicate penetration of the needle into the heart itself. If contrast appears in the cardiac chambers or if the needle encounters resistance and motion suggesting contact with or penetration into a cardiac chamber, it should be immediately but slowly retracted with constant aspiration and anticipation that the pericardial chamber may be entered retrograde. Contrast injections should be repeated at any time while the needle is being retracted if a serous or serosanguinous fluid is aspirated. If an effusion that is not grossly hemorrhagic is encountered during initial needle advancement and contrast injected at this time does not enter either the pericardium or the cardiac chambers, the effusion is likely to be pleural fluid, which accompanies pericardial effusions in many conditions. In such cases, the needle should be advanced further until its tip is evident in or near the pericardium or a new fluid pocket is encountered, in which case agitated saline should be injected again.

Any time that contrast is identified within the pericardial space, the syringe should be removed immediately and a guide wire threaded through the needle into the pericardial space. The guide wire should be threaded deeply within the pericardium under echocardiographic monitoring in order to "break up" any loculations that may be present, thereby optimizing the likelihood of complete drainage. Once the guide wire has been threaded into the pericardial space, the needle is removed, and a dilator is inserted over the wire to create a track sufficient for over-the-wire insertion of a drainage catheter with multiple side holes, which is threaded over the indwelling guide wire and advanced similarly deep within the pericardial space to dislodge loculations and thereby achieve greater pericardial drainage. The guide wire is then removed and the catheter attached to a drainage system consisting of large-bore connecting tubing, a three-way stopcock, and a drainage bag. The pericardium is first drained manually with the use of a large (60-mL) syringe. Fluid should be aspirated rapidly in patients with acute hemodynamic embarrassment (the contrast of the first syringe must be banked immediately for subsequent analysis). The pericardium is then drained to the fullest extent possible by aspiration. When drainage is limited at any given position, the catheter can be flushed with a very small amount of sterile injectable saline to remove potential clots for fibrinous material. If free flow is not restored, the catheter should be slowly and sequentially withdrawn at 2- to 3-cm increments under constant aspiration until free flow is reestablished while monitoring the volume of the effusion by echocardiography. Once the catheter has been withdrawn with only 20–30 cm remaining within the pericardium, further drainage may be enhanced by positioning the patient at a higher angle, which may move fluid toward the apex. Echocardiographic analysis is needed to define adequate reduction in the volume of pericardial fluid and increases in cardiac chamber volumes.

After maximal drainage has been accomplished, a decision must be made regarding whether to leave the catheter indwelling over 12 to 36 hr for drainage of recurrent effusions. Such decisions are predicated in part on the completeness of primary drainage and the suspected etiology of the effusion. Nonneoplastic, nonpurulent effusions that are completely drained on first catheterization attempts do not necessarily require indwelling catheters. A sterilely placed indwelling catheter in place for 18–24 hr, with repeat ultrasound to affirm lack of acute recurrence of effusion, is safe and may avoid the need for repeat pericardiocentesis. Incomplete initial drainage with substantial residual effusion is an indication for prolonged drainage. Evidence or suspicion of neoplastic effusion warrants an indwelling catheter. Echocardiographic documentation of incomplete drainage and/or early recurrence can be managed by installation of sclerosing agents, balloon pericardiotomy, or surgical subxiphoid pericardial window. Evidence of purulent effusion necessitates urgent surgical drainage as well as aggressive antibiotic therapy. Emergency pericardiocentesis for catheter or pacemaker cardiac perforation and induced tamponade (along with reversal of anticoagulation) often leads to hemodynamic stabilization and may be definitive. Even if complete drainage is accomplished and effusion does not recur promptly, cardiac perforations require indwelling catheter drainage for 24 hr, with repeat echocardiographic study over 1–4 hr be sure that hemostasis has been accomplished.

In many cases of perforation, pericardiocentesis is only a temporizing measure. If a bloody effusion reaccumulates 15–20 min after restoration of normal clotting, urgent surgical repair is required. This is the case in nearly all patients with traumatic effusions caused by penetrating injuries.

Long-term management of effusions is determined by the completeness of initial drainage and the underlying condition. In patients with recurrent effusions, surgical drainage by subxiphoid thoracotomy may be necessary. In expert hands, thoracoscopic procedures may be successful and less morbid. Balloon pericardiotomy is a newer catheter-based intervention employing standard pericardiocentesis techniques but utilizing a large valvuloplasty balloon catheter to "rupture" a hole in the pericardium. Although the limited experience with this procedure suggests that it may be successful in treating refractory effusions, its use has been associated with significant morbidity and some mortality. Further research is necessary to determine whether it should be employed widely, and if so, in which circumstances.

Long-term management of neoplastic effusions is particularly challenging. They are prone to early recurrence even after initial optimal catheter drainage. Such effusions tend to be large and compromising. Adjunctive measures including sclerotherapy (intrapericardial instillation of bleomycin or tetracycline) may diminish recurrences and be justified in severely ill patients with widespread metastases and limited longevity. Although advocates of primary balloon pericardiotomy or direct surgical windows argue that such measures may be definitive, they are employed only with appropriate reluctance because of their relatively high risk and often preterminal state of the patients. One strategy is to perform ultrasound after 24 hr of catheter drainage, following which, if the pericardium is dry, the catheter is removed and the patient reassessed clinically and by ultrasound in 1–2 weeks. If the effusion recurs, repeat pericardiocentesis with sclerotherapy can be employed. If substantial effusion persists after the initial 24 hr of drainage, a surgical window may be justified.

XIV. CONSTRICTIVE PERICARDITIS

Chamber-constrictive pericarditis occurs when a thick, inelastic pericardium encases the heart and restricts filling, resulting in chronic biventricular diastolic dysfunction, predominant right heart failure, and fatigue. It typically follows single or multiple episodes of acute pericarditis, giving rise to fibrocalcific thickening of parietal pericardium. The process is slowly progressive, occurring over months or years. It is often idiopathic. Common identifiable causes include irradiation pericarditis (typically at least 4000 rads to the chest mantle), hemorrhagic pericarditis, or hemopericardium (resulting from intense inflammation or, more commonly, from traumatic hemocardium developing postsurgically or from blunt chest trauma), and chronic inflammatory states including tuberculosis and uremia.

Constriction alters chamber compliance, resulting in biventricular diastolic dysfunction manifest clinically as predominant chronic right heart failure. However, in contrast to cardiac tamponade, the diastolic abnormalities are chronic and typically present as hepatic congestion or cirrhosis, ascites, and peripheral edema. Associated systolic impairment caused by restricted preload can result in easy fatigability. Whereas, in cardiac tamponade, pandiastolic resistance restricts ventricular filing, with constriction, early ventricular filling is resistance-free. However, as the ventricles rapidly fill, they meet the inelastic resistance of the stiff pericardium, at which time filling pressure rises rapidly to an elevated plateau. This hemodynamic pattern is manifest in the JVP and RA pressure waveforms as elevated mean filling pressure with both a sharp X descent, reflecting rapid atrial transport of blood into the stiff RV and pericardial shell, and associated accelerated atrial relaxation, with a sharp Y descent reflecting the initial rapid resistance-free early RV filling. The RV waveform is similarly distinctive, with a "dip and plateau" or "square root" pattern reflecting the rapid ventricular relaxation and a sharp increase in filling pressure as the expanding ventricle meets the constraints of the pericardium. The RA, RV, pulmonary capillary wedge, and LV filling pressures are elevated and equalized. The LV pressure waveform may exhibit a dip-and-plateau pattern similar to that seen in the RV.

In contrast to cardiac tamponade, in which intrathoracic pressures are transmitted through the pericardium and inspiratory augmentation of venous return and right heart filling are intact, in constrictive pericarditis, the inelastic pericardial shell does not allow inspiratory augmentation of right heart filling; therefore constrictive pericarditis does not result in a (pathological) paradoxical pulse. Instead, the inspiratory gradient created between the extrathoracic great vessels and intrathoracic but extrapericardial great vessels, combined with the increased intraabdominal pressure associated with deep inspiration, send blood rushing back to the thoracic cage. At the same time, augmentation of right heart filling is precluded by the constricted pericardium, resulting in an inspiratory increase in JVP, termed "Kussmaul's sign." A change in RV chamber shape with inspiration caused by the pericardium attached to the diaphragm by inflammatory tissue contributes. When pericardial effusions (particularly postsurgical, hemorrhagic ones) are coupled with constriction, effusive-constrictive hemodynamics may develop, with a hybridized hemodynamic state manifest as biventricular diastolic dysfunction with elevated and equalized filling pressures, with sufficient pericardial compliance to allow inspiratory augmentation of venous return and resulting in pulsus paradoxus and no Kussmaul's sign.

A. Physical Examination

Vital signs with the patient at rest are typically normal, with absence of dyspnea (unless the patient is in profound right heart failure, which results in reflex neurohormonal activation and sinus tachycardia). Lower-extremity edema, consistent with the magnitude of right heart failure, may be massive, extending to the buttocks and perineum. Upper extremities are not edematous but may share muscle wasting secondary to cardiac cachexia and malabsorption caused by bowel venous congestion. Clear lung fields, marked elevation of the JVP with a distinctive waveform (prominent A wave, sharp X descent, and—in contrast to tamponade—a sharp Y descent reflecting the fact that the first third of diastole is resistance-free) are typical. Kussmaul's sign is present in two-thirds of cases. The arterial pulse upstroke and amplitude are usually normal, although in severe constriction the amplitude may decline because of limited LV preload. (Pathological) pulsus paradoxus is seen in less than 30% of cases (i.e., those in which the pericardium though constricted, though sufficiently compliant for transmission of intrapleural pressure). The constricted pericardium typically results in a very quiet precordium. An auscultatory hallmark is a pericardial knock—a diastolic filling sound corresponding to the sudden cessation of ventricular filling that correlates with the end of the early "dip" in the RV pressure waveform. The first heart sound is typically normal. The second heart sound may be widely split, attributable to early aortic valve closure related to a decreased LV stroke volume, especially with inspiration. Ascites and marked hepatomegaly may be seen unless the chronic passive congestion leads to cirrhosis, in which case the liver may be small.

B. Noninvasive Diagnostic Studies

Chest x-ray reveals the cardiac silhouette on plain chest films. Pericardial calcification may be evident (especially on the lateral), particularly with tuberculous or posttraumatic constriction. The right superior mediastinum may be enlarged because of dilatation of the superior vena cava. Because the left atrium is not totally intrapericardial, its enlargement is not uncommon. Pleural effusions may be present (reflecting chronic severe right heart failure), but pulmonary densities typical of elevated pulmonary venous pressure are uncommon. The ECG may show diffuse low voltage with nonspecific ST-T changes. Atrial arrhythmias, including atrial fibrillation, may occur because of epicardial inflammation and calcification as well as left atrial dilatation.

Echocardiography demonstrates small ventricles and a preload-deprived right atrium. The left atrium (extrapericardial) may be enlarged because of impaired LV compliance. The LV contractility may be impaired and global ejection fraction depressed. Restricted filling early in diastole may be manifest as "bounce" of the interventricular septum and/or LV posterior wall. Echocardiographic images may demonstrate pericardial thickening, evident by M-mode as two parallel lines (representing two surfaces of the pericardium) separated by a clear space from the posterior wall of the LV and free wall of the RV. Alternatively, the pericardium may appear as multiple dense echos posterior to the LV free wall. Two-dimensional imaging may confirm thickening of the pericardial layers. Computed tomography and magnetic resonance imaging provide better images for calculating pericardial thickness. An abnormal contour at the reflection of the pericardium to the posterior left atrial wall may be evident. Dilatation of the inferior vena cava and hepatic veins, with blunted respiratory fluctuation ("plethora") is typical.

C. Differential Diagnosis

Constrictive pericarditis may present as chronic predominant right heart failure, hepatic failure, or cirrhosis. Conditions other than constriction that produce predominantly right heart failure must be considered, including superior vena cava constriction, tricuspid valve obstruction (tricuspid stenosis or RA or RV tumors), RV infarction, restrictive cardiomyopathy, dilated cardiomyopathy, and cor pulmonale. In those patients with constrictive or restrictive physiology in whom the pericardium is not thickened, assiduous search for infiltrative disease processes that result in restriction (e.g., amyloidosis, sclerodermas, hemochromatosis) sometimes leads to a thickened interatrial septum, which, evident on echocardiograms, will often identify underlying etiology. Rarely, endomyocardial biopsy will be helpful.

D. Management

Because of the indolent nature of the constrictive process, fatigability may be ignored or ascribed to nonspecific causes until right heart failure develops. Patients with mild right heart failure can be managed initially with diuretics and venodilators to relieve systemic venous congestion. However, most patients with substantial right heart failure ultimately require complete surgical resection of the pericardium, usually involving a median sternotomy with full cardiopulmonary bypass. Operative mortality approaches 7–10%. Many patients suffer postoperative low-output syndrome. However, the large majority exhibit improved hemodynamics and functional class.

16

Management of Patients with Supraventricular Arrhythmias

Management of Patients with Cardiac Arrhythmias   **286**
   I.   Sinus Rhythm   286
  II.   Sinus Tachycardia   286
 III.   Sinus Node Reentry   288
 IV.   Atrial Premature Depolarizations   290
  V.   Ectopic Atrial Tachycardia   293
 VI.   Junctional Escape Beats and Junctional Premature
       Depolarizations   296

Intraatrial Reentrant Arrhythmias   **299**
 VII.   Intraatrial Reentrant Tachycardia   300
VIII.   Atrial Flutter   303
  IX.   Atrial Fibrillation   305

Atrioventricular Nodal Reentrant Tachycardia   **311**
   X.   Pathology   311
 XI.   Electrocardiographic Characteristics   312
 XII.   Management Strategies   314

Accessory Pathway–Mediated Tachycardias   **318**
 XIV.   Manifest and Concealed Accessory Pathways   318
  XV.   Mechanisms Underlying Tachycardia   318
 XVI.   Mahaim Fibers   320
XVII.   Electrocardiographic Characteristics   321
XVIII.   Management   326

      Suggested Reading   330

Management of Patients with Cardiac Arrhythmias

James A. Reiffel, James Coromilas, J. Thomas Bigger, Jr., and Elsa Grace V. Giardina

I. SINUS RHYTHM

The dominant physiological rhythm in a normal heart originates in the sinus node. Normal sinus rhythm (NSR) is manifest by upright P waves in the inferior and lateral electrocardiographic (ECG) leads and rates of 60–100 beats/min with sedentary wakefulness in adults. Rates are higher in infants and children and decline with maturation. Although the intrinsic sinus node rate continues to decrease during adulthood, parasympathetic influence and alpha$_1$-receptor sensitivity does as well, with a net result of stable sinus rates.

The rate of NSR is not fixed, though the range it varies through is. The rate at any instant reflects intrinsic nodal function influenced by the modulating effects of many factors. Prime among these are parasympathetic and sympathetic input. Others include concentrations of adrenal catecholamines in blood, thyroid hormone, temperature, acid-base status, and electrolytes. Parasympathetic nervous system inhibition or adrenal medullary hormone release will, for example, increase sinus rates. If the rate exceeds 100 beats/min, the rhythm is considered to be sinus tachycardia.

II. SINUS TACHYCARDIA

Sinus tachycardia resulting only from vagal withdrawal will not exceed 120 bpm in normal adults, as has been shown by results after pharmacological parasympathetic blockade and by cardiac transplantation. In contrast, vagal withdrawal coupled with sympathetic activation or other metabolic or chemical stimulation will elevate sinus rates above 120 beats/min. In normal subjects, for example, aerobic exercise typified by parasympathetic inhibition and sympathetic stimulation increases sinus rate proportionately to the isotonic load until an age-related maximum is reached [approximately 220 minus age (in years) in beats/min]. Mechanical effects of atrial stretch and altered sinus node artery pulse pressure may influence the rates achieved with physiological sinus tachycardia through alterations in sinus node cellular electrophysiologic properties. With enhanced physiological training (conditioning), the maximal achievable sinus rate does not

286

change; rather, the rate of increase during aerobic exercise slows, so that exercise time preceding the point of reaching one's maximal sinus rate is prolonged.

Sinus tachycardia may be pathological as well as physiological. Uniquely among arrhythmias, it is a "red flag" demanding identification of a primary cause. Pathological sinus tachycardia is probably best defined by a rate over 100 beats/min, which is inappropriate for the level of physical activity. Most commonly, pathological sinus tachycardia results from enhanced adrenergic neuronal or adrenal catecholamine release, thyrotoxicosis, abnormal psychological states (e.g., anxiety), hypoglycemia, or the ingestion of an agent with sympathomimetic, vagolytic, or direct-stimulating effects. It may be a reflex response to hypotension, reduced cardiac output, or decreased vascular volume such as that seen with hemorrhage.

Pathological sinus tachycardia with or without hypotension may be orthostatic in the setting of autonomic neuropathy. Pharmacologically enhanced sympathetic input to the sinus node can result as a reflex response to the administration of hypotensive agents such as vasodilators—including nifedipine, hydralazine, or minoxidil. The ACE inhibitors and newer dihydropyridine calcium channel blockers (amilodipine and felodipine) are less apt to produce sinus tachycardia than are other vasodilators because of a variety of mechanisms. Centrally acting psychotropic drugs may increase sinus rate through vagolytic and other effects. Particularly vagolytic agents are the tricyclic antidepressants. Direct-acting and/or sympathomimetic agents include xanthine oxidase inhibitors (such as caffeine or theophylline), synthetic catecholamines with beta-agonist activity, exogenous thyroid hormone, and cocaine. Frequently, pathological sinus tachycardia is accompanied by other signs of catecholamine, thyroid, or stimulant excess, such as tremor, sweating, increased cardiac output, and uneasiness. The so-called hyperkinetic heart syndrome probably reflects such pathophysiology.

Less frequent causes of pathological sinus tachycardia include (a) sinus tachycardia following radiofrequency ablation of the atrioventricular (AV) node region, which is transient ($<$ 1 month) and probably results from altered intracardiac parasympathetic transmission, and (b) sinus node reentrant tachycardia, which is discussed below. Perhaps paradoxically, it results from impaired conduction rather than from enhanced automaticity. Occasionally, sinus tachycardia is idiopathic. As with other persistent tachyarrhythmias, tachycardia-induced cardiomyopathy is a risk of persistent idiopathic sinus tachycardia.

A. Electrocardiographic Characteristics

Sinus tachycardia is recognized electrocardiographically by a normal sinus P-wave contour but a rate of over 100 bpm beats/min. In the presence of a prolonged PR interval and/or at rates that result in the absence of a TP segment, however, the P-wave morphology may be difficult or impossible to discern, as the

P wave may merge with or be superimposed upon the T wave, where it can be distorted or unrecognizable. In such circumstances, sinus tachycardia may be inferred from a physiologically appropriate rate, a normal PR interval, the presence of some cycle-length variation (best seen at rapid ECG-paper speeds), and/or a gradual rather than abrupt increase and decrease in rate at the onset and offset of the tachycardia (if electrocardiographically captured) and/or with carotid sinus massage. Ectopic tachycardias, in contrast, particularly those that are paroxysmal, are more frequently extremely regular in their cycle length (except at tachycardia onset and offset), are usually abrupt in their onset and termination, and most typically have a prolonged PR interval, with an RP less than PR. In the infrequent nonsinus supraventricular tachycardias with late diastolic P waves, the abnormal P-wave vector easily allows differentiation from sinus tachycardia. On intracardiac electrograms, sinus tachycardia is typified also by the earliest atrial activation occurring in the SA nodal region of the high lateral right atrium.

B. Management

Physiological sinus tachycardia usually requires no management. In patients with high cardiac awareness, however, such that sinus tachycardia produces palpitation and anxiety (as is common in the mitral valve prolapse syndrome), management consists of slowing the sinus rate. Often this can be accomplished with a physical fitness conditioning program. In the extremely anxious patient, psychological counseling or pharmacotherapy may be required. Both short- and long-term symptomatic management can be achieved through the administration of beta blockers, verapamil, or occasionally diltiazem.

Pathological sinus tachycardia is best treated by therapy of the inciting cause, e.g., treatment of thyrotoxicosis, hypovolemia, heart failure, fever, orthostasis, hypoglycemia, withdrawal of the offending agent, and the like. When the cause is sinus node reentry, antiarrhythmic therapy is useful (see below). When no inciting cause is evident and empiric treatment with agents depressive to the sinus node (e.g., beta blockers, verapamil) fail and/or are contraindicated, modification of the sinus node through transcatheter radiofrequency ablation lesions can be considered. Though RF ablation can be extremely effective, with gratifying results, experience with it for sinus node arrhythmias remains limited. The risk of resultant sinus node dysfunction requiring permanent pacemaker implantation is real and must be considered justifable from the standpoint of the patient's symptoms and prognosis.

III. SINUS NODE REENTRY

A. Pathophysiology

Because the SA node shares many electrophysiological properties with the AV node, phenomena commonly associated with AV nodal physiology are seen in the

SA node as well. One of these is reentry. In both the AV and SA nodes, resting potentials less negative than those of Purkinje fibers or working myocardial cells, time-dependent recovery of excitability, substantial regions of slow channel dependent action potentials, and a structurally complex anatomy with areas of poor intercellular contact and inhomogeneous timing of activation all can promote slow intra- and perinodal conduction velocity and/or disparities in repolarization. In both nodes, manifestations of these properties are decremental conduction, inequalities in bidirectional conduction, and occasionally multiple pathway physiology. The presence of slow and decremental conduction with premature stimulation as well as the complex nodal anatomy can result in regions of conduction block. The existence of more than one functional pathway for conduction in the SA node, as in the AV node, enhanced by areas of slow conduction and areas of unidirectional block, provides conditions necessary to support reentry.

Sinus node reentry has been demonstrated in isolated atrial preparations as well as in hearts in vivo. Human sinus node reentry, however, is relatively infrequent. Wellens and colleagues reported that SA nodal reentry accounts for no more than 10% of supraventricular tachycardias seen in the clinical electrophysiology laboratory. Others have suggested a slightly higher incidence, but in our experience the incidence is less than 5%. Generally, sinus node reentrant PSVT is somewhat slower than PSVT caused by AV nodal reentry or reentry involving concealed or manifest bypass tracts. Rates of 110–150 beats/min are most common, and some cycle length variation is not unusual. Commonly, sinus node reentry tachycardia is unsustained. That is, at least in the clinical electrophysiological laboratory, induced sinus node reentry usually terminates spontaneously in 1 to 8 beats. How much of the reentrant circuit is within the sinus node and how much utilizes perinodal tissues is not yet resolved. The advent of curative radiofrequency ablation of sinus nodal tachycardias without uniform destruction of apparent sinus rhythm in several reported cases suggests that all of the node is not necessary for the generation or maintenance of such tachycardias.

B. Electrocardiographic Manifestations

Electrocardiographically, sinus node reentry may be manifest as single premature beats, salvos of premature beats, or sustained supraventricular tachycardias, all of which have P waves indistinguishable from those seen with NSR. The PR interval will be the same as or longer than the PR interval in NSR, and the RP/PR ratio will be greater than 1. For single sinus echoes, the postecho sinus cycle length will be shorter than that seen with interpolated APDs (unless a refractory wake is present) and the next sinus cycle length will be normal. Neither PR nor AH interval prolongation is a prerequisite for sinus node reentry, in contrast to the case of AV nodal reentry. In the electrophysiological laboratory, sinus node reentry, like other types of reentrant tachycardia, should be inducible and terminable by pacing or premature stimulation rather than exhibiting characteristics of automatic tachycardias.

289

C. Clinical Characteristics and Treatment

Sinus node reentry may be symptomatic or asymptomatic. When it is symptomatic, palpitations are the most common complaint. Symptoms indicative of hemodynamic impairment are only rarely present, given the relatively slow rates and brevity of the arrhythmia. When sinus node reentry is sustained, pharmacotherapy can be employed. However, as with AV nodal reentry, acute episodes can sometimes be terminated by maneuvers that enhance vagal tone. Thus, carotid sinus massage, facial ice-water immersion, and other "vagal" maneuvers should be tried before drug administration. When drug therapy is employed for a particular episode, adenosine, verapamil, diltiazem, beta blockers, and/or digitalis can be used. Long-term prevention with drugs is usually effective. On the basis of safety (proarrhythmic incidence and organ toxicity), convenience, and cost, digoxin, beta blockers, verapamil, and/or diltiazem should be considered initially. If necessary, class I or class III agents can be tried. In our experience, class IC agents may be particularly effective.

In patients with substantial and drug-refractory symptoms, radiofrequency transcatheter ablation can be attempted after adequate arrhythmia mapping confirms the location of the tachyarrhythmia. In most of the few reported cases to date, fractionated atrial electrograms are usually present, often in the posterior-superior aspect of the perinodal region. A major risk of catheter ablation for sinus node reentry is the potential for damage to the SA node, with subsequent sinus node dysfunction. Thus, RF ablation cannot yet be considered first-line therapy.

IV. ATRIAL PREMATURE DEPOLARIZATIONS

A. Pathophysiology

Like other ectopic impulses, atrial premature depolarizations (APDs) can arise secondary to automatic, reentrant, or triggered mechanisms. Clinical characteristics suggest that most are caused by reentry. Such APDs may arise in either the right or left atrium and may involve a portion of the AV node or sinoatrial node in the reentrant path.

B. Characteristics

Three ECG features of APDs are typical: (a) premature P wave; (b) a P-wave morphology differing from that of sinus P waves; and (c) a prolonged PR interval. The premature P wave is mandatory for the diagnosis. An alteration in P-wave morphology will be present except when the APD arises in the vicinity of the sinus node. The PR interval, although usually prolonged, need not be different from the PR interval present with sinus rhythm and may even be shortened. The PR interval is a reflection of the pathway taken through the atrium into the AV node as well as the state of refractoriness (and thereby conduction velocity) at the time the AV node is excited by the premature atrial depolarization.

Atrial premature depolarizations often occur early in the cardiac cycle because of the short effective refractory period of atrial tissue (160–200 msec). Atrioventricular function is still relatively refractory when an early APD occurs, and propagation of the impulse is delayed. Thus, an early APD always results in a prolonged PR interval. When APDs occur very early in atrial diastole and the AV node (refractory period generally much longer than that of atrial tissue) is absolutely refractory because of the preceding depolarization, APDs will block in the AV junction, producing a pause that mimics a sinus pause or sinus exit block. Differentiation between a nonconducted (or "blocked") APD and a sinus pause rests on recognition of the blocked P wave in one or more ECG leads. Typically, such early P waves are difficult to see because they are superimposed on the preceding T wave.

Most often, the QRS that follows an APD has a normal narrow configuration; however, the QRS may be distorted and wide (i.e., aberrant) when the His-Purkinje system or ventricular muscle has not completely repolarized. Under these circumstances, an APD can mimic a ventricular premature depolarization (VPD). Because the right bundle branch (RBB) usually has a longer refractory period than the left bundle branch (LBB), aberrant conduction of an APD usually has an RBB-block pattern, even in subjects without conduction system disease. However, aberrant conduction may have a LBB-block or alternating bundle branch block pattern, resembling multiform VPDs. Differentiation between an APD with aberrant conduction and a VPD rests on recognition of the premature initiating P wave.

Effects of APDs on the timing of subsequent sinus node depolarizations illustrate principles of conduction and refractoriness. The APDs may alter the postpremature depolarization in at least three ways, accounting for (a) reset of the sinus cycle length, (b) compensatory pauses, and (c) interpolated beats.

"Reset" of the sinus node occurs when an APD propagates retrogradely into and prematurely depolarizes the sinus node pacemaker, moving up the next sinus cycle. This is associated with a characteristic ECG finding in which the sum of the pre- and post-APD cycle lengths (PP′ + P′P) is less than twice the normal cycle length (PP interval); the pause after the APD is said to be "noncompensatory." This pattern is typical of midcycle APDs.

A compensatory pause occurs when an APD blocks in refractory perinodal and sinus node tissue and fails to reset the sinus node pacemaker tissue, leaving the basic sinus rhythm unperturbed. However, the emerging sinus node impulse is blocked also. The interval following the premature discharge is said to be a "compensatory pause." Under these circumstances, the sum of the pre- and post-APD cycle lengths (PP′ + P′P) is twice the normal sinus (PP) cycle length. This phenomenon occurs earlier in diastole than does the reset phenomenon. Compensatory pauses occur also with APDs late in diastole when the APD occurs simultaneously with spontaneous sinus node depolarization. The APD conducting retrogradely into the sinus node and the sinus node depolarization conducting out of the node toward the atria collide in the perinodal regional. Again, the atria are not activated by the sinus depolarization while the sinus node is not depolarized by the APD, and the next sinus beat, which will activate the atria normally, occurs on time.

Interpolated APDs occur when the interval following the APD is very short; the pre- and post-APD cycle lengths (PP + PP) are only slightly longer than or equal to one sinus cycle length. The interpolated APD does not alter the sinus impulse following the APD, though this sinus beat may be conducted with a slightly prolonged PR interval and/or aberrantly.

Frequently, it is difficult to diagnose APDs from a single ECG lead; therefore a 12-lead ECG is very useful. This is particularly true when sinus arrhythmia, sinus arrest versus a blocked APD, or VPD versus an APD with aberration complicate the differential diagnosis. Because the indications for treating APD differ from those applicable to sinus arrest and VPD, it is important that the diagnosis of APD be certain.

C. Epidemiology

Atrial premature depolarizations may occur in normal subjects as well as those with heart disease. Continuous ECGs in normal infants reveal that 12% have at least one APD in 24 hr. In the age group 10–11 years old, the incidence is 21%. The incidence of APDs in normal subjects increases with age, although their frequency does not appear to increase. For example, among healthy, active male medical students without heart disease, 56% have one or more APD during 24-hr ambulatory monitoring; however, fewer than 1% have 100 APDs. The incidence of APDs does not exhibit gender predilection. Frequency in women equals that in men. Healthy, active men 60–85 years old exhibit a substantial prevalence of supraventricular ectopic beats such as APDs.

D. Etiology

Although APDs are a normal phenomenon, they may result from infection such as viral myocarditis and pericarditis; myocardial ischemia or infarction; or thyroid disorder; they can also occur in association with stress, fatigue, and the use of stimulants such as coffee or tea, cigarettes, alcohol, and a variety of drugs including catecholamines and bronchodilators. Atrial premature depolarizations frequently accompany disease of the right or left ventricle as well as most intrathoracic insults (e.g., pulmonary disease) and may be precursors of more complicated arrhythmias, including paroxysmal supraventricular tachycardia, atrial flutter, and atrial fibrillation.

E. Treatment

Usually APDs are not associated with symptoms that require treatment; however, palpitations may be experienced. When treatment is considered to be necessary, beta blockers, digitalis, and occasionally calcium channel antagonists are useful. Antiarrhythmic agents with class IA action can be effective (procainamide, quinidine, and disopyramide). Trials with the class IC agents (propafenone, flecainide) indicate the usefulness of these agents for management of APDs as well. Amiodarone and sotalol, antiarrhythmic agents with class III properties, are also effective. Drug selection depends upon the severity of the symptoms, the presence or absence of underlying cardiac or pulmonary or thyroid pathology, and considerations of costs and potential side effects. Although class I and class III agents may be more effective than beta blockers, digoxin, or calcium channel antagonists, they are more expensive and more hazardous. None has FDA approval for the treatment of APDs.

V. ECTOPIC ATRIAL TACHYCARDIA

A. Pathophysiology

Automatic Atrial Tachycardia

This arrhythmia presents as a sustained or nonsustained episode of paroxysmal tachycardia. It occurs in all age groups, presumably because of enhanced automaticity. It can be caused by or associated with atrial surgery, myocardial ischemia and infarction, chronic lung disease, acute alcohol ingestion, or metabolic derangements including hypoxia and acidosis. The initiation of attacks usually occurs spontaneously and without a preceding premature complex, although sometimes it appears to be related to a late atrial premature complex.

Triggered Automaticity

Digitalis is a particularly important agent that may cause atrial tachycardia. In high concentrations, it enhances atrial automaticity and delayed afterdepolarizations. Digitalis-induced delayed after-depolarizations in vitro are considered to be responsible for some forms of ventricular tachycardia. In a similar fashion, triggered automaticity is a suspected mechanism of digitalis-induced atrial tachycardia. Atrial tachycardia caused by digitalis excess usually presents with AV block, often 2:1 or variable. The atrial rate increases gradually as digitalis is continued, often with associated prolongation of the PR interval. If the atrial rate is not excessive and AV conduction not significantly depressed, 1:1 conduction may persist. However, as the atrial rate increases or AV conduction is impaired, some degree of block follows. When the heart rate is high, it is occasionally difficult to distinguish paroxysmal atrial tachycardia (PAT) with block from atrial flutter.

293

Multifocal Atrial Tachycardia

Multifocal atrial tachycardia (MAT) occurs commonly in patients with chronic obstructive pulmonary disease, postsurgical patients, and those with metabolic abnormalities. It is frequently confused with atrial fibrillation or sinus tachycardia with atrial premature complexes. However, the varying P-wave configurations of MAT are important in the differential diagnosis. Multifocal atrial tachycardia often progresses to atrial fibrillation.

Because MAT is associated with hypoxemia, hypokalemia, digoxin, and all variables associated with delayed afterdepolarizations, it may be caused by triggered automaticity. Beneficial effects of verapamil and magnesium are consistent with this possibility.

B. Characteristics of the Electrocardiogram

Automatic Atrial Tachycardia

Automatic atrial tachycardias begin with a P wave identical to subsequent tachycardia P waves that characteristically accelerate during the first few cycles; average heart rate is 150–200 beats/min. An inferior and rightward or leftward axis or a distinctly different P-wave morphology from that with sinus rhythm suggests atrial tachycardia. Tachycardias originating in the region of the left superior pulmonary vein reportedly have a characteristic negative P wave in leads I, A_{VL}, and V_6.

AV Conduction Relationship

In the absence of digitalis, persistence of the atrial rhythm in the presence of AV block favors the diagnosis of automatic atrial tachycardia. Conduction may be variable (e.g., 3:2 or 2:1).

PR and RP Relationship

The relationship between the PR interval and the RP interval is useful in the diagnosis of atrial tachycardia. In regular atrial tachycardia, the PR interval is determined by the conduction properties of the AV node and the His-Purkinje system. The interval becomes prolonged as the atrial rate increases. The RP interval does not represent conduction time but is determined by the PP and PR intervals. With atrial tachycardia, the RP interval often exceeds the PR interval, in contrast to the case with paroxysmal supraventricular tachycardia caused by AV or AV node reentry, with which the PR usually exceeds the RP.

Vagal Intervention

In contrast to sinus and AV nodal arrhythmias, automatic atrial tachycardia is less reliably affected by vagal maneuvers. With atrial tachycardia, vagal maneuvers usually cause AV block to a greater extent than slowing of the atrial rate. Anticholinergic drugs such as atropine may shorten the PR interval without altering the atrial rates or, more commonly, increase the atrial rate.

C. Multifocal Atrial Tachycardia

Multifocal atrial tachycardia (MAT) is characterized by atrial rates between 100 to 150 beats/min with three or more variations in P-wave morphology and irregularly irregular PP intervals. Most of the P waves are conducted because the atrial rate is not excessively fast. Most often, the PR interval varies in association with the changing P-wave morphology.

D. Electrophysiological Studies

Electrophysiological studies may differentiate atrial tachycardia from sinus tachy-cardia if the atrial activation sequence varies from that seen with sinus rhythm. Atrioventricular reentrant tachycardias may be indistinguishable from atrial tachycardia in the absence of detailed atrial activation mapping. Such mapping is necessary to identify the site of origin of the atrial tachycardia before surgical or catheter ablation procedures. Initiation of the tachycardia with programmed electrical stimulation or pacing is often not reproducible with automatic atrial tachy-cardia in contrast to sinus node reentry. Reentry and triggered automaticity caused by delayed afterdepolarization may be possible or suspected as the mechanism of the tachycardia when it can be initiated and terminated by pacing. Close examina-tion of the behavior of the coupling intervals of the first tachycardiac beat to the programmed stimulus-coupling interval and/or MAP recordings may help to distinguish between the two. Other distinguishing considerations are that auto-matic tachycardias are reset by single premature complexes, whereas reentrant tachycardias may have a variable response, including reset, acceleration, or termi-nation. Overdrive pacing usually results in a prolonged escape cycle followed by acceleration to the prepacing cycle length over the next several cycles.

E. Specific Management Strategies

Automatic Atrial Arrhythmias

Only a few pharmacological options are available for the treatment of automatic tachycardia. Digoxin is of limited value because it usually does little to alter the tachycardia rate. It may produce clinically significant AV block if the atrial rate is rapid. Beta blockers may slow the tachycardia but usually do not suppress it. Verapamil, by prolonging AV conduction, may slow the ventricular response but is unlikely to terminate the atrial focus. Class I agents can be effective.

PAT with Block

PAT with block in a patient not being given digitalis is treated in the same way as it is in patients with other automatic atrial tachycardias. If excessive digitalis is not

295

suspected as a cause, digitalis may slow the ventricular rate. Then, a class IA, IC, or III agent, given after digitalis, may convert the tachycardia to NSR.

The special case of digitalis-induced PAT with block requires stopping digitalis immediately. Occasionally, a beta blocker, calcium channel blocker, or class IB drug (e.g., phenytoin) may be helpful in terminating the tachycardia. Hypokalemia (often a contributor) should be corrected. Rarely, antibody fragments against digitalis may be needed because of risk of refractory, potentially lethal ventricular arrhythmias. Electrical cardioversion is dangerous because of the risk of inducing ventricular tachycardia or fibrillation in this setting.

Multifocal Atrial Tachycardia

Because the atrial rate is often moderate, MAT is relatively well tolerated. Treatment of underlying chronic obstructive pulmonary disease or metabolic problems is usually required. Antiarrhythmic agents are not effective in slowing the rate of the atrial tachycardia and its ventricular response or converting MAT to sinus rhythm. Thus, careful attention to blood gases and electrolytes as well as treatment of infection and bronchospasm are critical. More specific therapy such as verapamil or magnesium may decrease the atrial and ventricular rate and increase AV block. Occasionally these two agents will terminate the arrhythmia. Beta blockers are frequently contraindicated because of the potential to induce bronchospasm in patients with pulmonary disease.

Surgery

Several surgical procedures—including localized resection, cryoablation, resection of sites in the atrial appendages—have been utilized; however, for the most part they are inadequate. A particular problem is that automatic atrial tachycardias are not consistently reproduced or induced by programmed stimulation and may be suppressed by general anesthesia. Atrial tachycardia may be associated with multiple discrete sites of origination.

Catheter Ablation

Electrode catheter ablation of automatic atrial tachycardia has been reported. Atrioventricular junctional electrode catheter ablation can alleviate the detrimental effects of rapid ventricular rates seen with atrial tachyarrhythmias, even though the atrial focus is not ablated.

VI. JUNCTIONAL ESCAPE BEATS AND JUNCTIONAL PREMATURE DEPOLARIZATIONS

A. Pathophysiology

Automaticity is a characteristic of the sinoatrial node, the atrioventricular junction, and the His-Purkinje system. The intrinsic rate of the sinus node is 60–75 depolarizations/min, usually sufficiently high to suppress the junctional and His-Purkinje pacemakers, which have an intrinsic rate of 40–60 depolarizations/min, respectively. The AV node is divided into AN, N, and NH regions (atrionodal, nodal, nodal-His), based on anatomic and electrophysiological considerations. The site of impulse initiation is thought to be in the NH region. However automaticity may be a property of the AN and N regions as well. Hyperpolarization of the AV nodal cells results in cessation of spontaneous depolarization. It is thought that electronic influence from more polarized atrial cells may prevent spontaneous depolarization of the AN and N regions of the AV node. The AV nodal pacemaker will spontaneously depolarize when input from higher pacemakers is absent. Thus, when the sinus node rate falls below the intrinsic rate of the AV node or when the sinus node–initiated depolarization fails to reach the AV node because of intraatrial or proximal AV nodal block, the AV junction will depolarize spontaneously, producing junctional escape beats. When the rate of the intrinsic pacemaker of the AV junctional region increases, junctional premature depolarizations (JPDs) occur. The mechanism is most likely an increase in physiological automaticity of the A, AN, or NH regions of the node. A reentry circuit within the AV junction may produce JPDs as well. This phenomenon can occur within the AV node or His-Purkinje tissue.

B. Electrocardiographic Characteristics of Atrioventricular Junctional Escape Complexes and Premature Depolarization

Atrioventricular junctional escape complexes are preceded by long sinus pauses, long RR intervals because of proximal AV block, or long pauses following an atrial or ventricular premature depolarization. The junctional escape or premature complex has the same QRS configuration as the sinus-initiated QRS complexes. When there is retrograde conduction of the junctional depolarization to the atria, a retrograde P wave may be seen. Depending on where in the AV junction the depolarization takes place and the time required for it to reach the atrium, the retrograde P wave may precede, follow, or be hidden in the QRS complex of the junctional escape complex. When the P wave precedes the QRS complex, the PR interval is shorter than the PR interval seen with sinus rhythm, and the P wave will usually be negative in the inferior leads. Junctional premature depolarizations are much less common than atrial or ventricular premature depolarizations.

The temporal position of the P wave is critical to the diagnosis. When the P wave follows the QRS complex or precedes the QRS complex with a PR interval that is less than 0.10 sec and is significantly shorter than the sinus PR interval, a diagnosis of a junctional premature complex can be made. When there is no visible P wave, the differential diagnosis includes a JPD with absent retrograde conduction, a junctional JPD with the retrograde P wave occurring in the QRS complex, or an atrial premature depolarization in which the premature atrial depolarization is not visible (hidden in the preceding T wave).

C. Management Strategies

Because junctional escape complexes often indicate an underlying disorder, treatment is directed toward treatment of the problem. Treatment of marked sinus bradycardia, prolonged sinus pauses, or AV block can be directed either toward discontinuation of drugs that have produced the disorder or implementation of a pacemaker if the bradycardia is symptomatic. In and of themselves, junctional escape beats require no therapy. Junctional premature depolarizations should be treated only if they are severely symptomatic. The choice of antiarrhythmic is purely empirical.

D. Nonparoxysmal Junctional Tachycardia

Junctional tachycardia can be divided into nonparoxysmal and paroxysmal junctional tachycardia. Paroxysmal junctional tachycardia is almost always caused by reentry within the junctional region or reentry involving a bypass tract in the retrograde direction. These paroxysmal arrhythmias are considered in the remaining parts of this chapter.

E. Pathophysiology

The mechanism underlying nonparoxysmal junctional tachycardia is not known with certainty. Enhanced automaticity in the NH region of the AV node is thought to be responsible. Delayed afterdepolarizations are good candidates for the etiology as well.

F. Electrocardiographic Characteristics of Nonparoxysmal Atrioventricular Junctional Tachycardia

The rate of nonparoxysmal AV junctional tachycardia is characteristically 70–130 beats/min. This tachycardia has a gradual onset and termination. Because the rate of the tachycardia is usually close to the sinus rate (especially at onset and termination), isorhythmic AV dissociation is often seen at the onset and termination of the tachycardia. The sinus P waves can be observed to "march into the QRS complex" at the onset of nonparoxysmal junctional tachycardia. The QRS complex is usually normal but may be slightly aberrant: there may be AV dissociation during the entire episode of nonparoxysmal junctional tachycardia, or there may be retrograde conduction through the AV node with capture of the atria. If so, the P waves may be positioned just before, during, or just after the QRS complex. Alternatively, the atria may be in atrial flutter or atrial fibrillation with nonparoxysmal junctional tachycardia, especially when the tachycardia is the result of digitalis that has been given to slow the transmitted rate of the atrial fibrillation (AF). Thus, "regularization" of the ventricular response to the AF is not really regularization but rather a double tachycardia that may be a sign of digitalis toxicity.

G. Epidemiology of Nonparoxysmal Atrioventricular Junctional Tachycardia

The occurrence of nonparoxysmal junctional tachycardia is most common in association with one of the following four conditions: (a) acute inferior myocardial infarction, (b) digitalis toxicity, (c) acute carditis, and (d) open heart surgery. It is almost always seen transiently in procedures leading to successful ablation or modification of the AV node by radiofrequency energy.

H. Management of Nonparoxysmal Atrioventricular Junctional Tachycardia

The treatment of nonparoxysmal AV junctional tachycardia should focus on the underlying condition. In acute MI or following open heart surgery, the tachycardia is usually self-limiting and requires no therapy. When nonparoxysmal AV junctional tachycardia is caused by digitalis excess, prompt management of digitalis toxicity should be initiated. If the arrhythmia is persistent and symptomatic, empirically chosen antiarrhythmic drugs may be tried; however, class IC agents should be avoided if underlying ischemia or other structural cardiac disorders are present because of the risk of proarrhythmia.

Intraatrial Reentrant Arrhythmias

Joseph M. Smith

Intraatrial reentry (reentrant electrical activation confined to the atria) is responsible for a subset of clinically separate though mechanistically related atrial tachycardias. Intraatrial reentrant tachycardia and atrial flutter are atrial tachycardias caused by a single, stable reentrant circuit within the atria. Atrial fibrillation is a result of the simultaneous presence of multiple reentrant circuits wandering throughout the area.

299

VII. INTRAATRIAL REENTRANT TACHYCARDIA

Intraatrial reentrant tachycardia typically presents as an atrial tachycardia with a rate of 120–200 beats/min and is most frequently seen in patients with previous cardiac surgery or complex congenital heart disease in whom atriotomy scars and/ or additional anatomic abnormalities serve as obstacles to conduction around which reentrant activity circulates. For a stable reentrant intraatrial circuit to exist, the relationship between the circumference of this circuit, the conduction velocity along the circuit, and the refractory period of each segment of the circuit must allow for a wavefront of excitation to traverse the entire circuit without ever impinging upon its refractory wake. Macroscopic, nonconductive barriers to conduction, together with slow conduction and/or short refractory period duration, provide the electrophysiological substrate for this arrhythmia.

A. Electrocardiographic Manifestations

The ECG obtained while intraatrial reentrant tachycardia typically shows an atrial rate of 120–200 beats/min with an unusual P-wave morphology and axis. The ventricular rate is usually the same as the atrial rate but may be lower in the setting of AV nodal Wenckebach or higher-degree AV nodal conduction block. The tachycardia is typically unaffected by intermittent AV conduction block or premature ventricular depolarization unless they occur very early or very late—i.e., in the excitable gap or interval in which some tissue in the circuit has recovered but has not yet been depolarized again by the reentrant wavefront.

B. Initial Treatment

Initial treatment of intraatrial reentrant tachycardia is selected depending upon the clinical presentation. Any evidence of hemodynamic instability, myocardial ischemia, or end-organ compromise should prompt restitution of normal sinus rhythm with DC cardioversion. When the rhythm is well tolerated, initial treatment may be directed instead at slowing the ventricular response, with subsequent efforts aimed at restoring sinus rhythm.

Controlling the ventricular response rate is most rapidly accomplished with intravenous administration of agents that impair AV nodal conduction (see Table 1). Treatment with parenteral calcium channel antagonists (e.g., diltiazem) or beta-adrenergic antagonists (e.g., metoprolol, inderal, esmolol) offers more rapid and titratable control of ventricular response than does treatment with digoxin.

Restoration of normal sinus rhythm can be accomplished with chemical agents that induce cardioversion (see Table 2), occasionally by atrial overdrive pacing (see "Atrial Flutter," below), and/or DC cardioversion (see "Atrial Fibrillation," below).

Table 1 Agents Used to Slow Ventricular Rate in Response to Atrial Arrhythmias

Drug	Load	Maintenance	Adverse reaction
Diltiazem	IV: 20–25 mg over 1–2 min	IV: 10–15 mg/hr	Hypotension (typically mild)
Verapamil	IV: 5–10 mg over 1–2 min	IV: 0.005 mg/kg/min	Hypotension (may be severe)
Metroprolol	IV: 5 mg q5′ × 3	PO: 50–200 mg/day in divided doses	Hypotension, bradycardia (typically mild)
Esmolol	IV: 0.5 mg/kg over 1 min	IV: 50–200 μg/kg/min	Hypotension, bradycardia, CHF
Propranolol	IV: 0.25–0.5 mg q 5 min	PO: 10–50 mg q6–8h	Hypotension, bradycardia (typically mild)
Digoxin	IV/PO: 1 mg divided doses over 1–4 hr	PO: 0.0625–0.25 mg qd	Digitalis toxicity

An important caveat to consider when restoring sinus rhythm is that other atrial arrhythmias caused by intraatrial reentry (atrial flutter and atrial fibrillation) are associated with an increased rate of thromboembolic events. The extent to which thromboembolic risk extends to patients with intraatrial reentrant tachycardia is not entirely clear, but, in the absence of specific contraindications, it is prudent to induce anticoagulation for 4 to 6 weeks before and after attempted restoration of sinus rhythm.

C. Long-Term Therapy

The efficacy of long-term medical treatment for the prevention of intraatrial reentrant tachycardia is limited; the anatomic substrate that contributes to the arrhythmia is unaltered by pharmacological therapy. Class IA, IC, and III agents may be used to decrease the number of episodes of tachycardia (see Table 1) and frequently have the effect of slowing the rate of the tachycardia by slowing atrial conduction velocity. Widespread use of these agents is limited by the risk of malignant proarrhythmia, particularly in patients with organic heart disease and/or diminished LV function. Class II and IV antiarrhythmic agents can be used to control (slow) the ventricular response rate (see Table 2) but usually have little effect on the mechanism underlying the arrhythmia.

Catheter-based ablative techniques have been employed to directly modify the anatomic substrate (scar) that often underlies the arrhythmia. By creating a nonconductive lesion that connects the initial obstacle to a natural border of the atrium, reentrant excitation around this obstacle can be prevented, in many cases providing a long-term cure.

Table 2 Antiarrhythmic Agents Useful in Chemical Cardioversion and Prevention of Recurrences of Atrial Fibrillation

	Load	Maintenance	Cardioversion	Prevention	Adverse reactions
Class IA					
Quinidine	PO: 600–1000 mg	PO: 300–600 mg q6h	+	+	Diarrhea, proarrhythmia
Procainamide	IV: 6–13 mg/kg @ 0.2–0.5 mg/kg/min PO: 500–1000 mg	IV: 1–4 mg/min PO: 350–1000 mg q3–6h	++	+	Lupuslike reaction, proarrhythmia
Disopyramide		PO: 100–400 mg q6–8h	+	+	Dry mouth, proarrhythmia
Class IC					
Propafenone	PO: 600–900 mg	PO: 150–300 q8–12h	++	++	Bradycardia, proarrhythmia
Flecainide	PO: 200–400 mg	PO: 100–200 mg q12h	++	++	Dizziness, proarrhythmia
Class III					
Amiodarone	PO: 800–1600 mg qd for 1–3 weeks	PO: 200–400 mg qd	+	+++	Pulmonary or hepatic toxicity
Sotalol		PO: 120–240 mg bid	+	?	TdP

VIII. ATRIAL FLUTTER

Atrial flutter, like intraatrial reentrant tachycardia, depends on a single stable reentrant circuit within the atria. It is distinguished from intraatrial reentry by the atrial rate, with atrial flutter having an atrial rate typically in excess of 260 beats/min. Atrial flutter occurs in two different forms.

Typical (type I) atrial flutter, usually associated with an atrial rate of 280 to 320 beats/min, results from a stable circulating wavefront that traverses down the free wall of the right atrium across the junction of the right atrium and the inferior vena cava through a narrow isthmus of tissue bounded by the inferior vena cava past the os of the coronary sinus; it then travels past the tricuspid annulus, up the intraatrial septum, and out to the left atrium. This form of atrial flutter may occur in the absence of organic heart disease.

Atypical (type II) atrial flutter, usually associated with atrial rates of 260–420 beats/min, reflects a single stable reentrant circuit that forms around other anatomic sites (including orifices of the vena cava, AV valves, and pulmonary veins) for functional obstacles to conduction. This form of atrial flutter is most often seen in association with organic heart disease and/or atrial fibrillation.

A. Electrocardiographic Manifestations

The ECG recording when typical (type I) atrial flutter is present exhibits the classic regular "sawtooth" baseline, with predominantly negative deflections in the inferior leads (II, III, and aV_F) occurring at a rate of approximately 300 beats/min (see Figure 1). The ventricular rate will vary depending on AV nodal conduction: 1:1 tracking of the atrial flutter rate resulting in a ventricular rate of nearly 300 beats/min is rare; 2:1 AV conduction is most common, resulting in a ventricular rate of 150 beats/min. In the setting of impaired AV conduction, either as a result of increased vagal tone, conduction system disease, or the actions of antiarrhythmic agents, the ventricular response may be much slower and variable. The ECG recorded when atypical (type II) atrial flutter is present exhibits regular atrial activity at a rate of 260–450 beats/min, with an unusual P-wave axis and morphology. As in type I flutter and intraatrial reentrant tachycardia, the ventricular rate will vary as a function of AV nodal conduction.

B. Initial Acute Treatment

Initial acute treatment of atrial flutter is dependent upon the clinical presentation. Any evidence of hemodynamic instability, myocardial ischemia, or end-organ compromise should prompt restitution of normal sinus rhythm with DC cardioversion. When the arrhythmia is well tolerated, initial therapy can be directed toward slowing the ventricular response rate, with subsequent efforts aimed at restoring sinus rhythm.

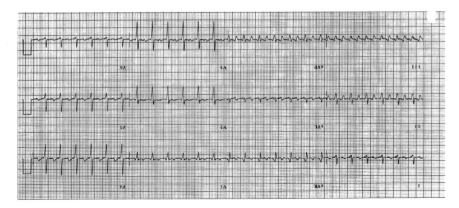

Figure 1   Classic 12-lead ECG of typical atrial flutter. The regular sawtooth pattern in the baseline of the inferior leads (II, III, avF) corresponds to an atrial rate of 300 bpm; 2:1 conduction block in the AV node results in a regular ventricular response at 150 bpm.

Controlling the ventricular response rate is most rapidly accomplished with the intravenous administration of agents that impair AV nodal conduction (see Table 1). Treatment with parenteral calcium channel antagonists (e.g., diltiazem) or beta-adrenergic antagonists (e.g., metoprolol, esmolol) offers more rapid and titratable control of ventricular response than does treatment with digoxin.

Restoration of normal sinus rhythm can be accomplished by atrial overdrive pacing, occasionally with chemical cardioversion (see Table 2) and/or DC cardioversion. Atrial overdrive pacing can be performed with the use of either an esophageal electrode, temporary (postcardiac surgery) epicardial pacing electrodes, percutaneously placed temporary atrial pacing electrode catheter, or permanent atrial pacemaker lead when the associated pacemaker generator is capable of rapid atrial pacing. Once the atrial cycle length has been measured, atrial overdrive pacing is performed by burst-pacing the atrium at a pacing cycle length 10 msec shorter than the flutter cycle length for 15–30 sec. If this is initially unsuccessful, the pacing cycle length is decreased in 10-msec intervals and the process is continued until the flutter circuit is interrupted, atrial fibrillation ensues, or a pacing cycle length of 150 msec is reached.

Regardless of the strategy employed for restoration of normal sinus rhythm, the risk of thromboembolic complications may increase during and immediately after cardioversion. If the clinical setting allows, it is prudent to assess the risks and benefits associated with 4 to 6 weeks of anticoagulant therapy both before and after attempting restoration of normal sinus rhythm and to implement anticoagulation in the absence of specific contraindications.

C. Long-Term Therapy

Long-term antiarrhythmic therapy for atrial flutter has limited efficacy. Class IA, IC, and III agents are only modestly efficacious for the prevention of recurrences, and their widespread use is limited by malignant proarrhythmia, particularly in patients with ischemic heart disease or left ventricular dysfunction. Class II and IV agents and/or digoxin are used to control the ventricular response rate, but long-term control with atrial flutter is made difficult by the extremely regular nature of the atrial arrhythmia. Subtle changes in AV nodal conduction characteristics can result in substantial changes in the ventricular response rate [i.e., a change in AV nodal refractoriness from 405 to 395 msec when the atrial flutter cycle length is 200 msec can result in a sudden change in the ventricular response rate from 100 beats/min (3:1 conduction) to 150 beats/min (2:1 conduction)]. Because autonomic influences and levels of circulating catecholamines substantially affect AV nodal conduction characteristics, a single measure of the ventricular rate at rest is a poor index of the adequacy of pharmacological control of the ventricular response rate. The ventricular rate response to exercise should be characterized with graded exercise testing. The integrated effects on ventricular rate response in the context of a patient's normal activities are best assessed with the use of 24-hr Holter monitoring.

(RF) catheter ablation has shown great promise in preventing recurrence (CU ring). It creates a nonconductive scar across the isthmus of tissue separating the tricuspid annulus from the os of the coronary sinus and/or the inferior vena cava. In atypical atrial flutter, the locus of the reentrant circuit responsible for the arrhythmia varies from patient to patient, and the efficacy of RF ablation may be limited by the technical constraints associated with accurate identification of the most susceptible portion of the circuit.

An increased incidence of thromboembolic events in patients with chronic or recurrent atrial flutter, particularly when it occurs in association with organic heart disease, makes it prudent to consider the risks and benefits associated with long-term anticoagulation and to implement it in the absence of specific contraindications.

IX. ATRIAL FIBRILLATION

Atrial fibrillation typically presents as an irregular, narrow complex tachycardia in patients with organic heart disease, but it may present as a manifestation of thyroid disease, pericardial disease, alcohol intoxication or withdrawal, catecholamine excess, electrolyte imbalance, and other conditions. It sometimes occurs in otherwise normal hearts. The incidence of atrial fibrillation increases with increasing age. It is seen in nearly 10% of subjects over age 75.

Mechanistically, AF results from the simultaneous presence of multiple reentrant wavelets that migrate over the surface of the atria. Unlike the case with intraatrial reentrant tachycardias and atrial flutter, anatomic obstacles do not appear to be primary factors in the pathophysiology of atrial fibrillation. Rather, derangements of the electrophysiological properties of atrial tissue that result in inhomogeneous refractoriness, short refractory period duration, and slow conduction promote the reentrant activity underlying the atrial fibrillation.

A. Electrocardiographic Manifestations

The ECG recorded while AF is present typically shows an irregular baseline without clearly identifiable P waves and normal or aberrantly conducted QRS complexes separated by irregularly irregular intervals. Because of the rate-related conduction properties of the right and left bundles of the His-Purkinje system, bundle branch aberration may occur with beats with short RR intervals, particularly those occurring after beats with relatively long RR intervals (Ashman phenomenon).

The rate of the ventricular response to AF in the absence of an accessory pathway is critically dependent on AV nodal function. In normal subjects, the ventricular response rate is between 100 and 160 beats/min. It may be considerably greater in the setting of excess catecholamines, vagolytic agents, theophylline, and other influences. A slow ventricular response rate may be seen in the setting of antiarrhythmic agents or other antidromotropic agents that slow conduction (e.g., beta-adrenergic antagonists, calcium channel antagonists, and digoxin).

B. Initial Treatment

Initial treatment of AF is selected on the basis of the clinical presentation. Any manifestations of hemodynamic instability, myocardial ischemia, or end-organ compromise should prompt restitution of normal sinus rhythm with DC cardioversion. When AF is well tolerated, initial efforts should be directed at identification and correction of any reversible cause of increased atrial irritability. The physical examination and results of initial screening studies identify or exclude hypertensive heart disease, thyroid disease, pericarditis, alcohol intoxication or withdrawal, excess endogenous or exogenous catecholamines, electrolyte abnormalities, or concomitant disorders (pneumonia, sepsis, and pulmonary embolism, among others). Initial therapeutic efforts in stable patients should concentrate on control of the ventricular response rate, with subsequent efforts directed toward identification of the presence and severity of organic heart disease. The risk of thromboembolism associated with AF mandates early consideration of systemic anticoagulation and its implementation in the absence of specific contraindications.

Controlling the ventricular response rate is most rapidly accomplished by intravenous administration of agents that slow AV nodal conduction (see Table 1).

Treatment with parenteral calcium channel antagonists (e.g., diltiazem) or beta-adrenergic antagonists (e.g., metoprolol, esmolol) offers more rapid and more titratable control of the ventricular response rate compared with treatment with digoxin.

Restoration of normal sinus rhythm occurs spontaneously in many patients with an acute episode of AF. For the remainder, except in those with chronic AF refractory to medical therapy or in whom echocardiography shows massively dilated atria (likely to entail a very high recurrence rate), restoration of sinus rhythm should be pursued. Timing of the cardioversion attempt is often complicated by the inability to date the onset of the arrhythmia precisely and the risk of stroke when sinus rhythm is restored in patients in AF for more than 72 hr without 4 to 6 weeks of previous anticoagulation. Echocardiography may identify clot within the left atrium, a harbinger of thromboembolic events in association with restoration of coordinated atrial contraction. The absence of identifiable clot within the left atrium has not proven useful in identifying patients at acceptably low risk from subsequent stroke related to restoration of sinus rhythm. Restoration of sinus rhythm may be accomplished by either pharmacological cardioversion (see Table 2) or DC cardioversion. DC cardioversion is outlined below. In patients with a first episode of an intraatrial reentrant arrhythmia, DC cardioversion is typically undertaken without concomitant antiarrhythmic therapy, such therapy being reserved for recurrence of the arrhythmia.

1. Whenever possible, it is recommended that 4 to 6 weeks of therapeutic anticoagulation with warfarin (sufficient to induce an increase in prothrombin time equivalent to an international normalized ratio (INR) of 2.0–3.0) both precede and follow any attempt at cardioversion.
2. Before elective cardioversion, all antiarrhythmic drug levels should be titrated to therapeutic range and digoxin levels should be measured to ensure exclusion of occult digoxin toxicity.
3. Informed consent should be obtained, reliable IV access should be established, and continuous monitoring of the ECG should be initiated, with a 12-lead ECG being obtained to confirm persistence of the index arrhythmia at the time of cardioversion.
4. Supplemental oxygen and equipment necessary for intubation and manual ventilation should be at hand.
5. Adhesive defibrillation pads (or paste-coated electrode paddles) should be positioned with the anterior pad or paddle just to the right of the sternum (overlying the right atrium) and the posterior pad or paddle to the left of the spine just below the left scapula (immediately posterior to the left atrium). Care should be taken to position electrodes at least 6 cm from indwelling pacemaker or defibrillator generators.
6. Amnesia should be induced with midazolam (1 mg/mL, 1–2 mg IV q 2

min to a maximum of 5 mg) or methohexital (25–75 mg IV) at doses sufficient to render the patient drowsy. Blood pressure and respirations should be monitored carefully. Ideally, an anesthetist should be available for optimal airway management.

7. Recommended initial energy settings for cardioversion are 50–100 J for atrial flutter, 100–200 J for AF.

8. The synchronization of the cardiovertor/defibrillator should be evaluated by visual confirmation of the presence of a synchronization artifact superimposed upon the QRS complex. If electrode paddles are being used, firm pressure should be applied to minimize contact impedance. Direct contact of personnel with the patient or the bed should be avoided. The cardioversion pulse should be provided at end-expiration so as to minimize transthoracic impedance. As a result of synchronization, the discharge may be delayed a short time; thus, the electrodes should be held in place until discharge occurs. If defibrillation attempts at the initial settings are unsuccessful, energy settings may be increased stepwise to 360 J. Should the arrhythmia terminate with a cardioversion attempt yet quickly recur, further attempts at DC cardioversion should be deferred, with adjunctive therapy considered first to facilitate later attempts.

C. Long-Term Therapy

Atrial fibrillation occurs in diverse clinical settings that significantly influence selection of long-term therapy. Atrial fibrillation may be chronic and persistent or may present in repeated self-limited paroxysms; it occurs in association with organic heart disease but also in the absence of other cardiovascular pathology. Symptoms may be related to a rapid ventricular response and to loss of AV synchrony (manifest as persistent symptoms despite excellent ventricular rate control). Rarely, in patients with intrinsic conduction system disease, AF may occur with a slow ventricular response rate, with symptoms secondary to bradycardia. In this case, permanent pacing is usually of great benefit. Either chronic or paroxysmal AF can occur without any symptoms. Even in patients with documented symptomatic episodes of AF, most episodes may be asymptomatic.

Lone Atrial Fibrillation

When AF occurs in persons under 65 years of age in the absence of organic heart disease, it is often referred to as lone AF. This clinical entity is associated with a relatively favorable prognosis, with therapy generally designed only to alleviate symptoms. If AF is chronic or occurs in rare, self-limited paroxysms and the symptoms relate to a rapid ventricular rate (i.e., symptoms abate with control of the ventricular rate response), long-term treatment with beta-adrenergic antagonists or calcium channel antagonists may be sufficient to control ventricular response. Assessment of the efficacy of rate control is best accomplished by observing the rate response to exercise during a graded exercise test and to the activities of daily living via Holter monitoring. If paroxysms of AF occur frequently, class IA and IC and less frequently class III agents may be sufficient by limiting incidence of recurrence. However, risks of noxious side effects and ventricular proarrhythmia are potentially serious. Thus, consultation with an electrophysiologist may be helpful to review the action and efficacy of available therapies in the context of patient-specific parameters. In patients with lone AF, aspirin is used often to reduce the already low rate of thromboembolic events even further.

Atrial Fibrillation and Organic Heart Disease

In patients in whom AF accompanies organic heart disease and in patients over 65 years of age with AF, the increased risk of stroke (with an incidence of 4–6% per year on average, significantly higher in the setting of severe LV dysfunction or congestive heart failure) dominates selection of therapy. Anticoagulation with warfarin, with a target of 2.0–3.0 is appropriate regardless of whether the AF is paroxysmal or sustained unless specific contraindications to anticoagulation exist.

For patients with organic heart disease and either chronic, drug-refractory AF or rare occurrences of AF with symptoms are related to a rapid ventricular response, beta-adrenergic antagonists, calcium channel antagonists, and digoxin may be used alone and if necessary cautiously in combination to control ventricular rate. Digoxin should seldom be used alone, because its effects are overcome readily by change in autonomic tone or circulating catecholamines that accompany exertion or stress. The efficacy of rate control is best assessed by observing the rate response to exercise and to the activities of daily living. When adequate rate control cannot be attained pharmacologically or in patients in whom such therapy is associated with intolerable side effects, radiofrequency ablation of AV nodal conduction and implantation of permanent pacing may afford long-term rate control and be justified.

For patients with AF associated with organic heart disease, antiarrhythmic therapy (class IA, IC, and III agents) may decrease recurrence. However, as the extent of LV dysfunction increases, the efficacy of antiarrhythmic therapy decreases and the risk of malignant proarrhythmic complications increases. For patients with severe LV dysfunction for whom preservation of sinus rhythm may offer the greatest hemodynamic benefit, antiarrhythmic therapy may be least effective and most likely to cause ventricular proarrhythmia. In this setting, consultation with an electrophysiologist is frequently helpful. Regardless of the antiarrhythmic agent chosen, absolute efficacy in terms of complete prevention of recurrences of arrhythmia over and extended interval is unlikely. Accordingly, antiarrhythmic therapy cannot be viewed as an alternative to anticoagulation.

Postoperative Atrial Fibrillation

New-onset AF complicates recovery from cardiac surgery in more than one-third of patients. It is associated with increased morbidity and prolonged hospitalization. Prophylactic administration of beta-adrenergic antagonists is very effective in preventing postoperative AF, reducing its incidence by as much as 75%. For patients who experience postoperative AF, antiarrhythmic therapy, if used, should be discontinued 6 weeks to 3 months after surgery, because the transient influences that predispose to the AF will probably have abated.

Chronic Atrial Fibrillation

The term "chronic" pertains to AF that is persistent (not self-remitting) or has recurred despite all appropriate therapeutic interventions. Therapy is limited to anticoagulation and rate control. Because of the implications and apparent finality of the decision to regard AF in any patient as chronic, a review of treatment in patients suspected of having chronic AF is critical and consultation with an electrophysiologist is often helpful.

D. Additional Therapeutic Considerations

Surgery

The refinement of surgical procedures for restricting the spread of electrical activation within the atria and thereby preventing AF (the so-called MAZE procedure) provides another therapeutic option for a limited subset of patients with AF. In patients with unrelenting symptoms in whom medical therapy is ineffective or intolerable, the MAZE procedure offers a very high likelihood or restitution of sinus rhythm without the need for long-term antiarrhythmic therapy. In patients with AF who are undergoing cardiac surgery for other indications, a concomitant MAZE procedure can be performed with little additional morbidity. For most patients, however, the considerable morbidity and potential mortality associated with this open-heart procedure limits its applicability.

RF Catheter Ablation and Atrial Fibrillation

Additional techniques will no doubt be developed to meet the challenge of replicating the effects of the MAZE procedure with the use of endocardial application of RF energy. For the near term, however, RF ablation in the management of patients with AF is limited to patients in whom medical therapy designed to control the ventricular response rate is ineffective or intolerable. RF ablation of the AV junction with implantation of a rate-responsive permanent pacemaker offers nonpharmacological control of the ventricular rate with preserved rate responsiveness to exercise or activity. Because this procedure effectively interrupts the

310

cardiac conduction system and leaves patients pacemaker-dependent, it should be viewed as a palliative one and reserved for a small minority of patients.

Implantable Atrial Defibrillators

Paralleling the development of the implantable ventricular defibrillator, implantable devices that recognize AF and can deliver low-energy synchronized cardioversion pulses to terminate it have been developed. However, their place in the management of patients has not yet been delineated.

Atrioventricular Nodal Reentrant Tachycardia

Michael E. Cain

Atrioventricular (AV) nodal reentrant tachycardia accounts for more than 50% of episodes of paroxysmal supraventricular tachycardia (SVT) that come to medical attention. It is the most common form of paroxysmal SVT in individuals without structural heart disease and affects patients of all ages. Analyses of data acquired during clinical electrophysiological studies and intraoperatively from patients undergoing arrhythmia surgery have provided substantial insights into the underlying mechanism as well as the location of the tissues critical to AV nodal SVT. Advances have permitted more intelligent use of antiarrhythmic drugs for patients with this arrhythmia and the development of nonpharmacological procedures, such as radiofrequency catheter modification of the AV node, that can "cure" AV nodal reentrant tachycardia. Because so much progress has been made, recognition of this arrhythmia and knowledge of treatment strategies are essential for optimal patient care.

X. PATHOLOGY

Supraventricular tachycardia caused by AV nodal reentry results from a microreentrant circuit having two functionally distinct pathways with different electrophysiological properties that incorporate, at least in part, the compact portion of the AV node. In contrast to the usual physiological linkage of phenomena in

311

electrically excitable tissues (fast conduction and rapid repolarization), the fast or beta limb conducts rapidly but repolarizes slowly. The slow or alpha pathway conducts slowly but recovers excitability quickly. Although dimensions of the microreentrant circuit are not yet completely delineated, the fast pathway is in the compact portion of the AV node and the slow pathway is made up, in part, of atrial tissue located in the atrial septum posterior to the compact portion of the AV node (Figure 2).

In sinus rhythm, the ventricles are activated by the preferential rapid conduction through the fast pathway. Parallel conduction in the slow limb is extinguished because the distal common limb is refractory from previous activation via the fast pathway. Under conditions such as those occurring when an atrial premature depolarization temporally engages the AV node before the fast pathway recovers but after the slow pathway has regained excitability, conduction blocks in the fast limb and proceeds slowly through the slow pathway to the ventricles. If the conduction time through the slow pathway is sufficiently prolonged, tissue in the fast limb can regain excitability and be activated retrogradely. If conduction time retrogradely in the fast pathway is sufficiently slow to permit recovery of the slow limb, the slow pathway will be reactivated antegradely to complete the microreentrant circuit. Thus, with the typical form of AV nodal SVT, anterograde conduction is through the slow pathway and retrograde conduction through the fast limb. Conduction time anterograde from the slow pathway to the ventricles is similar to conduction time retrograde in the fast pathway to the atria, resulting in near simultaneous (usually within 30 msec) activation of the ventricles and atria. In the atypical form of the arrhythmia, the effective refractory period of the fast pathway is short and that of the slow pathway long. Thus, with atypical AV nodal SVT, anterograde conduction occurs by the fast pathway and retrograde conduction by the slow pathway, resulting in more asynchronous activation of the atria and ventricles.

Because most of the reentrant circuit is confined to the AV node, conduction block in the AV node terminates the arrhythmia. Although uncommon, conduction block distal to the AV node at or below the His bundle can alter the usual 1:1 relationship between atrial and ventricular activation without terminating the arrhythmia.

XI. ELECTROCARDIOGRAPHIC CHARACTERISTICS

With sinus rhythm, the PR interval is normal reflecting anterograde conduction through the fast pathway. Atrioventricular nodal reentry initiates and terminates abruptly. The heart rate ranges from 150 to 250 beats/min. The RR interval is regular. The QRS complex is identical to that seen with sinus rhythm unless functional bundle branch block is present. If present, functional block in the right bundle is more common than block (aberration) in the left bundle branch. In the

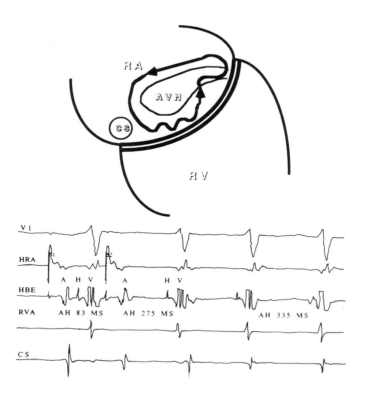

Figure 2 Top: Schematic representation of the fast and slow pathways that make up the microreentrant circuit responsible for AV nodal reentrant tachycardia. AVN = atrioventricular node; CS = coronary sinus; RA = right atrium; RV = right ventricle. Bottom: ECG lead V_1 and intracardiac electrograms from the high right atrium (HRA), His bundle (HBE), right ventricular apex (RVA), and coronary sinus (CS) recorded during the eighth beat (S_1) of an eight-beat atrial pacing drive, a programmed atrial extrastimulus (S_2), and AV nodal SVT. During S_1, AV conduction is through the fast pathway (AH interval, 83 msec). During S_2, conduction blocks in the fast limb and occurs through the slow pathway (AH, 275 msec) with reexcitation of the fast pathway and initiation of AV nodal SVT, characterized by simultaneous activation of the atria and ventricles. A = atrial electrogram; H = His bundle electrogram; V = ventricular electrogram.

313

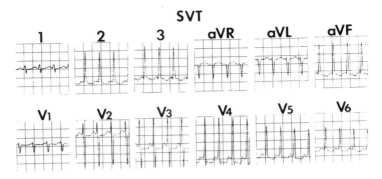

Figure 3 A 12-lead ECG recorded during typical AV nodal reentrant tachycardia. Anterograde conduction is through the slow pathway and retrograde conduction is through the fast pathway, resulting in near simultaneous activation of the atria and ventricles.

typical form of the arrhythmia (Figure 3), the P wave is concealed in the QRS complex (60% of patients) or distorts the terminal portion of the QRS complex (40% of patients). If detected, the retrograde P wave is negative in ECG leads 2, 3, and aV_F as a result of the nodal origin and the caudal-to-cephalad and septal-to-free wall sequence of atrial activation; the RP interval is less than 50% of the RR interval, reflecting the anterograde slow and retrograde fast AV nodal activation patterns. In contrast, ECGs recorded from patients with the atypical form of the tachycardia (Figure 4) show a P wave clearly preceding the QRS complex (short PR interval) and a long interval between the QRS complex and the next retrograde P wave. The rate of the SVT in these patients is slower (< 150 beats/min) and the tachycardia is often incessant.

With both typical and atypical AV nodal reentry, a 1:1 relation between P waves and QRS complexes is common. Conduction block in the fast or slow pathway, located at least in part within the compact portion of the AV node, terminates AV nodal SVT. Block of AV conduction occurs usually at the level of the AV node. Accordingly, ECG evidence of AV block, particularly in a Mobitz I pattern with persistence of an SVT, makes the diagnosis AV nodal SVT unlikely.

XII. MANAGEMENT STRATEGIES

In general, AV nodal SVT is recurrent but not life-threatening unless concomitant cardiac conditions such as coronary artery disease, valvular disease, or cardiomyopathy compromise the cardiovascular compensation. Because of progress in the development of antiarrhythmic drugs, antitachycardia devices, and surgical and catheter ablation techniques, management strategies in patients with AV nodal

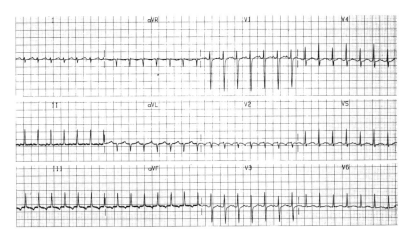

Figure 4 A 12-lead ECG recorded during atypical AV nodal reentrant tachycardia. Anterograde conduction is through the fast pathway and retrograde conduction is through the slow limb, resulting in a long RP and short PR pattern.

reentry can now be targeted to deal specifically with the needs of individuals. An ideal treatment is curative, safe, cost-effective, and free from end-organ damage. The mainstays of therapy are pharmacological or catheter modification of the AV node with the use of radiofrequency electrical energy. Antiarrhythmic drugs can be administered intermittently to terminate AV nodal reentry at the time of occurrence of arrhythmia or prophylactically to prevent episodes of SVT. Treatment with antiarrhythmic drugs, however, is only palliative. Modification of the AV node with radiofrequency energy can be curative.

Once a cause-and-effect relationship between AV nodal SVT and symptoms has been established, factors that influence the selection of therapy include the patient's age, underlying heart disease, the frequency and severity of symptoms, and the impact of occurrences of arrhythmia on lifestyle. For example, an individual without structural heart disease in whom AV nodal SVT occurs infrequently in association with tolerable symptoms, does not interfere with daily activities, and usually terminates spontaneously or after a Valsalva maneuver may not require continuous therapy. The patient may prefer infrequent visits to a medical facility for treatment with intravenous adenosine or verapamil if an episode is protracted or may benefit from intermittent oral administration of antiarrhythmic drugs in the form of a "drug cocktail." Conversely, a young individual with frequent episodes of SVT that interfere with participation in athletics or a patient with coronary artery disease in whom SVT produces angina would be more likely to benefit from modification of the AV node with radiofrequency energy.

315

A. Antiarrhythmic Drugs

Although AV nodal reentry is common, it is one of the most difficult paroxysmal SVTs to control with drugs, in part because of the profound nature of autonomic influences on the AV node. Because AV nodal SVT is recurrent and patients usually first develop symptoms as teenagers or young adults, it is unlikely that any drug will be successful long-term in totally preventing episodes of SVT. Among patients who experience some benefit from medical therapy, about 65% respond best to drugs that affect primarily the slow pathway (adenosine, verapamil, diltiazem, digoxin, beta blockers) or both the slow and fast limbs (propafenone, sotalol, amiodarone); the remaining 35% benefit from drugs that affect the fast pathway (procainamide, quinidine, disopyramide, flecainide). Rarely, a combination of both types of agents is effective, but generally such combinations compromise salutary effects of each individual agent.

Comparison of the relative efficacies of antiarrhythmic drugs for preventing recurrences of AV nodal SVT are summarized in Table 3. For patients with infrequent and well-tolerated SVTs, intermittent oral therapy with verapamil, diltiazem, and propranolol, alone or in combination, at the time of an episode is practical and effective if the drugs used have first been shown during the course of electrophysiology study to terminate the SVT without producing symptomatic bradycardia or AV conduction block. Long-term prophylaxis with digoxin, calcium channel blockers, or beta blockers is only modestly effective in preventing recurrences of SVT. Class IC drugs and sotalol are effective in up to 40% of patients and appear safe (proarrhythmia rate < 3%) and well tolerated when structural heart diseases is absent. Their use, however, in patients with cardiomyopathy or ischemic heart disease is associated with a higher risk of proarrhythmic events. The likelihood of end-organ damage with amiodarone, procainamide,

Table 3 Long-Term Efficacy of Antiarrhythmic Drugs for AV Nodal Supraventricular Tachycardia

Drug	Relative effectiveness	Drug	Relative effectiveness
Class IA		Class III	
Procainamide	+	Amiodarone	+ + + +
Quinidine	+	Sotalol	+ + +
Disopyramide	+	AV nodal	
Class IC		Digoxin	+
Flecainide	+ + +	Verapamil	+ +
Propafenone	+ + +	Diltiazem	+
		Beta blockers	+

and quinidine precludes their long-term administration, particularly in younger patients with a disorder that is not life-threatening. Other disadvantages of drugs include long-term administration, cost (approximately $65,000 over 40 years) and side effects (up to 50% in all drug trials).

B. Nonpharmacological Therapies

Modification of AV nodal conduction with the use of catheter-based radio-frequency electrical energy has had a dramatic impact on the management of patients with AV nodal reentry and has rapidly become the treatment of choice for patients with symptomatic SVT. Current approaches selectively alter or interrupt conduction in the slow pathway, maintain conduction in the fast limb, and prevent recurrent AV nodal SVT (i.e., cure the condition). The success rate is over 90%, with a 1% risk of inadvertent permanent AV conduction block. As judged from cumulative experience with thousands of patients, radiofrequency ablation procedures are associated with a rate of serious complications (perforation, tamponade) of less than 3% and mortality well below 0.5%. Advantages of the approach include (a) applicability to patients of all ages, (b) cost (approximately $5000); and (c) minimal time for recuperation (24–48 hr).

Atrioventricular nodal conduction has been selectively modified with the use of cryosurgical or direct dissection procedures. Although such surgical procedures are effective and safe, the cost (approximately $30,000), rehabilitation (approximately 6 weeks), and necessity for open-heart surgery have made them virtually obsolete for patients with AV nodal SVT.

Production of complete AV conduction block by catheter or surgical ablation of the His bundle and implantation of a permanent pacemaker is an alternative, palliative approach to reducing the symptoms of palpitations that is rarely if ever necessary because of the increasing availability of antiarrhythmic drugs and the proven success of catheter-based modification of AV nodal conduction.

Accessory Pathway–Mediated Tachycardias

Bruce D. Lindsay

XIV. MANIFEST AND CONCEALED ACCESSORY PATHWAYS

The Wolff-Parkinson-White (WPW) syndrome (preexcitation and tachycardias) is attributable to a congenital abnormality comprising strands of myocardium that bridge the annulus fibrosus. Such fibers, called accessory pathways, can be located on either side of the heart or within the septum. They may be capable of antegrade conduction from the atrium to the ventricle and retrograde conduction from the ventricle to the atrium or both. Accessory pathways are referred to as manifest or concealed based on whether or not their impulse transmission is evident on ECGs recorded when sinus rhythm is present. Figure 5 illustrates manifest accessory pathways detected by routine electrocardiography with a subject in sinus rhythm. Concealed pathways are never evident in this fashion. When sinus rhythm is present in patients with manifest accessory pathways, the ventricles are activated through both the normal conduction system and the accessory pathway. Because accessory pathways do not usually exhibit the conduction delay typical of the atrioventricular (AV) node, the ventricle is preexcited before propagation through the normal AV conduction system is complete. The eccentric preexcitation of the ventricle is responsible for a short PR interval, altered QRS morphology, and repolarization abnormalities that are characteristic of electrocardiograms recorded from patients with the WPW syndrome. The extent to which ventricular preexcitation is apparent on a randomly obtained ECG may vary from one recording to another.

In contrast to manifest accessory pathways, concealed accessory pathways can conduct only retrograde. Ventricular activation is normal in patients with concealed accessory pathways when sinus rhythm prevails. The electrocardiogram does not exhibit ventricular preexcitation.

XV. MECHANISMS UNDERLYING TACHYCARDIA

Patients with the WPW syndrome have electrophysiologic abnormalities and arrhythmias resulting from three different mechanisms of supraventricular tachycardia (SVT), as shown in Figure 6. Orthodromic SVT is the most common

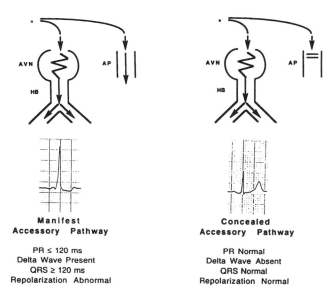

**Manifest
Accessory Pathway**

PR ≤ 120 ms
Delta Wave Present
QRS ≥ 120 ms
Repolarization Abnormal

**Concealed
Accessory Pathway**

PR Normal
Delta Wave Absent
QRS Normal
Repolarization Normal

Figure 5 Atrioventricular conduction patterns and QRS morphologies during sinus rhythm for manifest and concealed accessory pathways. AVN = atrioventricular node, HB = His bundle, AP = accessory pathway.

arrhythmia and accounts for 90–95% of those seen. It depends on a macro-reentrant circuit involving the atria, normal AV conduction system, ventricles, and an accessory pathway. With orthodromic SVT, antegrade conduction occurs through the AV node/His Purkinje system. Following activation of the ventricles, the wavefront of excitation continues retrogradely through the accessory pathway to the atria. The arrhythmia is terminated if conduction is blocked in either the AV node or the accessory pathway.

Antidromic SVT, which occurs spontaneously in only 5% of patients with WPW syndrome, depends on a macroreentrant circuit comprising the atria, accessory pathway, ventricles, and AV node/His bundle. The wavefront of activation conducts from the atria across the accessory pathway to the ventricles and proceeds retrogradely up the normal conduction system back to the atria. The arrhythmia can be terminated if conduction is blocked in the AV node or in the accessory pathway.

Approximately 30% of patients with the WPW syndrome experience atrial fibrillation. In many, orthodromic SVT develops first and degenerates into atrial fibrillation. In others, atrial fibrillation occurs de novo. When atrial fibrillation is present, the ventricles are activated through the normal conduction system, the

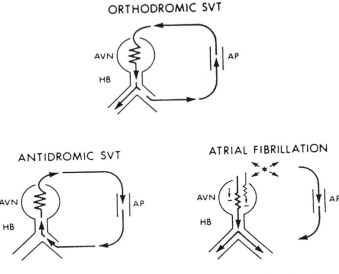

Figure 6 Schematic representation of the patterns of conduction through an accessory pathway (AP) and the normal conduction system (AVN-HB) during orthodromic SVT, antidromic SVT, and atrial fibrillation.

accessory pathway, or both. In patients with accessory pathways with short refractory periods, ventricular activation occurs predominantly through the accessory pathway, and heart rates exceeding 250 beats/min may occur. Thus, the arrhythmia can result in hypotension, degenerate into ventricular fibrillation, and be fatal.

Patients with concealed accessory pathways are prone to orthodromic SVT. Because concealed accessory pathways conduct only retrogradely, antidromic SVT cannot occur. Patients with concealed accessory pathways may, of course, experience atrial fibrillation, but if so, it is not associated with ventricular preexcitation. Thus, the ventricular rate and QRS morphology are comparable to those in patients without accessory pathways.

XVI. MAHAIM FIBERS

A distinctive variant of WPW syndrome is not associated with preexcitation in sinus rhythm but exhibits tachycardia invariably associated with preexcitation. The unique accessory pathways involved are Mahaim fibers. They can conduct only in an antegrade direction and exhibit long conduction times. Although Mahaim originally described a connection between the His fascicle and the right ventricle, the term is now applied to anomalous pathways that connect the AV node with the ventricle directly or the atrium with a distal portion of the right bundle branch.

Most Mahaim fibers are atriofascicular connections (Figure 7A) that originate from the free wall of the right atrium and insert into the apical portion of the right ventricular free wall, close to the distal components of the right bundle branch. Some fuse with the distal right bundle branch. Because of slow conduction through the proximal portion of the Mahiam fiber, the ECG recorded when sinus rhythm is present typically exhibits a normal PR interval and QRS complexes that do not provide evidence of ventricular preexcitation.

The mechanism underlying tachycardia in patients with Mahaim fibers is reentrant, but the components that make up the circuit are the subject of controversy. In some patients, dual AV nodal physiology is present, and AV nodal reentry may occur with the Mahaim fiber acting as a bystander that conducts impulses to the ventricle without being a critical component of the circuit. It is likely, however, that in most patients a macroreentrant circuit exists comprising the atria, Mahaim fiber, right ventricle, and conduction system (Figure 6A). When tachycardia is present, the wavefront of activation proceeds from the atria over the Mahaim fiber to the distal right bundle branch activating the ventricles; retrograde conduction occurs via the right bundle branch to the His bundle/AV node, which conducts the impulse back to the atria. The macroreentrant tachycardia requires 1:1 VA conduction and can be terminated by blocking conduction in either the Mahaim fiber or the AV node.

XVII. ELECTROCARDIOGRAPHIC CHARACTERISTICS

With orthodromic SVT (Figure 8) the QRS complex is normal in the absence of either aberration in the His-Purkinje system or other underlying heart disease. Atrial activation begins 70–110 msec after the onset of the surface QRS and requires 50–60 msec for completion. Consequently, the P wave occurs after the QRS complex and typically distorts the ST segment in the first half of the RR interval.

The effects of bundle branch block may provide clues regarding both the mechanism of the tachycardia and the location of the accessory pathway. Figure 9 shows a recording obtained while orthodromic SVT was occurring in a patient with a left-sided accessory pathway. The development of left bundle branch block was associated with prolongation of the tachycardia cycle length (decrease in rate). When accessory pathways are located in the free wall of either the left or right ventricle, conduction block in the ipsilateral bundle increases the distance over which the wavefront of activation must travel and thereby prolongs the cycle length of the tachycardia. No effect on the cycle length is observed when conduc-

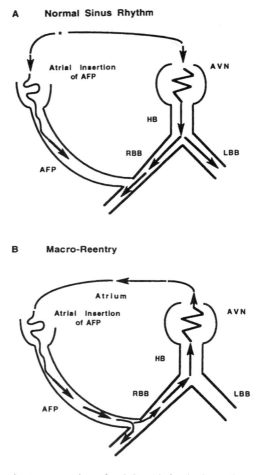

A   Normal Sinus Rhythm

B   Macro-Reentry

Figure 7   Schematic representation of a right atriofascicular pathway that originates in the right atrium and crosses the tricuspid annulus. The distal end of the atriofascicular pathway inserts into the distal right bundle branch. During sinus rhythm (A), the ventricle is activated by the atrioventricular node/His-Purkinje system because conduction through the proximal portion of the atriofasicular pathway is slow. During macro-reentry (B), the atriofascicular pathway functions as the anterograde limb and the His bundle is the retrograde limb of the circuit. AFP = atriofascicular pathway, RB = right bundle branch, AVN = atrioventricular node, HB = His bundle, LBB = left bundle branch.

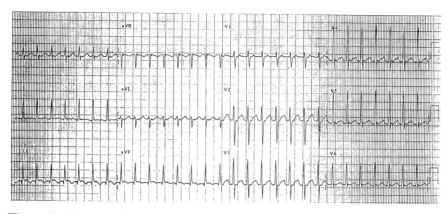

Figure 8 Electrocardiogram recorded during orthodromic SVT. The QRS complex is normal in the absence of aberration in the His-Purkinje system. During SVT, the P wave occurs after the QRS complex and typically distorts the ST segment in the first half of the RR interval.

tion block occurs in the contralateral bundle. Accordingly, left bundle branch block typically decreases the rate of orthodromic SVT mediated by a left-sided pathway, and right bundle branch block has the same effect on tachycardias mediated by right-sided pathways. The rate of tachycardias mediated by accessory pathways located within the septum is not affected by the development of either left or right bundle branch block.

An atypical form of orthodromic SVT is mediated by concealed accessory pathways characterized by slow retrograde conduction. The tachycardia may be nearly incessant. The ECG is characterized by a retrograde P wave that occurs near the midpoint or later in the RR interval. Figure 10 shows an ECG recorded from a patient who had an incessant tachycardia with these features. Activation of the atria began 280 msec after the onset of the QRS and is apparent in the second half of the RR interval.

With antidromic SVT, maximal preexcitation is present because ventricular activation occurs exclusively through the accessory pathway. As shown in Figure 11, ECGs recorded during antidromic SVT show a regular, wide, monomorphic QRS complex that resembles that seen in ventricular tachycardia. Retrograde P waves may be detectable during the first half of the RR interval, but they can be difficult to appreciate because of the marked repolarization abnormalities associated with preexcited complexes. When evident, P waves occur in a 1:1 relationship with respect to QRS complexes because block of conduction in either the accessory pathway or AV node would have terminated the tachycardia.

Figure 12 depicts an ECG recorded while atrial fibrillation was present in a

323

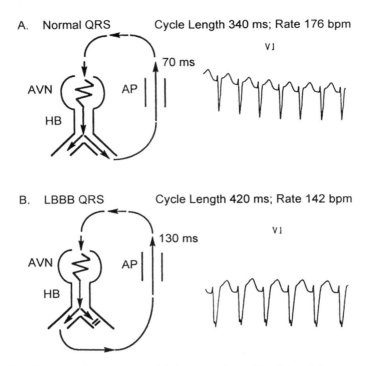

A. Normal QRS   Cycle Length 340 ms; Rate 176 bpm

70 ms

AVN   AP

HB

V I

B. LBBB QRS   Cycle Length 420 ms; Rate 142 bpm

130 ms

AVN   AP

HB

V I

Figure 9 Electrocardiograms recorded from a patient with a left-sided accessory pathway during orthodromic SVT with a normal QRS (A) and with LBBB (B). The development of LBBB resulted in a decrease in the rate of the tachycardia from 176 to 142 beats/min because the length of the circuit and the transit time of the wavefront was increased. Atrial activation occurred 70 and 130 msec after the onset of ventricular activation with a normal QRS and LBBB, respectively. AVN = atrioventricular node, HB = His bundle, AP = accessory pathway.

patient with a manifest accessory pathway. The ventricular rate is rapid, the RR intervals are irregular, and the QRS morphology varies depending on the extent to which the ventricle is activated via the accessory pathway or via the AV node. The irregular rate and QRS morphology differentiate this arrhythmia from antidromic SVT or monomorphic ventricular tachycardia. Patients with preexcited RR intervals shorter than 250 msec have accessory pathways with short refractory properties. It is these patients who are at an increased risk of atrial fibrillation inducing ventricular fibrillation because of the potential for rapid conduction over the accessory pathway.

As shown in Figure 13, tachycardias mediated by Mahaim fibers exhibit QRS morphology resembling the pattern with left bundle branch block. The QRS

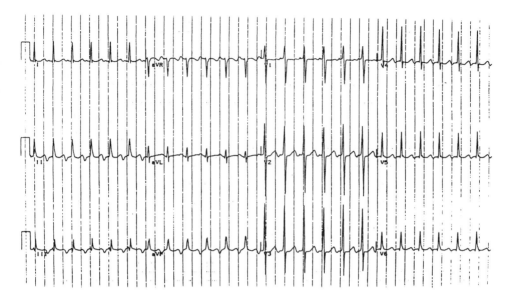

Figure 10   Electrocardiogram recorded from a patient with atypical orthodromic SVT caused by an accessory pathway with long retrograde conduction times. The retrograde P wave is located in the second half of the RR interval.

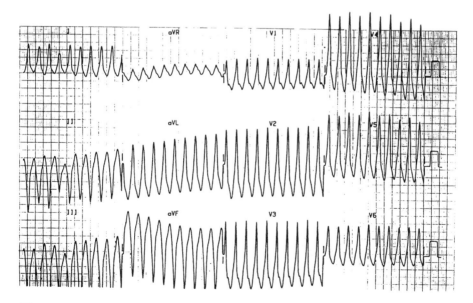

Figure 11   Electrocardiogram recorded during antidromic SVT. The QRS complex shows maximal preexcitation and the RR intervals are regular. When evident, P waves have a 1:1 relationship with the QRS, since AV or VA block would terminate the tachycardia.

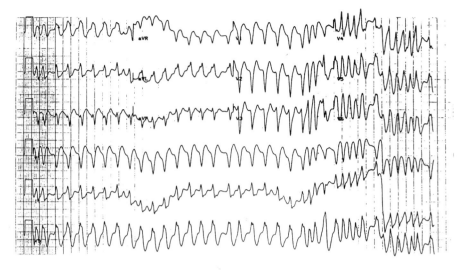

Figure 12 Electrocardiogram recorded during atrial fibrillation. The ventricular rate is rapid and the QRS is polymorphic because of varying degrees of fusion through the accessory pathway and normal AV conduction system.

axis is typically between 0 and $-75°$; QRS duration is 0.15 sec or less; an R wave is evident in limb lead I; an rS is seen in precordial lead V_1; and a transition is seen in the precordial leads with a predominantly negative QRS converting to a positive complex in leads V_4 to V_6.

XVIII. MANAGEMENT

Management should be determined by the need for treatment, relative risks and benefit of pharmacological and nonpharmacological interventions, and costs.

The approach to patients must be based on the natural history of preexcitation syndromes. The overall incidence of sudden death in patients with the WPW syndrome is 0.15% per patient year. For those with asymptomatic preexcitation detected on routinely obtained ECGs, the risk is negligible. Accordingly, the decision to evaluate and treat patients with ventricular preexcitation should depend on the presence and severity of symptoms. Most asymptomatic patients need not undergo electrophysiological evaluation or treatment. They should be advised to return for follow-up if symptoms develop, as is the case in 30% of patients who are asymptomatic initially. Asymptomatic patients who may warrant prophylactic measures include airline pilots, heavy machinery operators, truck drivers, competitive athletes, or others who could be endangered or endanger the lives of bystanders if an arrhythmia occurred.

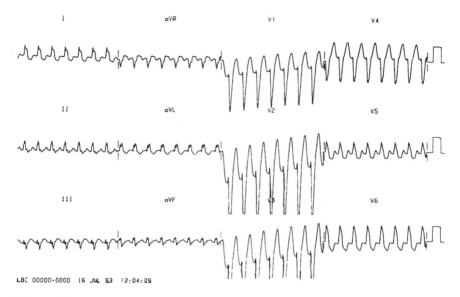

Figure 13 Electrocardiogram recorded during SVT mediated by a Mahaim fiber. The recording demonstrates a QRS morphology resembling left bundle branch block with a normal axis in the limb leads and delayed R-wave progression (V_5) in the precordial leads.

The alternatives for patients who require treatment include antiarrhythmic drugs, catheter-guided ablation of the accessory pathway, or surgery. Although antiarrhythmic medications have been used for many years, relatively few prospective studies have been performed; the duration of reported follow-up is brief; and for any particular drug, the number of patients studied is small. Figure 14 summarizes the relative efficacy of several long-term antiarrhythmic drug regimens as judged from published investigations and experience. In general, drugs associated with the lowest cost and toxicity tend to be the least effective. Those with greater efficacy are expensive and exhibit more adverse effects.

Digoxin and verapamil have been reported to provoke ventricular fibrillation when they are administered intravenously while atrial fibrillation is present in patients with the WPW syndrome. The incidence is uncertain when these drugs are administered orally or used over the long term.

Ventricular proarrhythmia can be anticipated in approximately 1% of patients treated with quinidine, procainamide, disopyramide, flecainide, propafenone, or sotalol.

Amiodarone is extremely effective in the treatment of preexcitation syndromes. However, its long-term toxicity is prohibitive for young patients.

327

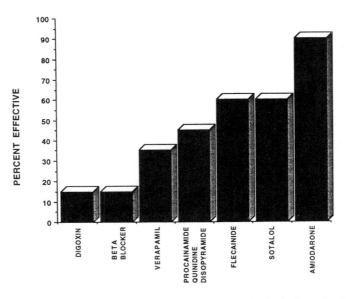

Figure 14   Comparison of the relative efficacies of antiarrhythmic drugs for the prevention of orthodromic SVT.

The inconvenience, cost, toxicity, and modest efficacy of antiarrhythmic drugs have greatly limited their role in the treatment of patients with the WPW syndrome and have provided a strong impetus for the development of nonpharmacological therapy.

The development of catheter-guided radiofrequency energy ablation of accessory pathways has radically changed management of patients with tachycardias mediated by accessory pathways. Thousands of patients with the syndrome have undergone ablation procedures with relatively high rates of success and infrequent complications. The procedure involves percutaneous insertion of several catheters positioned at selected locations within the heart. Recordings from the catheters are used to identify the location of the accessory pathway. A specially designed catheter is positioned at its site, and radiofrequency energy is applied for approximately 60 sec. Radiofrequency energy is alternating electrical current with a frequency of about 500,000 cycles/sec, which is beyond the range that stimulates muscles or nerves. Accordingly, most patients do not perceive any sensation when the accessory pathway is ablated. A small zone of tissue, approximately 5–7 mm in diameter, undergoes coagulation necrosis when the radiofrequency current is applied. Depending on the techniques used, either the atrial or ventricular insertion of the accessory pathway is destroyed selectively when ablation is performed. Conduction through the accessory pathway is therefore eliminated.

Successful ablation of accessory pathways is achieved in more than 90% of patients with the WPW syndrome. Among patients in whom the procedure is judged to be successful, recovery of accessory pathway function occurs in only 5–12%. Although relatively few patients have undergone ablation of Mahaim fibers, preliminary studies have demonstrated its feasibility.

The remarkable success of arrhythmia ablation procedures has encouraged many physicians to refer children and adults with supraventricular tachycardia for electrophysiological intervention as the first line of therapy. Ablation procedures are preferred to medical therapy because of the potential risks, expense, and inconvenience associated with long-term use of drugs. Ablation procedures are indicated for patients with life-threatening arrhythmias or those in whom treatment with antiarrhythmic medications is ineffective or not well tolerated. They provide an alternative for patients who wish to avoid lifelong therapy with drugs.

Enthusiasm for arrhythmia ablation techniques must be tempered by the recognition that these procedures do entail some risk. Cardiac perforation, vascular injury, valvular damage, stroke, and iatrogenic heart block can occur. The incidence is extremely low, but the risks must be considered strongly in patients whose arrhythmias are infrequent, associated with only mild symptoms, or easily controlled by medications that are well tolerated. Arrhythmia ablation procedures often require the prolonged use of fluoroscopy, which subjects patients to the potential long-term risks associated with radiation. Although radiation exposure during a procedure does not markedly increase the risk of developing of a fatal cancer or genetic defect that can be passed on to offspring, caution should be exercised to avoid subjecting patients to prolonged fluoroscopy when arrhythmias are difficult to ablate or require more than one procedure.

Surgical division of accessory pathways and Mahaim fibers has been largely replaced by catheter-guided ablation procedures. Surgery remains an option for patients with life-threatening or debilitating arrhythmias in whom ablation of the accessory pathway has failed. Successful division of the accessory pathway can be accompanied in more than 99% of patients without other forms of heart disease with an operative mortality of less than 1%.

In 1992, total costs of catheter-guided radiofrequency energy ablation of an accessory pathway were in the range of $10,000 to $11,000. This compares favorably with the total cost of arrhythmia surgery, which was approximately $55,000 in the same interval. In patients whose arrhythmias are not well controlled by medications, the cumulative expenses resulting from several emergency room visits per year would exceed the cost of an arrhythmia ablation procedure within 2 years. However, in patients whose arrhythmias are well controlled by medication, the cost of medical therapy might not exceed the cost of a radiofrequency ablation procedure for 15 years or more.

SUGGESTED READING

Management of Patients with Cardiac Arrhythmias

Dick A, Dominguez P. Nonparoxysmal A-V nodal tachycardia. Circulation 1957; 16:1022–1032.

Brugada P, Farre J, et al. Observations in patients with supraventricular tachycardia having a PR interval shorter than the RP interval: Differentiation between atrial tachycardia and reciprocating atrioventricular tachycardia using an accessory pathway with long conduction times. Am Heart J 1984; 107:558.

Fisch C, Knoebel SB. Junctional rhythms. Progr Cardiovasc Dis 1970; 13:141–150.

Gillette PC, Garson A. Electrophysiologic and pharmacologic characteristics of automatic ectopic atrial tachycardia. Circulation 1977; 56:571.

Goldreyer BN, Gallagher JJ. The Electrophysiologic Demonstration of Atrial Ectopic Tachycardia in Man. Am Heart J 1973; 85:205.

Gorgels AP, Beckman HD, et al. Extrastimulus related shortening to the first postpacing interval in digitalis induced ventricular tachycardia. J Am Coll Cardiol 1983; 1:840.

Josephson ME, Spear JF, et al. Surgical excision of automatic atrial tachycardia: Anatomic and electrophysiologic correlates. Am Heart J 1982; 1:1076.

Lown B, Wyatt NF, Levine HD. Paroxysmal atrial tachycardia with block. Circulation 1960; 21:129.

Reiffel JA. Normal sinus rhythm and its variants (sinus arrhythmia, sinus tachycardia, sinus bradycardia), sinus node reentry, and sinus node dysfunction (sick sinus syndrome): Mechanisms, recognition, and management. In: Podrid P, Kowey P, eds. Cardiac Arrhythmias: Mechanisms, Diagnoses, and Management. Baltimore, Williams & Wilkins, 1994.

Reiffel JA, Kuehnert MJ. Electrophysiologic testing of sinus node function: Diagnostic and prognostic application—Including updated information from sinus node electrogram. PACE 1994; 17:349–365.

Rosen MP, Fisch C, Hoffman BF, et al. Can accelerated atrioventricular junctional escape rhythms be explained by delayed afterdepolarization? Am J Cardiol 1980;

Scher DL, Asura EL. Multifocal atrial tachycardia: Mechanisms, clinical correlates and treatment. Am Heart J 1989; 85:205.

Atrioventricular Nodal Reentrant Tachycardia

Jackman WM, Beckman KJ, McClelland JH, et al. Treatment of supraventricular tachycardia due to atrioventricular nodal reentry by radiofrequency catheter ablation of slow-pathway conduction. N Engl J Med 1992; 327:313–318.

Josephson ME. Supraventricular tachycardias. In: Josephson ME, ed. Clinical Cardiac Electrophysiology: Techniques and Interpretation. 2d ed. Philadelphia: Lea & Febiger, 1993:181.

Kay GN, Epstein AE, Dailey SM, Plumb VJ. Selective radiofrequency ablation of the slow pathway for the treatment of atrioventricular nodal reentrant tachycardia: Evidence for involvement of perinodal myocardium within the reentrant circuit. Circulation 1992; 85:1675–1688.

Keim SG, Werner PH, Troup PJ, et al. Localization of the fast and slow pathways in atrioventricular nodal reentry tachycardia by intraoperative mapping. Circulation 1992; 86:919–925.

Lee MA, Morady F, Kadish A, et al. Catheter modification of the atrioventricular junction with radiofrequency energy for control of atrioventricular nodal reentry tachycardia. Circulation 1991; 83:827–835.

Lindsay BD, Chung MK, Gamache C, et al. Therapeutic endpoints for the treatment of atrioventricular node reentrant tachycardia by catheter-guided radiofrequency current. J Am Coll Cardiol 1993; 22:733–740.

Roden DM. Risks and benefits of antiarrhythmic therapy. N Engl J Med 1994; 331: 785–791.

Scheinman MM. North American Society of Pacing and Electrophysiology (NASPE) survey on radiofrequency catheter ablation: Implications for clinicians, third party insurers and government regulatory agencies. PACE 1992; 15:2228–2231.

Accessory Pathway–Mediated Tachycardias

Berkman NL, Lambe LE. The Wolff-Parkinson-White electrocardiogram: A follow-up study of five to twenty-eight years. N Engl J Med 1968; 278:492–494.

Calkins H, Sousa J, El-Atassi R, et al. Diagnosis and cure of the Wolff-Parkinson-White syndrome or paroxysmal supraventricular tachycardia during a single electrophysiologic test. N Engl J Med 1991; 324:1612–1618.

Cox JL, Gallagher JJ, Cain ME: Experience with 118 consecutive patients undergoing operation for the Wolff-Parkinson-White syndrome. J Thorac Cardiovasc Surg 1985; 90:490–501.

Jackman WM, Wang X, Friday KJ, et al. Catheter ablation of accessory atrioventricular pathways (Wolff-Parkinson-White syndrome) by radiofrequency current. N Engl J Med 1991; 324:1605–1611.

Kalbfleisch SJ, El-Atassi R, Calkins H, et al. Safety feasibility and cost of outpatient radiofrequency catheter ablation of accessory atrioventricular connections. J Am Coll Cardiol 1993; 21:567–570.

Klein GJ, Yee R, Sharma AD. Longitudinal electrophysiologic assessment of asymptomatic patients with the Wolff-Parkinson-White electrocardiographic patterns. N Engl J Med 1989; 320:1229–1233.

Lindsay BD, Crossen KJ, Cain ME. Concordance of distinguishing electrocardiographic features during sinus rhythm with the location of accessory pathways in the Wolff-Parkinson-White syndrome. Am J Cardiol 1987; 59:1093–1102.

Lindsay BD, Eichling JO, Ambos HD, Cain ME. Radiation exposure to patients and medical personnel during radiofrequency catheter ablation for supraventricular tachycardia. Am J Cardiol 1992; 70:218–223.

McClelland JH, Wang X, Beckman KJ, et al. Radiofrequency catheter ablation of right atriofascicular (Mahaim) accessory pathways guided by accessory pathway activation potentials. Circulation 1994; 89:2655–2666.

Munger TM, Packer DL, Hammill SC, et al. A population study of the natural history of Wolff-Parkinson-White syndrome in Olmsted County, Minnesota, 1953–1989. Circulation 1993; 87:866–873.

Scheinman MM. North American Society of Pacing and Electrophysiology (NASPE) survey on radiofrequency catheter ablation: Implications for clinicians, third party insurers, and government regulatory agencies. PACE 1992; 15:2228–2231.

17

Management of Patients with Ventricular Arrhythmias

Ventricular Premature Complexes   **333**
   I.   Epidemiology   334
  II.   Electrocardiography   336
 III.   Mechanisms of Ventricular Premature Complexes   338
 IV.   Treatment   340

Ventricular Tachycardia   **343**
   V.   Pathophysiologic Basis of Ventricular Tachycardia   344
 VI.   Electrocardiographic Features   345
VII.   Specific Types of Ventricular Tachycardia and Therapy   347

     Suggested Reading   370

Ventricular Premature Complexes

J. Thomas Bigger, Jr.

Ventricular premature complexes (VPCs) arise in the ventricles and may be asymptomatic or symptomatic. Many names have been used for VPCs: "ventricular premature contractions," "ventricular extrasystoles," "ventricular ectopic beats," "ventricular ectopic complexes," "ventricular ectopic depolarizations," and others.

I. EPIDEMIOLOGY

A. Ventricular Premature Complexes in Normal Persons

Infrequent VPCs are common even in young persons. Almost a thousand apparently healthy persons have been studied using long-term (24- to 48-hr) continuous electrocardiographic (ECG) recordings. Ventricular ectopy, ≥1 VPC per day, was found in about 30–55% of them. The prevalence of ventricular ectopy increases somewhat with age but does not differ significantly between genders. A frequency of VPCs ≥10/hr occurs in only about 1% of healthy young or middle-aged men or women but is found in about 7% of healthy older persons (age range 40–85 years). Continuous 24-hr ECG recordings show a low prevalence of complex VPCs in healthy persons. Multiform VPCs occur in about 10% of healthy young people studied with continuous 24-hr ECG recordings; the prevalence rises to about 30% in healthy persons over 70 years of age. The R-on-T phenomenon and repetitive complexes—i.e., paired VPCs and unsustained ventricular tachycardia (VT)—have an overall prevalence less than 1%, and the prevalence does not increase much with age. Sporadic VPCs in persons with normal hearts do not seem to affect outcome adversely. However, no longitudinal studies of the significance of VPCs have been done in unbiased samples of healthy individuals.

B. Ventricular Arrhythmias After Myocardial Infarction

Several studies have evaluated the prevalence of VPCs at about the time of discharge from hospital after myocardial infarction. At this time about 30% of the patients have 3 or more VPCs/hr, 20% have more than 10/hr, and 10% have more than 30/hr. About 10% have short runs of unsustained ventricular tachycardia. There is some increase in VPC frequency between 2–3 weeks and 12 weeks after myocardial infarction. Thereafter, the frequency of VPCs stabilizes. Patients who have frequent VPCs 2–12 weeks after myocardial infarction have a three to four times greater risk of dying over the subsequent 3–4 years. The risk predicted by VPCs is independent of any association with left ventricular dysfunction. Ventricular premature complexes found after full recovery from myocardial infarction also have prognostic significance.

C. Ventricular Arrhythmias to Hypertrophic Cardiomyopathy

24-hr electrocardiographic recordings have shown that 80% of the patients with hypertrophic cardiomyopathy have VPCs; 30% have ≥10 VPCs/hr, 50% have multiform VPCs, 35% have paired VPCs, and 25% have unsustained VT. There is no correlation between left ventricular outflow gradient and the presence or

334

severity of VPCs, but patients with septal thickness of greater than 20 mm have a higher prevalence of frequent VPCs and unsustained ventricular tachycardia. Only 10% of patients who report light-headedness during 24-hr ECG recordings have either atrial or ventricular arrhythmias associated with this symptom. The annual mortality attributable to premature death in a hospital-based referral population of patients with hypertrophic cardiomyopathy is about 2–3%. Most of these deaths are sudden and unpredictable and affect the young (under 30 years of age). The relatively high incidence of tragic sudden death in young persons with hypertrophic cardiomyopathy has led to a search for predictors and for treatment. The most promising predictor of subsequent sudden cardiac death is asymptomatic, unsustained VT detected by continuous 24-hr ECG recordings. The 3-year mortality is increased about sevenfold in patients who have unsustained VT compared with that in patients who do not have VT.

D. Ventricular Arrhythmias in Dilated Cardiomyopathy

Virtually all patients with dilated cardiomyopathy have VPCs. About 60% of patients with dilated cardiomyopathy and class III or IV congestive heart failure have ≥10 VPCs/hr and about 50% have unsustained VT. The available evidence on the prognostic significance of ventricular arrhythmias in dilated cardiomyopathy suggests that frequent and repetitive VPCs predict all-cause mortality and sudden cardiac death, just as they do after myocardial infarction. However, dilated cardiomyopathy has not been studied sufficiently to define clearly the relationships among left ventricular dysfunction, ventricular arrhythmias, and death. The available data suggest an independent role for ventricular arrhythmias.

E. Ventricular Arrhythmias in Mitral Valve Prolapse

Some workers found an association between ventricular arrhythmias and sudden death in mitral valve prolapse and proposed a casual relationship. Others have challenged this proposal. There are several controversial issues related to this argument: (a) the echocardiographic criteria for a diagnosis of prolapse, (b) the association between mitral valve prolapse and ventricular arrhythmias, and (c) the relationship between mitral valve prolapse and sudden death. It is not proven that the prevalence of ventricular arrhythmias is increased or that ventricular arrhythmias are associated with sudden cardiac death in mitral valve prolapse.

F. Ventricular Arrhythmias in Patients with Hypertension

The Framingham study showed that the ECG changes of left ventricular enlargement are associated with sudden cardiac death and coronary heart disease after statistical adjustment for blood pressure. Small but carefully controlled studies of patients with hypertension showed a strong relationship between the prevalence of ≥10 VPC/hr over a 48-hr period and ECG or echocardiographic evidence of left ventricular hypertrophy: normotensive controls, 2%; hypertension without ECG left ventricular hypertrophy, 10%; and hypertension with ECG left ventricular hypertrophy, 32%. The prevalence of unsustained ventricular tachycardia (≥3 consecutive VPCs at a rate > 120/min) for the three groups, 2%, 8%, and 28% respectively, is similar to the percentages for VPC frequency. Patients with ST-T wave changes as well as ECG voltage criteria for left ventricular hypertrophy had a 48% prevalence (of 21 patients) of unsustained ventricular tachycardia. The presence of frequent VPCs or unsustained ventricular tachycardia was not related to diuretic treatment or serum K^+ concentration. The relationship between left ventricular enlargement in patients with hypertension and ventricular arrhythmias is strong and relatively independent of other factors that might be involved. The significance of the relationship between left ventricular enlargement and ventricular arrhythmias in patients with hypertension is unknown with respect to prognosis. If ventricular arrhythmias do prove to be independently associated with increased mortality, it will still need to be proven that drug therapy can suppress the arrhythmias or reduce the risk of death.

II. ELECTROCARDIOGRAPHY

Ventricular premature complexes arise in the ventricles and depolarize the heart in an abnormal sequence. The QRS-T complex of VPCs is premature, wide, and often bizarre in its ECG appearance; the ST segment and T wave are opposite in direction to the QRS complex; and no premature P wave precedes the premature QRS complex. A VPC can be so premature that it occurs on the apex of the T wave of the previous QRS complex (R-on-T phenomenon). Conversely, the VPC may occur late enough to fuse with the subsequent sinus QRS (fusion complex). Typically, the VPC is followed by a fully compensatory pause (i.e., the RV interval plus the VR interval is equal to two RR intervals in sinus rhythm because the premature ventricular impulse conducts retrograde into the AV node, where it collides with the supraventricular impulse that is propagating toward the ventricle). The subsequent P wave conducts with a normal PR interval, making the pause perfectly compensatory. If the atrial rate is slow and the VPC quite premature, retrograde conduction of the ventricular impulse may capture the atrium.

Ventricular premature complexes may be *interpolated* between two successive sinus complexes. When sinus rhythm is slow, the VPC is quite premature and retrograde conduction blocks on the ventricular side of the AV node, the AV node may recover in time to conduct the next sinus impulse. When VPCs are interpolated, the retrograde conduction of the VPC into the AV node causes the PR interval of the subsequent sinus complex to prolong ("concealed" retrograde conduction).

Fixed or Variable Coupling of Ventricular Premature Complexes

In ECG rhythm strips, the coupling of VPCs to the QRS usually is "fixed," i.e., the (RV) interval varies less than 0.06 sec. Fixed coupling suggests that the mechanism responsible for VPCs is stable and involves a fixed conduction pathway with stable electrical properties. Variable coupling (RV) intervals can be caused by (a) ventricular parasystole, (b) instability in a reentrant circuit, or (c) multiple sites of origin in the ventricles.

Bi- or Trigeminy

Certain patterns of VPCs have special names. When every other QRS is a VPC, the pattern is termed *bigeminy*; a VPC every third QRS if termed *trigeminy*; and two successive VPCs is termed a *pair* or a *couplet*.

Multiform VPCs

Ventricular premature complexes may have a uniform appearance on an ECG or may have multiple configurations, i.e., be multiform. Multiform VPCs can occur when the site of origin varies or when the conduction pathway varies as the impulse propagates from a single site of origin.

Accelerated Idioventricular Rhythm

Accelerated idioventricular rhythm (AIVR) is defined as three or more consecutive QRS complexes of ventricular origin with a rate between 50 and 100. Some authors diagnose AIVR with rates as fast as 120/min. Because AIVR is slow, it is easy to determine that AV dissociation is present. Often, control of the ventricles switches back and forth between sinus rhythm and AIVR. Fusion QRS complexes often begin or end an episode of AIVR.

Ventricular Parasystole

Ventricular parasystole is an automatic rhythm in the His-Purkinje system that is reasonably independent of the dominant sinus rhythm. Parasystole has two cardinal features: variable coupling of VPC and a common denominator for interectopic intervals. Ventricular fusion complexes are common. Usually, ventricular parasystole is slower than the sinus rate. *Entrance block* is the key feature that permits parallel, independent activity in the ventricular focus even though the sinus rate is faster. Entrance block removes the parasystolic focus from the suppressant influence of the sinus impulses—i.e., overdrive suppression—permitting a stable automatic rhythm to emerge. When entrance block exists without exit block, the ectopic focus will activate the ventricle every time it fires unless the ventricle happens to be refractory from the previous sinus impulse.

Ventricular Premature Complexes Versus Aberrant Conduction

Aberrantly conducted supraventricular premature complexes can resemble VPCs. Ventricular premature contractions do not disturb sinus rhythm, whereas atrial premature depolarizations reset the sinus node so that the subsequent pause is not fully compensatory. In atrial fibrillation with occasional wide QRS complexes, the following features suggest a ventricular origin for the wide complexes rather than aberrant conduction: fixed coupling, short coupling intervals of the wide QRS complex followed by a pause, and a bigeminal sequence with alternating narrow and wide QRS complexes. Aberrant conduction in atrial fibrillation often results from the Ashman phenomenon—the aberrant complex terminates a short RR cycle which, in turn, follows a long cycle; also, the aberrant complex usually has a right bundle branch configuration.

III. MECHANISMS OF VENTRICULAR PREMATURE COMPLEXES

These complexes have been attributed to altered automaticity, reentry of the cardiac impulse, or some combination of these two mechanisms. More recently, afterdepolarizations and triggered activity have been proposed as possible mechanisms for VPCs.

A. Normal Automaticity

Normal Purkinje fibers can be automatic, i.e., they can spontaneously excite themselves. Pacemakers in the His-Purkinje system may control cardiac rhythm as escape pacemakers or when their automaticity is increased.

B. Abnormal Automaticity

Under abnormal conditions, e.g., soon after experimental myocardial infarction, Purkinje fibers can depolarize and become automatic. In markedly depolarized Purkinje fibers, the phasic current that is responsible for normal pacemaker activity is fully activated. Therefore, it is clear that this form of automaticity cannot be explained by the normal ionic mechanism.

C. Afterdepolarizations and Triggered Activity

Recently, afterdepolarizations and triggered activity have been recognized as potential mechanisms underlying cardiac arrhythmias. Two forms of afterdepolarizations (secondary depolarizations after repolarization has begun), i.e., early and late afterdepolarizations, have been described as important in initiating triggered activity. Triggered activity is not a form of automaticity because triggered activity is not self-excitatory but rather depends on a preceding action potential to initiate the process.

Early Afterdepolarizations

Early afterdepolarizations occur before the cell repolarizes, often arising from the plateau of the action potential. Early afterdepolarizations can occur in almost any type of heart cell, but they have been studied most extensively in cardiac Purkinje fibers. Early afterdepolarizations are likely to occur when repolarization is delayed—e.g., by hypokalemia, slow pacing rates, or drug toxicity. Early afterdepolarizations can trigger sustained rapid firing in Purkinje fibers. Because Purkinje fiber action potentials are much longer than those in adjacent ventricular muscle, ventricular muscle is likely to respond to early afterdepolarizations. There is substantial evidence to suggest that the torsades de pointes form of unsustained ventricular tachycardia results from early afterdepolarizations caused by hypokalemia, slow heart rate, congenital long QT syndrome, or long QT produced by drugs. Often several factors occur together, e.g., diuretic-induced hypokalemia in patients taking quinidine. Treatments that shorten action potential duration abolish experimental early afterdepolarizations and clinical torsades de pointes, e.g., rapid pacing, increasing extracellular K^+, and drugs that increase K^+ conductance.

Delayed Afterdepolarizations

Delayed afterdepolarizations are small depolarizations (10 mV or so) that occur after the cell has fully repolarized, usually immediately after maximum diastolic voltage is reached. This behavior can be seen in many cell types under abnormal conditions. Delayed afterdepolarizations are usually too small to reach the threshold voltage, but their amplitude varies dynamically with change in heart rate or firing pattern. Factors known to increase the amplitude of delayed afterdepolarizations include rapid pacing, premature activation, increased extracellular calcium $[Ca]_o$, increased catecholamine concentrations, and digitalis toxicity. As heart rate increases or stimulation become more premature, delayed afterdepolarizations become larger and larger until threshold voltage is reached and a run of rapid firing, i.e., triggered activity, is provoked. It is important to understand that triggered activity is *not* automaticity. Although triggered activity can be self-perpetuating, it is not self-initiating.

Digitalis Toxicity and Triggered Activity

Delayed afterdepolarizations develop in cardiac Purkinje fibers when they are exposed to toxic concentrations of digitalis and are associated with an abnormal current called "transient inward current." The abnormal current seems to result from the following sequence of events. Digitalis binds to the sarcolemmal Na^+,K^+-ATPase decreasing the activity of the Na^+ pump. As a result, the intracellular sodium concentration $[Na]_i$ increases. The intracellular calcium concentration $[Ca]_i$ increases as a result of Na^+/Ca^{2+} from the sarcoplasmic reticulum. Phasic increases in $[Ca]_i$ play an important role in generating the transient inward current. Some of the digitalis-induced ventricular tachycardias in humans have characteristics that are compatible with triggered activity. The digitalis toxic arrhythmias are the most convincing example of human arrhythmias that may be caused by delayed afterdepolarizations and triggered activity.

D. Reentrant Arrhythmias

Reentry has been proposed as a mechanism for cardiac arrhythmias for almost a century. The critical conditions for reentry are slow conduction and one-way block in some portion of a circuit. The one-way block may be permanent or dynamic. The exceedingly long refractory period of heart muscle makes reentry difficult to accomplish. Unless an impulse circulates for a very long time, cells in the circuit will still be refractory when the impulse returns to the site of one-way block. However, in disease states, conduction can slow sufficiently to permit reentry to occur even in fairly small circuits.

Experimentally, reentrant ventricular tachycardia can be initiated in subacute and chronically infarcted ventricles. A portion of the block is *static* due to barriers created by infarcted tissues and cell to cell uncoupling. However, in acute ischemia, part of the block is *dynamic* due to the abnormal behavior of ischemically damaged but surviving cells in the infarction zone. These and other mechanisms of reentrant excitation in the ventricle are discussed in Chapters 14, 16, and 17. It is not clear which or whether any of the mechanisms discussed above are responsible for the isolated VPC seen so often in normal human beings and in patients with heart diseases.

The mechanism or mechanisms underlying the common form of VPC, fixed coupled VPC, is unknown. Both reentry and afterdepolarizations have been proposed as mechanisms, but there is no substantive evidence for either.

IV. TREATMENT

A. Benign Ventricular Premature Complexes

Isolated VPCs in patients without heart disease are benign; i.e., they have no prognostic or hemodynamic significance. Therefore the only possible reason for treating VPC in patients without heart disease is to control significant symptoms. The best treatment for benign but symptomatic VPCs is to remove an aggravating factor—e.g., excessive use of caffeine-containing beverages or nicotine—or to remove drugs that may promote VPCs, such as diuretics, cocaine, and sympathomimetics given to treat asthma. If, in the judgment of the physician, drugs are indicated for VPCs in a normal person, beta-adrenergic blocking drugs are the first choice.

B. Prognostically Important Ventricular Premature Complexes

Drugs with Class I Antiarrhythmic Action

Isolated but frequent VPCs in patients with significant heart disease have prognostic significance independent of other cardiac risk factors. However, the pathogenesis of these arrhythmias and their mechanistic link to death are not known. Thus, there is uncertainty about how to respond to VPC in such patients. The findings of the Cardiac Arrhythmia Suppression Trial (CAST) showed that suppression of VPCs with several drugs with class I antiarrhythmic action (both class IC and IA) does not reduce mortality. Worse, for the drugs with class IC action, substantial harm was observed despite marked suppression of ventricular arrhythmias. Previous small clinical trials in patients after myocardial infarction, mostly with drugs having class IB antiarrhythmic action, showed no benefit from treatment, and the findings tended to indicate harm as well. Metaanalyses evaluating prophylaxis of atrial fibrillation and treatment of ventricular arrhythmias suggest that quinidine increases mortality more than twofold. As a result of these findings, drugs with class I antiarrhythmic action cannot be recommended for patients with asymptomatic but prognostically significant VPCs after myocardial infarction. No benefit has been shown for treatment of VPCs in any other form of heart disease either, although other groups have not been studied as extensively as patients after myocardial infarction. Accordingly, it is prudent to avoid treatment of patients with asymptomatic VPCs with drugs having class I antiarrhythmic action.

Drugs with Class II Antiarrhythmic Action

Beta-adrenergic blocking drugs have been shown to reduce arrhythmias and mortality after myocardial infarction and are the treatment of choice for patients with frequent asymptomatic VPCs after myocardial infarction. Patients with heart disease and prognostically significant ventricular arrhythmias who cannot tolerate beta-adrenergic blocking drugs can be treated with angiotensin converting enzyme inhibitors, agents that have been shown to reduce ventricular arrhythmias and mortality in patients with heart failure.

Drugs with Class III Antiarrhythmic Action

There is no definitive evidence that treatment of prognostically significant ventricular arrhythmias with amiodarone will improve survival. Two small randomized clinical trials done in patients with recent myocardial infarction showed a

341

trend toward improved survival for the amiodarone group. A large randomized clinical trial done in patients with congestive heart failure showed no effect of amiodarone on survival. There are at least two additional large-scale, randomized, controlled clinical trials under way to determine whether amiodarone improves survival after myocardial infarction. Until the results of these trials are available, we recommend that amiodarone or other drugs with class III action not be used to treat patients with asymptomatic, prognostically significant VPCs.

Adverse Effects on Mortality Are Not Detectable in Clinical Practice

The CAST study showed that it is almost impossible to detect harmful effects on mortality in uncontrolled clinical use of antiarrhythmic drugs because VPC suppression is an independent predictor of good outcome. Patients who do not respond to and those who do not tolerate antiarrhythmic drugs are not treated in clinical practice. The patients whose arrhythmias are suppressed and who tolerate the antiarrhythmic drugs are the ones treated long term, but these patients do well even without treatment. Thus, most patients who are treated with antiarrhythmic drugs have a relatively low risk of dying during follow-up. Because of the association between suppression of ventricular arrhythmias and good outcome, even patients treated with drugs that increase mortality considerably will appear to do well in a clinical practice setting. Randomized controlled trials with mortality as an endpoint are, therefore, essential to evaluate the effects of antiarrhythmic drug therapy on mortality rates.

Spontaneous Variability of Ventricular Premature Contractions and Treatment Goals

The physician may judge that symptomatic ventricular arrhythmias require treatment and choose Holter recordings to guide the choice of drug and drug dose. This approach has to contend with the large spontaneous day-to-day variability of VPCs. The sequence of drugs is the same as for asymptomatic ventricular arrhythmias, i.e., beta blockers are chosen first. Since control of symptoms is the primary objective of treatment, control of symptoms without much suppression of VPCs is a satisfactory response.

The approach to isolated VPCs is different from approaches to unsustained or sustained VT, entities that are discussed in the next section and Chapter 20.

Ventricular Tachycardia

Mark E. Josephson

Ventricular tachycardia (VT) can be life-threatening. Hypotension may be present because of the underlying heart disease. Accordingly, the recognition and differentiation of VT from supraventricular or tachycardia (SVT) are paramount. Several clinical clues point to VT when a rapid heart rate is the presenting sign, including (a) a somewhat slower rate than that with typical SVT, although some T is very rapid (160 more likely than > 180 beats/min), (b) intermittent cannon A waves visible in the jugular venous pulse, (c) variation in systolic blood pressure with breakthrough beats on auscultation, (d) variation in intensity of the first heart sound, and (e) multiple low-frequency heart sounds including split S_1 and S_2, right and left-sided S_3, and occasional atrial filling sounds. Thus, the heart sounds resemble hoofbeats on a muddy stream. Most of these phenomena are reflections of AV dissociation. The definitive diagnosis is, of course, based on electrocardiographic (ECG) and electrophysiological criteria. Ventricular tachycardia should be defined in terms of both its morphology and duration. Thus, VT may exhibit a single, uniform ECG morphology (monomorphic) or a constantly changing one (polymorphic). It may be nonsustained or sustained, lasting 30 sec or more or requiring termination before persisting for 30 sec because of circulatory collapse, myocardial ischemia, or degeneration into ventricular fibrillation, among other sequelae. Some clinicians might consider tachycardia exceeding 15 beats to be sustained.

More than 90% of VTs lasting for 15 beats also persist for 30 sec or require termination by external countershock. Tachycardias that cease spontaneously in 30 sec or less are classified as nonsustained. Most sustained and nonsustained arrhythmias, with accelerated idioventricular rhythm a striking exception, have a rate equal to or greater than 100 beats/min.

Although sustained VT usually occurs in association with structural heart disease, with coronary artery disease being the most common form, it occasionally occurs in the absence of structural heart disease. Nonsustained VT is more common and occurs with or without associated structural heart disease. Most sustained VTs are associated with symptoms that can be as mild as palpitations and as severe cardiac arrest and death. In contrast, most patients with nonsustained VTs are asymptomatic and most episodes of nonsustained tachycardia persist for only three to five beats. The incidence of ventricular tachycardias is difficult to determine because of the lack of symptoms with many nonsustained types.

Sustained VT occurs in approximately 3% of patients after myocardial infarction. It is rare in patients with coronary disease who have not sustained acute myocardial infarction and is uncommon in other forms of cardiac disease with the exception of arrhythmic right ventricular dysplasia.

V. PATHOPHYSIOLOGIC BASIS OF VENTRICULAR TACHYCARDIA

The mechanisms underlying VTs include derangements of impulse formation, impulse conduction, or both. Abnormal impulse formation may be caused by abnormal automaticity or triggered activity attributable to early or delayed afterdepolarizations. Abnormal automaticity occurs in injured myocardial cells that are partially depolarized and results from calcium-dependent phase 4 automaticity. This mechanism may be operative in accelerated idioventricular rhythm in the first 24 hr after myocardial infarction and in some tachycardias that are not inducible by programmed stimulation. Triggered activity attributable to delayed afterdepolarizations occurs in circumstances in which calcium overloading of the cardiac myocyte occurs, in turn leading to transient inward current that may nonspecifically carry sodium or induce sodium-calcium exchange. It can be initiated or exacerbated by catecholamines or digitalis. It is seen with specific disorders such as left ventricular hypertrophy, in which intracellular calcium overload is often present as well. Digitalis-induced tachycardias, exercise-related arrhythmias, and some arrhythmias after acute reperfusion may be a consequence of the same mechanism.

Tachycardias resulting from delayed afterdepolarizations are initiated at critical heart rates, usually between 90 and 120 beats/min. The triggering heart rate induces calcium loading of the cell, with subsequent development of delayed afterdepolarizations and tachycardia. The rate is relatively slow, from 90 to 160 beats/min. The arrhythmia can frequently be initiated by infusion of isoproterenol and rapid pacing and less reliably (for diagnostic purposes in an electrophysiology laboratory) by timed extrastimuli. The onset and initial rate of the tachyarrhythmia bears a direct relationship to the triggering rate.

Overdrive pacing frequently causes acceleration of the rhythm in proportion to the rate of the overdrive pacing. The faster the paced rate, the shorter the first return impulse of the ongoing tachycardia and the initial return cycles of the tachycardia. The tachycardia typically terminates spontaneously by gradual slowing except when digitalis is responsible.

Triggered activity caused by early afterdepolarizations is usually bradycardia-dependent and related to inward calcium transients following the plateau of the action potential. The phenomena are frequently associated with large humps at the end of the T wave that appear as U waves. Pause-dependent early afterdepolarizations are considered to underlie torsades de pointes; i.e., acquired polymorphic tachycardias associated with the long-QT syndrome. The relationship of early afterdepolarizations to the congenital long-QT syndrome associated with poly-morphic VT is unclear.

Reentry is the most common mechanism underlying paroxysmal ventricular arrhythmias, particularly sustained VT associated with coronary artery disease. Coronary artery disease with previous infarction is the primary pathological substrate leading to reentry. Viable muscle fibers, separated by connective tissue, result in uncoupling of the cells and very slow conduction, the critical requirement for arrhythmia. Ventricular tachycardia of this type is readily induced and can be terminated by programmed stimulation. Very slow conduction is also associated with VT seen in arrhythmogenic right ventricular dysplasia, but in this case the muscle fibers are separated by fatty tissue instead of scar. Although paroxysmal, sustained VT associated with other forms of heart disease is considered reentrant, the mechanism of reentry and the role of abnormalities of conduction and/or refractoriness are only poorly understood.

The ability to identify a reentrant arrhythmia by programmed stimulation permits not only characterization of the mechanism but also identification of the site of origin and evaluation of potential therapy. Fortunately, most sustained VTs, particularly those with uniform morphology, are attributable to reentry and can therefore be treated in a systemic way on the basis of results obtained in an electrophysiology laboratory.

VI. ELECTROCARDIOGRAPHIC FEATURES

The diagnosis of VT can be made accurately on the basis of the electrocardiogram in more than 90% of cases (Figure 1). Ventricular tachycardia is usually associated with QRS complex duration exceeding 0.14 sec. Occasionally, the width may be as narrow as 110 msec (particularly in young patients). Rarely, it will be as broad as 200 msec in the absence of drugs. Other causes of wide QRS complexes, such as preexistent bundle block, rate related bundle branch block (i.e., aberrant conduction), and preexcitation must be excluded. For practical purposes, wide-complex tachycardias in patients with established structural heart disease will be VT 85% of the time regardless of hemodynamic status. Thus, one should assume that all wide-QRS-complex tachycardias are VTs until proven otherwise.

Other criteria that can help detect VT are atrioventricular (AV) dissociation, fusion complexes or capture beats (rare), and specific characteristics of QRS morphology in leads V_1, V_2, and V_6. Ventricular tachycardia attributable to myocardial disease is associated with slow evolution of initial QRS forces, regardless of the site of origin or underlying disease state. Slurring of initial forces of the QRS complex is seen regardless of whether the configuration is of the right or left bundle branch block type. QR complexes in the precordial leads are particularly common and relatively diagnostic for VT with coronary artery dis-

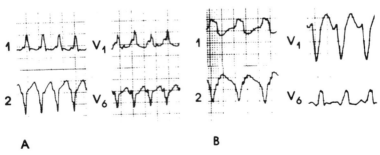

A   **B**

Figure 1 Electrocardiography in ventricular tachycardia. A and B show ventricular tachycardia with right bundle branch block and left bundle branch block configurations respectively. In A, during right bundle branch block tachycardia, AV dissociation is present, left axis is present, and RS ratio less than 1 in V_6 is seen. These are all characteristic of ventricular tachycardia. In B, during left bundle branch block tachycardia, a broad R wave equal to or exceeding 40 msec is seen in V_1, a delay from the onset of the QRS, delay in the S wave in V_1 exceeds 80 msec, and a broad Q wave is observed in lead V_6, all of which are diagnostic for ventricular tachycardia. (From Josephson ME, Tachyarrhythmias. Harrison's Principles of Internal Medicine. 12th ed. Wilson JD et al., eds. New York: McGraw-Hill, 1991.)

ease. Concordant positive or negative complexes have the same complication. In lead V_1, monophasic or biphasic R waves with the left peak greater than the right peak, or R.S < 1 in V_6, favors VT. When a left bundle branch block–like configuration is present, a broad initial R wave exceeding that seen in sinus rhythm, a notch of the downstroke of the S wave, or delay from the onset of QRS to the nadir of the S in leads V_1 or V_2 favors VT, as does a Q wave in V_6. The positive predictive value of the presence of these criteria exceeds 95% for left bundle branch block–like tachycardia. In the presence of preexisting bundle branch block and/or pharmacological agents, particularly those that block sodium channels, some of these morphological criteria become less predictive. In such instances, an electrophysiological study can provide a definitive diagnosis. Nonetheless, as long as one starts with the assumption that wide complex tachycardias are most often VTs, inappropriate therapy is less likely to be administered.

Polymorphic VT can occur in three varieties. The first is a tachycardia with multiple discrete QRS complexes separated by clear, isoelectric intervals. This is most commonly seen with nonsustained VT at relatively slow rates. Most polymorphic tachycardias have QRS morphologies that are difficult to distinguish as either positive or negative, with frequent changes, so that no more than three or four complexes in a row look even similar to one another. When the QRS complexes appear to be twisting around the baseline, the term "torsades de pointes" is frequently applied. This may be inappropriate, since the term should be reserved for a specific syndrome in which the VT is associated with an acquired long QT interval period.

VII. SPECIFIC TYPES OF VENTRICULAR TACHYCARDIA AND THERAPY

A. Ventricular Tachycardias Associated with Coronary Artery Disease

The initial therapy of sustained VT is similar regardless of underlying heart disease: DC cardioversion for tachycardias that produce severe cardiovascular symptoms or signs and pharmacological therapy with intravenous procainamide or antitachycardia pacing for those with ventricular arrhythmias that are well tolerated. Sustained VT associated with coronary artery disease frequently reflects previous myocardial infarction; nonsustained ventricular tachycardia does not. The exception is drug-induced VT (e.g., digitalis) or VT associated with an acquired long-QT syndrome, in which the offending agent must be discontinued and specific therapy initiated (see below).

Nonsustained VT may be paroxysmal with either uniform or polymorphic morphology (Figure 2). The incidence of nonsustained VT is difficult to ascertain because its rarity and high spontaneous variability. It can be observed in as many as 10% of patients within 2 weeks after acute myocardial infarction. However, the apparent incidence increases depending upon the extent of monitoring. With monthly 24-hr Holters, the likelihood of detection of at least one episode at the end of a year is equal to or greater than 50%.

The degree of myocardial dysfunction and extent of coronary disease are two factors that influence the frequency of occurrence of nonsustained VT. Although the rate, duration, and configuration (uniform or polymorphic) of non-sustained VT are believed by some to have prognostic implications, poor correlations between these characteristics and the incidence of subsequent sudden cardiac death have been found. Some have noted that the presence or absence of symptoms associated with nonsustained VT is not helpful in predicting risk of sudden cardiac death. One reason is the lack of relationship between nonsustained arrhythmias observed initially and subsequent sustained VT. In most instances, the nonsustained VT has a morphology different from that seen in the sustained VT. Accordingly, abolition of nonsustained arrhythmias may not confer protection against the occurrence of sustained arrhythmias.

One type of nonsustained VT seen with coronary disease and associated with a high incidence of death is the rapid polymorphic VT that typically occurs during the second week after extensive anterior infarction complicated by heart failure, particularly when ventricular aneurysm formation and right bundle branch block have supervened. Polymorphic VT of this type frequently leads to ventricu-

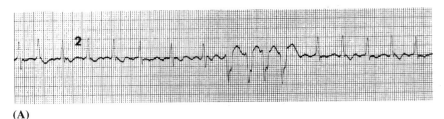

(A)

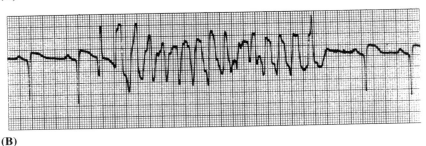

(B)

Figure 2 Sustained ventricular tachycardia. A: a four-beat run of uniform nonsustained ventricular tachycardia is shown during atrial fibrillation. Note the slight irregularity of the tachycardia. B: nonsustained polymorphic tachycardia in a patient with a prior myocardial infarction is shown. Note the early coupled initiating complex and the marked variability in the QRS morphology.

lar fibrillation and recurrent cardiac arrest. Cardiac surgery on an urgent basis is needed to improve outcome.

Therapy for Nonsustained Tachycardia

In some instances, nonsustained VT is an incidental electrocardiographic (ECG) finding in an asymptomatic patient. Routine efforts to suppress it are not warranted. Recent experience in the Cardiac Arrhythmia Suppression Trial (CAST) indicate that such efforts may, in fact, be deleterious and increase the risk of sudden death. If a patient is symptomatic with palpitations or syncope, antiarrhythmic therapy is justified. In general, the treatment chosen should be the simplest and safest possible sufficient to control symptoms. A documented relationship between the presence of the nonsustained arrhythmia and symptoms is essential. Long-term therapy for asymptomatic nonsustained VT remains of unproven value.

Patients with coronary artery disease who have nonsustained VT are at higher risk than those who do not; unfortunately, however, only because the arrhythmia is a marker of underlying heart disease. The percentage of patients dying suddenly among all who succumb (approximately 40–50%) is the same with or without nonsustained VT. The nonsustained VT simply identifies a subset of patients more likely to die but does not predict the mode of death. Patients with nonsustained VT, even if induced by exercise, with an ejection fraction equal to or greater than 40% appear to be at relatively low risk for sudden cardiac death. Even in the presence of multivessel disease, revascularization generally does not influence the incidence of the arrhythmias. Patients with nonsustained VT who have an ejection fraction below 40% are at a higher risk, which is compounded by the concomitant presence of an inducible sustained VT. the risk of sudden death in patients with both an ejection fraction below 40% and inducible, sustained uniform tachycardia approaches 30–50% over 2 years. The arrhythmia may thus be a target for therapy. Unfortunately, however, optimal management is unclear and is currently the subject of the Multicenter Unsustained Tachycardia Trial. It is not yet known whether antiarrhythmic agents, which may be proarrhythmic, can reduce mortality or whether they will cause increased mortality despite suppressing arrhythmia. Presently, it is prudent to avoid specific therapy in the management of nonsustained VT in order to prevent sudden cardiac death.

Sustained VT is attributable to reentry and may be either monomorphic or polymorphic (Figure 3). The type of arrhythmia, its morphology, and its cycle

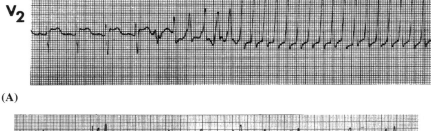

(A)

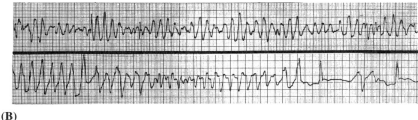

(B)

Figure 3 A sustained ventricular tachycardia in coronary artery disease. A: uniform sustained ventricular tachycardia. Note the tachycardia begins with a relatively late PVC, and once initiated and stabilized, remains uniform in morphology and regular in cycle length. B: Polymorphic tachycardia. Following the first sinus beat, two VPCs followed by a pause, and then another sinus complex. This is followed by a late PVC which initiates a tachycardia that has a continuously changing morphology. This polymorphic tachycardia frequently degenerates to ventricular fibrillation.

349

length depend upon the extent of slow conduction produced by previous infarction. Patients with well-tolerated tachycardias associated with coronary artery disease appear to have a significantly greater amount of myocardial scarring and abnormalities of endocardial activation (local and global) than do patients with nonsustained tachycardias or tachycardias that lead to cardiac arrest as demonstrated by endocardial mapping and body surface recordings. Signal averaged ECG exhibiting late high-frequency conduction abnormalities are seen in 85–90% of patients with inducible monomorphic ventricular tachycardia and previous infarction (Figure 4). Approximately 95% of patients with well-tolerated tachycardia exhibit replication of the clinical tachycardia with programmed stimulation (Figures 4, 5, and 6) and a standard stimulation protocol that includes up to three extrastimuli delivered to ventricular sites. Only 50% of patients with nonsustained VT and those resuscitated from cardiac arrest exhibit positive signal averaged ECGs.

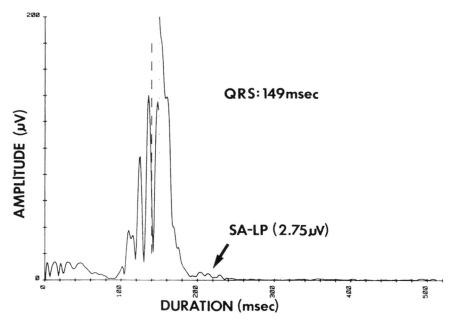

Figure 4   Signal-averaged ECG in a patient with ventricular tachycardia. An abnormal signal-averaged ECG is shown. The amplitude is shown in a vertical axis in microvolts and the duration is shown on the abcissa in milliseconds. The QRS duration of 149 exceeds the normal value of 120 msec. Note that the last 40 msec of the filtered QRS has a voltage of 2.75 μV and is called the signal-averaged late potential (SA = LP). Normal values for the last 40 msec are greater than 20 μV.

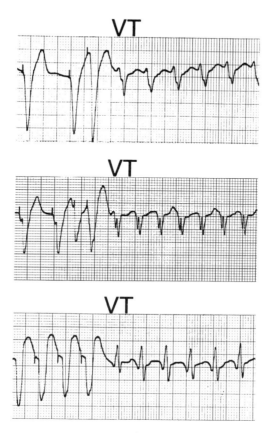

Figure 5 Initiation of ventricular tachycardia by programmed stimulation. Three panels are shown. From top to bottom, three different ventricular tachycardias are initiated by three different modalities. On top, a single extrastimulus delivered at a paced cycle length of 660 msec initiates ventricular tachycardia. In the middle panel, two closely coupled ventricular extrastimuli delivered at a drive cycle length of 500 msec initiate ventricular tachycardia, and in the lower panel, straight ventricular pacing at a cycle length of 375 msec initiates ventricular tachycardia.

Polymorphic tachycardia in patients with coronary artery disease can be mediated by at least two disparate mechanisms. One can be described as an insufficient substrate, in which the extent of endocardial abnormalities of propagation of impulse is less severe than that seen in uniform, well-tolerated VT. In such patients the reentry is so rapid that the rest of the ventricle cannot be captured electrophysiologically in a uniform and repetitive fashion. Accordingly, poly-

351

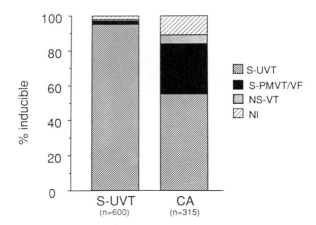

Figure 6 Inducibility of ventricular tachycardia associated with coronary artery disease. The percent of tachycardias that are inducible and types of ventricular tachycardia that are inducible in patients with sustained uniform ventricular tachycardia (S-UVT) and those presenting with cardiac arrest (CA) are shown in vertical bars. The types of inducible arrhythmias include sustained, uniform ventricular (S-UVT), sustained polymorphic ventricular tachycardia/ventricular fibrillation (S-PMVT/VF), nonsustained ventricular tachycardia (NS-VT), and no inducible ventricular tachycardia (NI-VT). In patients presenting with S-UVT, 96% can have the tachycardia replicated by programmed stimulation. In patients presenting with CA, 56% have an S-UVT inducible and 27% have S-PMVT/VF inducible. (From Josephson, ME, Clinical cardiac electrophysiology, 2d edition, with permission.)

morphic tachycardia results that can degenerate into ventricular fibrillation (VF). Frequently, drugs that slow conduction (Class IA, IC, amiodarone) can modify the arrhythmia such that it becomes a uniform tachycardia (Figure 7). The phenomenon of modification is diagnostic of reentry with insufficient substrate.

A second mechanism is acute ischemia. In this case no true anatomic substrate exists, but the polymorphic tachycardia occurs only with ischemia inducing functional derangements in conduction. Severe multivessel disease (usually without previous infarction) is present. Programmed stimulation rarely yields reproducible arrhythmia, although occasionally polymorphic VT/VF may be initiated. Revascularization is required to prevent recurrence, in sharp contrast to the case when an anatomic substrate is present that can be the target for therapy along with prevention or relief of ischemia. Electrophysiologic evaluation and cardiac catheterization are needed to define the actual mechanism responsible for such an arrhythmia so that appropriate therapy can be selected.

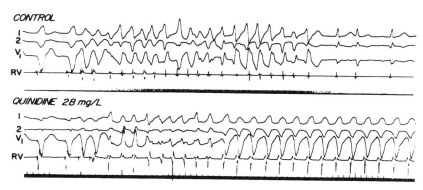

Figure 7 Change of polymorphic ventricular tachycardia to uniform ventricular tachycardia by drugs. Both panels are organized from top to bottom with surface leads I, II, and V_1, and intracardiac electrograms from the right ventricle (RV). In a control state, two ventricular extrastimuli induced a nonsustained polymorphic ventricular tachycardia. Following oral quinidine achieving a blood level of 2.8 mg/L, double extrastimuli initiate a uniform tachycardia with a left bundle left axis morphology. Note the onset of this tachycardia begins with a somewhat polymorphic VT which then stabilizes to a uniform morphology.

Electrocardiographic Features

The morphology of uniform (monomorphic) VT on the 12-lead ECG can provide information identifying the site of infarction and the site of origin of the arrhythmia. Ventricular tachycardia with left or right bundle branch block morphology can be seen in patients with anterior or inferior infarctions. Left bundle branch block tachycardias arise on or adjacent to the interventricular septum. In the case of inferior infarction, propagation proceeds from base to apex. This gives rise to R waves across the precordium in both left and right bundle branch block tachycardias. Positive concordance in precordial leads is always associated with a posterior origin of the arrhythmia. With anterior infarction, left bundle branch block tachycardias can arise on or adjacent to the septum, but apically in the region of infarction. Accordingly, the ECG forces are directed toward the viable, posterior myocardium, producing Q waves in the anterior leads. Negative precordial concordance may thus be observed in left bundle branch block–like tachycardias associated with anterior infarction.

When right bundle branch block tachycardias are associated with anterior infarction, Q waves appear early (V_1 or V_2) and often persist throughout the precordial leads. Because left bundle branch block tachycardias arise on or adjacent to the septum, they are easier to localize with a 12-lead ECG. Right bundle branch block tachycardias can arise from the septum or the free wall and are more difficult to localize. Atrioventricular dissociation is the rule in VT, although 1:1 VA conduction may be present and should not dissuade one from the diagnosis of VT. Nor should hemodynamic status. Patients with apparent VT may present in an emergency room with palpitations, stable blood pressure, and 1:1 VA conduction. A history of myocardial infarction should always make one assume that VT is present.

The clinical significance of sustained monomorphic VT is related to the circumstances in which it occurs. If tachycardia occurs early after infarction, the prognosis is ominous, particularly with anterior infarction. High early mortality resulting from recurrent heart attack, pump failure, and sudden cardiac death are likely. In patients who first develop tachycardia later, the prognosis is less ominous. The first episode of VT frequently occurs in the first year following infarction (median approximately 1 year). However, VT develops in 1–3% of patients per year. It is not unusual to see patients presenting with sustained monomorphic tachycardia 10, 20, and 30 years after a remote infarction.

The extent of coronary artery disease and depression of left ventricular function are the primary determinants of outcome. Patients with a very low ejection fraction but a single, occluded left anterior descending (LAD) lesion who present with a tolerated VT have a relatively good prognosis, and are unlikely to die suddenly. In contrast, patients with an ejection fraction that is less severely depressed (~ 30%) who have triple vessel disease have a significantly higher incidence of recurrence and sudden death. The choice and intensity of therapy depends on risk stratification.

Therapy for Sustained Ventricular Tachycardia

Patients with sustained uniform tachycardia can present with symptoms that are minimal, with cardiac arrest, and with signs and symptoms between these extremes. Treatment of cardiac arrest is considered in Chapter 20. Treatment of patients with palpitations, shortness of breath, increased heart failure, or chest pain requires termination of the arrhythmia and prevention of recurrence that can require repeat hospitalization, lead to debilitating heart failure, or result in sudden death (occurring 5–50% over 4 years), depending upon the extent of the coronary artery disease and the severity of impairment of myocardial function. It is usually not clear what triggers a recurrence of sustained VT in a particular case, although electrolyte imbalance, sympathetic discharge, heart failure, or ischemia are all capable of doing so.

Therapy of Monomorphic Ventricular Tachycardia

If a patient with monomorphic tachycardia is hemodynamically stable, intravenous pharmacological therapy can be initiated. The drug of choice is procainamide, with a total loading dose of 15 mg/kg to be infused at a rate of 25 to 50 mg/min under close supervision, to be slowed if the blood pressure falls more than

20 mmHg, or below an absolute value of 80 mmHg. Lidocaine, frequently the first drug employed, is only rarely successful in terminating uniform tachycardia associated with previous myocardial infarction. Although lidocaine is effective in terminating arrhythmias in which ischemia plays a prominent role in the underlying substrate, procainamide is five times more likely to be effective when the substrate of ischemia is absent, because the arrhythmia is usually caused by slow conduction produced by poorly coupled fibers rather than being due to inactivated sodium channels, as is the case with ischemia. Approximately 80–85% of patients with tolerated VT experience termination of the rhythm with intravenous procainamide infusion.

If a patient is acutely symptomatic with chest pain or heart failure, the patient should be treated by DC cardioversion. A synchronized shock should be delivered of at least 50 J, even though lower energies can sometimes convert VT to sinus rhythm. The reason for not using 1–25 J is that a higher incidence of acceleration of tachycardia and induction of VT can occur. Thus, the safest approach is with 50 to 100 J of energy.

Midazolam for conscious sedation or propafol for brief anesthesia are agents of choice when electrical cardioversion is to be implemented. An alternative mode of treatment for stable VT, particularly if the patient has eaten recently, is termination of the rhythm by overdrive pacing. This should be done by an electrophysiologist with expertise in catheter placement and with the use of a programmable stimulator.

Long-term treatment to prevent recurrences of VT and decrease the incidence of sudden death includes antiarrhythmic drugs, implantable cardioverter defibrillators, or ablation of the arrhythmogenic substrate by catheter-delivered energy or surgery. If pharmacological antiarrhythmic therapy is utilized, electrophysiologically guided use of antiarrhythmic agents is preferred. Although recent data from the ESVEM (Electrophysiologic Study Versus Electrocardiographic Monitoring) have suggested that Holter monitoring and electrophysiological testing methods are comparably effective, only 25–30% of patients with sustained VT exhibit a sufficient amount of spontaneous ventricular ectopic activity to permit delineation of efficacy of a specific agent. Furthermore, the CAST study demonstrated that abolition of ventricular arrhythmias detectable by Holter monitoring does not prevent sudden cardiac death. The ability to reliably initiate VT with standard electrophysiological protocols in up to 95% of patients favors the use of programmed stimulation as a method of choice to guide the selection of drug therapy. Additional advantages are that the mechanism of VT, the origin of VT, the potential for ablation, and the potential for an antitachycardia pacer to manage VT can be assessed.

Two endpoints are ascertained with electrophysiological testing relative to pharmacological therapy. The ideal endpoint is to find a drug that renders the tachycardia noninducible. This may take several trials of different antiarrhythmic

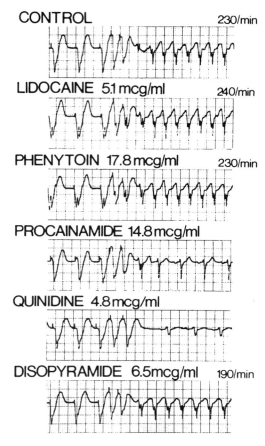

CONTROL 230/min

LIDOCAINE 5.1 mcg/ml 240/min

PHENYTOIN 17.8 mcg/ml 230/min

PROCAINAMIDE 14.8 mcg/ml

QUINIDINE 4.8 mcg/ml

DISOPYRAMIDE 6.5mcg/ml 190/min

Figure 8 Use of programmed stimulation to evaluate pharmacological therapy of ventricular tachycardia. The effect of a variety of antiarrhythmic agents on the ability to induce ventricular tachycardia is shown. In the control panel, two ventricular extrastimuli initiate a rapid uniform ventricular tachycardia. Lidocaine, phenytoin, tocainide, quinidine, and disopyramide are tested over a period of time. Note that lidocaine and phenytoin have virtually no effect on the tachycardia, while disopyramide slows the tachycardia. Procainamide and quinidine both prevent initiation of the tachycardia. Prevention of inducible ventricular tachycardia is associated with absence from recurrence. See text for discussion. (From Kastor et al: N Engl J Med 1981; 304:1004, with permission.)

agents (Figure 8). In general, if procainamide or another class IA agent fails to prevent initiation of VT, it is unlikely that any other sodium channel blocking drug will be successful. Thus, the sequence of serial drug trials should probably begin with a class IA agent, and if this fails, sotalol should be tried. Failure of sotalol can be followed by testing a combination of class IA and IB agents and/or amiodarone. Although it has been suggested that amiodarone can be given simply empirically, the response of tachycardias to amiodarone is unpredictable.

A second and acceptable endpoint is slowing of the tachycardia in order to render it better tolerated hemodynamically, such that if VT recurs, it will be less likely to compromise circulatory dynamics. The hemodynamic response to a drug can be assessed only by electrophysiological study as opposed to Holter monitoring.

Sodium channel blocking agents (class IA or IC) are the most effective in slowing a VT. Amiodarone, which has multiple ion channel effects, slows VT as well, but less predictably. The combinations of class IA agents and amiodarone are additive. The class IC agents are used less often because of the relatively high incidence of depression of myocardial contractility and a potential increase in heart failure produced by these drugs.

All of the class IA and IC agents are potentially proarrhythmic and can produce either incessant tachycardias or torsades de pointes. The incidence of proarrhythmia varies from 1–10% and is highest in those with overt congestive heart failure and low ejection fractions. Amiodarone has the lowest profile of proarrhythmia (~ 1%). Sotalol is prone to induce torsades de pontes because it prolongs the QT interval.

If VT is rendered noninducible, the incidence of recurrence over 2 years is 10–20%. If VT remains inducible, the rate is 50%. Of note, there is a good relationship between the tolerance of the tachycardia observed in the laboratory and that seen with a recurrence. If both noninducibility and improved tolerance of the tachycardia are considered desirable endpoints. A success rate for selecting therapy by electrophysiological testing of 50–60% is attainable.

Amiodarone is the one agent about which controversy persists regarding electrophysiological testing. Because the time for loading is so long, an accurate assessment of its long-term efficacy may not be provided even after 7 days of a loading dose. Although noninducibility of the arrhythmia seems to predict lack of recurrence with amiodarone, the incidence of noninducibility is only 10–15%. However, in most of the remaining patients, the tachycardia is significantly slowed. Thus, tolerance to the slowed tachycardia can be evaluated by electrophysiological study.

Because most reentrant VT can be terminated by a variety of pacing modalities, the use of an implantable antitachycardia pacer with defibrillator backup is an alternative form of therapy. The success in terminating VT by pacing is closely related to the VT rate. The slower the tachycardia, the more likely it can be terminated by pacing. The more rapid the rate of the arrhythmia, the more likely is

357

acceleration of the arrhythmia to ventricular flutter or induction of fibrillation by pacing. Thus, pacing must be performed with a device with defibrillation backup. At least two are currently available that have antitachycardia pacing and defibrillation capability. Implantation via a nonthoractomy lead system is possible. Such devices must be employed by electrophysiological specialists who can define the best mode of antitachycardia pacing termination and the lowest energy DC cardioversion required for optimal efficacy in a given patients. The devices are highly programmable and have a multitude of detection algorithms and therapeutic options. In some patients the use of an antiarrhythmic agent facilitates termination of the tachycardia by pacing and obviates the need for DC shocks that may be required in up to 50% of tachycardias with rates in excess of 200 beats/min.

An example of the efficacy of antitachycardia pacing with an implantable cardioverter/defibrillator (ICD) is shown in Figure 9. Because of the cost and invasiveness of the ICD, it is generally reserved for patients with tachycardias that produce significant symptoms (particularly those with > 200 beats/min) or those with recurrent VT despite the use of pharmacological agents that lead to multiple hospitalizations for elective external DC cardioversion. The role of the ICD in the

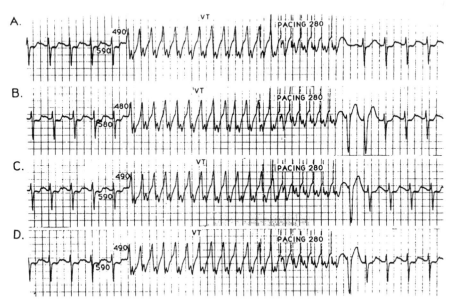

Figure 9 Termination of ventricular tachycardia by an ICD. A through D are lead-II rhythm strips. Ventricular tachycardia spontaneously occurs in all three panels and on each occasion the tachycardia is sensed and a burst of pacing at 280 msec reproducibly terminates the tachycardia.

future will depend on long-term outcome and cost-effectiveness analyses. However, prevention of recurrent hospitalization and the brevity of hospitalization required for implantation are promising.

Ablation of the arrhythmogenic substrate for sustained uniform tachycardia is the ideal option since it is curative. However, catheter ablation techniques are still in early evolution, although successful ablation can already be observed in nearly 50% of well-tolerated VT. This procedure is difficult and requires expertise in ventricular mapping. Changes in catheter design and energy delivery may increase the utility of this form of therapy in the near future. Surgical ablation is curative, rendering patients free of recurrences in more than 90% of cases over 5 years with less than a 3% incidence of sudden cardiac death. This remarkably favorable experience, however, carries with it a 5–15% operative mortality. Although the use of ICDs is associated with lower operative mortality and has largely replaced surgery, particularly in patients with low ejection fractions, surgery should be considered particularly for those with ventricular aneurysms, because ventricular function, tachycardia, and coronary artery disease can be addressed simultaneously.

Therapy of Polymorphic Tachycardia

Sustained polymorphic tachycardias invariably present with cardiac arrest or syncope. Specific treatment is discussed in Chapter 20, on cardiac arrest. Treatment and clinical significance depend on whether or not acute ischemia is the cause of the arrhythmia, as opposed to insufficient electrophysiologic substrate. Patients in whom a pathophysiological substrate or scar tissue underlies the arrhythmia require therapy directed toward that substrate in addition to treatment to correct ischemia if present. In those in whom ejection fraction is normal and where ischemia plays a primary role, therapy should be directed toward correcting ischemia by revascularization. A specific subset of patients requiring consideration is the group with polymorphic VT following large anteroseptal infarction. Extensive anterior wall damage, ejection fraction less than 35%, congestive heart failure, and right bundle branch block are often present. Prognosis is poor, with a 50–70% mortality rate in 1 year after infarction. Death is sudden in 50% of those who succumb. Revascularization, aneurysmectomy, and arrhythmia surgery provide the best long-term outlook. Unfortunately, polymorphic tachycardias cannot be mapped, and nonmapped attempts to destroy arrhythmogenic substrates must be employed. Often, however, the polymorphic tachycardia can be made uniform with the use of class I antiarrhythmic agents and the uniform tachycardia can be mapped, in which case map-guided therapy can be undertaken with remarkably good success.

Thus, therapy of sustained VT is necessary and best guided by electrophysiological testing to confirm the diagnosis, define the site of origin, elucidate the underlying substrate, and select therapy most objectively.

B. Ventricular Tachycardia Associated with Cardiomyopathy

Ventricular tachyarrhythmias are common in all forms of cardiomyopathy. Nonsustained VT is present in at least 50% of the patients with idiopathic dilated cardiomyopathy. It occurs often but somewhat less frequently in hypertrophic cardiomyopathy. As an isolated finding, however, the presence of nonsustained VT does not appear to predict the mode of death in patients who will succumb. In general, no form of treatment has been shown to improve survival. Thus, asymptomatic nonsustained VT associated with cardiomyopathic states should not presently be treated.

An exception may be patients with hypertrophic cardiomyopathy with nonsustained VT and syncope or near syncope and inducible sustained tachyarrhythmias who are at high risk for sudden death, especially if they have a family history of the disorder. In such patients, beta blockers or calcium channel blockers plus an ICD or surgery may be justified. Prospective studies, however, are needed to provide criteria for identifying those at highest risk for sudden death and to demonstrate efficacy of prevention.

Although sustained uniform VT is seen with diverse primary myocardial disorders, uniform VT is most closely associated with idiopathic dilated cardiomyopathy and arrhythmogenic right ventricular dysplasia. Most other cardiomyopathies present with cardiac arrest, which can be precipitated by a rapid monomorphic tachycardia or, more frequently, by polymorphic VT, degenerating to ventricular fibrillation (see Chapter 20, on cardiac arrest).

Uniform, sustained monomorphic VT in dilated cardiomyopathies can result from two different basic mechanisms. The first is a typical reentrant mechanism in which the reentrant circuit is presumed to be intramural myocardium. Such circuits may arise anywhere in the left or right ventricle but occur frequently in the interventricular septum. The morphological characteristics of the tachycardia depend on its site of origin. As with coronary artery disease, when tachycardias arise within the interventricular septum, left bundle branch block tachycardias are possible. Localization of a tachycardia on the basis of QRS morphology seems to be more accurate in such patients than in patients with coronary artery disease because of less distortion of propagation of impulses by scar tissue and hence closer correlation between QRS morphology and the site of origin of the tachycardia. In most cases the spontaneous VT can be replicated by an induced programmed stimulation, although this may, perhaps, be less reproducible than it is in patients with coronary disease. However, there is currently no proof that antiarrhythmic drug therapy guided by electrophysiological studies in idiopathic cardiomyopathies or those associated with a known pathogen elicits predictable long-term benefit. Because the patients are at high risk for sudden death, an ICD should be used. Drugs that slow the tachycardia may be useful in facilitating termination by the antitachycardia pacing function of the ICD, but the efficacy of antiarrhythmic therapy alone in the management of VT is unproven. Even when pharmacological agents have prevented inducibility of VT, sudden death has often occurred. Although the ICD can prevent deaths from ventricular fibrillation, 3- to 5-year mortality remains high (50%). Empiric use of amiodarone has been suggested as the best mode of therapy for such patients, but its overall benefit is uncertain. Cardiac transplantation is an alternative, particularly for young patients who suffer from heart failure as well as the arrhythmia.

Another form of VT associated with cardiomyopathies, particularly dilated cardiomyopathies, is bundle branch reentry. It usually occurs in patients who have preexisting conduction disturbances, usually with incomplete left bundle branch block or apparent left bundle branch block morphology associated with sinus rhythm. Such patients usually have idiopathic dilated cardiomyopathy, but they may have myopathic ventricles as a result of hypertensive or valvular heart disease. In such cases, a reentrant arrhythmia that utilizes the bundle branches can produce a rapid, uniform VT. If the tachycardia circuit uses the right bundle branch in the antegrade limb and the left bundle branch in the retrograde limb, it will exhibit left bundle branch block and left axis deviation morphology and will resemble aberration with rapid initial forces because ventricular activation proceeds through the right bundle branch. Such a tachycardia will therefore exhibit the characteristics of left bundle branch block aberration in which the impulse proceeds down the right bundle branch in activating the ventricles. Bundle branch reentrant VT is readily inducible by right ventricular stimulation.

Rarely, the reentrant circuit may be reversed and antegrade conduction may proceed over one of the major limbs of the left bundle branch, with retrograde conduction over the right bundle branch or another limb of the left bundle branch. In such cases, the morphology will resemble that seen with aberrant conduction of one of the fascicles of the left ventricle.

Bundle branch reentrant tachycardia with the left bundle branch block morphology is impossible to distinguish from rapid SVT with left bundle branch block aberration except for presence of AV dissociation, usually observed with bundle branch reentry. Antiarrhythmic therapy guided by electrophysiological testing can be used to treat bundle branch reentry, with class IA agents and amiodarone usually the agent of choice. Class IC agents and sotalol often cannot be utilized because of the poor left ventricular function already present. Catheter ablation may be effective because destruction of one of the bundle branches will prohibit completion of the reentrant circuit. Ablation of either the right bundle branch or the proximal left bundle branch can be employed. Two factors should be considered that limit the efficacy of ablation as sole treatment. First, abolition of the right bundle branch system exposes an already diseased left ventricular conducting system as an Achilles' heel. Permanent pacing may therefore be necessary, particularly if antiarrhythmic agents are required to treat other arrhythmias (e.g., atrial fibrillation) often present as well. Second, in at least 50–60% of patients additional myocardial VT are present. Because ablation of these arrhythmias is not possible at this time and drug therapy is often unreliable, the use of an ICD in such patients seems most appropriate. Catheter ablation to eliminate bundle branch reentry may decrease the incidence of bundle branch reentry and prevent the possibility of the device initiating bundle branch reentry when it is targeting another arrhythmia. Thus, the ablative procedure may be a useful adjunct.

One form of cardiomyopathy that requires specific treatment for arrhythmias is arrhythmogenic right ventricular dysplasia. This is a primary myopathy generally involving only the right ventricle. Occasionally the left ventricle may be involved as well. The free wall of the right ventricle is diffusely diseased, with myocardium replaced by fatty infiltration and some fibrous tissue, in contrast to a scar after myocardial infarction, in which little fat is seen. The three areas of right ventricular dysplasia seen typically include outflow tract, the apex, and the base near the tricuspid valve. In all cases, free wall is the site primarily involved. The disorder, which usually present in patients with VT between 20 and 40 years of age, can be best diagnosed by cardiac magnetic resonance imaging. The typical ECG shows T-wave inversion in the right precordial leads and delayed activation, (epsilon waves) on the surface ECG (Figure 10). The late potentials (epsilon waves) are more readily seen on a signal-averaged ECG (Figure 11), an important diagnostic procedure when this disorder is being considered.

Arrhythmogenic right ventricular dysplasia should be suspected in any young patient without apparent ventricular dysfunction who presents with VT having a left bundle branch block morphology with a superior or a normal axis or with multiple VTs having a left bundle branch block morphology. The presence of left bundle branch block tachycardia of any morphology and a positive signal-averaged ECG should suggest right ventricular dysplasia as well. In its early stages, the tachycardia may be provoked by exercise. Later initiation occurs more often and spontaneously. Extensive fatty infiltration produces markedly slowed conduction, which underlies the reentrant arrhythmias.

Right ventricular dysplasia can be hereditary but is generally sporadic. It may account for some episodes of sudden death in athletes. In the electrophysiology laboratory, the arrhythmia can be initiated reliably and terminated by programmed stimulation. Endocardial mapping of the free wall of the right ventricle shows extensive abnormalities of slow conduction that correlate well with the signal-averaged ECG.

Therapy includes antiarrhythmic drugs, surgery, ICDs, and catheter ablation. Drugs should be selected on the basis of programmed stimulation, but their efficacy declines as the disease progresses. Sotalol and amiodarone appear to be the best agents for prevention of VT and sudden death. In those patients with

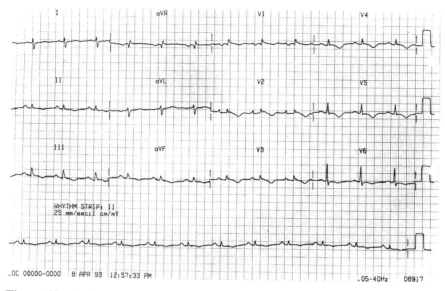

Figure 10   Arrhythmogenic right ventricular dysplasia. A typical ECG in a patient with arrhythmogenic right ventricular dysplasia is shown. Incomplete right bundle block with T-wave inversion in the right precordial leads is obvious. In addition seen best in lead V_2 are terminal deflections called epsilon waves, which represent late activation over the dysplastic right ventricle.

recurrent VT despite antiarrhythmic drugs, surgical or catheter ablation or an ICD can be employed.

Catheter ablation, first developed with the use of DC shocks, was initially abandoned because of rupture of the thin-walled right ventricle. Radiofrequency ablation, a modification that is effective and safer, is helpful in selected patients with single tachycardia. Unfortunately, the extensive arrhythmogenic substrate makes catheter ablation techniques unsuitable for those with multiple arrhythmias. Surgery is occasionally used but is a massive undertaking that involves disarticulating the free wall of the right ventricle from the remainder of the heart and then reattaching it. Although the tachycardia may persist in the isolated right ventricle, the remainder of the heart is brought under the control of the sinus node. The procedure is effective but morbidity is high. Attempts at more localized ventriculotomies have been less successful. Because of the high surgical morbidity, ICDs are used in patients with arrhythmias that recur despite antiarrhythmic therapy. As in the treatment of patients with sustained monomorphic

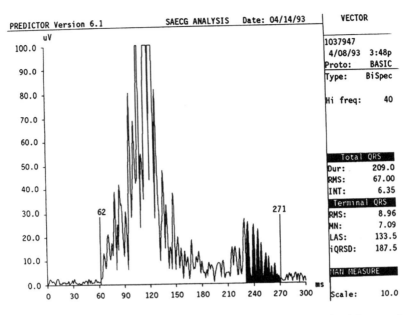

Figure 11 Signal-averaged ECG in a patient with arrythmogenic right ventricular dysplasia and recurrent ventricular tachycardia. The duration of the filtered QRS is 209 msec (normal ≤120 msec), root mean square voltage of the terminal 40 msec of the QRS of 8.96 μV (normal >20 μV) and the duration of the terminal voltage below 40 μV is 133.5 msec (normal <38 msec). Marked delayed activation is a hallmark of right ventricular dysplasia.

tachycardia and coronary disease, the ICDs are used primarily as antitachycardia pacemakers with defibrillator backup. The latter is especially important in young patients who have exercise-induced VT and who are at high risk of sudden death.

C. Ventricular Tachycardia in Patients Without Overt Organic Heart Disease

Occasionally patients without overt organic heart disease have VT. Nonsustained VT is rare; when it does occur, it is usually asymptomatic and does not require treatment. One form, however, known as repetitive monomorphic tachycardia, is characterized by frequent runs of monomorphic VT, typically with left bundle branch block inferior axis morphology (Figure 12). The runs can be nearly incessant and can disappear for prolonged periods of time. More often than not, they are present during the daytime and exacerbated by exercise. Sleep and the recumbent position often result in their cessation. Vagal maneuvers, beta blockers,

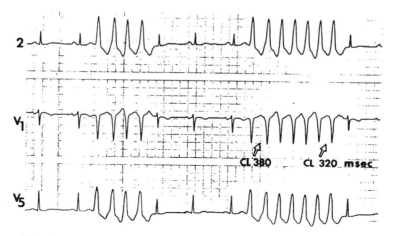

Figure 12 Repetitive monomorphic tachycardia. Leads II, V_1, and V_5 are shown. Repetitive bouts of nonsustained ventricular tachycardia have a left bundle branch block, inferior axis morphology. Note, the smooth upstroke of these complexes and gradual acceleration followed by termination of the arrhythmia. See text for discussion.

and adenosine can temporarily stop these arrhythmias, which are increased not only by exercise but also by infusion of isoproterenol. The natural history of this arrhythmia is relatively benign, although in rare cases incessant tachycardias can lead to dilatation of the right ventricle (just as prolonged rapid pacing can elicit heart failure after cessation of exogenous stimulation in laboratory animals). When they are symptomatic, the arrhythmias should be treated with beta blockers, calcium blockers, or occasionally sotalol.

A related arrhythmia is sustained monomorphic tachycardia that arises from the right ventricular outflow tract in the absence of overt organic heart disease. Instead of repetitive, brief episodes of nonsustained VT, affected patients have occasional VPCs and episodes of nonsustained VT that are punctuated by sustained episodes of VT that are exercise-related. The ECG in the absence of tachycardia and results of noninvasive and invasive evaluations show entirely normal ventricles and coronary arteries. QRS morphology during tachycardia is left bundle and either right or left inferior axis. Although the tachycardias arise in the outflow tract of the right ventricle, anatomic abnormalities are not evident. Exercise provokes the arrhythmia and, not uncommonly, isoproterenol can induce it as well. In the electrophysiology laboratory, programmed stimulation or rapid pacing can only infrequently initiate the arrhythmia but can often alter facilitation by isoproterenol (Figure 13). Long-term prognosis is good.

In contrast to the case of right ventricular dysplasia, endocardial mapping

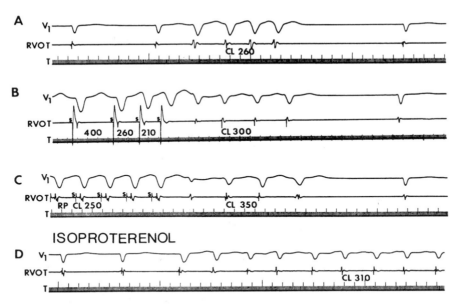

Figure 13   Right ventricular outflow tract tachycardia. Panels are arranged as V_1 and an electrogram from the RV outflow tract (RVOT), and time line (T). During sinus rhythm, spontaneous nonsustained ventricular tachycardia is seen (A). Programmed stimulation (B) and rapid pacing (C) produce only nonsustained ventricular tachycardia. Following Isoproterenol, sustained ventricular tachycardia occurs spontaneously.

and signal-averaged ECGs show no abnormalities. Both this sustained arrhythmia and repetitive monomorphic nonsustained VT can be terminated by vagal maneuvers, calcium channel blockers, beta blockers, and adenosine, suggesting that the mechanism underlying them is catecholamine-induced, adenyl cyclase–mediated triggered activity.

Initial treatment of this left bundle branch block inferior axis tachycardia requires recognition of its mechanism. Carotid sinus pressure can occasionally terminate the arrhythmia and therefore should be performed first. If the tachycardia is known to be ventricular and is arising from the right ventricular outflow tract in an otherwise normal person, a drug that has prompt onset and a short duration of action that can terminate the arrhythmia is adenosine. It should be given as a 6- to 12-mg bolus IV. If it fails to terminate the arrhythmia, intravenous verapamil usually does. Long-term management of this arrhythmia can involve either drugs or catheter ablation. The drugs that are most effective are beta blockers or sotalol (a beta blocker with class III properties); the latter is often better tolerated than other beta blockers, which frequently have to be used in very high doses often in combination with calcium channel blockers. With recent advances in catheter ablation, it is now used widely. Many of the patients affected are young and do not elect long-term antiarrhythmic drug therapy. Potential cure by catheter ablation may make it a first-line option. Map-guided catheter ablation can successfully prevent recurrence in 90% of affected patient.s Long-term effects of radiofrequency ablation have yet to be elucidated definitively, although they are expected to be modest.

Another tachycardia seen in patients without overt organic heart disease is one with a classic right bundle branch block pattern that arises in the left ventricle. It occurs frequently in young men and is not typically exercise-related. The QRS morphology shows a right bundle branch block pattern with a relatively narrow duration (between 0.12 and 0.14 sec) and a left or right superior axis. The signal-averaged ECG is normal. Transesophageal echocardiography may show one or more muscular bands connecting the region of the posterior papillary muscle to the adjacent interventricular septum (seen in as many as 90% of patients). The region appears to be the site of origin of the tachycardia. The most common presentation is sudden onset of palpitations with few or no other symptoms. Prognosis is generally excellent except for the need for recurrent admissions for treatment of episodes. In the electrophysiology laboratory, tachycardia can be reproducibly initiated by programmed stimulation, suggesting a reentrant mechanism. Unlike the left bundle branch block normal axis tachycardia described above, this tachycardia cannot be terminated by beta blockers or adenosine; however, it is terminated reliably by verapamil or procainamide. The explanation for the response to verapamil is not clear but may reflect part of the conducting system being involved.

Initial therapy is intravenous verapamil, to which almost 100% of the patients are responsive. Intravenous procainamide is an alternative. For long-term suppression, oral verapamil and a variety of other agents (class IA and IC drugs, sotalol, and amiodarone) can be used. This choice is best made by demonstrating prevention of inducibility by programmed stimulation. Catheter ablation has been employed as well.

The tachycardia appears to arise from the midseptum, at the junction of the septum and the papillary muscle, or in the inferior papillary muscle itself. Ablation guided by mapping procedures currently undergoing rapid evolution is successful in 75–80% of affected patients. Although the risk is less than 1%, rare acute complications of radiofrequency ablation, such as tamponade or embolization, must be considered and sometimes require emergency interventions during performance of the procedure.

D. Polymorphic Ventricular Tachycardia Associated with Long QT Intervals

Polymorphic tachycardia associated with long-QT intervals may be acquired or congenital. Here we consider the polymorphic tachycardias associated with the prolonged-QT syndrome in contrast to polymorphic VT associated with coronary artery disease, which usually is associated with normal QT intervals when sinus rhythm prevails (Figure 13). Torsades de pointes was initially described as a polymorphic tachycardia associated with a long-QT interval with sinus rhythm often associated with transient phenomena including use of antiarrhythmic agents such as quinidine; electrolyte imbalance, specifically hypokalemia; and brady-arrhythmias. Following its initial description three decades ago, the lists of anti-arrhythmic agents and conditions that can induce this disorder has become exten-sive. Any antiarrhythmic agent that can affect potassium channels can be responsible, most commonly quinidine, disopyramide, procainamide (particularly *N*-acetyl procainamide), sotalol, bepridil, and amiodarone (Figure 14). The inci-dence of induction of torsades is probably highest with quinidine, with which it appears as an idiosyncratic non-dose-related reaction, and with sotalol, as a dose-related phenomenon. With doses of sotalol exceeding 320 mg a day the incidence of torsades de pointes may exceed 5%, slightly higher than that seen with qui-nidine. With quinidine-induced torsades de pointes, the arrhythmia is seen fre-quently after conversion of atrial fibrillation to sinus rhythm in a patient with heart failure who is taking digitalis as well, especially in women. Some 50% of episodes occur in the first 3 days after initiation of drug therapy. Whether or not digitalis is actually involved in the genesis of the arrhythmia is unknown.

Phenothiazines, tricyclic antidepressants, antihistamines (e.g., Seldane), anti-fungals (e.g., ketoconazole), liquid protein diets, and many other agents can cause the problem. It is now apparent that this rhythm is a major cause of sudden death in people with heart block (Stokes-Adams syndrome) and that pacemaker implanta-tion may not only prevent congestive heart failure, light-headedness, and syncope but also prevent sudden death otherwise resulting from bradycardia-dependent torsades de pointes.

The mechanism underlying this arrhythmia is believed to be triggered activity attributable to early afterdepolarizations associated with action potential prolongation facilitated, in turn, by bradycardia rhythms. Potassium channel

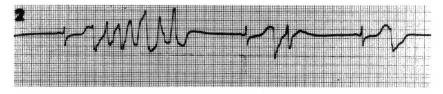

Figure 14 Torsades de pointes. Lead II is shown. Following a sinus complex, nonsus-tained polymorphic ventricular tachycardia is observed. The QT interval of this sinus complex and other sinus complexes exceed 600 msec in response to quinidine.

blocking drugs as well as antihistamines and phenothiazines produce QT prolongation that reflects action potential prolongation and associated with early afterdepolarizations or calcium transients probably mediated through the L-type calcium channel. The initiating sequence is typical: the patient with a long QT interval initially develops VPCs that produce pauses, followed by sinus rhythm and more VPCs. The short-long-short sequence facilitates further prolongation of the QT interval, with development of giant U waves and the initiation of torsades de pointes (Figure 14). The arrhythmia may be responsible for nearly 20% of the sudden deaths seen in patients being treated for VTs. It is often an iatrogenic condition that can be prevented.

The treatment of torsades de pointes involves cessation of the causative drug, correction of the electrolyte imbalance, or treatment of the bradyarrhythmia. If the arrhythmia is diagnosed appropriately, class IA agents or other agents can and should be avoided. Initial treatment should be bolus administration of magnesium sulfate, 2 g delivered over 1 to 2 min, repeated every 5 to 10 min until hypotension occurs or the arrhythmia stops. Isoproterenol or pacing to increase heart rate are alternatives. Potassium should be given to induce slightly hyperkalemic to shorten action potential duration. Once the acute episode has been interrupted, prevention of subsequent episodes is of paramount importance. Insertion of a pacemaker to maintain adequately high heart rates—with atrial pacing being preferred over ventricular pacing—repletion of depleted electrolytes, and washout of all potentially offending agents can be undertaken. Patients affected may have a propensity for developing this disorder with diverse conditions. Thus, careful evaluation must be undertaken any time medications are given.

The congenital long-QT syndrome is a disorder that may be familial (with or without hearing loss) or sporadic. Although several genetic markers have been recognized, no specific gene abnormality presently explains all the disorders. In families with a genetic marker, overlap in QT interval duration is common between carriers and noncarriers. Thus, additional factors appear to be involved in the full-blown syndrome beyond those related to the genetic markers of QT interval duration per se. Presently, the best way to identify subjects at risk involves measurement of the QT interval and acquisition of family history.

The pathogenesis of congenital long-QT-interval syndrome remains controversial. Overactivity of the left or underactivity of the right cardiac sympathetic nervous system appears to be involved leading to disparities in sympathetic input to the heart. Because the arrhythmias associated with this disorder are often triggered by heightened sympathetic tone and can be prevented by sympathectomy, many have thought the disorder to be a primary dysautonomic condition. However, primary dysfunction of potassium channel activity has been implicated recently. A decrease in potassium conductance would lead to prolonged action potential duration and the development of early afterdepolarizations. In experimental animal preparations in which bradyarrhythmias, potassium channel blocking, drugs, and catecholamines have been combined, polymorphic tachycardia associated with the long QT interval syndrome have been simulated.

Regardless of the mechanism responsible, affected patients present early in life with syncopal episodes precipitated by emotion or extreme exercise. Usually the first episode takes place between age 5 and 15 years. A history of inappropriate bradycardia before episodes is common. Markers that portend a bad outcome are (a) T-wave abnormalities (notched, multiple hump, biphasic T waves in V_2 to V_5); (b) corrected QT intervals greater than 480 msec; (c) T-wave alternans; (d) physiologically inappropriate sinus bradycardia; and (e) abnormal systolic function of the inferobasal left ventricle.

Acute treatment of episodes of torsades de pointes includes beta blockers and pacing. Magnesium is not as effective as it is in the congenital long-QT syndrome in the acquired forms. In general, large doses of beta blockers are required, coupled with temporary pacemaker support for overdrive pacing if needed. After the acute episode, beta-blocker therapy is given in maximally tolerated doses. This approach has decreased the mortality of symptomatic patients from 70 to 6%. Because approximately 50% of the patients affected will have nonspecific EEGs , phenytoin or a barbiturate is given in addition to the beta blocker. Continued episodes despite beta blocker therapy are usually dealt with by implantation of a permanent pacemaker. If recurrences persist, a left thoracic sympathectomy or ICD may be indicated. The youth of these patients discourages use of an ICD, but it may be a treatment of last resort when multiple recurrences remain refractory. Standard left cervical thoracic sympathectomy often leaves a residual Horner's syndrome, which young people find disfiguring. A posterior approach or a pure thoracic sympathectomy will prevent this difficulty. Of interest is the fact that successful treatment (i.e., prevention of recurrent torsades), whether with beta blockers alone or drugs followed by thoracic sympathectomy, is associated with a persistent prolongation of the QT interval in at least 50% of patients, underscoring our lack of complete understanding of the pathogenesis of this disorder and the relationship between QT prolongation to the mechanism underlying the arrhythmia.

SUGGESTED READING

Ventricular Premature Complexes

Bigger JT Jr. Cardiac arrhythmias. In: Wyngaarden JB, Smith LK Jr, Bennett JC, eds. Cecil Textbook of Medicine, 19th ed. Philadelphia: Saunders, 1994.

Bigger JT. Identification of patients at high risk for sudden cardiac death. Am J Cardiol 1984; 54:3D–8D.

Bigger JT Jr. Ventricular premature complexes. In: Kastor JA, ed. Arrhythmias. Philadelphia: Saunders, 1993:310–335.

Bigger JT Jr, Fleiss JL, Kleiger R, et al. The relationships among ventricular arrhythmias, left ventricular dysfunction, and mortality in the 2 years after myocardial infarction. Circulation 1984; 69:250–258.

Bigger JT Jr, Rolnitzky LM, Merab J. Epidemiology of ventricular arrhythmias and clinical trials with antiarrhythmic drugs. In: Fozzard HA, Haber E, Jennings RB, et al, eds. The Heart and Cardiovascular System. New York: Raven Press, 1986:1405–1448.

Coplen SE, Antman EM, Berlin JA, et al. Efficacy and safety of quinidine therapy for maintenance of sinus rhythm after cardioversion: A meta-analysis of randomized controlled trials. Circulation 1990; 82:1106–1116.

Cranefield PF. The Conduction of the Cardiac Impulse—The Slow Response and Cardiac Arrhythmias. Mt Kisco, NY: Futura, 1975.

Echt DS, Liebson PR, Mitchell LB, et al. Mortality and morbidity in patients randomized to receive encainide, flecainide, or placebo in the Cardiac Arrhythmia Suppression Trial. N Engl J Med 1991; 324:781–788.

Hine LK, Laird NM, Hewitt P, Chalmers TC. Meta-analysis of empirical long-term anti-arrhythmic drug therapy after myocardial infarction. JAMA 1989; 262:3037–3040.

Hoffman BF, Cranefield PF. Electrophysiology of the Heart. New York: McGraw–Hill, 1960.

Morganroth J. Premature ventricular complexes: Diagnosis and indications for therapy. JAMA 1984; 252:673–676.

Morganroth J, Goin JE. Quinidine-related mortality in the short-to-medium-term treatment of ventricular arrhythmias: A meta-analysis. Circulation 1991; 84:1977–1983.

Noble D. The Initiation of the Heartbeat. Oxford: Claredon Press, 1975.

Zipes, DP. Specific arrhythmias: Diagnosis and treatment. In: Braunwald E, ed. Heart Disease. Philadelphia: Saunders, 1992.

18

Management of Patients with Bradycardias

Abnormalities of Impulse Formation and Atrioventricular Conduction **373**

   I.   Sinus Node Dysfunction   374
   II.   Carotid Sinus Syndrome   377
   III.   Malignant Vasovagal Syncope   379
   IV.   Disturbances of Atrioventricular Conduction   380
   V.   Cardiac Pacing for Bradycardias   387

Intraventricular Conduction Abnormalities **393**

   VI.   Electrocardiographic Diagnosis   394
   VII.   The Role of Electrophysiology Study   394
   VIII.   Management of Intraventricular Conduction Abnormalities   394

Abnormalities of Impulse Formation and Atrioventricular Conduction

A. John Camm and Josef Kautzner

Bradycardias, defined as rhythms characterized by slowing of the heart rate below 50–60 beats/min, may represent either normal cardiac rhythm or a manifestation of a wide spectrum of abnormalities such as sinus node dysfunction, carotid sinus hypersensitivity and other neurally mediated disorders, and/or impairment of atrioventricular conduction. They are common, and their treatment often involves long-term cardiac pacing.

I. SINUS NODE DYSFUNCTION

Dysfunction of the sinoatrial (SA) node, often known as "sick sinus syndrome" (SSS), accounts for more than half of all pacemaker implantations in developed countries. In most cases, the etiology of SSS is unknown. Among conditions that may disturb the physiology of the SA node, local fibrosis or ischemia, rheumatic heart disease, cardiomyopathies, systemic disease such as collagen diseases, metastatic involvement, and amyloidosis are the most frequent. In some SSS patients, symptomatic sinus bradyarrhythmias may be exaggerated by paroxysmal increases in vagal tone. This may also occur when SSS and carotid sinus hypersensitivity coincide. Symptomatic bradyarrhythmias can be promoted by a variety of drugs, such as digitalis, beta blockers, or calcium channel blockers. Sometimes, SSS is associated with abnormalities of atrioventricular (AV) node function which may be manifest merely as a slow ventricular response during atrial fibrillation in the absence of drugs with negative dromotropic effect.

The transient or intermittent nature of symptoms attributable to sinus node dysfunction and their low specificity often makes the diagnosis and electrocardiographic (ECG) documentation of the condition difficult. Because the sinus rate is controlled largely by the autonomic nervous system with predominant resting vagal tone, it is not rare that significantly slow resting heart rates (about 30 beats/min) or long sinus pauses approaching 2.5 sec can be detected in normal subjects without any symptoms. For this reason, assessment of the persistence and inappropriateness of bradyarrhythmias in the absence of reversible causes, such as drug effects, is essential, together with evaluation of the relationship between symptoms and ECG abnormalities.

A. Symptoms

Sinoatrial node dysfunction provokes symptoms as a result of the associated decrease in cardiac output (e.g., fatigue, dizziness, syncope, or near syncope) or pulmonary congestion (i.e., dyspnea). However, in a substantial proportion of SSS patients, syncope may not be related to bradyarrhythmia but be vasodepressor in origin. On the other hand, sinus node dysfunction appears to enhance the cardioinhibitory reflex. Patients with SSS may also suffer from paroxysmal or sustained atrial tachyarrhythmias, and this is the basis of the bradycardia/tachycardia syndrome. Tachyarrhythmias usually manifest themselves by palpitations, occasionally by angina pectoris or syncope. Sick sinus syndrome may present with subtle disturbances such as personality changes and memory loss. Symptoms related to systemic embolism are not uncommon.

B. Electrocardiographic Diagnosis

The electrocardiographic (ECG) manifestations of SSS include the following patterns: (a) persistent and inappropriate sinus bradycardia, (b) intermittent sinus arrest with escape atrial or junctional rhythm, (c) long periods of sinus arrest with failure of subsidiary pacemaker escape rhythm, (d) episodes of sinoatrial exit block, (e) sinus pauses following termination of supraventricular tachyarrhythmias, and (f) chronic or paroxysmal atrial fibrillation, flutter, or tachycardia. Concomitant bundle branch block can be seen in 15–20% of the patients, and AV conduction abnormalities can be demonstrated in 50–60% of patients with SSS.

Sinoatrial blocks are classified into three categories based on their severity. First-degree SA block produces no ECG changes unless intermittent when an ECG pattern similar to sinus arrhythmia is seen. Second-degree SA block type I presents with gradual shortening of the PP interval over a sequence of three or more P waves with a subsequent longer pause equal to or less than twice the shortest PP interval. Second-degree SA block type II is defined as an intermittent interruption in sinoatrial conduction, which is seen on the ECG as a missed PQRS complex with a pause equal to twice the length of the preceding (or following) PP interval. Third-degree SA block manifests as sinus arrest, a pause without P waves which continues until an escape rhythm appears or sinus rhythm is restored. The pauses due to SA block are approximate multiples of the normal PP interval, but no such relationship can be demonstrated in sinus arrest.

As already discussed, the diagnosis of SSS requires documentation of a bradyarrhythmia coincident with symptoms. Therefore, the primary diagnostic tool is long-term ECG monitoring (Figure 1), either by telemetry in the hospitalized patient or by ambulatory ECG monitoring. Transtelephonic monitoring of the use of various ambulatory event recorders can be helpful in patients with sporadic symptoms. Various provocative maneuvers can be attempted to elucidate

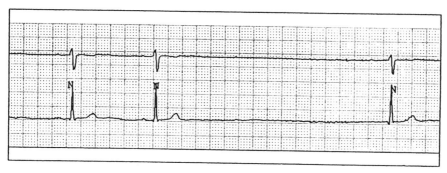

Figure 1 Ambulatory ECG from a patient with sick sinus syndrome showing a 3.3-sec-long pause due to sinus arrest. Note that the pause is terminated by junctional escape beat.

the cause of symptoms in patients with suspected SSS. These include assessment of the ECG response to exercise or autonomic blockade, carotid sinus massage, and head-up tilt test. Chronically enhanced vagal tone may ultimately be distinguished from abnormalities in intrinsic heart rate by total autonomic blockade, accomplished with propranolol 0.2 mg/kg body weight, and atropine sulfate 0.04 mg/kg. Normally, the value of the intrinsic heart rate should approximate that calculated by the formula $117.2 - (0.53 \times$ age in years).

C. The Role of Electrophysiology Study

Although an electrophysiology study can help to document the presence of SA node, it generally cannot help to find any relationship between such dysfunction and the symptoms. It may be helpful in cases of isolated sinus bradycardia or when no bradyarrhythmia is detected in patients with clinically suspected SSS. Among the most useful measures of overall sinus function is the sinus node recovery time (SNRT). A prolonged SNRT is defined as a pause greater than 1600 msec following atrial pacing. The corrected SNRT, defined as the SNRT minus the preceding sinus cycle length, should not normally exceed 550 msec. The use of these high upper-normal values for SNRT makes the test less sensitive but reasonably specific. Sinoatrial conduction time (SACT) is another SA nodal functional parameter, advocated to assess conduction to and from surrounding atrial tissue. However, SACT is even less sensitive than SNRT and therefore is not considered helpful in the assessment of SSS patients. At the time of electrophysiology study, the assessment of AV nodal function should be performed. A normal HV interval and preserved 1:1 AV conduction in response to atrial pacing rates in the range of 140 beats/min may favor long-term atrial pacing rather than dual chamber pacing.

D. Management of Sinus Node Dysfunction

Therapy for SSS should always be individualized. Because atropine or isoproterenol may provide only temporary improvement of SA nodal function, permanent cardiac pacing is the treatment of choice. Several basic principles must be followed: (a) SSS is a generally benign condition and therefore therapy is needed only in symptomatic patients; (b) in some patients with the bradycardia/tachycardia syndrome, pacing may be required to enable treatment of tachyarrhythmias with antiarrhythmic drugs; (c) pacing may prevent or reduce the incidence of atrial fibrillation in bradycardia/tachycardia syndrome; and (d) atrial or dual-chamber pacing should be used, while ventricular pacing is generally contraindicated.

Some recent clinical data show that syncopal episodes in patients with SSS or sinus bradycardia may be a result of an abnormal neural reflex, being reproducible during head-up tilt testing. This reflex seems to be unrelated to the severity of sinus node dysfunction, although the latter may exaggerate the cardioinhibitory response to head-up tilt test. In that case, pharmacological treatment for pro-phylaxis of neurally mediated syncope may be preferable to cardiac pacing.

II. CAROTID SINUS SYNDROME

Carotid sinus syndrome (CSS) is often considered as a paradigm of the neurally mediated syncopal syndromes, reflecting an abnormally exaggerated carotid sinus reflex. However, despite the fact that carotid sinus hypersensitivity can be demon-strated relatively often, the frequency with which this hypersensitivity is respon-sible for spontaneous syncopal symptoms is low (in approximately 5–20% of hypersensitive patients). The relation of CSS to SSS is unclear, but the clinical features of both conditions can be associated in approximately 25% of cases. Nevertheless, there are some data demonstrating clinical differences that justify a distinction between the two syndromes.

A. Symptoms

CSS is characterized mainly by symptoms resulting from the associated decrease in cardiac output (e.g., dizziness, syncope, or near syncope) caused by cardio-inhibition or vasodepression. Unlike the normal carotid sinus reflex, which is a physiological reaction to activation of the carotid baroreceptors by external pres-sure, the response is pathological in patients with CSS. The cardioinhibitory component of the reflex consists of an increased parasympathetic response that manifests as sinus bradycardia, sinus arrest, sinoatrial block and/or high-degree atrioventricular block. The vasodepressor component is reflected by a significant drop in blood pressure. The etiology of the decrease in peripheral vascular resistance is not known. The vasodepressor component may not be evident until atropine or atrial pacing are used to prevent heart rate changes during carotid sinus massage. In a mixed type of response, both components are manifest. Although these symptoms are similar to those of SA nodal dysfunction, there is a signifi-cantly higher prevalence of syncopal episodes among patients with CSS compared to those with SSS.

B. Carotid Sinus Massage

Diagnosis and identification of different types of CSS is based on the response of heart rate and blood pressure to carotid sinus massage. Testing by unilateral digital massage (after checking that no carotid bruits are present) should first be done with gentle and brief pressure with the patient supine. Subsequently, rotatory pressure is applied on the right and then left side for 10 sec. The cardioinhibitory response is arbitrarily defined as the development of ventricular asystole lasting equal to or greater than 3 sec or a more than 30% decrease in heart rate compared to the baseline heart rate (Figure 2). The vasodepresor response is usually defined

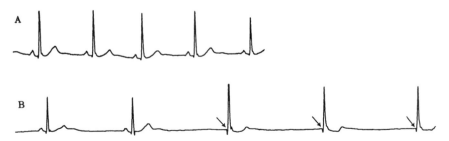

Figure 2   An ECG obtained before (A) and during (B) carotid sinus massage in a patient with the cardioinhibitory response. Sinus bradycardia at a rate of 41 beats/min is followed by junctional escape rhythm (arrows) at a rate of 37 beats/min.

as a decrease in systolic blood pressure of 30–50 mmHg or to below 80 mmHg (Figure 3). However, there is neither a standardized method of carotid sinus massage nor a universally accepted definition of responses. As the cause-and-effect relation between the hypersensitive carotid sinus reflex and the dpatient's symptoms should always be established, some authors recommend performing carotid sinus massage even with the patient in the erect position. The testing should be avoided in patients with known or suspected cerebrovascular disease. It

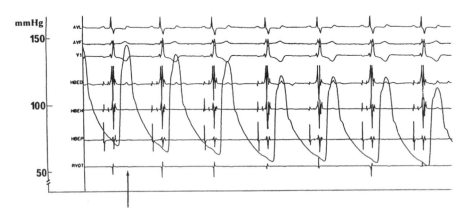

Figure 3   A composite recording of blood pressure, three surface ECG leads (aV$_1$, aV$_F$ and V$_1$), three His bundle electrograms (HBED, HBEM, and HBEP), and the right ventricular outflow tract (RVOT) electrogram during carotid sinus massage (arrow marks the beginning of massage) in a patient with the vasodepressor response. Blood pressure falls from 145 to 105 mmHg without significant change in heart rate.

should also be noted that administration of drugs like digoxin, beta blockers, and alpha-methyldopa may accentuate the response to carotid sinus massage.

C. Management of Carotid Sinus Syndrome

In general, precipitating factors such as tight collars should be avoided. There may be a beneficial response to mineralocorticoids (fludrocortisone acetate 50–300 μg daily). In more severe, recurrent cases, cardiac pacing is considered a method of choice. There is overall agreement that pacing is therapeutically most effective for the cardioinhibitory form of CSS. On the contrary, conventional pacing is ineffective in the isolated or predominant vasodepresor form of the syndrome. Positive rate hysteresis (i.e., pacing at a fast heart rate) may, however, prove useful. As ventricular pacing often fails to control symptoms, dual-chamber pacing is essential.

III. MALIGNANT VASOVAGAL SYNCOPE

Neurally mediated vasovagal episodes are the most common cause of syncope, accounting for the vast majority of isolated events. But in only a small proportion of patients with neurally mediated syncope does significant bradycardia or asystole cause the symptoms. This condition has been termed "malignant vasovagal syncope (MVVS)." In Europe, this term is also frequently used to describe individuals who have severe, recurrent episodes of neurally mediated syncope, usually refractory to drug therapy.

The identification of patients prone to develop neurally mediated episodes of hypotension and/or bradycardia has been substantially improved by head-up tilt testing. Although the pathophysiology of both hypotensive and bradycardic components of the neurally mediated response to head-up tilt has been a subject of considerable interest, current theories remain rather controversial. The most accepted theory proposes that the major trigger for afferent neural signals from cardiovascular receptors is a reduction in central blood volume elicited by upright posture in conjunction with marked elevation of circulating catecholamines (especially epinephrine). Ventricular mechanoreceptors are stimulated by a vigorously contracting left ventricle in response to the surge of sympathetic activation. Epinephrine-induced peripheral vasodilatation seems to play a causative role in hypotension, whereas the cardioinhibitory component is vagally mediated. Therefore, the hypotension appears to be essentially independent of heart rate. However, when bradycardia occurs hypotension is further accentuated and the process is self-perpetuating.

A. Symptoms

Individuals presenting with syncope but no other apparent illness and no structural heart disease or documented arrhythmia are ideal candidates for head-up tilt

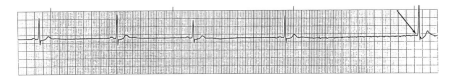

Figure 4 An ECG recorded during a head-up tilt test which reproduced clinical syncope. Gradual slowing of sinus rate is followed by a 3.5-sec pause terminated by a junctional escape beat (arrow).

testing. As convulsive activity may occur with interruption of cerebral blood flow, the presence of seizures should not abate suspicion of neurally mediated syncope. In addition, head-up tilt testing may also help to evaluate patients with vertigo of unknown origin or reproduce symptoms in elderly patients with "transient ischemic attacks."

B. Head-up Tilt Test

As already mentioned, the advent of the head-up tilt test has changed diagnostic algorithms in patients with syncope of unknown origin. Head-up tilt testing is usually performed after an overnight fast in a quiet room with dimmed lights. Although some institutions use supplemental intravenous hydration, this may decrease the sensitivity of testing. The patient is usually tilted to 60–80° for 30–60 min, while heart rate (ECG) and blood pressure are monitored at 1- or 2-min intervals until symptoms occur or a predetermined time period is reached (Figure 4). When the test is negative, repeat testing during isoproterenol infusion may be considered. However, isoproterenol infusion decreases the specificity of the test.

C. Management of Malignant Vasovagal Syncope

Although treatment of neurally mediated syncope primarily consists of drug therapy, cardiac pacing has an role in the treatment of the malignant variant. Dual-chamber pacing with a positive rate hysteresis appears to be preferable in those patients with predominant cardioinhibitory response who are refractory to pharmacological therapy. Otherwise the indications for this treatment modality are controversial (Figure 5).

IV. DISTURBANCES OF ATRIOVENTRICULAR CONDUCTION

Atrioventricular (AV) conduction abnormalities are common indications for permanent pacing. For this reason, understanding the mechanisms, clinical manifestation and management of different types of AV block is important.

380

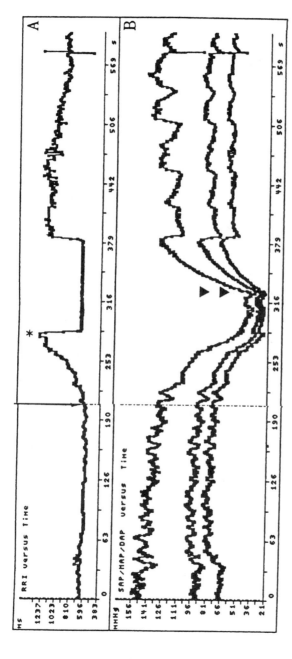

Figure 5 An example of simultaneous recording of instantaneous heart rate (A), expressed as a sequence of RR intervals in time, and systolic, mean, and diastolic blood pressures (B) in millimeters of mercury during head-up tilt test in a patient with neurally mediated syncope. Note that blood pressure gradually decreases before the heart rate change (arrow). Continuous fall in blood pressure and loss of consciousness is not prevented by dual-chamber pacing at cycle length 600 ms (*). A rapid increase in blood pressure occurs immediately after detilting (▼).

Table 1   Causes of Atrioventricular
Block

Ischemic heart disease
Myocarditis
Congenital
Infection (e.g., Lyme disease)
Iatrogenic (e.g., surgery, catheter ablation)
Neuromuscular (e.g., muscular dystrophy)
Infiltrative

The term "AV block" describes a condition in which electrical impulses generated in the SA node or in subsidiary atrial pacemakers fail to conduct to the ventricles. Since the function of the AV node and the His-Purkinje system are the major determinants of AV conduction, heart block is virtually always secondary to AV nodal or His-Purkinje disease. Although lesser degrees of AV block often occur in the absence of structural heart disease, higher degrees are almost invariably organic in origin (Table 1). The exception may be the cases of AV block in endurance athletes. Congenital heart block occurs either sporadically or in families. In some patients, selective degenerative or inflammatory changes can be found in the AV node or His bundle region. For instance, Lenegre's disease is characterized by selective noninflammatory degeneration of either region, while Lev's disease is due to destructive scarring associated with local degeneration or inflammation.

In principle, the approach to patients with AV conduction abnormalities is based on the analysis of symptoms, and estimation of the severity (i.e., degree) and location of the block. Although the management is primarily focused on the relief of symptoms, the prognosis is dependent mainly on the site of block—i.e., block within the AV node (proximal) implies a more favorable prognosis, whereas block in the His-Purkinje system (distal) tends to progress to a higher degree and may become life-threatening. Therefore, in some cases prophylactic pacing may be considered, regardless of symptoms.

A. Symptoms

Patients with abnormalities of AV conduction may be asymptomatic or experience symptoms of varied severity. Bradyarrhythmias related to AV conduction abnormalities are usually manifested as hypotension or low cardiac output. Bradyarrhythmias often cause confusion, dizziness, near syncope, or syncope. A Stokes-Adams attack is caused by a transient cardiac arrest, usually related to AV block (Figure 6), with spontaneous recovery. Other symptoms vary from shortness of breath or angina on exercise to resting dyspnea, based on the balance between

382

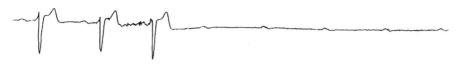

Figure 6   An ECG recording during Stokes-Adams attack showing ventricular standstill for 6.2 sec.

the severity of bradyarrhythmia and the associated pathology of the cardiovascular system.

B. Electrocardiographic Diagnosis

The ECG usually provides enough information to make appropriate decisions concerning the management of patients with AV conduction abnormalities. Besides the diagnosis of AV block itself, the surface ECG is often helpful in locating the site of block. This can be inferred from the appearance of QRS complexes and by the discharge frequency of the escape pacemaker. A narrow QRS complex suggests proximal block (i.e., in the AV node) when the escape rate is usually 40–60 beats/min. When complete heart block is due to more distal block, the QRS complex is wide and the ventricles are controlled by distal His-Purkinje pacemakers with intrinsic heart rates lower than 40 beats/min. Autonomic maneuvers may improve the noninvasive assessment of the site of the block. There is abundant innervation to the AV node compared with the distal conduction system, and vagotonic maneuvers tend to worsen AV nodal block but not distal block. On the other hand, maneuvers that increase sympathetic tone may improve AV nodal block, especially in 2:1 second-degree AV block. The same holds for the use of drugs such as isoproterenol or atropine.

Traditionally, AV conduction abnormalities have been classified into three types based on severity: first-, second- and third-degree (complete) heart block. So called high-degree block is AV block with a 2:1 or higher AV ratios (i.e., 3:1) and maintained AV synchrony.

> *First-degree AV block* results in prolongation of the PR interval beyond 0.20 sec on the surface ECG (0.22 sec in the elderly); normal sinus rhythm is otherwise present. In this case, the impulse conduction from atria to ventricles is prolonged but 1:1 transmission is preserved.
>
> *Type I second-degree AV block (Mobitz type I or Wenckebach block)* is progressive prolongation of the PR interval until an atrial depolarization fails to conduct to the ventricles. Occasionally, an atypical periodicity may simulate Mobitz type II block if the last two or three cycles have a relatively constant PR. However, comparison of the last PR interval with the first PR interval in the sequence demonstrates a clear prolongation prior to the dropped beat.

383

Type II second-degree AV block (Mobitz type II block) is characterized by periodic loss of AV conduction without preceding progressive AV delay. The PR interval remains constant and bundle branch block or bifascicular block is usually present, suggesting distal location of the block.

High-degree AV block that is 2:1 (Figure 7) may be either type I or II second-degree AV block, and it is therefore difficult to localize the site of block from the surface ECG. However, location of block within the His-Purkinje system can be expected when bundle branch block or bifascicular block is present in conducted beats, no AV nodal blocking drugs have been used, and no changes in conduction occur after atropine administration.

In *complete heart block (third-degree AV block)*, the atria and ventricles beat independently. The ventricular rhythm is usually slower than the sinus rhythm, and the frequency depends on the site of the subsidiary pacemaker (idioventricular or junctional). It is usually 20–60 beats/min. The atria may be controlled by sinus depolarization or by atrial fibrillation (or flutter).

C. The Role of Electrophysiology Study

As precise localization of the block is only possible by recording His bundle activity, an electrophysiology study may be needed when it provides therapeutically important information regardless of the patient's symptoms. Such recordings may also differentiate between a primary conduction disorder and ectopic activity, such as concealed junctional extrasystoles, which impair subsequent AV conduction. His bundle recordings (Figure 8) allow delineation of four levels of block: (a) intraatrial, (b) intra AV nodal, (c) intra-His, and (d) infra-His.

As conduction delay in the AV node is the most common cause of *first-degree AV block*, the AH interval is typically prolonged. Intra-His conduction delay is relatively rare and is characterized by prolonged H deflection duration (beyond 25 msec) or by the presence of split His potentials. Infra-His conduction delay or HV interval >55 msec is almost always associated with a prolonged QRS complex because of inhomogenous impairment of intraventricular conduction. Although a significantly prolonged HV interval is unlikely in the presence of a PR

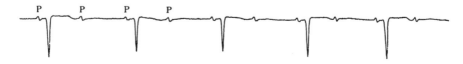

Figure 7   2:1 AV block. Every other P wave is not conducted to the ventricles.

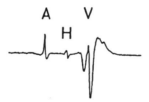

Figure 8 The His bundle electrogram in a normal individual. The A deflection represents atrial depolarization, the H spike reflects the depolarization of the His bundle, and the V deflection corresponds with the depolarization of the adjacent ventricular myocardium.

interval below 0.16 sec, the PR interval itself is a poor predictor of the HV interval duration.

With *type I second-degree AV block*, the characteristic feature is a progressive prolongation of the AH interval until conduction is blocked in the AV node. This may be a pathological process or a physiological response to increased vagal tone. Wenckebach type AV block in the His bundle is uncommon but may occur in the presence of a narrow or wide QRS complex. In this situation, progressive delay can be recorded between the two components of a split His potential, with eventual failure of conduction to the site of recording of the distal potential. Block in the His-Purkinje system is characterized as progressive prolongation of the HV interval until block below the His bundle occurs.

The occurrence of *Mobitz type II block* with normal QRS complexes (i.e., originating in the AV node) remains questionable, but this pattern may be caused by concealed His bundle extrasystoles. Infra-His block is defined by intermittent conduction between the proximal and distal His bundle potentials. In the vast majority of cases, the location of block is below the His bundle. Infra-His block usually occurs without gradual HV prolongation.

Complete heart block in the AV node is relatively common. Intracardiac study demonstrates atrial deflections dissociated from His bundle and ventricular activation. The escape rhythm usually originates in the proximal His-Purkinje system, and the QRS complex is preceded by a His bundle deflection. Infra-His block, which is the most common site of complete heart block in adults, is characterized by dissociation of the AH intervals from V deflections (Figure 9).

D. Management of Atrioventricular Conduction Abnormalities

Permanent ventricular pacing (with ventricular or dual-chamber pacemaker) is currently the only practical treatment for AV conduction disorders. Patients considered for pacemaker therapy can be grouped as follows: (a) sustained or inter-

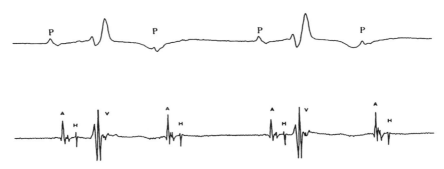

Figure 9 Surface ECG and His bundle recording in complete infra-His AV block. H spikes follow each A deflection without any relationship to ventricular escape complexes. Not resulting AV dissociation on the surface tracing.

mittent documented AV block associated with symptoms, (b) unexplained intermittent symptoms due to suspected paroxysmal AV block, and (c) no symptoms but risk of dangerous AV block.

Although the decision to implant a pacemaker in the first group is very straightforward, regardless of the site of the block, indication for pacemaker insertion in other groups is more complicated. In the second group of patients, therapeutic decisions depend primarily on the evidence of a possible electrophysiological substrate and on the probability that the symptoms are cardiac in origin. In the third group, the therapeutic approach is the most difficult and controversial (Table 2). In patients with first-degree AV block caused by delay in the His-Purkinje system, no therapy is usually required. However, when HV intervals exceed 100 msec, prophylactic pacing is recommended regardless of symptoms. Pacemaker implantation should also be considered in asymptomatic

Table 2 Recommended Indications for Cardiac Pacing in Asymptomatic Patients with AV block

	Site of AV block	
Degree of AV block	Proximal	Distal
First Degree	No	No[a]
Second Degree	No	Yes
Third Degree	No	Yes

[a]Unless HV interval ≥100 msec.

type I second-degree AV block at intra-His or infra-His levels. In type II second-degree AV block, progress to complete heart block is common and permanent pacing is generally recommended.

Specific criteria apply for management of AV conduction abnormalities following myocardial infarction. The need for temporary pacing in the acute phase of infarction does not necessarily constitute an indication for permanent pacing. For instance, type I second-degree AV block within the AV node is usually a temporary phenomenon associated with acute inferior wall infarction, which reflects the common source of blood supply to the AV node and inferior wall myocardium. This conduction abnormality may be treated either by administration of atropine or by temporary pacing when the ventricular rate is below 40 beats/min or congestive heart failure or ventricular arrhythmias are present. Even third-degree AV block in inferior infarction is often reversible. However, in anterior myocardial infarction, AV block occurs more rarely and reflects extensive myocardial injury. In these cases, AV block is usually distal and the prognosis is poor despite pacing. Therefore, unlike many other indications for permanent pacing, the criteria in patients with myocardial infarction and AV block do not necessarily depend on the presence of symptoms. A pacemaker is indicated in patients with advanced second-degree AV block or complete heart block with block in the His-Purkinje system or in those with transient advanced AV block and associated bundle branch block.

Complete heart block, typically with block proximal to the His bundle, may occur as a congenital lesion and is widely regarded as benign. The prognosis depends mainly on any associated structural heart disease, which may be present up to 30% of cases. Those without underlying heart disease probably have a good prognosis, but some patients develop symptoms or die suddenly during follow-up. Permanent pacing should be considered in those patients with risk factors such as a nodal escape rhythm below 50 beats/min, poor chronotropic response to exercise, long periods of asystole, broad QRS complexes, or repetitive ventricular ectopy. Permanent pacing is recommended in all symptomatic patients.

V. CARDIAC PACING FOR BRADYCARDIAS

Cardiac pacing has become the dominant treatment modality for bradycardias; long-term artificial pacing is usually indicated.

A. Permanent Pacing

Implantable pacemakers are classified according to the NASPE/BPEG generic (NBG) five-letter code, which describes the site of pacing electrode(s) and other characteristics of the pacemaker system (Table 3). The first letter indicates the chamber paced [A = atrium, V = ventricle, D = dual (i.e., atrium and ventricle),

Table 3 The NASPE/BPEG[a] Generic Five-Letter Pacemaker Code

Letter position	1	2	3	4	5
Category	Chamber(s) paced	Chamber(s) sensed	Response to sensing	Programmability, rate modulation	Anti-tachyarrhythmia function(s)
	0 = None	0 = None	0 = None	0 = None	0 = None
	A = Atrium	A = Atrium	T = Triggered	P = Simple programmable	P = Pacing (anti-tachyarrhythmia)
	V = Ventricle	V = Ventricle	I = Inhibited	M = Multi-programmable	S = Shock
	D = Dual (A+V)	D = Dual (A+V)	D = Dual (T+I)	C = Communi-cating	D = Dual (P+S)
				R = Rate modulation	

[a]NASPE = North American Society of Pacing and Electrophysiology, BPEG = British Pacing and Electrophysiology Group.

0 = none] the second letter indicates the chamber in which electrical activity is sensed, the third letter indicates the response to the sensed electrical signal [I = inhibited, T = triggered, D = dual (i.e., inhibited and triggered), 0 = no sensing], the fourth letter expresses special features such as rate responsiveness (R) or programmability. The last letter, which describes antitachycardia functions, is not relevant to pacing for bradycardia.

Generally, selection of a particular pacing mode should reflect an attempt to reproduce normal sinus rhythm as closely as possible. To accomplish this, the atrium should be paced (and preferably sensed) unless contraindicated, the ventricle should be paced in case of AV block or threatened AV block, chronotropic incompetence in an active patient may be overcome by adaptive rate pacing, and hysteresis may be beneficial if the bradycardia is intermittent. In addition, in selecting the optimal pacing mode, the patient's overall condition and associated medical problems should be taken into consideration.

B. Mode of Pacing?

There are two basic types of pulse generator: single- and dual-chamber.

Atrial single-chamber (AAI) pacing refers to a pacing mode with both pacing and sensing in the atrium and with inhibition of pacing when an intrinsic atrial beat is sensed. The hemodynamic advantage of this pacing mode in patients with SSS and intact AV conduction is well established and is related mainly to preserved AV synchrony. There is a significantly lower morbidity and mortality in patients treated with AAI compared to VVI pacing. The latter suffer more frequently from atrial fibrillation, congestive heart failure, and systemic embolization. Long-term survival is higher in those treated by AAI pacing. However, the presence of minor abnormalities of AV conduction or bundle branch disease generally favors implantation of a dual-chamber pacemaker. AAI pacing is more widely used in Europe. In the United States, it constitutes only a very small proportion of pacemaker implants (about 1%).

Ventricular single-chamber (VVI) pacing was the most commonly used pacing mode for many years, not only for AV block but also for patients with SSS. Indications for VVI pacing include symptomatic bradycardias associated with the lack of an atrial hemodynamic contribution (persistent atrial fibrillation or markedly enlarged atria) or bradycardias where pacing simplicity is of primary interest (senility or limited locomotor function, very rare bradycardia, etc.).

Dual-chamber (DDD) pacing allows pacing and sensing in both the atrium and the ventricle, inhibition of atrial or ventricular output by sensed atrial or ventricular activity, and triggering of ventricular output by sensed atrial activity. The principal advantage of this pacing mode and its variants (e.g., VDD or DDI) is maintenance of AV synchrony over a wide range of rates. Therefore, these modes are preferred in active patients without chronotropic incompetence or in those clearly benefiting from the atrial hemodynamic contribution.

C. Rate-Adaptive Pacing?

The lack of a physiological chronotropic response in paced patients may be overcome by the implantation of a pulse generator with an adaptive-rate function. These pacemaker systems are equipped with one or more sensors that monitor physical activity or physiological parameters which change with metabolic needs, such as a piezo-crystal sensing body activity or sensors detecting the QT interval duration, the central venous blood temperature, oxygen saturation, or respiration/minute ventilation. Several pacing systems are available that can facilitate a chronotropic response irrespective of intrinsic sinus node activity. This modality is designated by the letter "R" in the fourth position of the generic pacemaker code. Thus, for instance, the code for an adaptive-rate ventricular demand pacemaker is "VVIR". Use of more than one sensor—such as the combination of a fast-response "activity sensor" with a delayed proportional-response QT interval sensor—can overcome the inherent theoretical limitations of individual sensors but has not yet proved helpful in clinical situations.

In selecting pacemakers with or without adaptive-rate functions, several factors—such as the AV conduction abnormality, the presence of angina pectoris or left ventricular dysfunction, the level of anticipated activity, and the presence of associated diseases—should be considered. For instance, angina may be precipitated during rate-adaptive pacing or rapid ventricular pacing may worsen congestive heart failure or precipitate ventricular arrhythmias. The primary indication for rate-adaptive pacing is chronotropic incompetence. The major disadvantage of rate-adaptive pacing is the complexity of its programming.

D. Rate Hysteresis?

This programmed feature allows prolongation of the first pacemaker escape interval after a sensed beat and therefore allows a longer period for the patient's intrinsic escape beat to occur before pacing at the programmed rate starts. For instance pacemaker programmed at a cycle length 1000 msec (60 beats/min) at a hysteresis of 1500 msec (40 beats/min) offers a period of 1500 msec before initiation of pacing at 60 beats/min. This prevents unnecessary pacing when bradyarrhythmia is only intermittent.

Another available feature is positive hysteresis, which allows pacing at a faster rate than the sensing rate. This appears to be especially beneficial in patients with carotid sinus syndrome or malignant vasovagal syncope. For example, pacing at 80 pulses/min with a hysteresis rate of 55 means that the pacemaker is inhibited until the spontaneous heart rate falls below 55. However, being activated by slower heart rate, the pacemaker starts to pace at rate 80 pulses/min and this may help to prevent further fall in cardiac output in patients with neurally mediated syncopal episodes.

A list of the most important pacing modes, together with their indications and contraindications, is given in Table 4. In selecting the optimum type of pacemaker for an individual patient, the answers to several simple questions are helpful (Figure 10).

1. *"Is atrial pacing possible?"* If not—for instance, because of chronic atrial fibrillation or the presence of giant atria—AAI or DDD pacing are contraindicated and the VVI mode is recommended.
2. *"Is AV conduction preserved?"* If so, for example in isolated SA nodal dysfunction, AAI pacing can be used rather than DDD pacing.
3. *"Is synchronized AV contraction necessary?"* If needed, for instance in patients with a hypertrophic or noncompliant left ventricle, the DDD pacing mode should be selected. Otherwise, VVI pacing is appropriate.
4. *"Is there chronotropic incompetence?"* If present, the selected pacing modes should incorporate rate-adaptive algorithms.

E. Temporary Pacing

There are currently three treatment modalities available for temporary treatment of bradycardias.

Table 4 Indications for Different Pacing Modes

Pacing mode	Indication	Contraindication
AAI	Symptomatic SA block or sinus arrest with preserved AV or intraventricular conduction and no chronotropic incompetence	AV conduction abnormalities, poor intracavitary atrial complexes, chronic supraventricular tachyarrhythmias such as atrial fibrillation
AAIR	As above, when chronotropic incompetence is present and physical activity is anticipated	As above
VVI	Symptomatic bradycardias with no expected significant atrial contribution (chronic atrial fibrillation, giant or silent atria), pacing in terminally ill patients or those with limited locomotion	Need for atrial hemodynamic contribution, sinus node dysfunction, carotid sinus syndrome, malignant vasovagal syncope, known pacemaker syndrome
VVIR	As for VVI, when chronotropic incompetence is present and physical activity anticipated	As for VVI, retrograde VA conduction (angina pectoris of CHF likely to be aggravated at faster pacing rates)
DDD	Symptomatic bradycardias when there is a need for AV synchrony or when pacemaker syndrome is known or anticipated	Chronic supraventricular tachyarrhythmias, inadequate atrial sensing
DDDR	As for DDD, when chronotropic incompetence is present	As for DDD (angina pectoris or CHF likely to be aggravated at faster pacing rates)
VDD(R)	AV block with normal sinus node function, especially when atrial contribution is mandatory (an adaptive-rate component improve this mode of pacing)	SA node dysfunction, inadequate atrial sensing, intact VA conduction, paroxysmal supraventricular tachyarrhythmias
DDI(R)	As for DDD, when frequent supraventricular arrhythmias are present, malignant vasovagal syncope (an adaptive-rate component improve this mode of pacing)	Chronotropic incompetence, chronic supraventricular tachyarrhythmias

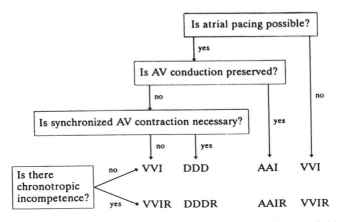

Figure 10   Algorithm for determining the optimum pacing mode for an individual patient.

Transesophageal Pacing

This technique may be useful for temporary atrial pacing or for assessment of sinus node dysfunction, and for differential diagnosis and treatment of supraventricular arrhythmias. The advantage is a low complication rate. However, this technique is not used for reliable ventricular pacing.

Temporary Transvenous Pacing

Ventricular atrial or dual-chamber pacing may be accomplished using pacing leads introduced percutaneously and connected to an external pulse generator. It is important to maintain atrioventricular synchrony with temporary pacing in critically ill patients. The indications for temporary pacing include bradycardia, which is likely to be a short-term problem, or symptomatic bradycardia in patients awaiting a long-term implantation. Another indication is acute failure of a permanent pacemaker. Temporary pacing is often necessary in acute myocardial infarction. Dual-chamber temporary pacing may be useful in pacemaker syndrome due to VVI pacing or when there is severe hemodynamic impairment in the setting of acute myocardial infarction.

Temporary Transcutaneous Pacing

This treatment modality constitutes a reliable alternative for the emergency management of unexpected bradycardias. Recent improvements make it feasible, even in conscious patients, as a standby modality. The pacemaker may function in the demand mode with a maximum output of 150 mA. Transcutaneous pacing appears to be less useful in the termination of supraventricular arrhythmias.

Intraventricular Conduction Abnormalities

A. John Camm and Josef Kautzner

The ventricles are activated under physiological conditions by synchronous conduction over the distal His-Purkinje system. Abnormalities in this process result in intraventricular conduction disturbances. Since the upper portion of the intraventricular system is the terminal part of the AV conduction system, intraventricular and AV block may occur as well. Intraventricular conduction disturbances usually indicate the presence of underlying cardiac disease, and patients with conduction abnormalities of this type have a higher incidence of cardiac mortality, sudden death, ventricular arrhythmias, and complete AV block.

The intraventricular conduction system consists of three separate fascicles: the right bundle branch and both the anterior or posterior fascicles of the left bundle branch. Right bundle branch block (RBBB) results in activation of the ventricles via the left bundle branch. Block in only one of the fascicles of the left bundle branch is known as left fascicular block, either anterior (LAFB) or posterior (LPFB). Left bundle branch block (LBBB) is caused by a conduction defect either in the main bundle or in both individual fascicles. Trifascicular block during 1:1 AV conduction is rare and occurs usually in the presence of alternating RBBB and LBBB or RBBB with alternating LAFB and LPFB.

The combination of RBBB and LAFB is the most common form of bifascicular block, seen in about 1% of hospitalized patients. Progression to AV block is estimated in up to 6% cases per year. RBBB plus LPFB is seen much less frequently but is a more serious conduction abnormality. A high mortality, often from sudden death, is known to be associated with trifascicular block and syncope. The progression to complete heart block is frequent in this type conduction abnormality. The presence of LBBB indicates conduction defect in the main left bundle or in individual fascicles. The incidence of complete heart block in patients with LBBB appears to be lower than in patients with RBBB and LAFB or LPFB. RBBB is often recorded in acute pulmonary embolism, and its incomplete form is common in atrial septal defect of the ostium secundum type. Incomplete right bundle branch block together with left anterior fascicular block suggests the presence of atrial septal defect of the ostium primum type or common atrioventricular canal.

393

VI. ELECTROCARDIOGRAPHIC DIAGNOSIS

Specific intraventricular conduction defects can be recognized by an altered pattern of ventricular activation on the surface ECG. In the case of fascicular block, ventricular activation occurs without significant delay, and the QRS complex remains of normal width. However, changes in the activation sequence shifts the mean frontal axis. In LAFB, the ventricles are activated through the posterior fascicle and the frontal axis shifts upward and to the left ($< -45°$). LPFB may be diagnosed only after exclusion of right ventricular hypertrophy, pulmonary disease, and an extreme vertical heart position. When it is present, activation spreads via the opposite fascicle and the frontal axis is shifted downward and to the right ($> +110°$). Bundle branch block indicates conduction delay or block resulting in activation of the ventricles via the opposite bundle. Therefore, initial septal activation occurs from the non-blocked bundle branch. Subsequently, both normal (intact bundle) and delayed abnormal (blocked bundle) ventricular activation occurs. Abnormal ventricular activation is followed by an abnormal repolarization with the ST segment and a T wave of opposite polarity to the terminal deflection of the QRS complex.

VII. THE ROLE OF ELECTROPHYSIOLOGY STUDY

In asymptomatic subjects with chronic bifascicular block or bundle branch block, the clinical usefulness of routine electrophysiology studies is not established. It has been documented that although the presence of these abnormalities suggests a higher risk of sudden death, the risk is not related to the HV interval per se, nor does pacemaker implantation change mortality. However, in those patients with transient neurological symptoms (near syncope, syncope, etc.) and an inconclusive noninvasive workup, an electrophysiology study is usually indicated. The methods of assessing His-Purkinje reserve include measurement of baseline HV interval, incremental atrial pacing to stress the conducting system, programmed atrial stimulation with the extrastimulus technique, and provocative drug studies (acute administration of procainamide, ajmaline, disopyramide, or flecainide). Because of the relatively high incidence of ventricular tachycardia in patients with bundle branch block and syncope, a complete electrophysiology study including programmed ventricular stimulation should be performed in order to assess possible tachyarrhythmic cause of syncope.

VIII. MANAGEMENT OF INTRAVENTRICULAR CONDUCTION ABNORMALITIES

Although the prognostic significance of left anterior or left posterior fascicular block is minimal, recognition of a bundle branch block pattern is clinically

Table 5 Indications for Permanent Pacing in Intraventricular Conduction Block

Pacemaker indicated	Pacemaker probably indicated
Symptomatic patients with bundle branch block or bifascicular block with intermittent complete heart block	Patients with bundle branch block or bifascicular block presenting with syncope that is not proved to be due to complete heart block and other possible causes are not identifiable
Symptomatic patients with trifascicular block and 1:1 AV conduction: (a) alternating LBBB and RBBB, (b) RBBB and alternating LAFB or LPFB	Asymptomatic patients with trifascicular block and 1:1 AV conduction: (a) alternating LBBB and RBBB, (b) RBBB and alternating LAFB or LPFB
Asymptomatic patients with bundle branch block or bifascicular block with intermittent type II second-degree AV block	Symptomatic patients with markedly prolonged AH interval ($>$100 msec), pacing-induced infra-His block at atrial paced rates of $<$150 beats/min or infranodal block or doubling of the HV interval following administration of drugs

important. Whereas right bundle branch block may occur in otherwise healthy individuals, left bundle branch block is a relatively reliable indicator of cardiac disease. Because of the trifascicular nature of the His-Purkinje system, the presence of right bundle branch block and either of the left fascicular blocks implies a more extensive conduction defect, reflecting the extent of the underlying cardiac involvement. General criteria for pacemaker implantation in patients with different types of intraventricular conduction abnormalities are listed in Table 5.

Bifascicular blocks occur in about 13% of patients with acute myocardial infarction, usually due to extensive anteroseptal or anterolateral infarction. The incidence of complete AV block in these patients varies from 10–50%, and in-hospital mortality doubles, mostly because of heart failure. Therefore, the appearance of bifascicular block in a patient with acute myocardial infarction is considered to be a warning sign for an imminent complete AV block. Patients in whom it occurs should undergo prophylactic temporary pacing. The prophylactic use of a permanent pacemaker is accepted in patients who develop bifascicular block and transient second-degree type II block or third-degree block during acute myocardial infarction.

19

Cardiac and Pulmonary Arrest

I.	Ventricular Tachycardia	399
II.	Ventricular Fibrillation	399
III.	Pulseless Electrical Activity	400
IV.	Brady-Asystolic Arrest	400
V.	Additional Considerations	401

Allan S. Jaffe

The primary determinants of success in the management of cardiac or cardio-pulmonary arrest are the rapidity with which cardiopulmonary resuscitation (CPR) is initiated and the rapidity of definitive therapy to correct underlying pathophysiology. An obvious example is early defibrillation in patients with primary ventricular fibrillation. When early defibrillation is possible, as many as 30–40% of outpatients with cardiac arrest survive without severe neurological sequelae. Prompt assessment of the rhythm and immediate defibrillation are mandatory. In the absence of ventricular fibrillation, when an organized rhythm is present but no pulse is detectable (pulseless electrical activity or PEA, also called electrical mechanical dissociation), or when severe bradycardia (brady-asystolic arrest) is present, therapy must be directed toward reversal of the underlying pathophysiology that led to the arrest. Adequate basic life support (BLS) is essential until the necessary definitive measures can be implemented. Often airway management is less than optimal during CPR and the cause of adverse outcomes. Accordingly, scrutiny of the adequacy of ventilation is essential. In general, CPR must be learned, practiced regularly, and reinforced with periodic retraining.

The usual component of BLS for an apparent victim of cardiac arrest include, in sequence:

1. A call for help. Additional paramedical or medical personnel are of inestimable help. The 911 number should be used if available.
2. Shake the victim by the shoulders and loudly call his or her name to determine whether the victim is conscious.
3. If there is no response, attempt to open the airway with the chin lift maneuver (Figure 1).
4. If spontaneous respirations are not present, ventilate the victim with two long breaths. Observe chest expansion to verify that the breath has been delivered successfully.

   If the victim cannot be ventilated, abdominal thrusts (the Heimlich maneuver) should be repeated 6–8 times in an attempt to clear the airway. Subsequently, another attempt at ventilation should be made. This sequence should continue until adequate ventilation is achieved.
5. Next, check for a carotid pulse.
6. If no pulse is present, begin chest compressions with the hands in the midsternal line one hand above the xiphoid. When only one rescuer is present, 15 compressions at a rate of 80–100 compressions/min should be performed followed by two ventilations. When two rescuers are available, five compressions should be performed at a rate of 80–100 compressions/min followed by one ventilation. The sequence should be

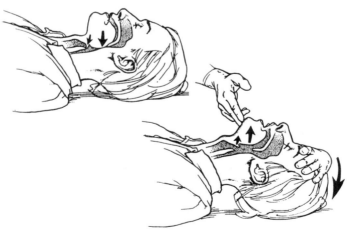

Figure 1 Opening the airway. Top, Airway obstruction by tongue and epiglottis. Bottom, Relief by head tilt with chin lift. (© Copyright American Heart Association. Reproduced with permission from Textbook of advanced cardiac life support, 1994.)

continued until equipment necessary for additional interventions is made available.

When specific arrhythmias are present, they should be managed as follows:

I. VENTRICULAR TACHYCARDIA

Immediate electrical cardioversion is the optimal treatment. A shock of 100 J of energy is usually adequate. When a pulse is present, synchronized cardioversion is indicated if and only if synchronization can be accomplished expeditiously. Otherwise, the advantage of a prompt shock, even if not synchronized, should be exploited.

If sustained ventricular tachycardia (VT) is present with normal blood pressure and no signs or symptoms of hemodynamic compromise or ischemia, lidocaine 1 mg/kg may be helpful. If the VT abates, cardioversion can be avoided. However, if hemodynamic compromise ensues, electrical cardioversion should be implemented immediately.

Recurrent runs of VT may compromise hemodynamics and may require electrical cardioversion. Adjunctive lidocaine 1 mg/kg as an initial bolus followed by three additional boluses of 0.5 mg/kg every 15 min followed by a constant intravenous infusion of 2 mg/min may be helpful in preventing episodes. Procainamide, up to 30 mg/min to a full loading dose of 1 g is an alternative or can be used if lidocaine is ineffective. The loading dose should be followed by a 2 mg/min intravenous infusion. Careful monitoring of the QT interval and QRS duration is essential. Substantial widening of either (greater than 50%) of hypotension should lead to immediate reduction or discontinuation of the infusion.

Torsades de pointes, a variant of ventricular tachycardia, characterized by intermittent alteration of the QRS complex amplitude yielding a "swirling appearance" on the electrocardiogram (ECG) associated with QT prolongation on the basal ECG often responds to magnesium sulfate 2 g given as a slow IV infusion over 5 min or to lidocaine. An isoproterenol infusion may be effective as well.

Short nonsustained runs of ventricular tachycardia do not require treatment in the absence of hemodynamic compromise.

Ventricular tachycardia associated with a pulseless state should be treated in the same way as ventricular fibrillation (VF) is treated.

II. VENTRICULAR FIBRILLATION

The presence of this rhythm requires immediate defibrillation. The paddles must make firm contact with the chest and an appropriate conductive gel or pads must be used. One paddle should be placed in the second to third right intercostal space and one lateral to the midclavicular line. The initial energy setting should be 200 J.

Additional shocks of 300 or 360 J are warranted in rapid succession if VF persists. If a defibrillator is not immediately available, "thump-version" (a firm blow to the chest) may occasionally interrupt VF.

Advanced cardiac life support should be implemented, as with brady-asystolic arrest and pulseless electrical activity. It should include placement of intravenous lines for administration of pharmacological agents, administration of epinephrine 1 mg intravenously every 3 to 5 min, and intubation with vigorous hyperventilation with 100% oxygen. For most purposes, peripheral intravenous lines are adequate. Delivery of pharmacological agents to the central circulation can be enhanced by injecting a bolus of 20–30 mL of saline after administration of each drug to clear dead space in the intravenous line. In the absence of an intravenous conduit, epinephrine can be administered via an endotracheal tube, in which case the dose should be doubled. A central venous line is necessary only if initial resuscitative efforts fail.

Antiarrhythmic drugs are often used when electrical defibrillation alone fails to abolish VF. Lidocaine 1.5 mg/kg is the drug of choice. If VF persists or recurs, bretylium 5 mg/kg and subsequently 10 mg/kg can be administered. After each dose of an antiarrhythmic drug, electrical defibrillation should be attempted again at 300–360 J. Beta blockers and magnesium have been tried in these circumstances as well.

Recurrent ventricular fibrillation with intermittent rhythms associated with a pulse requires loading with procainamide with doses as high as 50 mg/min to a maximum dose of 1 g followed by 2 mg/min via IV infusion. Careful monitoring of the QT interval and QRS duration is mandatory. More than a 50% increase in the QT interval requires reduction or discontinuation of the infusion, as does severe hypotension. Intravenous amiodarone may be helpful as well.

III. PULSELESS ELECTRICAL ACTIVITY

This disturbance, previously called electrical mechanical dissocation, involves slow or fast rhythm with no pulse. The most common correctable abnormalities include pulmonary embolism, cardiac tamponade, pneumothorax, hypovolemia, drug overdose, hyperkalemia, hypothermia, and hypoxia. While the possible presence of these factors is being ascertained, intubation and ventilation with 100% oxygen, frequent doses of intravenous epinephrine (at least 1 mg every 3 to 5 min), as well as basic life support are essential. If a tension pneumothorax or cardiac tamponade is suspected, immediate insertion of a needle into the pleural or pericardial space is required for decompression.

IV. BRADY-ASYSTOLIC ARREST

End-stage heart disease and high mortality accompany this condition often. Pacing often fails once asystole has occurred but can be effective in preventing the progression of bradycardia to arrest. Either transvenous or external pacing should be implemented.

Once asystole has occurred, pharmacological agents are rarely effective. Atropine in 1 mg aliquots to a maximum dose of 0.04 mg/kg may be helpful. Atropine can be administered via an endotracheal tube, in which case the dose should be doubled. Aminophylline 250 mg, given as a slow intravenous bolus, may restore an effective rhythm. Definitive correction of underlying abnormalities is critical. Hypoxia, hyperkalemia, drug overdose, or hypothermia may be responsible; if so, it must be corrected expeditiously.

V. ADDITIONAL CONSIDERATIONS

1. Hyperventilation can vasodilate cerebral vessels. Therefore, modest hyperventilation after restoration of spontaneous circulation is desirable.
2. Transient hypertension can increase cerebral perfusion and can be induced pharmacologically during the first 20–30 min of restored, spontaneous circulation.
3. An FIO_2 of 100% is continued until measurements (by co-oximetry or blood gas determination) verify safe, gradual reduction without compromise of PaO_2.
4. Catecholamines administered to correct hypotension may induce arrhythmias. Thus, careful observation of the blood pressure for 1–3 min after the return of spontaneous circulation is prudent before initiating them and cautious initial titration is essential.
5. Acidosis is common after the return of spontaneous circulation. Hydrogen ions—which have been trapped in tissues and in the venous circulation because of reduced pulmonary perfusion—enter the systemic circulation. Buffers such as bicarbonate are not necessary and may be detrimental by decreasing cardiac performance. The generation of CO_2 in blood may paradoxically exacerbate intracellular acidosis.
6. After arrests attributable to ventricular tachycardia or fibrillation, lidocaine is used often to prevent recurrences. The dose is the same as that used for the treatment of ventricular tachycardia.
7. The underlying cause of the arrest (e.g., myocardial ischemia, hypoxia, electrolyte imbalances, and numerous others) should be identified and corrected.

401

Evaluation and Management of the Survivor of Cardiac Arrest

I.	Evaluation of Survivors of Cardiac Arrest	406
II.	Noninvasive Laboratory Studies	407
III.	Invasive Laboratory Studies	412
IV.	Therapeutic Approach to the Survivor of Cardiac Arrest	416
V.	Conclusion	420
	Suggested Reading	420

Mark E. Josephson

There is, perhaps, no more demanding need in the care of patients with cardio-vascular disease than the need to properly categorize and treat survivors of a cardiac arrest and to identify subjects at high risk of this tragic event so that prevention can be accomplished. The extensive information that must be considered requires judgment on the part of the primary care physician as well as the specialist, predicated on principles and phenomena elucidated only recently. Accordingly, we shall devote considerable attention to the topic and some of its technical considerations as well.

Among the more than 300,000 people who suffer cardiac arrest yearly, only a minority survive sufficiently long to permit hospitalization and only a subset of those who do can leave the hospital functionally intact. Although public education has improved awareness of the phenomenon and increasing availability of para-medical support has improved outcome, no more than 5–15% of such victims are presently resuscitated such that they can ultimately leave the hospital. Thus, identification of patients who are at particularly high risk of developing cardiac arrest is essential so that it can be prevented.

For the nearly 35,000 successfully resuscitated victims of cardiac arrest, the main contributions of the physician are identification of the cause of the cardiac arrest, correction of underlying contributing factors, and development of effective regimens to prevent recurrence. Thus, the physician must understand the pathophysiological substrate and mechanisms responsible for cardiac arrest.

Cardiac arrest can be defined as an instantaneous loss of pump function leading to immediate loss of consciousness and death within 1 hr. Although there are many potential causes (e.g., pulmonary embolism, aortic dissection, cardiac rupture, pulseless electrical activity—often called electromechanical dissociation), most episodes are attributable to arrhythmias. Lethal arrhythmias include ventricular tachyarrhythmias and bradyarrhythmias and/or asystole. Rarely supraventricular tachycardias with rapid ventricular responses can cause cardiac arrest either directly or because of progression to ventricular fibrillation secondary to compromised cardiac function.

Tachycardias are responsible for 80–85% of arrhythmic cardiac arrests. Bradyarrhythmias, usually associated with electromechanical dissociation and heart failure, comprise the remainder. Holter monitoring data obtained at the time of arrests have generally demonstrated rapidly accelerated uniform or polymorphic tachycardia precipitating ventricular fibrillation (Figures 1 to 3). When arrest is caused by ventricular tachycardia, the rates of success of resuscitation and

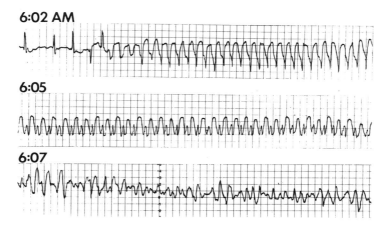

Figure 1   Holter recording from a patient with spontaneous cardiac arrest. Cardiac arrest is initiated at 6:02 A.M. by rather late coupled extrasystoles which initiate a uniform ventricular tachycardia. The tachycardia widens after 3 min (middle strip) and subsequently degenerates to ventricular fibrillation at 6:07 A.M.

404

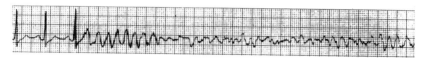

Figure 2 Cardiac arrest induced by rapidly accelerating polymorphic tachycardia. Following three beats of sinus rhythm, a very short coupled PVC initiates a rapidly accelerating polymorphic tachycardia that within a few seconds degenerates to ventricular fibrillation. (From Harrison's Principles of Internal Medicine. 12th ed. Wilson JD et al., eds. New York: McGraw-Hill, 1991, Fig. 185-12.)

subsequent survival are highest. Bradyarrhythmias are usually seen in patients with severe myocardial dysfunction. Asystole or electromechanical dissociation are causes of approximately 50% of the deaths in patients with class IV heart failure.

The most common underlying structural heart disease in patients suffering cardiac arrest is coronary artery disease, present in 75% of patients. Among these, 75% have significant coronary artery disease; 75% of patients with coronary artery disease have prior infarction, two-thirds have greater than 75% stenosis of three vessels, 70–75% harbor a recent thrombus (30% of which produce greater than 75% occlusion). However, total occlusion of a vessel is rare. Acute myocardial infarction is present in only 10–20%; recurrent arrest is rare in such patients.

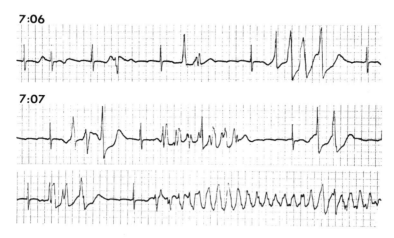

Figure 3 Cardiac arrest induced by torsades de pointes. In the top panel, during atrial fibrillation, a markedly long QT interval is readily seen, which is exacerbated following long pauses. Multiple ventricular premature contractions (VPCs) are followed by pauses, which initiate runs of longer VPCs, ultimately culminating in a polymorphic VT producing cardiac arrest, seen in the bottom panel.

Significant ST-segment changes compatible with ischemia occur in only 10–15% of victims of cardiac arrest as judged from Holter data. Thus, although ischemia may be present and may trigger the event, it does not appear to be the dominant factor.

A trend of increasing heart rate and increasing frequency of ventricular premature contractions (VPCs) often precedes the fatal event, even if no arrhythmias had been noted earlier or on Holter recordings. Thus, an autonomic change may be associated with predisposition to an acute event. Cardiac arrest occurs with the same circadian variability as myocardial infarction. Its peak incidence is in the midmorning hours.

Some 5–10% of patients suffering cardiac arrest have no structural heart disease, especially young subjects. In such patients, electrolyte abnormalities, proarrhythmic drug effects, substance abuse, the long-QT syndrome, or preexcitation with atrial fibrillation–induced ventricular fibrillation may be responsible. In patients less than 30 years of age, hypertrophic cardiomyopathy is an important underlying abnormality. Ventricular hypertrophy seems to be an important independent risk factor for sudden cardiac death at all ages.

I. EVALUATION OF SURVIVORS OF CARDIAC ARREST

Survivors of cardiac arrest require careful evaluation of factors that could have contributed to the initiation of the arrest, the pathophysiological mechanisms of an arrhythmia that could have produced the arrest, and definition of the type and extent of underlying cardiac pathology that could have been responsible for the arrest and will influence the prognosis following the arrest. The history, physical exam, and electrocardiogram (ECG) can provide insight into underlying heart disease responsible for the cardiac arrest. The presence of coronary artery disease with previous infarction and/or angina at the time of the arrest, congestive heart failure, or a family history of sudden death are particularly important factors to identify. A positive family history often provides a clue to familial disorders associated with sudden cardiac death, such as hypertension, hypertrophic cardiomyopathy, and a congenital long-QT syndrome, each of which is a relatively more common cause of cardiac arrest in young patients. The physician exam can point toward aortic stenosis, hypertrophic cardiomyopathy, congestive heart failure, or pulmonary embolism. The ECG can document previous infarction, hypertrophy, ventricular preexcitation, a long QT interval (particularly in excess of 0.50 sec) and arrhythmogenic right ventricular dysplasia. Arrhythmogenic right ventricular dysplasia, suggested by T-wave inversion in the anterior precordial leads, is associated with small deflections (at the end of the QRS) termed "epsilon waves" that represent delayed activation over the right ventricle (Figure 10 in Chapter 17).

Electrolyte abnormalities may play a role in the genesis of some of lethal arrhythmias, but a cause-and-effect relationship of the arrhythmia to the electrolyte abnormality is difficult to prove. Hypokalemia may be present in patients after arrest because of the impact of endogenous or exogenous catecholamines, which shift potassium into cells. It can be exaggerated by hyperventilation-induced respiratory alkalosis during resuscitation. The presence of a long QT interval and giant U waves suggests that hypokalemia *may* have played a causative role. Hyperkalemia is an important cause of cardiac arrest and is frequently iatrogenic. Its ECG manifestations include a widened QRS, loss of the ST segment, peaked T waves, and a slow heart rate often associated with severe ventricular dysfunction and a "sine wave–like" ventricular tachycardia. Often, such findings are secondary to the arrest rather than causal. A history of diabetes, renal failure, or use of angiotensin converting enzyme (ACE) inhibitors in combination with potassium supplements or potassium-sparing diuretics points toward true, hyperkalemic arrest. A toxic screen should be performed, particularly when ECG abnormalities are present (e.g., long-QT or T-wave abnormalities) for drugs with proarrhythmic effects. Digoxin, antiarrhythmic agents, tricyclic antidepressants, phenothiazines, cocaine, antihistamines, and numerous other agents may be implicated.

II. NONINVASIVE LABORATORY STUDIES

Noninvasive studies can define anatomic and physiological factors that could trigger or perpetuate arrhythmic causes death and identify the cardiac structural disorders potentially responsible. The single strongest predictor of recurrent cardiac arrest and reduced long-term survival is impaired left ventricular function. Although left ventricular ejection fraction is the standard variable used to judge left ventricular function, functional capacity is at least as important. For example, a left ventricular ejection fraction of 15% produced by an isolated large ventricular aneurysm in a patient with single-vessel disease and New York Heart Association (NYHA) class I to II functional capacity is associated with a better prognosis than a 30% ejection fraction in a patient with angina and NYHA class III congestive heart failure.

A. Echocardiography

Echocardiography provides information delineating both systolic and diastolic ventricular function, specific structural or anatomic abnormalities that may be cause of cardiac arrest, and the presence or absence of hypertrophic cardiomyopathy or dilated cardiomyopathy, which signify a poor prognosis. Valvular disorders and specific entities such as cardiac amyloidosis can be recognized. Regardless of etiology, the worse the ejection fraction, the worse the outcome.

Although echocardiography can provide information about left ventricular ejection fraction, until three-dimensional echocardiography becomes generally available, the accuracy of assessment of ejection fraction by echocardiography will be limited. However, assessment of wall motion during exercise or infusion of dobutamine to induce physiological stress if helpful. Depression of left ventricular function in response to either type of stress defines high risk.

Exercise nuclear ventriculography provides better assessment of ejection fraction at rest and with exercise than does echocardiography, but it does not provide as much structural information. Depressed left ventricular function at rest and during exercise, detected by this method, is an independent predictor of long-term survival after cardiac arrest. Because the echocardiogram provides structural information as well, it is a better guide to subsequent evaluation and treatment.

B. Exercise Testing and Nuclear Imaging

In addition to providing information about left ventricular function, exercise testing is most often used to detect the presence and severity of coronary artery disease, usually with thallium or sestamibi. Both tracers require assessment at rest and during exercise for acquisition of information relative to the extent of scar tissue and reversible ischemia. In patients in whom exercise is not possible, dipyridamole or adenosine may be given with thallium to assess effects of vasodilation in response to these agents on myocardial perfusion. The combination of left ventriculography with thallium or sestamibi scintigraphy provides complementary information regrading the functional significance of coronary disease. Should extensive coronary disease be present, it may be difficult to define significant heterogeneity in myocardial perfusion. However, exercise-induced lung uptake and/or decreased left ventricular ejection fraction are hallmarks of three-vessel coronary artery disease. Such findings may be seen also with myopathic ventricles. Exercise scintigraphy is helpful in patients with relatively normal ejection fractions at rest in whom detection of large regions of reversible ischemia may be a major clue that the cardiac arrest was secondary to myocardial ischemia. Of note, however, is the fact that malignant arrhythmias are rarely induced during an exercise test.

In the absence of significant ventricular dysfunction and previous infarction, a patient surviving a cardiac arrest who has a large reversible defect by thallium scintigraphy can be treated successfully by revascularization alone. Newer procedures such as magnetic resonance imaging (MRI) and positron emission tomography (PET) may be useful in individual cases to detect specific abnormalities, either physiological or anatomic, but they are too expensive and are not widely enough available to be commonly or routinely employed. One specific indication for MRI is suspicion of arrhythmogenic right ventricular dysplasia, because of its power to characterize myocardial tissue and differentiate fatty degeneration of the right ventricular wall, characteristic of arrhythmogenic right ventricular dysplasia, from thinned myocardium. Positron emission tomography may be especially useful in distinguishing viable myocardium that is dysfunctional because of ischemic, hibernating, but still viable myocardium from zones of infarction and fixed, irreversibly damaged myocardium from zones of reversible insult.

C. Holter Monitoring

Recent information has demonstrated marked limitations of Holter monitoring for the assessment of patients at risk for recurrent cardiac arrest. In the first week after arrest, high-grade ectopy, nonsustained ventricular tachycardia, and recurrent cardiac arrest are not uncommon. They reflect instability secondary to the arrest as well as the persistence of an inciting mechanism (i.e., ischemia, hypokalemia, proarrhythmia, etc.). Once a patient is stable and has been discharged from the hospital, Holter monitoring provides far less valuable information than does assessment of left ventricular function. In the absence of left ventricular dysfunction, the presence of arrhythmias on Holter monitoring has little prognostic significance.

The use of spontaneous ectopy as a surrogate endpoint for the prevention of sudden cardiac arrest is at best controversial. Two important facts highlight its limitations. First, even in those studies indicating that suppression of arrhythmias may improve survival, neither the risk imposed by ventricular ectopy nor the effect of pharmacological suppression of the ectopy to prevent sudden death were independent of left ventricular dysfunction. Thus, spontaneous ectopy may be a reflection of the underlying cardiac dysfunction without any direct impact on the mechanism of death, sudden or nonsudden. In fact, several studies have shown that the presence of ventricular ectopy (simple, complex, or nonsustained ventricular tachycardia), myocardial infarction may often be associated with a high risk of sudden death. However, the same features are markers of high risk of nonsudden death. Thus, the ratio of deaths that are sudden compared to total deaths is independent of the presence or frequency of spontaneous ectopy. Ectopy remains a marker for both ventricular dysfunction and a high risk for dying, but it is not sufficiently specific to portend how the patient will succumb.

The most telling argument against the use of Holter monitoring to identify the high-risk subject and thereby prevent sudden cardiac death is based on the Cardiac Arrhythmia Suppression Trial (CAST) results, in which suppression of ventricular ectopy in a relatively low-risk patient population with coronary artery disease was associated with a nearly threefold increase in sudden cardiac death compared with the incidence in patients in whom suppression of ectopy was not attempted. Although this dichotomy may be related to induction of proarrhythmia by the agents used in the study, it nonetheless demonstrates that abolition of ectopy is not a criterion of reduced risk of sudden death and that the presence of ectopy does not imply a poor outcome. Thus, Holter monitoring to assess risk and guide therapy in patients who have been resuscitated from sudden cardiac death is controversial.

Nevertheless, Holter monitoring may be useful in patients after myocardial infarction; in those with recurrent asymptomatic ST-segment changes (silent ischemia), which appears to be associated with a higher mortality, both sudden and nonsudden; and, accordingly, in those who do not have angina but are still at high risk. Such findings indicate the need for further evaluation to delineate the extent and physiological consequences of coronary artery disease.

D. Autonomic Testing

Another more recent use of Holter monitoring is in the assessment of heart rate variability as a measure of autonomic tone. Heart rate variability grossly reflects changes in mean heart rate throughout the day, which, in turn, is a reflection of the influence of parasympathetic and sympathetic forces on the sinus node. Patients with low heart rate variability (< 50-msec difference in RR intervals) have a threefold higher mortality than those with heart rate variabilities exceeding 100 msec. Such data apply to patients who have survived a remote myocardial infarction and those with congestive heart failure. Even brief periods of Holter monitoring may be sufficient to gather such information. Breakdown of heart rate variability into its frequency components (assessment of the power spectra) does not appear to provide significant additional descriptors for the risk of sudden death.

The absence of heart rate variability reflects enhanced sympathetic tone and withdrawal of parasympathetic tone, either primarily or secondarily. Abnormal autonomic tone detected by other measurements is commonly associated with impaired heart rate variability. Thus, the autonomic abnormality may be primary. Baroreceptor reflex sensitivity in experimental animals and in patients is a valuable prognostic indicator after myocardial infarction. Both impaired heart rate variability and baroreceptor reflex sensitivity portend an increased risk of death after acute myocardial infarction. However, their value for risk assessment after resuscitation from cardiac arrest is unclear.

In patients suffering cardiac arrest while being monitored with a Holter recorder, an increase in heart rate and an increase in ectopy often occurs before the lethal arrhythmia. Thus, sympathetic tone may increase in the moments immediately preceding cardiac arrest. The circadian occurrence of cardiac arrest (higher incidence in the midmorning hours) correlates with the periodicity of increased sympathetic activity.

E. Signal-Averaged Electrocardiography

In the setting of coronary artery disease, signal-averaged electrocardiography elucidates the extent of abnormalities of slow conduction that form a substrate for malignant ventricular arrhythmia. In the absence of bundle branch block, criteria for abnormal late potentials include (a) a filtered (> 40 Hz) QRS duration exceeding 120 msec; (b) mean voltage in the last 40 msec of less than 20 uV; and (c) a duration of a terminal signal that is less than 49 uV for more than 38 msec. Such abnormalities have been found in 20–30% of patients within 1 month of acute myocardial infarction. Unfortunately, they have a positive predictive value of only 15–25% for the development of ventricular tachycardia or sudden cardiac death. The negative predictive value exceeds 95% (i.e., the *absence* of a positive signal averaged ECG correlates with subsequent freedom from such arrhythmic events). Improvement in the positive predictive value of this test can be accomplished by adding assessment of left ventricular function. Several studies have demonstrated that the combination of a low ejection fraction (< 40%) and an abnormal signal-averaged ECG has a predictive accuracy of about 35% for development of sudden cardiac death or ventricular tachycardia in the first year after myocardial infarction. The absence of left ventricular dysfunction coupled with a normal signal-averaged ECG is associated with nearly 100% freedom from these events.

In survivors of cardiac arrest secondary to coronary artery disease, a positive signal-averaged ECG is present in only approximately 50–60%, compared with 85% of patients presenting with sustained monomorphic ventricular tachycardia. This reflects a lesser extent of abnormalities of conduction in patients with cardiac arrest, a finding compatible with the shorter cycle lengths of arrhythmias producing cardiac arrest. Nevertheless, the presence of an abnormal signal-averaged ECG in a patient resuscitated from cardiac arrest is highly associated with the potential for induction of a sustained tachycardia. Thus, survivors of cardiac arrest with positive signal-averaged ECGs have more than an 80% chance of having an inducible sustained monomorphic ventricular tachycardia. By contrast, those with a normal signal-averaged ECG rarely exhibit an inducible monomorphic ventricular tachycardia. In such patients, induction of either no arrhythmia or polymorphic ventricular tachycardia/ventricular fibrillation is much more likely.

The value of signal-averaged electrocardiography in patients without coronary artery disease, particularly those presenting with dilated or hypertrophic cardiomyopathy, is uncertain. A positive signal-averaged ECG may be seen in idiopathic dilated cardiomyopathy at high risk of sudden death, and its absence may predict freedom from sudden cardiac death caused by tachyarrhythmias. However, the fact that sudden death in patients with severe heart failure may be due to bradyarrhythmias, as a reflection of end-stage pump failure, and the poorly understood mechanism of ventricular arrhythmias associated with heart failure, may account for the inconsistency of results that have been reported. Positive signal-averaged ECGs have been found in nearly 20% of patients with hypertrophic cardiomyopathy, but the predictive value of this finding with respect to sudden cardiac death is unknown.

Patients without apparent heart disease rarely have a positive signal-averaged ECG, but false positives can occur in as many as 10–15%. A markedly abnormal signal-averaged ECG in a patient with apparently normal left ventricular function may be a clue to the presence of arrhythmogenic right ventricular dysplasia. In such patients, the signal-averaged ECG is profoundly abnormal.

III. INVASIVE LABORATORY STUDIES

All patients without a documented precipitating cause for cardiac arrest should undergo complete cardiac catheterization and an electrophysiological study to clarify both the underlying anatomic and functional substrates present (which determine the propensity for recurrence) and to guide pharmacological and/or nonpharmacological therapy.

A. Cardiac Catheterization

In patients suspected of having coronary artery disease and potentially having had ischemia-mediated cardiac arrest, cardiac catheterization is undertaken to assess left ventricular function and the extent of coronary artery disease, both of which are critical determinants of overall survival. Left ventricular dysfunction and reduced ejection fraction are the most predictive risk factors for recurrent events in the first 6 months following resuscitation, with a threefold increase of risk of sudden death when ejection fraction is less than 30%. Approximately 75% of patients who have experienced cardiac arrest will have coronary artery disease, and two-thirds of these will have triple-vessel disease. Left ventricular aneurysms will be present in 20–40% of patients. Although coronary anatomy and the presence of an aneurysm are not specific predictors of recurrent cardiac arrest, failure to induce revascularization is an important predictor of recurrence. The Coronary Artery Surgery Study (CASS), comprising nearly 20,000 patients, clearly demonstrated that the incidence of overall cardiac death and sudden cardiac death is reduced by coronary revascularization, particularly in patients with impaired left ventricular function. The coronary anatomy, however, is not distinctly different in patients who die suddenly compared with those who do not.

Right and left ventriculography should be performed. If a primary myopathic process is implicated, ventricular biopsy may be useful. The presence of acute inflammation suggesting active myocarditis may shed light on the mechanism of the cardiac arrest. Whether or not anti-inflammatory or immunosuppressive agents influence outcome is unclear.

Rare congenital anomalies of the coronary arteries or focal wall motion abnormalities missed by echocardiography may be recognized during cardiac catheterization. The presence of severe coronary artery disease mandates therapy targeted toward that coronary disease, even though the coronary disease may not be the precipitating mechanism of the arrhythmia. A favorable long-term prognosis depends on prevention of progression of coronary disease and congestive heart failure. Patients with important coronary artery disease and normal ejection fraction should undergo thallium exercise testing. Documentation of severe ischemia suggests that the cardiac arrest was primarily attributable to ischemia and that recurrence can be prevented by revascularization.

B. Electrophysiological Evaluation

Unless the specific cause of the arrest has been documented, all patients suffering a cardiac arrest should undergo a *complete* electrophysiological study in order to (a) identify patients with inducible sustained ventricular tachyarrhythmias, (b) identify an arrhythmogenic substrate in patients without inducible arrhythmias, (c) identify other arrhythmic mechanisms (e.g., supraventricular tachyarrhythmias) responsible for cardiac arrest, and (d) guide pharmacological or nonpharmacological choices of therapy.

Because the most common mechanism of cardiac arrest is a sustained ventricular tachyarrhythmia, the first objective of the electrophysiology study is to determine whether protocol, which involves at least three ventricular extrastimuli delivered from at least two sites using at least two different basic drive cycle lengths, 40–85% of patients (depending on patient population) will exhibit a sustained uniform or polymorphic ventricular tachycardia induced. In the setting of coronary artery disease, sustained tachyarrhythmias can be induced in 55–85% of patients. The incidence of inducibility depends on the substrate. In patients with previous infarction, the incidence approaches 85%. In those without a history of infarction, the incidence is lower. Although the induction of uniform sustained monomorphic tachycardia is a considered to be a highly specific response and can be treated as such, controversy about the specificity of polymorphic ventricular tachycardia–ventricular fibrillation (VT-VF) induction remains. The induction of polymorphic VT-VF is considered to be a nonspecific response in patients without a history of cardiac arrest or in those who present with sustained uniform ventricular tachycardia, a higher incidence of induction of this arrhythmia, occurring with less aggressive programmed stimulation, occurs in patients who survive cardiac arrest. Although the induction of sustained ventricular arrhythmias with cardiac arrest requires triple extrastimuli in nearly two-thirds of patients, the induction of monomorphic ventricular tachycardia is never seen in normal subjects regardless of the number of extrastimuli; and the induction of sustained polymorphic ventricular tachycardia with comparable stimulation protocols is one-fifth to one-tenth as common as that observed in patients resuscitated from cardiac arrest. Thus, in patients who present with a cardiac arrest, suppression of induction of polymorphic VT-VF *may* be a meaningful target for therapy.

In the absence of coronary artery disease, the value of programmed stimulation, in terms of induction of ventricular arrhythmias, is uncertain. Although patients presenting with uniform sustained ventricular tachycardia and cardiomyopathy can have their tachycardia replicated, the success of treatment of this arrhythmia does not predict outcome, which is generally poor. However, bundle branch reentry may be a cause of cardiac arrest in patients with dilated cardiomyopathies or valvular heart disease and is a treatable form of arrhythmia by radiofrequency catheter ablation (see Chapter 16). Programmed stimulation in patients with arrhythmogenic right ventricular dysplasia is useful also because of the high specificity of induced arrhythmia in relation to clinical events in this condition. Thus, in patients who have a well-defined substrate such as previous infarction or arrhythmogenic dysplasia, programmed ventricular stimulation is an important tool for ascertaining the mechanism underlying the cardiac arrest.

If sustained arrhythmias are inducible, their suppression may be used as targets for therapy. The significance of induction of nonsustained ventricular arrhythmias or no ventricular arrhythmias is unknown. Although it had previously been felt that a survivor of cardiac arrest with no inducible arrhythmia was at low risk, it is now clear that patients with cardiomyopathy or even those with no structural heart disease have a high recurrence rate (10–40%) within 2 years.

In the patient with coronary artery disease who has no inducible arrhythmia, a sinus rhythm map of the left ventricle should be performed to assess the presence and extent of abnormal electrograms on the endocardial surface. Fragmented electrograms represent an abnormally slow propagation through fibers separated by scar tissue, the characteristic arrhythmogenic substrate. Although extensive regions with locally abnormal electrograms are often reflected in an abnormal signal-averaged ECG and extensive infarction may be reflected by abnormal 12-lead surface ECGs, sometimes the surface markers are inapparent. Under these conditions, mapping can document the substrate. If no substrate is present and the patient has significant coronary artery disease, the likely mechanism of the arrest (assuming that the remainder of the electrophysiology study is normal) is ischemia, and therapy should be directed toward that alone. If, however, extensive regions of abnormal conduction are observed, the risk of recurrence is high and an antifibrillation device should be implanted.

In addition to induction of ventricular arrhythmias, electrophysiologic studies may demonstrate other causes of cardiac arrest. Occasionally patients will have preexcitation that may or may not be evident on the surface ECG but is associated with cardiac arrest and can be documented by an electrophysiologic study, typically the case in patients with left-sided bypass tracts, particularly when accompanied by intraatrial conduction defects. In such patients, atrial fibrillation should be induced and the potential for developing ventricular fibrillation assessed (Figure 4). In such patients, who are almost always young, ablation of the bypass tract is curative.

414

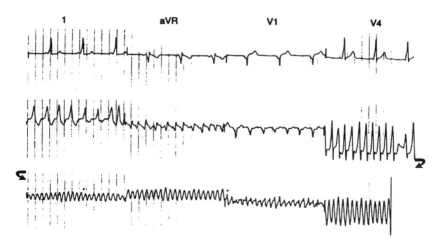

Figure 4 Wolff-Parkinson-White syndrome producing ventricular fibrillation. Leads I, aV_R, V_1, and V_4 are shown in the top in sinus rhythm. In the middle panel, atrial fibrillation develops and the ventricular response clearly accelerates and degenerates to ventricular fibrillation in the bottom panel.

Rarely, such patients may manifest flutter with 1:1 conduction, which can precipitate cardiac arrest. The identification of this rhythm mandates ablative therapy to eliminate the flutter or induction of AV block and the implantation of a permanent pacemaker, particularly if the ventricular rate cannot be slowed easily with antiarrhythmic agents.

In patients with hypertrophic cardiomyopathy, atrial arrhythmias may be an important cause of cardiac arrest. Supraventricular tachyarrhythmias occur in nearly 15% of such patients. Conduction system abnormalities, producing brady-cardias or occasionally associated with bundle branch reentry, can be seen in 33%. Sustained ventricular tachycardias, the vast majority of which are polymorphic, can be precipitated in patients with hypertrophic cardiomyopathy. These arrhyth-mias appear to be markers of risk only when the patient has presented with cardiac arrest or syncope. As with coronary disease, the polymorphic VT-VF may be relatively specific as a marker of risk. However, in patients with hypertrophic cardiomyopathy who have no symptoms, induction of such arrhythmias does not seem to entail increased risk.

Programmed stimulation is useful in guiding antiarrhythmic therapy. The capacity of a pharmacological agent to prevent inducibility of a sustained ven-tricular tachycardia correlates with its capacity to decrease incidence of recur-rence of that arrhythmia. Persistent inducibility of arrhythmias is associated with poor prognosis compared with rendering the arrhythmia noninducible. However,

415

the clinical impact of the difference depends on the extent of left ventricular function. In patients with ejection fraction greater than 30%, rendering the tachycardia noninducible by drugs is associated with a good prognosis, with about 90% survival at 3 years. However, if a patient has an ejection fraction of less than 30% and the arrhythmia is suppressed by pharmacological agents, the 3-year mortality remains high (i.e., 40%). Although survival is significantly better than that in patients with low ejection fractions in whom ventricular tachyarrhythmias remain nonsuppressed (3-year mortality of > 50%), the absolute mortality (40%) may be unacceptably high. Thus, alternative therapies, particularly in young people, may be needed, such as use of an implantable cardioverter/defibrillator (ICD).

Overall, persistent inducibility of an arrhythmia entails a fourfold risk of sudden death. A low ejection fraction entails a threefold risk of sudden death. The combination of both increases risk of death tenfold.

The capability of pharmacological agents to slow a poorly tolerated tachycardia so that it is hemodynamically better tolerated has been associated with a reduced incidence of sudden death, although recurrent ventricular tachycardia may occur in nearly 50% of such patients within 3 years. In contrast, lack of slowing of ventricular tachyarrhythmia by pharmacological agents has been associated with a 50% greater increased risk of sudden death. In general, it appears that if a tachycardia can be rendered hemodynamically stable, even though the patient is likely to have a better prognosis, the risk of recurrent cardiac arrest will remain approximately 20% within 2 years.

There is not drug which has been proven to be uniquely superior for prevention of cardiac arrest. Several drugs, including class IA and III agents, including sotalol and amiodarone, may be used. Combination of drugs may also be tried. If three drug trials fail to either prevent the initiation of the arrhythmia or to slow it to a tolerable rate, nonpharmacological therapy is likely to be required.

IV. THERAPEUTIC APPROACH TO THE SURVIVOR OF CARDIAC ARREST

The first objective in managing the survivor of a cardiac arrest is to correct all potentially reversible causes or contributors to that arrest. Plasma electrolyte concentrations should be normalized. Heart failure and ischemia must be treated. If surgical revascularization is necessary, the potential role of an electrophysiological abnormality in the setting of coronary artery disease must be considered, so that surgical ablation can be implemented, if necessary, at the time of revascularization. In a patient who has sustained cardiac arrest in the setting of acute myocardial infarction, workup other than risk stratification is not indicated. Cardiac arrest in this setting does not carry with it, per se, any increased risk of recurrence.

Because most patients with cardiac arrest have coronary artery disease and because electrophysiological studies will usually demonstrate an inducible arrhythmia in most, initial therapy can be directed by the electrophysiological study. Because patients with low ejection fractions ($< 30\%$) have a poor prognosis with pharmacological therapy, even if it renders the tachycardia noninducible, nonpharmacological approaches to prevention of recurrent sudden death should be undertaken, including revascularization and the use of an implantable ICD (Figure 5). In selected patients who have uniform monomorphic sustained tachycardia induced as a cause of their cardiac arrest, map-guided surgical ablation of the arrhythmia can be curative. This approach is, in fact, preferable to other forms of therapy, because the arrhythmogenic substrate and potential precipitating causes (ischemia and heart failure) can be addressed in one procedure. Despite the fact that surgery entails considerable mortality (15%), long-term gains are considerable, with improvement in left ventricular function, reduction of ischemia, and freedom from arrhythmia being the best seen with any form of treatment.

In centers where this procedure is not available and in patients who are at excessively high risk, ICD implantation, preferably with a nonthoracotomy lead system, should be employed after revascularization. Although an epicardial lead system can be implanted at the time of surgery, such systems are associated with a complicated postoperative course and add to the morbidity of subsequent revascularization procedures.

In patients who have polymorphic ventricular tachyarrhythmia, an ICD and

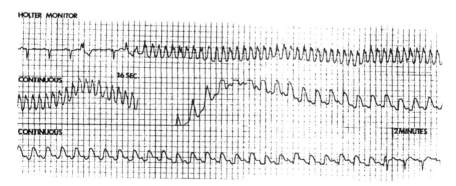

Figure 5 Successful termination of ventricular tachycardia by automatic defibrillator. A Holter recording is shown obtained during a spontaneous cardiac arrest. In the top panel, a rapid ventricular tachycardia is initiated: a short-long-short sequence. The tachycardia is uniform in morphology with a rate of approximately 250 beats/min. The patient lost consciousness and had cardiac arrest, which was aborted after 16 sec by a discharge from the automatic implantable defibrillator, resulting in sinus rhythm. ST elevation noted immediately after conversion resolved within 2 min (lower right-hand panel).

417

revascularization with optimization of heart failure should be implemented. In patients who have an ejection fraction greater than 30%, the prognosis with successful pharmacological therapy is excellent. Thus, serial drug testing of diverse pharmacological agents can be accomplished with programmed stimulation, and the drug that renders the tachycardia noninducible or hemodynamically stable is acceptable. Revascularization, if necessary, should be undertaken.

An ICD provides an additional option in patients in whom tachycardia remains inducible and rapid or in those who prefer this approach to programmed stimulation and multiple drug trials.

In patients with coronary artery disease who have no inducible arrhythmia, the therapeutic approach depends on the nature and extent of the anatomic substrate. If coronary artery disease is severe but no electrophysiological substrate can be defined—as judged from the absence of a positive signal-averaged ECG, lack of evidence of Q-wave infarction in three adjacent surface leads, and lack of abnormalities of conduction in more than 30% of the endocardium—cardiac arrest can be assumed to be a result of ischemia. This interpretation is supported further by a positive exercise test. In such patients, revascularization should be the primary therapy. In a patient with no inducible arrhythmia but with evidence of an arrhythmogenic substrate, revascularization plus use of an ICD is preferred because of the lack of specific targets with which to judge the efficacy of pharmacologic therapy.

In patients without coronary artery disease or arrhythmogenic right ventricular dysplasia, including those with idiopathic dilated cardiomyopathy, hypertrophic cardiomyopathy, or idiopathic ventricular fibrillation, there is no objective means by which to assess therapy directed toward prevention of ventricular tachyarrhythmias. In such patients, the ICD is a mainstay of therapy to prevent sudden cardiac death. In patient with arrhythmogenic right ventricular dysplasia, pharmacologic agents can be used as in patients with coronary artery disease. If sustained monomorphic tachycardia is induced with or without drugs, a surgical procedure requiring disarticulation of the right ventricle can be employed to prevent clinically important arrhythmias, despite the high morbidity of the procedure. An ICD is an appropriate alternative.

Several specific disorders require individualized treatment. In patients whose electrophysiological study has demonstrated the presence of Wolff-Parkinson-White syndrome with life-threatening arrhythmias caused by the bypass tract, radiofrequency catheter ablation of the bypass tract can prevent recurrences. In the small percentage of patients in whom radiofrequency ablation is not successful, pharmacological or surgical therapy can be employed. In patients in whom supraventricular arrhythmias without bypass tracts cause cardiac arrest, ablative techniques and permanent pacemaker implantation can be employed to either destroy the arrhythmogenic focus or prevent a rapid ventricular response by the inducing heart block. These are important alternatives to pharmacological ap-

418

proaches, which may be undertaken as well. Such patients usually require class IA or IC agents or amiodarone to control the ventricular response or the arrhythmia itself. In a small group of patients, heart block may lead to the development of torsades de pointes and cardiac arrest. In them, pacemaker implantation can prevent recurrent torsades de pointes and hence cardiac arrest (Figure 6). They should be distinguished from patients in whom torsades de pointes is a proarrhythmic manifestation of an antiarrhythmic agent.

The possibility of a drug-induced arrhythmia should always be considered in patients with polymorphic tachycardias associated with long QT intervals. In such patients, removal of the offending agent and substitution of an agent that does not result in QT prolongation is preferred.

Patients with the idiopathic, congenital long-QT-interval syndrome should be treated with maximally tolerated doses of beta blockers. If marked (> 0.50 sec) QT prolongation still persists, particularly if QT prolongation is exacerbated by exercise, the patient is considered to be at high risk. A left thoracic sympathectomy or use of an ICD may be helpful. However, recurrent shocks with an ICD for nonsustained episodes may occur over several decades, with profound psychological and social stress. Accordingly, thoracic sympathectomy (which is not complicated by Horner syndrome, in contrast to the case with cervical sympathectomies) is appropriate. If the QT interval shortens on exercise but the patient has

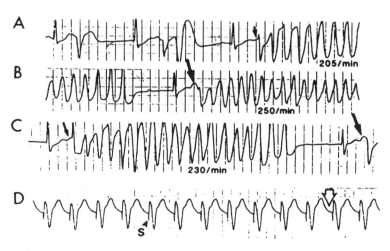

Figure 6 Ventricular pacing to prevent torsades de pointes. Drug-induced torsades de pointes is demonstrated in A, B, and C. The terminal portion of the QT interval is noted by the arrows. In D, ventricular pacing at a rate of 100 beats/min totally prevents torsades de pointes. (From M.E. Josephson, Clinical Cardiac Electrophysiology Techniques and Interpretations, with permission.)

419

recurrent episodes of prolongation, atrial pacing coupled with the use of a beta blocker may be employed to maintain the shortened QT interval. Genetic testing is employed to identify patients at risk of having this disorder, but whether or not prophylaxis can be helpful remains uncertain.

V. CONCLUSION

Cardiac arrest is responsible for more than 300,000 deaths per year. Survivors of this tragic event make up only a small minority (perhaps only 10%). Although they are at high risk for recurrence, much work is needed to identify patients at high risk who have not yet had an event. In patients who have survived cardiac arrest and can be discharged from a hospital, removal of all potential inciting causes of the arrest followed by careful definition of anatomic and electro-physiological substrates responsible can lead to effective prevention of recurrence and improvement of survival.

SUGGESTED READING

Bigger JT Jr, Fleiss JL, Steinman RC, et al. Frequency domain measures of heart period variability and mortality after myocardial infarction. Circulation 1992; 85:164–171.

Buxton AE, Fisher JD, Josephson ME, et al. Prevention of sudden death in patients with coronary artery disease: The Multicenter Unsustained Tachycardia Trial (MUSTT). Prog Cardiovasc Dis 1993; 36:215–226.

Callans DJ, Josephson ME. Future developments in implantable cardioverter defibrillators: The optimal device. Prog Cardiovasc Dis 1993; 36:227–244.

CAST Investigators. Preliminary report: Effect of encainide and flecainide on mortality in a randomized trial of arrhythmia suppression after myocardial infarction. N Engl J Med 1989; 321:406–412.

CAST-II Investigators. Effect of the antiarrhythmic agent moricizine on survival after myocardial infarction. N Engl J Med 1992; 327:227–233.

Greene HL, Roden D, Katz RJ, et al. The Cardiac Arrhythmia Suppression Trial: First CAST ... then Cast-II. J Am Coll Cardiol 1992; 19:894–898.

Marchlinski FR, Flores BT, Buxton AE, et al. The automatic implantable cardioverter-defibrillator: Efficacy, complications, and device failures. Ann Intern Med 1986; 104:481–488.

Wilber DJ, Garan H, Finkelstein D, et al. Out-of-hospital cardiac arrest: Use of electro-physiologic testing in the prediction of long-term outcome. N Engl J Med 1988; 318: 19–24.

Wilber DJ, Olshansky B, Moran JF, et al. Electrophysiological testing and nonsustained ventricular tachycardia: Use and limitations in patients with coronary artery disease and impaired ventricular function. Circulation 1990; 82:350–358.

Heart Disease in Special Settings

The astute clinician will well recognize that any kind of heart disease can occur in virtually any setting. However, the natural history of a given disorder, its implications for the patient, and decisions regarding its treatment will often be influenced by the setting in which the disorder occurs. Furthermore, in certain settings physical findings, subjective phenomena, and laboratory observations that would be indicative of heart disease in other settings may simply be normal variants. For example, in a well-trained athlete the resting electrocardiogram may show prodigious QRS complexes that would be indicative of pathological left ventricular hypertrophy in a nonathlete of the same age and gender, bizarre arrhythmias attributable to slowing of the sinus rate and nodal and ventricular escape beats that are not indicative of organic heart disease, and markedly altered ST segments and T waves. Alternatively, in a pregnant woman with pulmonary artery dilatation evident on the chest x-ray and dyspnea as well as a loud P_2 (potentially confused with an opening snap), misdiagnosis of mitral stenosis is always a possibility, particularly because the high cardiac output can produce a diastolic rumble.

It is in this context that the following part of this book addresses the presence or absence of heart disease in special settings. In many instances, reference is made to material detailed elsewhere in the text addressing the specific disease entity. Certain challenges in patient management resulting from the use of novel therapeutic interventions such as antitachycardia devices are considered because, in fact, the therapy creates a potentially new "disease" that must be recognized and managed just as the underlying condition being treated must be recognized and managed. The appropriate management of patients with heart disease in special settings and the appropriate recognition of normal variations in special settings is as much an art as a science. It is above all, a gratifying challenge for the astute clinician.

21

Cardiac Findings in Athletes with and without Heart Disease

I.	Athletic Heart Syndrome	423
II.	Cardiac Arrhythmias in Athletes	427
III.	Management of Specific Arrhythmias	427
IV.	Preparticipation Screening	431

A. John Camm and Josef Kautzner

Assessment of the importance of cardiac arrhythmias in an athlete and consideration of his or her eligibility for physical competition is a difficult task, especially in the context of malignant or prognostically significant ventricular arrhythmias. Both screening for the risk of sudden death and the clinical evaluation of those presenting with symptomatic arrhythmias are complicated by difficulties in establishing criteria of abnormality. Regular exercise produces physiological changes in both hemodynamics and cardiac electrophysiology that may be misinterpreted as abnormal findings. To avoid overinterpretation and inappropriate attribution of disease in evaluating a population of athletes, the range of reported physiological changes in the cardiovascular system, known as the "athletic heart syndrome," should be understood.

I. ATHLETIC HEART SYNDROME

The heart of the athlete undergoes morphological and functional adaptation that differentiates it from the hearts of sedentary people. Increased demands for cardiac output are principally accomplished by alterations of heart rate and contractility. The resulting adaptation responses differ according to the prevailing pressure or volume overload and thus, depend on the degree of dynamic or isometric exercise. Pressure overload (in isometric athletes such as weight lifters) leads to both septal and free wall thickening, thus reducing systolic wall stress. Chronic volume overload (in isotonic athletes such as runners) is characterized by a proportional increase in end-diastolic volume and wall thickness, allowing the athlete to cope with increased end-diastolic and systolic wall stress.

Regular physical training changes cardiac electrophysiology in an adaptive process. Increased baroreceptor sensitivity reflects augmented vagal efferent activity and the resulting sinus bradycardia allows optimization of ventricular filling at rest. Exercise itself is then characterized by less vagal withdrawal, and subsequent changes in sympathovagal balance. The adaptation tends to counterbalance its electrophysiological effects that may either facilitate or suppress cardiac ectopic activity and influence impulse conduction. These complex relationships are shown in Figure 1. Prevailing sympathetic neural activity and increases in circulating catecholamines during exercise may provoke ectopic activity by accelerating the rate of phase 4 depolarization in the Purkinje system. This enhances spontaneous depolarization and promotes automaticity. Increased sympathetic activity also stimulates delayed afterdepolarizations and triggered activity. Increase in sympathetic tone is the main determinant of repetitive responses. On the other hand, exercise-related sinus tachycardia may suppress arrhythmias by inhi-

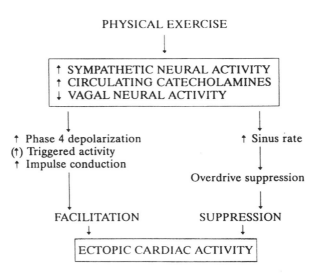

Figure 1   Scheme of the electrophysiological changes during physical exercise.

bition of an ectopic focus before its intrinsic discharge reaches threshold potential (overdrive suppression).

On physical examination, the pulse is slow and its volume is increased as a result of the higher resting stroke volume. These changes are more pronounced in isotonic athletes than in isometric athletes. Auscultation usually reveals a normal first sound, although S_2 may be split in inspiration, and a third sound is commonly present, reflecting an increased rate of diastolic filling. The significance of a fourth sound is unclear, albeit this sound is detectable in 20–50% cases, especially when myocardial hypertrophy is apparent. In addition, systolic ejection murmurs (grade I–II) have been reported in 30–50% of endurance athletes.

Echocardiographic evaluation of the athlete's heart confirms left ventricular hypertrophy, usually concentric, with a normal septal-to-free-wall ratio (< 1.3). The calculated left ventricular (LV) mass increases, especially in isotonic athletes with some degree of eccentric hypertrophy, while in isometric athletes, the increase in LV mass is usually proportional to the lean body mass. In some cases the septal-to-free-wall ratio may increase beyond the normal limit. When differentiation from hypertrophic cardiomyopathy is very difficult, even myocardial biopsy may not give the correct answer. The ratio of septal wall thickness to the LV end-systolic diameter is a useful parameter, a value of ≥ 0.48 suggests that hypertrophy occurs at the expense of the LV cavity size. This is not the case in athlete's heart. Increased left atrial or right ventricular dimensions have been reported, but there is less information regarding the implications of these measurements.

The resting ECG may show a variety of changes that are abnormal in untrained individuals. The reported incidence of these abnormalities is presented in Table 1. The most prevalent findings, especially in isotonic athletes, are sinus

Table 1 Comparison of the Incidence of Different Types of Arrhythmias on Resting ECG in the General Population and Athletes

Type of arrhythmia	General population, percent	Athletes, percent
Sinus bradycardia	23.7	50–85
Sinus arrhythmia	2.4–20	13.5–69
First-degree AV block	0.65	6–33
Second-degree AV block		
Mobitz I	0.003	0.13–10
Mobitz II	0.003	Not available
Third-degree AV block	0.0002	0.017
Junctional rhythm	0.06	0.031–7
Ventricular preexcitation	0.1–0.15	0.15–2.5
Atrial fibrillation	0.004	0–0.06

Source: Adapted from Huston et al., N Engl J Med 1985; 13:24–32.

bradycardia and respiratory arrhythmia at rest. They have been attributed to an increase in vagal tone or to changes in sympathovagal balance, presumably a decrease in resting sympathetic tone. However, pharmacological blockade in athletes demonstrates significantly lower intrinsic heart rates when compared with the normal population. Athletes have more frequent or longer sinus pauses and a higher incidence of both first- and second-degree atrioventricular block. Even third-degree atrioventricular block appears to be significantly more prevalent among athletes. Incomplete right bundle branch block is frequently seen in athletes in an incidence as high as 15%. Not surprisingly, ECG evidence of LV hypertrophy is common (14–85%). ST- and T-wave changes (namely J point and ST segment elevation with peaked or inverted T waves, ST segment depression with depressed J points, juvenile T waves or T wave inversion in lateral leads) are frequently present and are sometimes difficult to differentiate from pathological changes seen with organic heart disease (Figure 2). Disappearance of these changes with exercise or after administration of isoproterenol and limited effects of atropine, suggest that decrease in sympathetic tone may be an underlying cause.

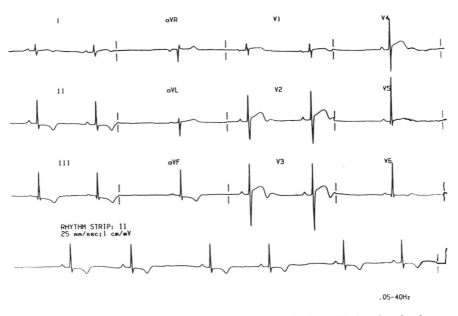

Figure 2 Resting ECG of a 28-year-old top-level squash player. Notice sinus bradycardia with pronounced respiratory arrhythmia, a prolonged PQ interval (0.22 sec) and abnormalities of the ST segment and T wave (J point and ST segment elevation, inverted and biphasic T waves).

II. CARDIAC ARRHYTHMIAS IN ATHLETES

The incidence of supraventricular arrhythmias in athletes varies markedly. Although isolated supraventricular extrasystoles can be found in approximately 40–60% of competitive athletes, paroxysmal supraventricular tachycardias are not reported any more frequently than in untrained subjects. In contrast, atrial fibrillation appears to be more prevalent in competitive athletes. This may reflect the purely functional basis (e.g., sympathovagal imbalance) for lone atrial fibrillation, whereas most supraventricular tachycardias require an anatomic substrate. Left atrial enlargement, especially seen in endurance athletes, may contribute to the occurrence of atrial fibrillation. Supraventricular tachyarrhythmia is generally not prognostically important except in association with ventricular preexcitation. The occurrence of atrial fibrillation in this setting may result in a very rapid ventricular activation via the accessory pathway, with subsequent degeneration of the ventricular rhythm into ventricular fibrillation. However, in certain sports involving high speed, even the occurrence of supraventricular arrhythmias may put the athlete at risk of serious injury or death related to transient loss of control due to impaired concentration or consciousness.

The incidence of ventricular ectopic activity in athletes is uncertain because studies have differed with respect to the selection of the study group (e.g., isotonic or isometric athletes, or professional athletes versus amateurs), the length of ECG monitoring, and the definition of the control group. On average, isolated ventricular premature beats have been reported in one-third of the athlete population evaluated by 24-hr ambulatory monitoring. Although some studies have documented a higher occurrence of ventricular arrhythmias in endurance athletes, the prognostic value of this finding remains unclear. The frequency of ventricular arrhythmias observed during actual sporting activity is underestimated by treadmill testing. This underlines the necessity for long-term recording during training. In addition, mental stress during competition may influence cardiac electrophysiology and the occurrence of arrhythmias. It should be kept in mind that an increased frequency of arrhythmias may, in occasional athletes, reflect the abuse of drugs, either "recreational" or "performance enhancing." Although complex forms of ventricular arrhythmias are relatively infrequent, they should not be considered as a normal characteristic of athlete's heart. Their detection should always lead to comprehensive cardiologic evaluation, as they may often represent latent cardiovascular disease.

III. MANAGEMENT OF SPECIFIC ARRHYTHMIAS

Current management strategies for cardiac arrhythmias in athletes as well as guidance on further participation in competitive sports reflect our uncertainty about the definition of what is normal in the spectrum of exercise-related rhythm disturbances. Although, in the majority of the cases, complex forms of ventricular arrhythmias and/or significant conduction abnormalities are related to underlying, often inapparent structural heart disease, instances with no other detectable organic abnormality beyond the athlete's heart syndrome are not exceptional. Arrhythmias may be associated with the presence of "physiological" ventricular hypertrophy per se. They may represent effects of exercise-related adaptive changes in autonomic balance and cellular electrophysiological properties. They may relate to the hemodynamic burden of vigorous sporting activity or stem from transient silent ischemia of hypertrophied myocardium during peak activity or during the early recovery phase, when hypotension occurs because of peripheral vasodilatation.

Many recommendations extrapolated from observations obtained in non-athletes are not supported by firm scientific data. However, some anecdotal data show the disappearance of prognostically significant arrhythmias with detraining, suggesting that in some instances these arrhythmias may be caused by the sporting activity.

A. Premature Beats

When premature supraventricular complexes occur in the absence of evidence suggestive of structural heart disease and in the absence of significant symptoms, detailed evaluation is not necessary, and athletes may participate in all sporting activities. In the case of premature ventricular complexes, even when the evidence to suggest the presence of structural heart disease is weak, an echocardiographic study and 24-hr Holter recording is advised. Irrespective of evidence of structural heart disease, an increase in the number of premature complexes during exercise warrants further evaluation. Those athletes without structural heart disease but an increase in the frequency of premature ventricular complexes with exercise can participate in low-intensity competitive sports and cautiously in moderate-intensity sports. Those with structural heart disease who are in high-risk groups (such as individuals with aortic valve disease, coronary artery disease and cardiomyopathies) should be excluded from high- to moderate-intensity competitive sports.

B. Supraventricular Arrhythmias

Because the occurrence of *atrial fibrillation* or *flutter* may reflect the presence of structural heart disease, echocardiography is always recommended. Other causes, such as latent hyperthyroidism, should be excluded. Determination of the ventricular response to an exercise test may be useful in order to assess the potential for rapid ventricular rates. In individuals without structural heart disease and an appropriate range of ventricular rates on or off medical treatment can participate in all competitive sports. Beta blockers are, however, banned for use in some competitive sports. Those with structural heart disease with a controlled ventricular rate may participate in sports according to the severity of the underlying disease. Analogous measures can be applied to athletes suffering from *atrial tachycardias* or *sinus node reentrant tachycardia*. However, in these cases catheter ablation of the arrhythmia substrate could be considered. When *nonparoxysmal atrioventricular junctional tachycardia* is diagnosed, the appropriateness of exercise should be assessed by changes in ventricular heart rate during exercise. Provided there is no structural heart disease and the ventricular rate is controlled, no restrictions are necessary. Incompletely controlled ventricular rates or the presence of underlying disease limit exercise to low levels of activity. Individuals presenting with *paroxysmal supraventricular tachycardia* should be evaluated and treated as recommended for the nonathletic population. Those asymptomatic or minimally symptomatic athletes in whom prevention of recurrences has been achieved by antiarrhythmic drugs or by catheter ablation may participate in all competitive sports. Those with syncope, near syncope, or significant palpitations or individuals with structural heart disease should not participate in any competitive sport until they have been adequately treated for more than 6 months. Athletes with structural involvement can then participate only in such sports as are appropriate for a subject with the underlying heart disease.

Asymptomatic subjects presenting with *ventricular preexcitation* on the surface ECG should undergo 24-hr ECG recording during athletic activity, an exercise test, and echocardiographic evaluation. Those with no structural abnormalities are at relatively low risk of sudden death. However, before participating in sports, particularly of moderate or high intensity, assessment of the electrophysiological properties of the accessory pathway, especially its refractory period and its change with rapid stimulation, is advisable. Athletes with conduction over the pathway at a rate greater than 240 beats/min should be considered for catheter ablation. This therapeutic alternative may be considered in all individuals, based on the type of sport, localization of the pathway, and the patient's preference. In symptomatic patients, electrophysiological testing and catheter ablation should be recommended. When an athlete refuses an ablation procedure, an assessment of the functional properties of the accessory pathway should be mandatory before deciding on participation in competitive sports, especially in those with episodes of atrial fibrillation. Symptomatic individuals with rapid conduction over the pathway should not participate in moderate- or high-intensity sports. Following successful ablation of the accessory pathway, those who are asymptomatic and have no inducible arrhythmia during repeat electrophysiology study and/or no recurrence for 3 to 6 months can participate in all competitive sports.

C. Ventricular Arrhythmias

Ventricular tachycardia is always a potentially serious problem that merits complete clinical evaluation. This is described in detail in Chapter 17. The most difficult task in athletes is to differentiate "athlete's heart" from structural abnor-

429

malities. Temporary detraining (for approximately 3 months) may help in some borderline cases to differentiate adaptive ventricular hypertrophy from hypertrophic cardiomyopathy. Whether detraining may also decrease the risk of ventricular arrhythmias remains unanswered.

A majority of those subjects with ventricular tachycardia in the absence of detectable structural heart disease, such as those with tachycardias originating in the right ventricular outflow tract, may be successfully treated by radiofrequency ablation or drugs. Provided that there are no other clinical recurrences and tachycardia is not inducible by exercise or during electrophysiological study, all competitive sports may be permitted in these individuals. For athletes with structural heart disease and recently diagnosed sustained or nonsustained ventricular arrhythmias, moderate- and high-intensity exercise is generally contraindicated despite the fact that tachycardia is suppressed by treatment. These individuals should not engage in any competitive spots during the first 6 months after the diagnosis is made. Anecdotal data show that continuing sporting activity represents one of the major causes of sudden cardiac death in this population. Survivors of *cardiac arrest*, irrespective of the presence of structural heart disease, should not be allowed to participate in any moderate- to high-intensity competitive sports. Athletes with the diagnosis of *congenital long-QT syndrome* are at particular risk for exercise-related sudden death and should be restricted from all competitive sports.

D. Bradyarrhythmias

Asymptomatic sinus arrhythmias—including sinus arrest of less than 3sec duration or first degree or type I second-degree atrioventricular block—are significantly more frequent in athletes than in the normal population. Similarly, second-degree Mobitz type II atrioventricular block and complete heart block are more common in athletes, but their occurrence may suggest the presence of structural heart disease. The same holds for inappropriate bradycardia, sinus arrest with long pauses, exit block, and bradycardia-tachycardia syndrome. Although incomplete right bundle branch block is relatively frequent in athletes, complete right bundle block may represent structural disease. Left bundle block is considered an abnormal finding.

Individuals with *sinus node dysfunction* whose bradyarrhythmia produces no symptoms and that does not worsen with physical activity can participate in all competitive sports. They should be reassessed periodically to determine the influence of training on the bradycardia. Those with arrhythmia-related symptoms should be appropriately treated, usually by cardiac pacing, and if they are then asymptomatic for 3 to 6 months, no restrictions are necessary. Athletes with a pacemaker should not engage in sports where body collision and trauma are likely to damage the pacemaker system. The management of symptomatic *bradycardia/ tachycardia syndrome* should follow the same guidelines.

430

Those with *type I second-degree atrioventricular block* appearing or worsening with exercise should be evaluated further and may require pacemaker therapy. *Type 2 second-degree atrioventricular block* as well as *acquired complete heart block* should be treated with pacing before any sporting activity is allowed. Athletes with *congenital complete heart block* should be evaluated and an exercise testing should be included. Those who are asymptomatic, with a structurally normal heart and an escape rhythm with narrow QRS complexes and who respond appropriately to exercise should not be restricted. However, those with symptoms should have a pacemaker. Patients with an abnormal heart and symptomatic bradyarrhythmias should not participate in any competitive sport without a pacemaker. The intensity of the exercise should be inversely proportional to the severity of cardiac impairment.

The mere presence of *complete right bundle block* without any arrhythmias and symptoms does not require any restriction in sporting activity. In young athletes with *left bundle branch block*, an invasive electrophysiological study should be performed, and those with abnormal conduction (HV interval >100 ms or His-Purkinje block) should be considered for pacing. Older athletes without structural heart disease, detectable arrhythmias, or symptoms can participate in all competitive sports.

Athletes with *syncope* or *presyncope* should not participate in competitive sports until the cause has been established and treated. The possibility of associated ventricular tachyarrhythmias should be considered. The diagnostic value of head-up tilt testing, which is otherwise a useful tool for the evaluation of patients with syncope of unknown origin, is handicapped by its lower specificity in the athletic population.

IV. PREPARTICIPATION SCREENING

Although the incidence of sudden cardiac death in the athletic population is very low compared with the large number of participants in sport, possible prevention of these tragic events is important. Data available have shown that the yield from large-scale comprehensive screening studies is very low and that the cost of such screening is enormous. Therefore, the most acceptable screening method remains history and physical cardiac examination. The history should focus on identification of symptomatic individuals and those with a family history of congenital heart disease or sudden cardiac death. The basic cardiac physical examination should detect a large proportion of athletes with congenital or valvular heart disease, Marfan syndrome, and some hypertrophic cardiomyopathy. This simple, cost-effective approach restricts further diagnostic workup to the majority of individuals at risk of sudden cardiac death.

22

Pregnancy

Management of Cardiac Disease in Pregnancy   **434**
    I.   Cardiac Physiology Associated with Pregnancy   434
    II.   Cardiac Evaluation   434
    III.   Laboratory Findings   435
    IV.   Common Reasons for Cardiac Consultations in
        Pregnant Subjects   435
    V.   Valvular Heart Disease   437
    VI.   Mitral Valve Prolapse   437
    VII.   Congenital Heart Disease   438
    VIII.   Hypertrophic Cardiomyopathy   438
    IX.   Peripartum Cardiomyopathy   438
    X.   Pregnancy in Patients with Prosthetic Valves   439
    XI.   Medical Conditions Associated with Increased Risk
        to the Mother   439

Management of Arrhythmias in Pregnancy   **442**
    XII.   Pharmacological Management   443
    XIII.   Class I Antiarrhythmic Drugs   446
    XIV.   Class II Antiarrhythmic Drugs   449
    XV.   Class III Antiarrhythmic Drugs   449
    XVI.   Class IV Antiarrhythmic Drugs   450
    XVII.   Other Antiarrhythmic Drugs   451
    XVIII.   Nonpharmacological Management   452
    XIX.   Management of Specific Arrhythmias   452

Management of Cardiac Disease in Pregnancy

Uri Elkayam

Pregnancy and the peripartum period are associated with significant hemo-dynamic changes in the patient with cardiovascular disease. These changes may lead to deterioration of hemodynamics and symptoms appearing for the first time in the patient's life or exacerbation of symptoms in an already symptomatic patient.

I. CARDIAC PHYSIOLOGY ASSOCIATED WITH PREGNANCY

Pregnancy is associated with a significant increase in blood volume (plasma volume peaking at 32 weeks), averaging 40%. This change starts early and progresses gradually to a maximum at term. Changes in blood volume lead to a substantial increase in stroke volume and cardiac output. In addition, a physiologi-cal increase in heart rate of about 10–20 beats/min occurs. Systemic arterial pressure begins to fall during the first trimester, with a maximum decrease in midpregnancy and a return toward baseline before term. The reduction in diastolic pressure is greater than that in systolic blood pressure, leading to a widening of pulse pressure. A substantial fall in systemic vascular resistance is seen.

The emotional stress, pain, and uterine contraction at the time of labor and delivery lead to substantial hemodynamic changes, with an increase in cardiac output, blood pressure, and heart rate. Thus, labor and delivery may entail in-creased risk in a patient with heart disease. Abdominal delivery or a cesarean section may prevent such changes. However, the intubation and anesthesia in-volved may be hemodynamically deleterious in their own right.

After delivery of the fetus and because of an increase in venous return to the heart, intracardiac pressures often increase, with subsequent clinical deterioration even after successful labor and delivery.

II. CARDIAC EVALUATION

Because of anatomic and functional changes, physical examination detects phe-nomena that can be misleading. Rapid and shallow respiration normally seen in pregnancy can be attributed to respiratory embarrassment; distension of jugular veins secondary to an increase in blood volume and lower-extremity edema commonly seen late in pregnancy can be misinterpreted as manifestations of congestive heart failure. The systemic pulses are bounding and collapsing, like those in patients with aortic regurgitation or a patent ductus arteriosus; the left ventricular impulse is often hyperactive, brisk, unsustained, and somewhat displaced to the left. A right ventricular heave is commonly palpated in second- and third-trimester subjects, and closure of the pulmonic valve can often be palpated. Auscultation demonstrates increased intensity of heart sounds with exaggerated splitting of both of the first and the second heart sounds. A functional systolic murmur can be heard in most women during the later part of gestation, usually midsystolic, with an intensity at 1–2/6 located at the left sternal border and over the pulmonic area, often radiating to the suprasternal notch and the left side of the neck. Rarely, a functional diastolic rumble may be audible and be misconstrued to be indicative of mitral stenosis. A venous hum can be misdiagnosed as the continuous murmur of a patent ductus.

Normal pregnancy can give rise to hyperventilation, fatigue, a decrease in exercise tolerance, and inability to lie flat in bed, especially in the later phase. All of these phenomena can easily be misinterpreted as changes related to heart disease. Accordingly, it is often necessary to acquire clinical information astutely in conjunction with definitive and objective means when cardiac status is ambiguous.

III. LABORATORY FINDINGS

The electrocardiogram (ECG) is generally normal. However, a slight QRS axis shift to either the left or the right is not uncommon, and transient ST-segment depression and T-wave changes are often seen. A small Q wave and an inverted P wave in lead III, both of which may vary with respiration, as well as increased R wave amplitude in lead V_2 are often present. The chest x-ray may demonstrate straightening of the left upper cardiac border. The heart may seem to be slightly enlarged because of its horizontal positioning secondary to elevation of the diaphragm. Increase in lung markings may be seen, and pleural effusion occurs often in the early postpartum period. Echocardiograms often show mild enlargement of cardiac chambers and a small pericardial effusion. Doppler examination often shows mild tricuspid, mitral, and pulmonary regurgitation.

IV. COMMON REASONS FOR CARDIAC CONSULTATIONS IN PREGNANT SUBJECTS

The most common reasons are listed in Table 1. *Evaluation of a murmur* is probably highest on the list. The functional murmurs of pregnancy should be differentiated from murmurs secondary to organic heart disease, especially those seen with a bicuspid aortic valve, atrial septal defects, and ventricular septal defects. Because the characteristics of functional murmurs of pregnancy are

435

Table 1 Common Reasons for Cardiac
Consultations in Pregnant Subjects

1. Evaluation of a murmur
2. Palpitations
3. Arrhythmias
4. Congenital heart disease
5. Rheumatic and other valvular disease

variable, especially in terms of intensity, and because other findings such as increased loudness of heart sounds and wide splitting of the two components of both heart sounds are so common, echocardiographic evaluation may be needed to exclude organic heart disease in some patients.

Palpitation is a common complaint in pregnancy. Frequently, important cardiac arrhythmias or other cardiac abnormalities are absent. However, sinus tachycardia and a high incidence of atrial or ventricular premature beats and sometimes nonsustained supraventricular and ventricular tachycardia have been found in many women presenting with this complaint. The presence of such arrhythmias in patients without other signs of cardiac disease does not constitute a sign of an adverse effect on either maternal or fetal outcome. The incidence of the arrhythmias usually decreases markedly after delivery.

In the evaluation of a pregnant patient with cardiac arrhythmia during pregnancy, underlying heart disease must be excluded because of the fact that patients with organic heart disease have a higher incidence of arrhythmias when pregnant. In patients with cardiac arrhythmia during pregnancy but no other evidence of cardiovascular disease, other causes of arrhythmia—including pulmonary disease, electrolyte abnormalities, thyroid disease, arrhythmogenic drugs, alcohol, caffeine, cigarette smoking, and drug abuse—should be considered. If found, such conditions should be corrected. Antiarrhythmic drug therapy should be considered only after such efforts fail to correct the arrhythmia. In patients without identifiable cause for arrhythmia, reassurance should be the first measure. Antiarrhythmic drug therapy, preferably beta blockers, should be considered only for relief of disturbing symptoms or treatment of hemodynamically important arrhythmias. In the patient with organic heart disease, development of arrhythmias during pregnancy often represents progression of the underlying condition. For this reason, the first step should be stabilization of underlying cardiovascular disease to the maximal extent possible. If this approach fails, antiarrhythmic drug therapy should be considered.

When antiarrhythmic drugs are being considered, the lowest therapeutically effective doses should be used. Drugs given should be those known to be safe for the fetus. The indication for drug therapy should be reevaluated periodically.

V. VALVULAR HEART DISEASE

In general, regurgitant lesions, including mitral and aortic regurgitation, are well tolerated during pregnancy, most likely because of the substantial reduction in systemic vascular resistance and the resulting unloading of the left ventricle. However, stenotic valvular lesions are potentially hazardous during pregnancy. Ideally a patient with significant aortic stenosis (aortic valve area $\leqslant 1.0$ cm^2) should be operated upon before pregnancy. The incidence of complications in patients with aortic stenosis during pregnancy has been thought to be high. However, recent experience indicates that pregnancy in a patient with hemodynamically important aortic stenosis can be managed effectively provided that diagnosis is established early and close follow-up, initiation of cardiovascular therapy if necessary, and hemodynamic monitoring during labor and delivery are implemented.

Because of the increase in blood volume, acceleration of heart rate, and arrhythmias that may lead to atrial fibrillation, the patient with mitral stenosis is likely to become more symptomatic during pregnancy. Ideally, hemodynamically important mitral stenosis should be repaired, either surgically or by balloon techniques, before conception. In the patient with mitral stenosis who becomes pregnant, therapy focuses on reduction of heart rate and decreasing blood volume with diuretics if necessary. Hemodynamic monitoring is helpful during labor, delivery, and the puerperium in every patient with mitral stenosis who is symptomatic during pregnancy. Epidural anesthesia is the anesthesia of choice because of its favorable hemodynamic effect and induced lowering of pulmonary venous and arterial pressures. In patients who become severely symptomatic during pregnancy and do not respond to medical therapy, balloon valvuloplasty can be performed to improve hemodynamics and symptoms. However, to minimize the risk of radiation, appropriate shielding of the fetus and referral of patients to operators and medical centers with substantial experience in technique are needed.

VI. MITRAL VALVE PROLAPSE

The prevalence of mitral valve prolapse in women of childbearing age is approximately 1%. Pregnancy may be associated with reduction in the incidence of prolapse-related auscultatory and echocardiographic changes because of the increase in left ventricular volume. In general, this condition is well tolerated during pregnancy. The most important clinical issue concerns the need for antibiotic prophylaxis during labor and delivery. Because the development of bacteremia during delivery cannot always be predicted, antibiotic prophylaxis should be employed in patients with mitral valve prolapse caused by myxomatous degeneration reflected by thickening of the mitral valve and the presence of mitral regurgitation.

VII. CONGENITAL HEART DISEASE

The simple forms of congenital heart disease—including atrial septal defect, ventricular septal defect, and patent ductus arteriosus—are generally well tolerated during pregnancy. Although coarctation of the aorta had been thought to carry a high risk of aortic dissection in pregnancy, recent experience has not confirmed this. Complications such as hypertension, congestive heart failure, and angina may occur. Accordingly, correction of aortic coarctation before pregnancy is warranted. In patients who become pregnant, management focuses on control of blood pressure. However, because of the potential for reduction in fetal perfusion, blood pressure should not be reduced too aggressively and should be lowered only if systolic blood pressure exceeds 180 mmHg.

Cyanotic congenital heart disease is associated with a high incidence of complications during pregnancy. Thus, if at all possible, corrective surgery should be performed before conception. In general, in pregnant patients with cyanotic congenital heart disease a decrease in functional class, hematocrit above 60%, arterial oxygen saturation below 80%, right ventricular hypertension, and syncopal episodes, are all signs of poor prognosis.

VIII. HYPERTROPHIC CARDIOMYOPATHY

Patients with hypertrophic cardiomyopathy may exhibit worsening of symptoms during pregnancy. Chest pain, palpitations, dizzy spells, syncope, and shortness of breath are common. Although the risk of sudden death does not appear to be generally increased with pregnancy, isolated cases of malignant arrhythmias and observed activation of implanted defibrillators have been described that may be indicative of an increase in risk of serious arrhythmias during gestation.

In the symptomatic patient with obstructive hypertrophic cardiomyopathy, blood loss during delivery should be corrected promptly. In addition, vasodilation and sympathetic stimulation during anesthesia should be avoided. Because of the risk of infective endocarditis, antibiotic prophylaxis should be implemented for labor and delivery.

IX. PERIPARTUM CARDIOMYOPATHY

This dilated cardiomyopathy of unknown etiology often presents with symptoms of heart failure during the last month of pregnancy or the first month postpartum. Typically, symptoms of congestive heart failure, chest pain, palpitations, and occasionally peripheral or pulmonary embolization appear. Congestive heart failure should be treated conventionally with diuretics, digoxin, and vasodilators. The use of angiotensin converting enzyme (ACE) inhibitors before delivery is inadvisable because of potential fetal complications.

Approximately 50% of women will exhibit spontaneous improvement in left ventricular function as well as symptoms. Some 20–30% will continue to manifest severe heart failure with possible clinical deterioration and even death. The remainder will exhibit partial or no improvement in left ventricular function and develop chronic congestive heart failure with its associated increased incidence of morbidity and mortality. Cardiac transplantation should be considered in the patient with severe left ventricular dysfunction who fails to respond to medical therapy with demonstrable improvement in cardiac function. The value of immunosuppressive agents has not been established.

X. PREGNANCY IN PATIENTS WITH PROSTHETIC VALVES

The risk of pregnancy in women with artificial heart valves is multifactorial. Hemodynamic and symptomatic deterioration may occur because of the increased circulatory burden, thromboembolic events, risks inherent in the use of anticoagulants, and risks associated with fetal exposure to cardiovascular and other drugs. Patients with mild to moderate symptoms of heart failure and those with normal or near normal cardiac function tolerate the hemodynamic load of pregnancy quite well. Although pregnancy is associated with changes in the concentration of coagulation and fibrinolytic system proteins in blood and a hypercoagulable state, the incidence of thromboembolic events in patients with heart disease treated appropriately with anticoagulants is acceptably low. Because oral anticoagulants entail an increased incidence of fetal complications related to their teratogenic effects and an increased risk of fetal intracranial bleeding and central nervous system complications, oral anticoagulation should be avoided during the first trimester except for high-risk patients (old generation valves in the mitral position). In all others heparin should be used during the first trimester and during the last 2 to 4 weeks of pregnancy. When the patient goes into labor on oral anticoagulation, cesarean section should be performed.

XI. MEDICAL CONDITIONS ASSOCIATED WITH INCREASED RISK TO THE MOTHER

Cardiac conditions during pregnancy that entail considerable risk to the mother are listed in Table 2.

A. Cyanotic Congenital Heart Disease

A substantial increase in maternal complications is likely during pregnancy. Worsening of symptoms such as chest pain, exacerbation of heart failure, and arrhythmias are often seen. Complications such as pulmonary embolism, systemic

439

Table 2 Pregnancy Associated Cardiac Conditions with Major Maternal Complications

Cyanotic congenital heart disease
Marfan syndrome
Peripartum cardiomyopathy with persistent left ventricular dysfunction
Primary pulmonary hypertension
Eisenmenger's syndrome

embolization, and bacterial endocarditis increase mortality. Fetal outcome continues to be poor, with a high incidence of fetal death, growth retardation, and congenital heart disease.

B. Marfan's Syndrome

Risks are twofold: (a) a high incidence of aortic dissection in the mother and (b) transmission of the disease to the fetus in 50% of the cases. The incidence of aortic dissection and death during gestation is high in patients with preexisting cardiovascular manifestations, especially aortic root dilatation. In patients without such manifestations, pregnancy may be uneventful. A successful outcome, however, cannot be guaranteed. The size of the aortic root is the most reliable descriptor for the risk of complications. Thus, patients with Marfan's syndrome should be evaluated by transesophageal echocardiography before they become pregnant.

Beta blockers may delay or prevent cardiovascular complications in patients with Marfan's syndrome and should be prescribed throughout pregnancy. Serial echocardiographic evaluations of the aortic root dimension should be performed during pregnancy to detect progressive dilation that may justify (depending on effect) either surgery or abortion in an early stage of pregnancy. In the patient with a dimension equal to or greater than 5.5, prophylactic replacement of the aortic root should be considered. In women with aortic dilatation, abdominal delivery by cesarean section is preferred to prevent potentially deleterious effects of straining during labor.

C. Primary Pulmonary Hypertension

Maternal mortality associated with primary pulmonary hypertension in pregnancy is approximately 40%. Exacerbation of symptoms may occur in the second trimester, with fatigue, dyspnea, syncope, and chest pain. Right ventricular failure and death may occur during late gestation or in the early postpartum period. Because of the poor maternal outcome, pregnancy is contraindicated. In patients who become pregnant, early abortion is warranted. If the patient elects to continue pregnancy, physical activity should be restricted. Anticoagulation is appropriate throughout pregnancy. During labor and delivery, hemodynamic monitoring should be performed and volume depletion secondary to blood loss should be minimized. Segmental epidural anesthesia and intrathecal morphine are safe and effective for analgesia. Because of the risk of right ventricular dysfunction, anesthetics with negative inotropic effects should be avoided. Most patients can tolerate vaginal delivery, but hemodynamic monitoring should be continued for 24 to 48 hr after delivery to facilitate early detection and prompt treatment of complications.

D. Peripartum Cardiomyopathy with Residual Left Ventricular Dysfunction

Clinical deterioration and death often occur in patients who become pregnant after an episode of peripartum cardiomyopathy with residual left ventricular dysfunction. Thus, pregnancy should be discouraged or early abortion considered. If a patient elects to continue a pregnancy, close follow-up and management of congestive heart failure with diuretics, digoxin, and vasodilators such as hydralazine and organic nitrates are needed. Angiotensin converting enzyme inhibitors are contraindicated because of the risk they entail for fetal complications.

E. Eisenmenger's Syndrome

Eisenmenger's syndrome (pulmonary hypertension and right-to-left shunting as a result of any communication between the systemic and pulmonary circulation) is associated with approximately 50% mortality in pregnancy. Most maternal deaths occur during delivery or in the first week postpartum. In addition to the unfavorable maternal outcome, pregnancy with Eisenmenger's syndrome is associated with a high rate of fetal loss, prematurity, and fetal growth retardation. Thus, pregnancy is contraindicated in women with Eisenmenger's syndrome. For afflicted women who become pregnant, early abortion should be considered. Women who insist on continuing the pregnancy should be hospitalized if any sign or symptom of hemodynamic instability appears. Anticoagulation is indicated throughout the third trimester. In hemodynamically stable patients, vaginal delivery is preferred. Spontaneous labor is better tolerated than induction. Prolonged postpartum hospitalization is recommended to detect and vigorously treat complications.

Management of Arrhythmias in Pregnancy

A. John Camm and Josef Kautzner

Cardiac arrhythmias are among the most common reasons for cardiac consultation during pregnancy. Pregnant women are exposed to the same risk of cardiac arrhythmias as the nonpregnant population of the same age group. Arrhythmias may appear for the first time during pregnancy or may continue to occur in patient with a previous history of various rhythm disturbances. In addition, anecdotal reports and common clinical experience support the view that pregnancy may provoke arrhythmias. On the other hand, some arrhythmias are suppressed by pregnancy.

Multiple mechanisms may explain the increased propensity to various arrhythmias during pregnancy. These include hemodynamic, autonomic, hormonal, and emotional changes occurring in the period of gestation. Increased left end-diastolic volume and remodeling in response to physiological volume overload may lead to an increased ventricular irritability. An accelerated heart rate may promote cardiac arrhythmias through modification of conduction velocity, refractoriness, and its dispersion. Hormonal influences may also be arrhythmogenic or cardiotoxic, predominantly because of modulations of hormone or neurotransmitter receptors in various tissues. Enhanced sympathetic tone or increased catecholamine sensitivity may increase automaticity in ventricular myocardium or promote triggered activity. In addition, shifts in electrolyte levels or physical stress and anxiety during pregnancy may contribute to arrhythmogenesis.

As with those who are not pregnant, the initial evaluation of patients with apparent or suspected arrhythmias should focus on documentation of the arrhythmia. The 12-lead electrocardiogram (ECG), ambulatory ECG, and event monitor are all valuable. In some cases, exercise testing may reveal the relationship between adrenergic tone and arrhythmia. In parallel, the presence of underlying structural cardiac disease should be addressed. Compared with their use in the nonpregnant population, the value of various diagnostic techniques must be weighed against any extra risk for the pregnant woman or the fetus. All diagnostic techniques involving ionizing radiation should be avoided. Management should include a search for reversible precipitating factors such as caffeine or alcohol, anemia, electrolyte imbalances, and hyperthyroidism.

Specific treatment of cardiac arrhythmias in pregnancy should be guided by the severity of symptoms, the presence or absence of underlying heart disease, the knowledge of pregnancy-related changes in the pharmacokinetics of antiarrhythmic drugs, and the potential hazards to the fetus. Basic principles of the approach to the pregnant patient with arrhythmias are shown in Figure 1. In general, a conservative approach should be followed, and if applicable, nonpharmacological interventions should be employed before medications. In cases refractory to pharmacotherapy or in situations of hemodynamic deterioration, synchronized electrical cardioversion may become necessary and should not be postponed. Nevertheless, drug therapy remains the mainstay of arrhythmia management in pregnancy.

XII. PHARMACOLOGICAL MANAGEMENT

The approach to pharmacological antiarrhythmic therapy in pregnancy is, in principle, analogous to that in nonpregnant patients. There are, however, some special considerations. As no antiarrhythmic drug is completely safe, selection of the drug should be made with respect to its therapeutic efficacy and its proven relative safety during pregnancy. Because of limited information on the effects of antiarrhythmic agents on the fetus and the possible changes in therapeutic re-

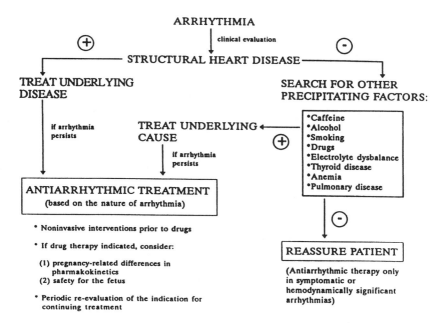

Figure 1. The approach to the pregnant patient with cardiac arrhythmia.

Table 3 Overview of the Use of Antiarrhythmic Drugs in Pregnancy

Drug	Route of administration	Therapeutic concentration	Fetal/ Maternal ratio	Milk/ Plasma ratio	Clinical indication	Use in pregnancy	Comment
Quinidine	Oral	3–6 µg/mL	0.24–1.4	0.71	Prophylaxis of SVT and ventricular arrhythmias	Relatively safe	Rarely, precipitation of premature labor, potential cause of eighth-nerve damage in fetus
Procainamide	Oral or parenteral	4–8 µg/mL	0.28–1.32	~1.0	Acute termination and prophylaxis of ventricular arrhythmias	Relatively safe	Relatively high incidence of maternal lupuslike syndrome during chronic therapy
Disopyramide	Oral or parenteral	2–4 µg/mL	0.39	0.9	Prophylaxis of ventricular arrhythmias	Probably safe	Negative inotropic effects, drug-induced uterine contractions
Lidocaine	Parenteral	1.5–5 µg/mL	0.5–0.6	~1.0	Acute termination of ventricular arrhythmias	Safe	Neonatal toxicity following high doses of drug
Mexiletine	Oral	0.5–2 µg/mL	1.0	0.78–1.89	Prophylaxis of ventricular arrhythmias	Probably safe, insufficient data	
Phenytoin	Parenteral	10–20 µg/mL	0.8–1	0.18	Digitalis-related refractory ventricular arrhythmias	Avoid if possible	Teratogenic effects in the first trimester, bleeding disorders

Drug	Route	Therapeutic level			Indication	Safety	Comments
Flecainide	Oral or parenteral	<0.2–1 µg/mL	0.7–0.83	1.57–2.18	Acute termination and prophylaxis of ventricular arrhythmias	Probably safe	
Propafenone	Oral or parenteral	0.2–3 µg/mL	0.14–0.20	0.14–0.20	Acute termination and prophylaxis of ventricular arrhythmias	Probably safe	
Beta blockers	Oral or parenteral	Variable	Variable, generally ~1.0	Variable	Termination and prophylaxis of SVT and ventricular arrhythmias, rate control in chronic AF	Relatively safe	Chronic administration may be associated with fetal growth retardation, risk of neonatal hypoglycemia
Amiodarone	Oral or parenteral	1–2.5 µg/mL	0.09–0.14	2.25–10.25	Treatment and prevention of refractory ventricular arrhythmias or SVT	Probably safe	Risk of neonatal hypothyreoidism
Sotalol	Oral or parenteral	1.5–4 mg/L	1.05–1.18	2.43–5.64	Treatment and prevention of refractory ventricular arrhythmias or SVT	Probably safe	See beta blockers
Verapamil	Oral or parenteral	15–30 ng/mL	0.17–0.4	0.23–0.94	Termination and prophylaxis of SVT, rate control in chronic AF	Probably safe	Rapid IV injection may cause maternal hypotension and fetal distress
Adenosine	Parenteral	N/A	No data	No data	Termination of SVT	Probably safe	
Digoxin	Oral or parenteral	1–2 ng/mL	1.0	0.6–0.9	Paroxysmal SVT, rate control in chronic AF	Safe	

sponse of the pregnant patient, general pharmakokinetic principles and clinical judgment are very important. Several specific points should be emphasized.

1. Cardiovascular adaptation of the mother to pregnancy may complicate drug disposition. The most important differences are as follows: (a) Decreased motility of gastrointestinal tract may affect absorption of certain drugs, while increased maternal intravascular and extravascular fluid volumes may lead to lower serum concentrations during the acute administration of a single dose of a drug. (b) Decrease in plasma protein concentration leads to reduction in drug protein binding and thus increase the level of free drug that is pharmacologically active. (c) Increase in renal blood flow and glomerular filtration influence clearance of those drugs excreted primarily by the renal route.

2. The selection of a particular antiarrhythmic drug should be made with regard to placental drug transfer. Although the vast majority of drugs may cross the placenta by simple diffusion, the rate of diffusion may significantly vary due to fat solubility and ionization of the drug, its molecular weight, plasma concentration, and the pH of maternal and fetal fluids. Only that fraction of the drug not bound to the plasma proteins is subject to placental transfer.

3. The sensitivity of the embryo or fetus to the toxic effects of drugs varies during the course of pregnancy, with the greatest susceptibility during the first trimester. Congenital malformations may occur in this period. Interference with normal fetal growth and development is the major risk of drug administration in the second and third trimesters. Because of the possibility of teratogenic effects, antiarrhythmic drugs should be administered only if the benefit of drug therapy clearly outweighs its potential risks to the fetus.

4. The choice of an antiarrhythmic drug with respect to breast feeding should be considered. The level of the drug in human milk depends on similar factors to those which determine placental transfer. Therefore, nonionized, fat-soluble drugs with minimal protein binding diffuse readily into the milk. Nevertheless, the amount of drug appearing in milk is rarely more than 1–2% of the dose administered to the mother and, with the exception of amiodarone, is usually not hazardous.

Detailed discussion of all antiarrhythmic drugs is beyond the scope of this chapter. Therefore, only specific aspects relevant to the use of antiarrhythmics in pregnancy are addressed (see also Table 3).

XIII.   CLASS I ANTIARRHYTHMIC DRUGS

A.   Quinidine

Quinidine is an effective drug for the treatment of both supraventricular and ventricular arrhythmias and for the maintenance of sinus rhythm after cardioversion of atrial fibrillation or flutter. Despite its extensive use in obstetric practice for more than half a century, teratogenic or other adverse fetal outcomes have not been documented. The drug crosses the placenta readily and also diffuses into breast milk, with a milk–plasma ratio of 0.7. The dose excreted in breast milk is considered safe for breast-feeding neonates. Because the drug potentiates uterine contractions, premature labor may occasionally be precipitated at therapeutic doses. Rarely, fetal thrombocytopenia has been reported. When high concentrations of the drug cross the placenta, quinidine may also be a potential cause of eighth-nerve damage to the fetus. Therefore, adequate monitoring of the maternal serum concentrations is required. The risk of proarrhythmia related to chronic administration of quinidine has reduced the use of quinidine in both pregnant and nonpregnant patients.

B. Procainamide

Procainamide, which has electrophysiologic properties similar to those of quinidine, is used primarily for the treatment of ventricular arrhythmias, especially for the acute termination of ventricular tachycardias. There is ready placental transfer of the drug because it is a small molecule and is not highly bound to plasma proteins. Both procainamide and its active metabolite N-acetylprocainamide pass into breast milk, reaching concentrations up to five times higher than those in the maternal serum. However, the daily amounts of both substances consumed by the neonate appear to be clinically negligible. Procainamide has not been shown to have teratogenic effects, even when used in the early stages of pregnancy. It can, therefore, be regarded as a drug of choice for the chronic therapy of maternal ventricular arrhythmias. Nevertheless, the potential risk of drug accumulation as well as a relatively high incidence of lupuslike syndrome associated with chronic procainamide therapy should be kept in mind.

C. Disopyramide

Although disopyramide may be useful in subset of patients with ventricular tachycardia, its negative inotropic effects, significant placental transfer, and drug-induced uterine contractions preclude clinical use of this drug in pregnancy unless absolutely necessary. Data about the safety of the drug for breast-feeding mothers are insufficient to recommend its use.

D. Lidocaine

This antiarrhythmic agent is used predominantly for the acute termination of ventricular arrhythmias. Information on the use of lidocaine during pregnancy is relatively limited, and most of the pharmakokinetic data were collected when it was used as a maternal anesthetic during labor. Lidocaine enters the fetal circulation rapidly after maternal intravenous administration, reaching approximately

55% of the maternal plasma level of the drug. Lidocaine has no adverse effects on the fetus. However, anecdotal reports have demonstrated neonatal toxicity following local anesthesia for the mother. Transfer of the drug to breast milk appears to pose minimal or no hazard to the newborn. Lidocaine at the smallest effective dose is considered safe for the treatment of acute ventricular arrhythmias during pregnancy and lactation.

E. Mexiletine

Mexiletine is structurally similar to lidocaine and is absorbed from the gastrointestinal tract. The drug crosses the placenta freely and enters breast milk. In this respect, adequate controlled studies have not been performed in pregnant women. Although the drug has been used safely in individual cases, current data do not provide a basis for recommending its use during pregnancy.

F. Phenytoin

This drug is teratogenic and should not be used during the first trimester of pregnancy. The fetal hydantoin syndrome is characterized by growth and mental retardation, craniofacial and limb abnormalities, and cardiac defects. The use of the drug as an antiarrhythmic agent in later stages of pregnancy should be limited strictly to the acute treatment of digitalis-induced ventricular arrhythmias, refractory to other drugs. Concentrations of the drug in the breast milk are low, reaching approximately 40% of the maternal serum levels. No adverse effects have been documented in the infants of nursing mothers taking phenytoin.

G. Flecainide

This is a potent antiarrhythmic drug for management of atrial, junctional, and ventricular arrhythmias. The drug passes readily across the placenta, and about 70–80% of the drug reaches the fetus. The documented milk to maternal plasma ratios range from 1.5 to 2.2. However, no data are available about the influence of the drug on the infant. Teratology studies in animals as well as clinical data suggest that flecainide administration during pregnancy is safe. However, in pregnant women with structural heart disease, the application of flecainide must be considered with caution.

H. Propafenone

This drug, which is similar to flecainide, has low bioavailability (20%) due to extensive hepatic first-pass metabolism. Very high protein binding of the drug may influence its pharmacokinetics in pregnancy. Both drug and its active metabolites cross the placenta to a limited extent (30–40%). Milk to maternal plasma concentration was found higher for the metabolite compared to the drug itself (0.50

448

versus 0.20), which probably corresponds to a difference in the maternal protein binding of the two components (75% for the metabolite compared to 95% for the drug). Intake from breast milk is estimated to be very low.

XIV. CLASS II ANTIARRHYTHMIC DRUGS

The clinical use of beta blockers for the treatment of arrhythmias is based mainly on their inhibitory effects of sympathetic excitation of the heart. They are effective in the management of atrial and ventricular extrasystoles, the control of rapid ventricular rate in patients with supraventricular arrhythmias, and the prevention of malignant ventricular arrhythmias in patients with structural heart disease, such as hypertrophic cardiomyopathy or mitral valve prolapse. Beta blockers increase uterine activity in pregnant women. Despite easy placental crossing, no beta blocker has been shown to cause any fetal malformation. Although anecdotal reports have suggested that beta blockers cause intrauterine growth retardation, bradycardia, apnea, hypoglycemia or hyperbilirubinemia, results of placebo-controlled studies have not confirmed these complications. Only mild growth retardation appears to be related to the treatment. Because of the theoretical possibility of fetal hypoglycemia or bradycardia, cardioselective beta blockers or those with intrinsic sympathomimetic activity are often recommended. This holds true particularly for acebutolol, oxprenolol, and pindolol. Most of the beta blockers are secreted into breast milk at concentrations about five times higher than in maternal plasma. This is supposed to be a result of "ion trapping" due to the lower pH of milk compared to blood. Beta blockers, which are mostly weak bases, are more readily trapped in the milk. However, the amount of the drug transmitted to the child with normal renal and hepatic function is of no clinical significance.

Recently, the short acting beta-blocker *esmolol* has been used for acute management of supraventricular arrhythmias in pregnancy. Because of its short elimination half-life (under 10 min), there is relatively little transplacental passage of the drug. However, experimental data show that even low levels of the drug may adversely influence fetal hemodynamics. Because there is only very limited information about clinical use during pregnancy, the drug cannot be widely recommended.

XV. CLASS III ANTIARRHYTHMIC DRUGS

These agents generally block potassium channels and prolong repolarization. They are potent antiarrhythmic drugs, effective in terminating and preventing most of the supraventricular and ventricular arrhythmias. Of the whole group, amiodarone and sotalol are the most frequently used.

A. Amiodarone

Amiodarone has been successfully used for recurrent, life-threatening supra-ventricular and ventricular tachyarrhythmias at various stages of pregnancy. Transplacental passage of amiodarone and its metabolite desethylamiodarone is relatively low (about 10 and 25%, respectively). Nevertheless, there are major concerns about the high concentration of iodine and its effects on the fetus, such as neonatal goiter. Although initial reports showed no teratogenicity and few adverse effects, some later reports described neonatal hypothyroidism with growth retar-dation or premature delivery. The incidence of neonatal hypothyroidism has been estimated at about 9%, a proportion similar to that reported for the adult popula-tion treated with amiodarone. On the other hand, experimental studies have found no adverse effects of the drug on the gestation period. Both amiodarone and its metabolite are readily excreted into breast milk, with a milk-to-plasma ratio between 2.3 and 9.2. For this reason, administration of amiodarone during the lactation period cannot be recommended. With respect to other potentially nega-tive effects, the use of amiodarone must be restricted only to cases resistant to other antiarrhythmics.

B. Sotalol

Besides its class III effects, racemic (d,l) sotalol is a noncardioselective beta-blocker. As a result of rapid placental transfer, the mean maternal-to-fetal plasma concentration ratio is 1.05. The milk-to-plasma ratio ranges from 2.4 to 5.6, and the breast-fed neonate may receive up to 20% of the maternal dose. Clinical experience with sotalol is rather limited, although no adverse effects of the drug on the fetus have been reported. Therefore, sotalol should be administered with caution.

XVI. CLASS IV ANTIARRHYTHMIC DRUGS

Calcium antagonists exert their antiarrhythmic effect by blocking slow calcium channels. Of the whole group, certain experience exists with the use of verapamil and diltiazem during pregnancy.

A. Verapamil

Verapamil is effective for the acute treatment of paroxysmal supraventricular tachycardia and for slowing the ventricular response during atrial fibrillation or flutter. Negative mutagenic studies in animals and clinical studies indicate the relative safety of verapamil administration during pregnancy. This drug has also been used safely in the management of preeclampsia or premature labor. The toco-lytic effects of verapamil appear to be mild compared with those of diltiazem.

After 6 to 12 weeks of therapy, levels of the drug in the fetal circulation reach 35–40% of maternal serum levels. Rapid intravenous injection has occasionally been shown to precipitate maternal hypotension with fetal distress. Reports about the passage of the drug into breast milk are inconclusive. Extensive clinical experience suggests that verapamil may be used safely for the acute termination of paroxysms of supraventricular tachycardia with a narrow QRS complex during pregnancy.

B. Diltiazem

The clinical use of diltiazem is analogous to that of verapamil. However, diltiazem suppresses spontaneous uterine contractions, and animal studies in which high doses of the drug were used resulted in fetal deaths, decreased neonatal survival, and skeletal abnormalities. Little is known about the passage of the drug into breast milk. Therefore, current data do not provide a basis for recommending its use during pregnancy.

XVII. OTHER ANTIARRHYTHMIC DRUGS

A. Adenosine

Adenosine is an endogenous metabolite used for diagnostic purpose as well as for acute therapy of supraventricular tachyarrhythmias. The overall efficacy of the drug is analogous to that of verapamil. However, because adenosine is a naturally occurring nucleotide and has a very short half-life (less than 10 sec), it can be used safely during pregnancy. However, during pregnancy, the serum concentration of the adenosine-degrading enzyme, adenosine deaminase, is only 25% of the normal value. On the other hand, the distribution volume of adenosine is increased in the pregnant woman. Thus, plasma levels of adenosine do not differ substantially from those in nonpregnant subjects. The clinical safety of adenosine in pregnancy has been reported repeatedly and it appears to be the drug of first choice for the acute treatment of supraventricular tachyarrythmias.

B. Digoxin

Digoxin is used mainly for prophylaxis and acute management of supraventricular tachyarrhythmias or for the control of the ventricular rate in atrial fibrillation and/or flutter. Normal dosing with the drug in pregnant women results in relatively low maternal serum concentrations, probably because of increased blood volume and glomerular filtration. Digoxin crosses the placenta freely, and its concentrations in the fetus have been reported to be similar to or higher than maternal concentrations. Despite extensive use of digoxin in pregnancy, no significant adverse effects have been reported when therapeutic levels of the drug were administered. The drug is excreted into breast milk in concentrations similar to or even lower than those in maternal serum under steady-state conditions. Therefore, digoxin can be used in lactating women.

XVIII. NONPHARMACOLOGICAL MANAGEMENT

Electrical cardioversion can be performed safely in all stages of pregnancy, both electively and in emergency settings. Even multiple DC cardioversions with energies of 400 J have been reported in the course of the same pregnancy without an adverse effect on the fetus. The risk of inducing fetal tachyarrhythmia appears to be minimal. However, as there are scarce data about transient fetal arrhythmias during maternal DC cardioversion, fetal heart monitoring, when feasible, is advisable during elective procedures. Similarly, because of the potential risk of embolism, anticoagulation with heparin should be considered before cardioversion of atrial fibrillation in mitral valve disease. Cardiopulmonary resuscitation during pregnancy follows the same principles as in other circumstances. In principle, resuscitation in the earlier stages of pregnancy (up to 24 weeks) is mainly focused on saving the mother's life. After this period, emergency delivery of the fetus by cesarean section should be considered when maternal resuscitation is unsuccessful within 15 min.

XIX. MANAGEMENT OF SPECIFIC ARRHYTHMIAS

A. Premature Beats

In the absence of organic heart disease, the occurrence of supraventricular or ventricular premature beats is of no clinical importance and should be managed by reassuring the patient. When these benign rhythm disturbances become troublesome for the woman, precipitating factors such as hyperthyroidism, alcohol, caffeine, or cigarette smoking should be identified and eliminated. Administration of minor tranquilizers may be beneficial for some patients with no underlying heart disease or precipitating factors but with bothersome symptoms. In these patients, antiarrhythmic drugs should be restricted for the management of significant symptoms or hemodynamic instability. In patients with organic heart disease, beta-blockers are preferred.

B. Supraventricular Tachyarrhythmias

Paroxysmal supraventricular tachycardia may occur commonly in the third trimester of pregnancy. The incidence of hemodynamic compromise is relatively low, because of the young age of the patients and the low incidence of organic heart disease. Nonpharmacological interventions such as vagal maneuvers should be tried first. Propranolol, verapamil, and adenosine are useful for the acute termination of supraventricular tachycardias. Among these drugs, adenosine is preferred because of its rapid action, few side effects, and probable lack of placental transfer. Blood pressure and the ECG should be monitored during pharmacological interventions.

In patients with atrial fibrillation, therapy is cardioversion or control of the ventricular rate. In the majority of patients, digoxin is chosen traditionally. In patients with thyrotoxicosis, beta blockers are preferable. When digoxin is insufficient to control ventricular rate, verapamil may be added.

C. Ventricular Tachyarrhythmias

Ventricular tachycardia may occur in association with organic heart disease, such as coronary heart disease, hypertrophic cardiomyopathy, or mitral valve prolapse. As in the nonpregnant population, ventricular tachycardia occurs also in the absence of detectable structural cardiac abnormalities. Hemodynamically tolerated tachycardia may be cardioverted with intravenous lidocaine. Beta blockers or sotalol should be used for ventricular tachycardia in the absence of structural heart disease. Verapamil is effective for most patients with idiopathic tachycardias arising from the left ventricle (right bundle branch block morphology with left axis deviation). Torsades de pointes should be managed conventionally by correcting any causal factor, especially hypomagnesemia or hypokalemia and by accelerating sinus rate. DC shock should be used if hemodynamic compromise occurs during ventricular tachycardia or for the treatment of cardiac arrest. Long-term prophylactic antiarrhythmic treatment should be determined individually. The management strategies are similar to those used in nonpregnant patients. However, the choice of antiarrhythmic drug is critical (Table 3).

D. Bradyarrhythmias

High-degree conduction abnormalities occur occasionally in pregnancy. They are usually congenital in origin or related to underlying structural heart disease. Despite the presence of atrioventricular block, most women remain asymptomatic during the whole pregnancy. In symptomatic patients, implantation of a pacemaker should be considered—also in asymptomatic patients when the rhythm is unstable. Data relating to sinus node abnormalities in pregnancy are sparse, but in principle, a similar strategy should be followed. Pregnant patients with bundle branch block should be evaluated for detection of underlying cardiac disease. Pacemakers do not interfere with the normal course of pregnancy and fetal development.

Chronic Pulmonary Disease

I.	Arrhythmias in Chronic Pulmonary Disease	456
II.	Management of Specific Arrhythmias	458

A. John Camm and Josef Kautzner

Most of the information about the incidence of cardiac arrhythmias in patients with a pulmonary pathology is related to chronic obstructive pulmonary disease (COPD). Because of the high prevalence of COPD, it provides prominent insights pertinent to evaluation of the effects of impaired pulmonary and respiratory function on the rhythm of the heart.

In patients with stable COPD, there is no clear relationship between the frequency or severity of arrhythmias and the extent of hypoxemia, functional pulmonary impairment, right atrial or pulmonary artery pressure elevations, or right ventricular hypertrophy. Arrhythmias often reach their maximum during sleep, especially in those patients with significant nocturnal hypoxemia. This implies that severe nocturnal hypoxemia, which is often related to periods of obstructive sleep apnea and increase in sympathetic nervous activity, is associated with increasing ventricular ectopy. In patients with acute deterioration of chronic respiratory failure, hypoxemia and metabolic derangements appear to promote the occurrence of both supraventricular and ventricular arrhythmias. The arrhythmogenicity of various bronchodilator drugs or their combinations is a special area of concern, especially because of the suggested association between death from asthma and the use of inhalation of beta-agonist bronchodilators and/or aminophylline administration.

Aminophylline/Theophylline

Despite documented fatal reactions to intravenous aminophylline and experimental data demonstrating a reduction of the fibrillatory threshold after the administration of these drugs, clinical evidence and trial data suggest that there is little danger from aminophylline, maintained at therapeutic blood levels (i.e., 10–20 μg/mL). Nevertheless, its administration increases heart rate by activating the sympathetic system leading to increased levels of circulating catecholamines. The relative safety of aminophylline in combination with beta-mimetic drugs has been documented in recent studies, some of which evaluated patients with COPD and concomitant ischemic heart disease.

Beta-Mimetic Agents

The administration of beta$_2$-selective bronchodilatory drugs may lead to a higher frequency of ventricular arrhythmias, but detailed studies have shown no such effects, except for the provocation of sinus tachycardia. Although these drugs dilate peripheral vessels and consequently increase cardiac output and heart rate, the resulting sinus tachycardia is usually very mild (approximately 5–10 beats/min). Hypokalemia, observed after the administration of larger doses of beta$_2$-mimetic drugs, can play a more specific role in arrhythmogenesis. In addition, other factors, such as the toxicity of halogenated hydrocarbon propellants used in metered-dose inhalers, can lead to proarrhythmic effects. These propellants are not completely inert, sensitizing myocardium to the arrhythmogenic effects of sympathomimetic drugs. However, clinical data do not support the hypothesis that propellants in doses inhaled during treatment are particularly arrhythmogenic.

Digitalis

Digoxin is a minor cause of arrhythmias in patients with COPD. The association between paroxysmal supraventricular arrhythmias with atrioventricular block and digitalis toxicity implies that this arrhythmia, which is seen relatively frequently in patients with COPD, is related to the use of digitalis. In contrast, the occurrence of multifocal atrial tachycardia, which can be seen in patients with serious pulmonary diseases, is not associated with digitalis treatment.

I. ARRHYTHMIAS IN CHRONIC PULMONARY DISEASE

Estimates of the incidence of cardiac arrhythmias in patients with pulmonary disease vary considerably. Some of these differences can be attributed to the variety and severity of the underlying lung disease, the presence or absence of respiratory failure with acid-base or metabolic disturbances, the use of various cardiovascular and bronchodilator drugs, the presence of concomitant cardiovascular disease, the length of observation, and the method of recording. Accordingly, it is difficult to draw simple conclusions from these few clinical studies which are available.

Although patients with COPD and mild to moderate functional impairment exhibit a frequency of cardiac arrhythmias comparable to that in the normal population, cardiac arrhythmias can be detected in more than 75% of patients with stable but severe COPD. However, the majority of these arrhythmias consist of isolated premature beats, which are not frequent. For instance, data from the Nocturnal Oxygen Therapy Trial, conducted on a well-defined population of patients with severe COPD and hypoxemia (Pa_{O_2} <55 mmHg), showed that ventricular premature beats occurred in 83%, ventricular bigeminy in 68%, paired ventricular premature beats in 61%, and nonsustained ventricular tachycardia in 22%. More frequent ventricular premature beats (>25/hr) were seen in only a relatively small proportion of the patients (35%). Similar data were found in a large group of patients with severe COPD during exercise, with the occurrence of potentially significant arrhythmias in only 12%.

Patients with COPD and acute respiratory failure appeared to have predominantly supraventricular arrhythmias. However, the many initial studies demonstrating this used only the standard resting ECG. A more recent study using a 72-hr period of monitoring in hospitalized COPD patients, among whom many had respiratory failure, demonstrated that premature atrial contractions occurred in the same frequency as premature ventricular beats—i.e., in approximately two-thirds of the subjects studied. Paroxysmal atrial tachycardia occurred in 7 and ventricular tachycardia in 5 of 35 patients. More important, among the 16 patients with respiratory failure, 15 had arrhythmias. Therefore, the data suggest that respiratory failure associated with severe hypoxemia promotes the occurrence of both supraventricular and ventricular arrhythmias. Nevertheless, the prognostic value of this finding remains unknown.

Multifocal Atrial Tachycardia

This arrhythmia, which typically occurs in seriously ill patients, appears to be almost specific for pulmonary disease with oxygen desaturation. As it is associated with an increased mortality (the average mortality rates vary between 29 and 62%), multifocal atrial arrhythmia (MAT) is often considered as a harbinger of an adverse outcome. Compared with other arrhythmias, MAT occurs relatively infrequently with an incidence of 0.13–0.36% in hospitalized patients. The mean age of those patients presenting with MAT is greater than 70 years, with male predominance. Clinically important pulmonary disease can be identified in at least 60% of cases; often an acute exacerbation of COPD is the apparent precipitating factor. Although coronary artery disease has been found in a large proportion of MAT patients, a causal relationship has not been established. In some studies, MAT has been linked to the postoperative state, especially when complicated by pneumonia

457

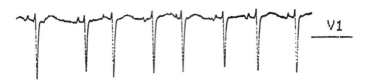

Figure 1   An ECG of multifocal atrial tachycardia from a patient with chronic obstructive pulmonary disease and recent lung resection because of cancer. Notice the irregularity of the rhythm and multiform P-wave morphology.

or pulmonary embolism. From the pathophysiological point of view, it appears that MAT is associated with an excess of circulating plasma catecholamines, especially in response to hypoxia. In addition, many patients take methylxanthine derivatives, which may contribute the hyperadrenergic state. Hypokalemia or hypomagnesemia are other factors that may play a role in the pathogenesis of MAT, promoting triggered activity in the atrial myocardium.

Electrocardiographic characteristics of MAT are an atrial rate greater than 100 beats/min, the presence of P waves of multiple morphologies (at least three) in a single ECG lead with an isoelectric baseline between them, and variation in PR intervals (Figure 1). The ventricular rate is usually irregular, often lower than the atrial rate. Because of these characteristics, a 12-lead ECG should be used to establish the correct diagnosis, especially when differentiating MAT from atrial fibrillation.

II. MANAGEMENT OF SPECIFIC ARRHYTHMIAS

The management of cardiac arrhythmias in patients with chronic pulmonary disease is notoriously difficult, being influenced by the many factors noted above. The following considerations should be kept in mind: (a) Significant pulmonary disease leading to hypoxemia imposes an additional burden on the cardiovascular system. Thus, any compromise of the compensatory mechanisms may lead to profound tissue hypoxia and metabolic acidosis. For this reason, a decrease in cardiac output secondary to various arrhythmias, even when the arrhythmias themselves are otherwise benign, can be particularly deleterious for patients with pulmonary disease. (b) It is not known whether ventricular premature beats are prognostically significant, as in the postmyocardial infarction population. Nevertheless, the sparse epidemiologic data available suggest that patients with chronic obstructive pulmonary disease are probably at a much lower risk of sudden cardiac death.

Hemodynamically compromising or imminently life-threatening arrhythmias should be treated promptly, with established regimens of antiarrhythmic drugs or electrical cardioversion. However, less confidence exists about the optimal management of other, less urgent arrhythmias associated with chronic pulmonary disease. Therapy with conventional antiarrhythmic drugs is usually less effective in these conditions than are general measures, such as the correction of hypoxemia and other underlying metabolic or electrolyte abnormalities (Figure 2). Therefore, management of the underlying pulmonary disease and correction of associated hypoxemia are essential for the control of both supraventricular and ventricular arrhythmias. Adjustment of bronchodilator treatment may prove effective in eliminating certain arrhythmias. Administration of antiarrhythmic drugs should be considered only when the arrhythmia is not responding to these measures, causes significant symptoms, or impairs cardiac hemodynamics. Atrial fibrillation or flutter with a rapid ventricular response is controlled optimally by digoxin and/or calcium channel blockade. Selective beta blockers should be considered cautiously because of the potential for worsening airway function, especially during episodes of acute exacerbation of the lung disease. The mainstay of therapies for MAT is correction of predisposing causes and treatment of the underlying disease. With improvement in oxygenation and correction of electrolyte disturbances, spontaneous cardioversion to sinus rhythm can be achieved in many patients. When MAT hemodynamically compromises the seriously ill pa-

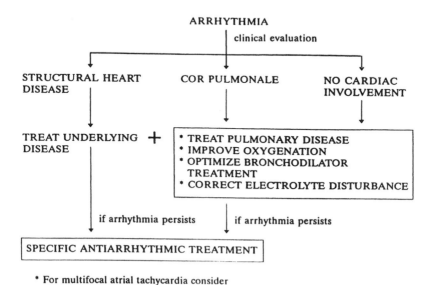

Figure 2 The approach to the management of arrhythmias in pulmonary disorders.

tient, specific antiarrhythmic drugs should be administered. Unlike many other drugs, both metoprolol and verapamil have recently proved to be successful. Apart from cardioversion to sinus rhythm, both drugs also decrease the ventricular rate, rendering the tachycardia more tolerable. Comparisons of metoprolol and verapamil suggest better efficacy for beta blockade. Several studies have demonstrated that metoprolol can be given cautiously to most COPD patients without inducing clinically important adverse effects. For ventricular arrhythmias, both cardioselective beta blockade and antiarrhythmic drugs may be needed.

Diagnosis and Management of Arrhythmia in Patients with Cardiomyopathy

I.   Hypertrophic Cardiomyopathy   461
II. Dilated Cardiomyopathy   464

William J. McKenna and Perry M. Elliott

I. HYPERTROPHIC CARDIOMYOPATHY

Arrhythmias of both supraventricular and ventricular origin are frequent in patients with hypertrophic cardiomyopathy (HCM) (Table 1). They are important symptomatically and have prognostic implications.

A. Supraventricular Arrhythmias

Paroxysmal supraventricular arrhythmias occur during the course of ambulatory electrocardiographic (ECG) monitoring in 30–50% of patients with HCM. In a small minority of patients, these may be associated with accessory atrioventricular pathways, but resting ECG abnormalities make the diagnosis of Wolff-Parkinson-White syndrome from the surface ECG difficult in patients with HCM.

Treatment is usually not indicated for episodes that are asymptomatic and self-limiting. If episodes are sustained (> 30 sec) and/or associated with symptoms, then specific medical therapy should be instituted. Amiodarone in low doses (1000–1400 mg weekly) or beta blockers with class III action (e.g., sotalol) are effective in maintaining sinus rhythm and in controlling the ventricular rate during

Table 1   Incidence of Arrhythmia at the Time
of Initial Diagnosis of Hypertrophic
Cardiomyopathy

	Age (years)				
	≤15	16–30	31–45	46–60	>60
AF	0	0	4%	10%	5%
SVT	7%	14%	30%	29%	36%
VT	2%	17%	21%	31%	23%

Source: Adapted from McKenna WJ, Watkins HC: Hyper-
tropic cardiomyopathy. In: Scriver RC et al, eds. The
Metabolic and Molecular Bases of Inherited Disease. 7th
ed. New York: McGraw-Hill, 1995:4353.

breakthrough episodes. The role of other drugs (e.g., class I agents) is uncertain.
Anticoagulation is indicated if episodes are frequent or prolonged.

Atrial fibrillation (AF) is present in 5% of patients at the time of diagnosis of
HCM and develops in a further 10% over the subsequent 5 years. Predisposing
factors include left atrial enlargement and marked left ventricular (LV) hypertrophy.

In general, most patients tolerate AF as long as the ventricular rate is
controlled. In a small subset of patients, the loss of atrial systole associated with
the onset of AF may result in rapid hemodynamic deterioration requiring urgent
DC cardioversion. The risk of thromboembolism is high (particularly in the
presence of left atrial enlargement) and anticoagulation is mandatory.

B. Ventricular Arrhythmias

Sustained ventricular tachycardia is uncommon in HCM. The occurrence is
largely confined to patients with LV aneurysms. They are managed conventionally
with either empirical therapy or treatment guided by electrophysiological drug
testing.

Nonsustained Ventricular Tachycardia

Nonsustained ventricular tachycardia (NSVT) is defined as three or more consecutive ventricular extrasystoles with a mean rate of ≥ 120 beats/min lasting for less
than 30 sec. It occurs during the course of 48-hr ambulatory monitoring in 25% of
adults with the disease. It is usually asymptomatic, multiform, relatively slow, and
occurs predominantly during periods when vagal activity is relatively high (e.g.,
sleep). The presence of NSVT in adults is associated with a sevenfold increase in
the incidence of sudden death, making it the best noninvasive marker of risk

Table 2 Relation of Nonsustained Ventricular Tachycardia Evident During the Course of Ambulatory Monitoring and the Risk of Sudden Death in Patients with Hypertrophic Cardiomyopathy

Nonsustained Ventricular Tachycardia	
Sensitivity	69 (%)
Specificity	80
Positive predictive accuracy	22
Negative predictive accuracy	97

Source: Pooled data from Maron et al. (Am J Cardiol 1981; 48:252) and McKenna et al. (Br Heart J 1981; 46:168).

(Table 2). Its positive predictive accuracy is, however low (22%), reflecting the fact that most patients with NSVT do not die suddenly.

Invasive Electrophysiological Testing in Patients with Hypertrophic Cardiomyopathy

The annual mortality from HCM is 4–6% in the young and less (1–2%) in adults. In children and adolescents, recurrent syncope and a family history of sudden death are highly specific markers of the risk of sudden death, but most deaths occur in their absence.

Conventional electrophysiological (EP) testing demonstrates multiple abnormalities, including sinus node/His-Purkinje conduction abnormalities, accessory atrioventricular (AV) pathways (5%), atrial tachycardia (10%), and atrial fibrillation (55% with previously documented AF and 7% without). The prognostic importance of inducible ventricular arrhythmias in HCM remains uncertain, and aggressive stimulation protocols are not without risk. At present the routine use of conventional EP testing for risk stratification cannot be recommended. Results of recent studies suggest that an alternative approach using multiple recording electrodes to determine the degree of "fractionation" of the right ventricular ECG may be a more accurate method of defining the risk of ventricular fibrillation.

C. Management of "High-Risk" Patients

Amiodarone is the only drug to date that has been shown to reduce mortality in patients with HCM. Its serious side effects (thyroid and pulmonary toxicity, among others) can be minimized by using the lowest effective dose and maintaining plasma levels of the drug at less than 1.5 mg/L. An increasing number of patients are being treated with implanted cardioverter defibrillators, but further studies are required to identify those patients for whom this treatment modality is mandated or appropriate.

II. DILATED CARDIOMYOPATHY

Dilated cardiomyopathy (DCM) is associated with an annual mortality of 20–30% per year. The majority of deaths are attributable to progressive heart failure, but a significant number are sudden and presumed to be secondary to arrhythmia. Atrial and ventricular arrhythmias are common in DCM (Table 3) but of limited prognostic value. The first priority of medical therapy should be the treatment of heart failure with angiotensin converting enzyme inhibitors (in maximal tolerated doses), digoxin, and diuretics.

Table 3   Incidence of Arrhythmia in Patients with Dilated Cardiomyopathy

Reference	Number	AF (%)	VE > 30/hr (%)	Couplets (%)	NSVT (%)
[1]	35	7 (20)	29 (83)	26 (74)	21 (60)
[2]	69	12 (17)	19 (28)	—	15 (22)
[3]	74	14 (19)	30 (41)	15 (20)	36 (49)
[4]	124	18 (15)	70 (56)	70 (56)	48 (39)
[5]	73	12 (16)	40 (54)	73 (100)	31 (42)
[6]	110	38 (35)	—	94 (85)	49 (45)

Abbreviations: AF = atrial fibrillation; VE = ventricular ectopic beats; NSVT = nonsustained ventricular tachyardia.
[1] Huang SK, Messer JV, Denes P. Significance of ventricular tachycardia in idiopathic dilated cardiomyopathy: Observation in 35 patients. Am J Cardiol 1983; 51:507–12.
[2] Unverferth DV, Magorien RD, Moeschberger ML, Baker PB, Fetters JK, Leier CV. Factors influencing the one year mortality of dilated cardiomyopathy. Am J Cardiol 1984; 54:147–52.
[3] Meinertz T, Hofmann T, Kasper W, Treese N, Bechtold H, Steinen U, Pop T, Leitner ER, Andresen D, Meyer J. Significance of ventricular arrhythmias in idiopathic dilated cardiomyopathy. Am J Cardiol 1984; 53:902–7.
[4] Stewart RA, McKenna WJ, Oakley CM. Good prognosis for dilated cardiomyopathy without severe heart failure or arrhythmia. Quart J Med 1990; 275:309–18.
[5] Olshausen KV, Steinen U, Schwarz F, Kubler W, Meyer J. Long term prognostic significance of ventricular arrhythmia in idiopathic dilated cardiomyopathy. Am J Cardiol 1988; 61:146–51.
[6] Hofmann T, Meinertz T, Kasper W, Geibel A, Zehender M, Hohnloser S, Steinen U, Treese N, Just H. Mode of death in idiopathic dilated cardiomyopathy: a multivariate analysis of prognostic determinants. Am Heart J 1988; 116:1455–63.

A. Atrial Fibrillation

Restoration and maintenance of sinus rhythm in patients with DCM is rarely successful. The drugs of choice for control of the ventricular rate are digoxin and/ or low-dose beta blockers and calcium antagonists because the negatively inotropic effects of most other agents preclude their general use. All patients with AF should be anticoagulated in the absence of specific contraindications.

B. Ventricular Arrhythmias

Most patients with DCM have ventricular premature beats (VPBs), repetitive multiform VPBs, and NSVT. However, noninvasive testing (ambulatory ECG monitoring, signal-averaged ECG, QT dispersion) does not reliably identify patients at risk of sudden death. Only 50% of patients with clinical VT or VF have inducible monomorphic VT as judged from results with conventional EP protocols. However, a lack of inducibility does not imply a benign prognosis.

There is no evidence that treatment with class I antiarrhythmic drugs improves prognosis. There is increasing interest in the role of amiodarone because it does not exert negative inotropic effects, has antiadrenergic activity, homogeneously prolongs repolarization, and raises VF thresholds. It is effective in suppressing ventricular ectopic activity in patients with DCM. Ongoing trials are assessing its influence on prognosis. Patients who survive sudden cardiac death are being treated increasingly with implantable cardioverter/defibrillators (ICDs). These devices may prevent sudden death but are unlikely to influence progression of disease. They may have a role as a "bridge" to cardiac transplantation.

25

Management of Congenital Heart Disease in Adults

I.	Mechanism of Cyanosis and Age of Onset	467
II.	Associated Abnormalities	468
III.	Management of Hypoxemia in Acquired Heart Disease	470
IV.	Management of Congenital Heart Disease in the Adult	471
V.	Anatomic Defects (Shunt Lesions)	471
VI.	Postoperative Congenital Heart Disease	473
VII.	Associated Defects	474
VIII.	Endocarditis	474
IX.	Pregnancy	478
X.	Activity	479
XI.	Cyanosis	479
	Suggested Reading	479

William E. Hopkins

I. MECHANISM OF CYANOSIS AND AGE OF ONSET

Cyanosis in patients with congenital heart disease results from three primary mechanisms—parallel circulations, reduced pulmonary blood flow, and mixing of arterial and venous blood. Parallel circulations occur in patients with transposition of the great arteries and are almost never encountered in adults. Reduced pulmonary blood flow occurs in patients with anatomic obstruction to pulmonary blood flow and a defect that allows for a right-to-left shunt (i.e., tetralogy of Fallot). Decreased pulmonary blood flow can also occur in patients with markedly elevated pulmonary vascular resistance and a right-to-left shunt (Eisenmenger's syndrome), especially during exertion. Mixing of arterial and venous blood occurs in patients with a single ventricle and in those with Eisenmenger's syndrome secondary to bidirectional shunting.

In evaluating an adult with cyanotic congenital heart disease, an attempt should be made to determine the age at which cyanosis was first present. A history of cyanosis in the neonatal period or infancy invariably means that the adult patient has anatomic obstruction to pulmonary blood flow. The central pulmonary arteries are usually seen to be small on chest x-ray, though some patients exhibit poststenotic dilatation. Depending on the defect type, previous surgery, and co-morbid conditions, the adult may still be amenable to definitive repair or a shunt procedure to increase pulmonary blood flow.

Onset of cyanosis in childhood or adolescence is most often secondary to a nonrestrictive ventricular septal defect or patent ductus arteriosus and the super-vention of Eisenmenger's syndrome (secondary to increased pulmonary arterial resistance). The central pulmonary arteries seem to be large on chest x-ray, and surgery is not possible because of the presence of severe pulmonary vascular occlusive changes.

Onset of central cyanosis in adulthood is generally secondary to an atrial septal defect with Eisenmenger physiology. Once again, the central pulmonary arteries seem to be large on chest x-ray, and surgical repair is not possible because of the severe pulmonary vascular occlusive changes.

II. ASSOCIATED ABNORMALITIES

Physicians who care for adults with cyanotic congenital heart disease should be aware of specific problems that arise in this patient population. In addition, preventive care should be emphasized, such as the yearly administration of influenza vaccine, avoidance of high altitude or dehydration, and prophylaxis for bacterial endocarditis.

A. Erythrocytosis

Persistent hypoxemia in adults with cyanotic congenital heart disease results in a secondary erythrocytosis. Most patients have compensated erythrocytosis with a stable hemoglobin and hematocrit. Hyperviscosity symptoms are absent or mini-mal (fatigue, lassitude, headache, dizziness, visual changes, and myalgias). De-compensated erythrocytosis (continually rising hematocrit with significant hyper-viscosity symptoms) is unusual. Phlebotomy results in a transient lowering of the hematocrit and iron deficiency if performed on a regular basis. Iron deficiency results in nondeformable, microcytic red blood cells and, ultimately, a paradox-ically greater increase in viscosity as erythrocytosis occurs. Repetitive phle-botomy also depletes the patient of hemoglobin necessary to carry oxygen and can deplete skeletal muscle of iron necessary for energy metabolism. Phlebotomy can virtually always be avoided despite erythrocytosis, even in patients with hemoglobins as high as 24–25 g/dL and hematocrits as high as 74%.

Many of the more symptomatic adults with cyanotic congenital heart disease are, in fact, iron-deficient. Iron replacement must be performed cautiously, as patients may have a brisk reticulocytosis and symptoms related to the relatively abrupt increase in hematocrit. One should replace iron vigorously only until the reticulocytosis begins and then advance slowly.

Patients with erythrocytosis must avoid dehydration associated with fever, diarrhea, vomiting, or sweating, because volume depletion can lead to hyperviscosity.

B. Bleeding Diathesis

Patients with hematocrits above 65% tend to have a bleeding diathesis secondary to abnormal platelet and coagulation function. In fact, preoperative phlebotomy is helpful in patients with hematocrits above 65% to improve hemostasis. The phlebotomized blood can be stored and used for an autologous transfusion, if necessary. Aspirin, nonsteroidal anti-inflammatory medications, and warfarin should be avoided in these patients unless a specific indication is present. Acetaminophen is a safe choice for analgesia. Salsalate can be used as an anti-inflammatory agent because it does not inhibit platelet function.

C. Hyperuricemia/Gout

Hyperuricemia is common in adults with cyanotic congenital heart disease and is secondary to abnormal renal tubular handling of urate rather than the increased red cell mass. Hyperuricemia itself need not be treated. One must be cautious when treating gout. Because of the increased risk of bleeding, nonsteroidal anti-inflammatory medications should be used cautiously or not at all (see above). Diarrhea secondary to colchicine can lead to volume depletion and hyperviscosity.

D. Paradoxic Emboli

Right-to-left shunts in patients with cyanotic congenital heart disease put them at risk for paradoxic embolus. For this reason intravenous catheters should be used with extreme caution and placed only when absolutely necessary. Filters should be used to prevent infusion of air or particulates.

E. Gallstones

Because of the increased red blood cell mass, adults with cyanotic congenital heart disease have an increased incidence of bilirubin-rich gallstones. The possibility should be considered whenever such patients complain of abdominal pain.

F. Hemoptysis

The incidence of hemoptysis is increased in cyanotic patients with Eisenmenger's syndrome and in patients with bronchial collaterals and is likely secondary to friable, thin-walled vessels. Therapy is often only supportive bed rest and oxygen. Patients with more severe hemoptysis require aggressive management (bronchoscopy, selective intubation, and embolization) because the hemoptysis can be severe enough to cause death.

G. Acne

Acne is, of course, common in adolescents and often seen in adults with cyanotic congenital heart disease. It is important to inform patients that manipulation of the lesions can result in bacteremia, endocarditis, and death.

H. Noncardiac Surgery

Patients with cyanotic congenital heart disease are at high risk with noncardiac surgery. Decreased systemic cardiac output because of volume depletion or depression of myocardial contractility can decrease mixed venous oxygen saturation and therefore worsen arterial hypoxemia. A reduction of the systemic vascular resistance can increase the net right-to-left shunt and significantly worsen hypoxemia. It may require the temporary administration of pressor agents. Significant blood loss can lead to dangerous reductions in volume and hemoglobin. Hemostasis can be improved by preoperative phlebotomy if the hematocrit is greater than 65%. Foley catheters and intravenous lines should be minimized to reduce the risk of endocarditis and paradoxic emboli.

III. MANAGEMENT OF HYPOXEMIA IN ACQUIRED HEART DISEASE

Hypoxemia associated with acquired heart disease is most often secondary to pulmonary edema. Therapy consists of administration of oxygen and treatment of the primary pathophysiological process (e.g., acute valvular insufficiency or myocardial infarction). Hemodynamics should guide the intensity of arterial and venous vasodilation, relief of bronchospasm, diuresis, use of agents with positive inotropic effects, circulatory support, and, rarely, surgical intervention.

Hypoxemia can occur occasionally in patients with a significantly increased right atrial pressure (primary pulmonary hypertension, pulmonary embolus, tricuspid regurgitation, right ventricular infarction) secondary to right-to-left shunt through a patent foramen ovale. The presence of right-to-left shunt can be determined by contrast echocardiography. Supplemental oxygen does not increase the arterial oxygen saturation under these conditions, and treatment should be directed toward the underlying pathophysiological abnormality.

IV. MANAGEMENT OF CONGENITAL HEART DISEASE IN THE ADULT

A. Overview

Congenital heart disease presents both an intellectual and management challenge for most adult physicians, including cardiologists. It is estimated that there are more than 500,000 adults with congenital heart disease in the United States. In addition, there are approximately 25,000 infants born with a congenital heart defect each year of whom more than 80% are expected to reach adulthood. Most physicians treating adult patients are unfamiliar with the unique hemodynamic derangements, specialized nomenclature, constellation of associated defects, and postoperative sequelae in such patients. A comprehensive view of all of congenital heart disease is beyond the scope of this book. Our goal is to help physicians understand specific aspects of congenital heart disease in adult patients. Some specific matters are covered in the section of Chapter 2 that deals with dyspnea and congenital heart disease; Chapter 6, "General Observations"; Chapter 22, "Pregnancy"; and Chapter 28, "Infective Endocarditis." A review of basic malformations and their implications in adult patients is provided in the suggested reading.

V. ANATOMIC DEFECTS (SHUNT LESIONS)

A. Basic Principles

Shunt lesions comprise a significant proportion of congenital heart defects encountered in adults. They can occur at the level of the atria (atrial septal defects), ventricles (ventricular septal defects), and great arteries (most commonly patent ductus arteriosus). A nonrestrictive defect implies that the communication is large enough that there is no pressure drop from one chamber or artery to another. A nonrestrictive atrial septal defect results in equalization of right and left atrial pressure; a nonrestrictive ventricular septal defect results in equalization of right and left ventricular pressure; and a nonrestrictive patent ductus arteriosus results in equalization of aortic and pulmonary artery pressure. A restrictive defect is smaller in size and results in a pressure drop across the defect. The smaller the defect, the greater the pressure difference.

B. Atrial Septal Defect

Atrial septal defects are the most common shunt lesions first diagnosed in adulthood and occur more commonly in women than men. Secundum type atrial septal defects (defect within the fossa ovalis) are much more common than either primum type atrial septal defects, sinus venosus defects, or coronary sinus defects. The classic hemodynamic manifestations of an atrial septal defect occur in those patients with nonrestrictive defects (defects > 1.0–1.5 cm in diameter) and are

471

similar in all defect types. The magnitude and direction of shunt is determined predominantly by the relative compliance of the left and right ventricles. Because the right ventricle is usually significantly more compliant than the left ventricle, the shunt is left to right. This results in volume loading of the right ventricle (hence right ventricular dilatation) and increased pulmonary blood flow (pulmonary artery dilatation and shunt vascularity seen on chest x-ray). The left-to-right shunt at the atrial level results in an underfilled left ventricle and decreased systemic cardiac output. Smaller, restrictive atrial septal defects generally do not result in significant left-to-right shunt unless the left atrial pressure is increased secondary to mitral regurgitation or stenosis.

The most common symptoms in patients with atrial septal defect are exertional dyspnea, fatigue, and palpitations. The classic physical findings include a right ventricular lift, pulmonary artery tap, and the so-called fixed split second heart sound. No matter how dysfunctional the right ventricle, signs of right heart failure (jugular venous distention, hepatic engorgement, and peripheral edema) are rarely present because the right atrium can be decompressed through the interatrial defect. Classic electrocardiographic (ECG) findings include right axis deviation and an rSR' pattern in lead V_1. With advancing age, right axis deviation is less common because of evolving left ventricular abnormalities that shift the axis leftward (e.g., with myocardial infarction or systemic hypertension). Unrepaired atrial septal defects result in a decreased life expectancy, with 90% mortality by age 60. With advancing age, the pulmonary vascular resistance often increases, pulmonary arterial hypertension ensues, and the right ventricle becomes progressively more dysfunctional. Atrial arrhythmias are more prevalent with advancing age. Atrial fibrillation and flutter occur in up to 50% of patients over age 40. Eisenmenger's syndrome, defined as severe pulmonary vascular occlusive changes with reversal of the previous left-to-right shunt and hypoxemia, occurs in less than 5% of patients with an atrial septal defect. (see section III.D. Cyanosis/Clubbing).

The presence and type of atrial septal defect, pulmonary artery pressure, and the direction and magnitude of shunts often can be determined by echocardiography (transthoracic and transesophageal). Treatment of an atrial septal defect requires surgical closure. Life expectancy is normal in patients who have an atrial septal defect repaired before age 20 to 25 years. Older patients who undergo repair of an atrial septal defect, including those above age 60, can expect an improvement in symptoms and increased survival. The rare patient with severe pulmonary vascular occlusive changes, especially those with Eisenmenger's syndrome, have a markedly increased surgical mortality. Surgical repair of an atrial septal defect does not eliminate (cure) atrial arrhythmias in those patients with preoperative atrial arrhythmias. In fact, the incidence of atrial fibrillation or flutter may be as great as 50% in patients in whom repair is undertaken after age 40, even if no previous clinical history of atrial arrhythmias is present.

C. Ventricular Septal Defect

The ventricular septum is composed of distinct anatomic regions consisting of the muscular system (inlet, outlet, trabecular and atrioventricular septum) and the fibrous membranous septum. Most ventricular septal defects involve the membranous septum. Hemodynamically, ventricular septal defects can be classified as small, moderate, or large in size. Small, restrictive ventricular septal defects do not result in significant shunts and therefore do not require surgical repair or restriction of activity. The major risk is that of endocarditis. A precordial thrill and loud holosystolic murmur (Rogers) are present in many patients with a small restrictive defect. Moderate-sized defects result in a significant left-to-right shunt (pulmonary/systemic flow of 2 or greater), with volume loading of the left ventricle, but they are almost never seen in adulthood because of previous surgical repair or spontaneous closure in infancy. Large, nonrestrictive ventricular septal defects result in biventricular volume loading and heart failure in infancy. Adults with large, nonrestrictive ventricular septal defects invariably have Eisenmenger's syndrome and are cyanotic. (see section III.D. Cyanosis/Clubbing).

The mortality associated with closing a ventricular septal defect surgically in patients with Eisenmenger's syndrome is quite high. Ventricular septal defects in adults, then, almost never require surgical repair because they are either small and hemodynamically insignificant or large and associated with a secondary Eisenmenger's syndrome.

D. Patent Ductus Arteriosus

Patent ductus arteriosus, like ventricular septal defects, can be classified as small, moderate, or large in size. Small, restrictive shunts are often silent by physical exam and do not require surgical repair. They do entail a risk of endocarditis. Moderate-sized shunts (pulmonary/systemic flow of 2 or greater) result in volume loading of the left ventricle (hence left ventricular dilatation). The classic physical finding is a continuous murmur (Gibson 5) at the left infraclavicular area. The therapy is surgical ligation. Large, nonrestrictive patent ductus arteriosus in adults is associated with Eisenmenger's syndrome and therefore unrepairable. The continuous murmur is no longer present. The classical physical finding is differential cyanosis (see Chapter 6, "General Observations").

VI. POSTOPERATIVE CONGENITAL HEART DISEASE

Many adults with congenital heart disease have had a previous cardiac surgical procedure. However, the surgical nomenclature and long-term implications of specific procedures are often unfamiliar and even intimidating to physicians who care for adults. Optimal management of adults with congenital heart disease requires some understanding of the surgical procedure, possible postoperative residua, and the potential long-term sequelae following specific surgical interventions. Examples include recurrent stenosis or regurgitation after a valvular procedure; conduit obstruction after repair of truncus arteriosus; arrhythmias, and right ventricular failure secondary to pulmonary insufficiency or recurrent outflow tract obstruction in patients with repaired tetralogy of Fallot. Many adult patients alive today had cardiac surgery in an era when intraoperative myocardial preservation was less adequate and surgical techniques were less refined. Both right and left ventriculotomies were more commonly performed in the repair of defects such as tetralogy of Fallot or ventricular septal defect. Because surgery was generally performed with patients at greater age, the heart was subjected to longer periods of hypoxemia, pressure overload, and/or volume overload. Consequently, unexplained ventricular systolic dysfunction in an adult with an adequately repaired congenital heart defect may be secondary to fibrosis from previous ventricular volume and/or pressure overload, previous cyanosis, poor intraoperative myocardial preservation, and/or a surgical ventriculotomy. Table 1 shows the more common surgical procedures used in patients with congenital heart disease. The column headed "sequelae" is included to alert physicians who care for adults to potential long-term sequelae after a specific procedure.

VII. ASSOCIATED DEFECTS

Optimal management of adults with congenital heart disease requires knowledge of associated defects. For instance, an adult who had a coarctation of the aorta repaired during infancy or childhood is at risk for aortic valvular disease, type B dissection, and endocarditis if he or she has a bicuspid aortic valve. Table 2 lists some of the more common congenital heart defects and the associated abnormalities physicians of adults should be aware of. Included are a few of the more common syndromes associated with congenital heart defects that may be encountered.

VIII. ENDOCARDITIS

Endocarditis is a risk in both operated and unoperated adults with congenital heart disease. Obstruction to flow (intracardiac, valvular, or arterial), valvular insufficiency, prosthetic valves, surgical shunts from systemic artery to pulmonary artery, and shunt lesions at the great artery or ventricular level (especially small communications) all entail risk for endocarditis. Atrial septal defects, whether repaired or unrepaired, are not associated with endocarditis unless an associated abnormality is present (see Table 2). Repaired patent ductus arteriosus and ventricular septal defects do not require antibiotic prophylaxis unless residual shunting or another defect persists. Likewise, repaired coarctation of the aorta with minimal or no gradient does not require antibiotic prophylaxis unless an associ-

474

Table 1 Surgical Procedures for Patients with Congenital Heart Disease

Procedure	Description	Purpose	Sequelae
Arterial switch	"Switching" the aorta and pulmonary artery (PA) and reimplanting the coronary arteries.	Normalize the circulation in patients with transposition of the great arteries (TGA).	PA stenosis can occur. Long-term outlook regarding the aorta and coronary arteries still unknown.
Blalock-Hanlon atrial septectomy	Creation of an atrial septal defect.	Increase mixing of blood at the atrial level in patients with TGA.	
Blalock-Taussig shunt (classic)	End-side anastomosis of the sub-clavian artery to the PA.	Increase pulmonary blood flow in patients with anatomic obstruction to PA blood flow (i.e., tetralogy of Fallot).	Markedly diminished or absent arm pulses on the side of the shunt. Usually performed on the opposite side of the aortic arch.
Blalock-Taussig shunt (modified)	Side-side anastomosis of the sub-clavian artery to PA using an interposed conduit graft.	Increase pulmonary blood flow in patients with anatomic obstruction to PA blood flow (i.e., tetralogy of Fallot).	Diminished pulses on the side of the shunt
Coarctation repair	A. End-end anastomosis. B. Subclavian flap technique—use of the left subclavian artery to enlarge the coarctation site. C. Prosthetic graft material.	All techniques enlarge the coarctation site and relieve the stenosis.	Recurrent coarctation more common in infant repair. Persistent hypertension more common in later repairs. Markedly diminished or absent left arm pulses in subclavian flap repair. Aortic aneurysms at the site of repair occasionally occur when prosthetic graft material used. Increased incidence of type B aortic dissection.

Table 1 (Continued)

Procedure	Description	Purpose	Sequelae
Fontan shunt	Multiple variations, all of which result in right atrial (RA) to PA flow.	Allows for segregation of the venous and systemic circulations in patients with tricuspid atresia or single ventricle.	Sick sinus syndrome, atrial fibrillation and flutter are common. Pulmonary arterio-venous malformation (AVM), and protein losing enteropathy occasionally occur.
Glenn shunt (classic)	End-side anastomosis of the superior vena cava (SVC) to the right (R)PA. The RPA is ligated and therefore disconnected from the main PA and left (L)PA.	Increase pulmonary blood flow.	Pulmonary AVMs occasionally occur
Glen shunt (bidirectional)	Same as the classic Glenn shunt but the RPA is not ligated.	Increase pulmonary blood flow.	Pulmonary AVMs occasionally occur
Mustard atrial baffle Senning atrial baffle	Intraatrial baffle using pericardium or prosthetic material.	Normalizes the circulation in patients with TGA. Diverts systemic venous blood into the left ventricle (LV) and out the PA. Diverts pulmonary venous blood into the right ventricle (RV) and out the aorta.	Bradyarrhythmias more common than atrial tachyarrhythmias. Occasional baffle obstruction or leak. Systemic ventricular failure (morphologic RV) and systemic atrioventricular (AV) valve regurgitation (tricuspid valve) can occur.
Potts-Smith anastomosis	Side-side anastomosis of the descending thoracic aorta and the LPA.	Increase pulmonary blood flow in patients with anatomic obstruction to PA blood flow (i.e., tetralogy of Fallot)	Often creates too much pulmonary blood flow, resulting in pulmonary vascular obliterative changes (Eisenmenger reaction)

Pulmonary artery band	Obstructive band placed on the main PA.	Decrease pulmonary blood flow in patients with large ventricular septal defect (VSD).	The previously banded segment of the PA occasionally becomes stenotic.
Rastelli procedure	Conduit from the RV to PA and closure of VSD.	Create a two ventricular system in patients with truncus arteriosus, complex forms of double outlet RV, or TGA with VSD.	Conduit obstruction after 5–10 years is quite common.
Ross procedure	Aortic valve replacement using the native pulmonary valve. A pulmonary homograft is then placed in the pulmonary position.	Aortic valve replacement for stenosis and/or insufficiency.	PA stenosis can occur. Long-term outlook still unknown.
Transannular patch	Incision in the RV outflow tract extending across the pulmonary valve into the main PA and placement of a patch to enlarge the area.	Relief of infundibular, valvular, and PA stenosis in patients with tetralogy of Fallot.	Significant pulmonary insufficiency is common. RBBB pattern on ECG. Occasional RV outflow aneurysms.
Valvotomy (surgical or balloon)	Enlargement of a stenosed valve. Most commonly aortic or pulmonic.	Relief of stenosis.	Aortic valvotomy: stenosis often recurs; significant insufficiency may result.
Waterston shunt	Side-side anansomosis of the ascending aorta to the RPA.	Increase pulmonary blood flow in patients with anatomic obstruction to PA blood flow (i.e., tetralogy of Fallot).	Often creates too much pulmonary blood flow, resulting in pulmonary vascular obliterative changes. Often causes distortion (kinking) of the right pulmonary artery

Abbreviations: AV = atrioventricular; AVM = arteriovenous malformation; LPA = left pulmonary artery; LV = left ventricle; PA = pulmonary artery; RA = right atrium; RBBB = right bundle branch block; RPA = right pulmonary artery; RV = right ventricle; SVC = superior vena cava; TGA = transposition of the great arteries; VSD = ventricular septal defect.

Table 2 Associated Defects

Primary defects	Associated defects/abnormalities
Atrial septal defect	
Primum type	Cleft mitral valve with regurgitation.
Secundum type	Mitral valve prolapse (~25%).
Sinus venous	Ectopic atrial rhythm.
Bicuspid aortic valve	Type A aortic dissection.
Coarctation of the aorta	Bicuspid aortic valve (>50%), aortic dissection occasional.
Congenitally corrected transposition (L-transposition, ventricular inversion)	Heart block, systemic AV valve (tricuspid valve) regurgitation, systemic ventricular (morphological RV) dysfunction are all common.
Ebstein's anomaly of the tricuspid valve	Secundum ASD or PFO common.
Tetralogy of Fallot	Anomalous coronary arteries (5–10%) (LAD arising from RCA most common); secundum ASD occasional (pentalogy of Fallot).
Ventricular septal defect (membranous and outlet)	Aortic insufficiency (<10%).
Syndromes:	
Down's	~50% incidence of congenital heart defects. Endocardial cushion defects, especially complete AV canal, are most common. ASD, VSD, PDA also common.
Noonan's	Pulmonic stenosis and hypertrophic cardiomyopathy most common.
Turner's	Coarctation of the aorta and bicuspid aortic valve occur commonly. Ascending aortic aneurysms or dissection occasionally occur.

Abbreviations: ASD = atrial septal defect; AV = atrioventricular; LAD = left anterior descending coronary artery; LV = left ventricle; PDA = patent ductus arteriosus; PFO = patent foramen ovale; RCA = right coronary artery; RV = right ventricle; VSD = ventricular septal defect.

ated bicuspid aortic valve is present. Patients should be made aware that manipulation of acneiform lesions or biting of nails can be associated with bacteremia, endocarditis, and even death (see Chapter 28, "Infective Endocarditis").

IX. PREGNANCY

Pregnancy is a major issue because many patients with congenital heart disease now survive into adulthood. Briefly, normal pregnancy results in a 50% increase in maternal blood volume, increased heart rate, decreased pulmonary and systemic vascular resistance, relative anemia, increased risk of thromboembolic events (all maximal at approximately 32 weeks), and the potential for blood loss during delivery and the early postpartum period. The highest-risk group includes women with severe pulmonary arterial hypertension (pulmonary artery systolic pressure $> 75\%$ systemic arterial pressure, maternal mortality approximately 50%). It includes women with Eisenmenger's syndrome and primary pulmonary hypertension. Data on the risk of moderate to moderate-severe pulmonary artery hypertension (pulmonary artery systolic pressure 50–75% of systemic arterial pressure) are lacking. A recent report on pregnancy in women with cyanosis but without Eisenmenger's syndrome demonstrated very low maternal mortality, although postpartum cardiac signs and symptoms were common. An increased incidence of spontaneous abortions, stillbirths, and low-birthweight infants was seen.

Other phenomena that increase maternal risk are ventricular failure, obstructive valvular lesions and Marfan's syndrome. In general, the worse a woman's prepregnancy condition, the greater the risk of pregnancy. No matter what primary defect is present, women in New York Heart Association class 3 or 4 have a much worse prognosis than those in class 1 or 2. Women with Marfan syndrome have an increased risk of aortic dissection during pregnancy. Women with hypertrophic cardiomyopathy or atrial septal defects generally do well. Women with defects that place them at risk for endocarditis should receive antibiotic prophylaxis before delivery (see Chapter 22, "Pregnancy").

X. ACTIVITY

Because most adults with congenital heart disease are young, restriction of activity may affect quality of life markedly. The recommendations of the 26th Bethesda Conference of the American College of Cardiology (see suggested reading) are comprehensive. It is important to keep in mind that a patient with dramatic findings on physical examination may not require any restriction of activity (i.e., a patient with a small, restrictive ventricular septal defect with a distinct precordial thrill and a loud systolic murmur).

XI. CYANOSIS

Cyanotic adults with congenital heart disease require special care as outlined in Chapter 6, "General Observations."

SUGGESTED READING

Liberthson RR. Congenital heart disease in the child, adolescent, and adult. In: Eagle KA, Haber E, DeSanctis RW, Austin WG, eds. The Practice of Cardiology: The Medical and Surgical Cardiac Units at the Massachusetts General Hospital. 2d ed. Boston: Little Brown, 1989; 1091–1281.

Perloff JK. The Clinical Recognition of Congenital Heart Disease in Adults. Philadelphia: Saunders, 1991.

Perloff JK, Marelli AJ, Miner PD. Risk of stroke in adults with cyanotic congenital heart disease. Circulation 1993; 87:1954–1956.

Perloff JK, Child JS. Congenital Heart Disease in Adults. Philadelphia: Saunders, 1991.

Perloff JK, Rosove MH, Child JS, Wright GB. Adults with cyanotic congenital heart disease: Hematologic management. Ann Intern Med 1988; 109:406–413.

26th Bethesda Conference: Recommendations for Determining Eligibility for Competition in Athletes with Cardiovascular Abnormalities, January 6–7, 1994. J Am Coll Cardiol 1994; 24:845–899.

Territo MC, Rosove MH, Perloff JL. Cyanotic congenital heart disease: Hematologic management, renal function, and urate metabolism. In: Perloff JK, Child, JS, eds. Congenital Heart Disease in Adults. Philadelphia: Saunders, 1991:93–103.

26

Evaluation and Management of Patients with Ischemic Heart Disease Undergoing Noncardiac Surgery

I.	Evaluation	481
II.	Recommended Evaluation	483
III.	Management	483
	Suggested Reading	487

Allan S. Jaffe

I. EVALUATION

Patients with serious cardiac dysfunction are at a 25–50% increased risk for cardiovascular complications associated with noncardiac surgery. Thus, both noncardiac and cardiac risk factors, which are additive or even synergistic, must be characterized prospectively when elective noncardiac surgery is contemplated.

Noncardiac risk factors include the following:

1. Age, with up to a tenfold increase in mortality in patients > 70 years of age. Physiological rather than chronological age is the critical determinant.

2. Type of procedure, with intrathoracic, upper abdominal, and vascular surgical procedures (except carotid endarterectomy) associated with greater morbidity and mortality. The incidence of myocardial infarction increases if the surgical procedure is prolonged (> 3 hr).

3. Urgent as opposed to less urgent procedures, with greater risk (2.5–

4-fold increase) associated with emergency procedures, in part because of the lack of time available to treat other medical problems before surgery.

4. Nutrition, with malnourishment increasing risk for infection and respiratory failure. Conversely, extremely obese patients are at increased risk for pulmonary embolism, wound infections, and atelectasis with or without pneumonia.

5. Type of anesthesia, with spinal anesthesia probably safer than general anesthesia because of a reduced likelihood of postoperative congestive heart failure in view of the vasodilating properties of spinal anesthesia.

Cardiac risk factors include:

1. Previous myocardial infarction. In the past, surgery during the 6 months after a myocardial infarction was associated with a very high incidence of recurrent infarction (25–50%) and high case fatality rate (approximately 70%) with recurrent infarction. Presently, the risk of recurrent infarction is in the range of 2.5–5% with a 30–35% risk of mortality associated with recurrence.

2. Coronary artery disease. The presence of symptomatic coronary artery disease increases risk. In general, the more stable the coronary symptom complex, the less risk is increased.

   Because coexisting disease can obscure symptoms of severe coronary arterial disease by limiting activity (e.g., in patients undergoing vascular surgery and those with severe pulmonary disease), stress testing may be helpful. Eagle and coworkers defined five risk factors that seemed to differentiate high-risk from low-risk groups: absence of Q waves on the ECG, age below 70 years, absence history of angina, absence of VPCs, and absence of diabetes mellitus were associated with low risk for complications during surgery. If three or more of the factors are present, high risk is implicated, requiring preoperative cardiac catheterization and treatment of the coronary disease delineated. For the intermediate-risk subset, pharmacological stress testing is appropriate to further define risk.

3. Coronary bypass surgery. Patients who have undergone coronary bypass surgery tolerate noncardiac surgical procedures with little additional risk. Results after angioplasty are likely to be similar.

4. The presence of congestive heart failure markedly increases risk. Mortality in patients in New York Heart Association class 3 or 4 is 25% and 67% compared with 4% and 1% for class 1 or 2. Worsening or newly appearing heart failure, infection, and respiratory failure are encountered often after noncardiac surgery. An abnormal electrocardiogram (ECG) may presage newly appearing failure. Valvular heart disease and

the presence of significant chronic obstructive pulmonary disease increase the risk of postoperative heart failure. Hemodynamic monitoring is helpful in all patients with moderate to severe heart failure and reasonable for many high-risk patients without frank, antecedent failure as well.

5. Supraventricular arrhythmias, especially atrial fibrillation. These are associated with a high operative risk, in part because of their association with advanced age or structural heart disease. In Goldman's series, mortality was 18% in patients with supraventricular arrhythmias (predominantly atrial fibrillation) compared with 1.9% overall. If underlying structural disease is implicated, echocardiography is helpful for identifying it definitively.

6. Ventricular arrhythmias. Frequent ventricular premature contractions (VPCs) are associated with increased risk, in part because they may be indicative of underlying structural heart disease, often identifiable by echocardiography.

II. RECOMMENDED EVALUATION

Goldman and associates presented a useful risk factor profile system in 1977 in which the risk factors were assigned point values (Table 1) and in which the overall score appears to provide a good estimate of risk (Table 2).

III. MANAGEMENT

Preoperative care is required for:

1. Previous myocardial infarction. Although increased risk associated with previous infarction has declined, complacency is not warranted. Part of the decline is attributable to the increased detection of smaller infarcts. Whenever possible, surgical procedures that can be deferred for 6 months or more after infarction should be delayed. Conversely, essential noncardiac surgery can be accomplished relatively safely with proper care and diligence, especially in a patient whose coronary disease is asymptomatic and who has a negative stress test.

2. Coronary artery disease without infarction. Patients with unstable angina usually require coronary angiography. Many will require mechanical revascularization before surgery. It is likely that coronary bypass surgery or angioplasty in high-risk patients will reduce risk. However, it does not appear that patients with stable coronary disease require coronary interventions before most operations.

In general, patients with coronary artery disease tolerate noncardiac surgery well if care is taken to preclude or minimize increases in myocardial oxygen demand (e.g., secondary to tachycardia, hypertension, or congestive heart failure)

Table 1 Scoring System for Cardiac Risk Factors in Noncardiac
Surgery

Criteria	Points
1. History	
Age >70 years	5
Myocardial infarction in past 6 months	10
2. Physical examination	
S_3 gallop or jugular venous distention	11
Significant aortic stenosis	3
3. Electrocardiogram	
Rhythm other than NSR or PACS on preoperative ECG	7
>5 VPSc/min detected preoperatively	7
4. General condition	
$P_{O_2} < 60$ or $P_{CO_2} > 50$ mmHg	3
$K < 3.0$ or $H_{CO_3} < 20$ mEq/L	
Abnormal AST, signs of chronic liver disease or patient	
bedridden from noncardiac causes	
5. Operation	
Intraperitoneal, intrathoracic or aortic	3
Emergency procedure	4
Total possible points: 53	

Source: Modified from Braunwald E (ed.). *Heart Disease.* 4th ed. W. B. Saunders 1991:
1717.

or reductions in myocardial oxygen supply (e.g., secondary to hypotension or
anemia). Parenteral anti-ischemic agents should be used if GI surgery is anticipated because it is desirable to continue anti-ischemic medications. Hemodynamic monitoring is helpful when ventricular function is markedly impaired or
unstable.

    3. Congestive heart failure. Optimally, patients with congestive heart fail-
ure should be treated aggressively before surgery. Because they often benefit from
hemodynamic monitoring during surgery, Swan-Ganz catheterization initiated on
the day before surgery and then continued is useful to guide preoperative treatment and facilitate intraoperative monitoring. Vasodilators such as intravenous
nitroglycerin are the drugs of choice when oral agents cannot be continued
because of the type of surgery contemplated or contraindicated because of low
arterial blood pressure. Diuretics are often useful, but digitalis should be avoided
to avoid arrhythmogenic effects. However, it may be useful in preventing atrial
fibrillation preoperatively in patients with a history of this arrhythmia. In the
patient who cannot be managed successfully with these agents alone, dobutamine
and amrinone may be helpful. However, agents with positive inotropic effects are
not indicated "routinely" to increase cardiac output during surgery.

Table 2   Relationship of Score (see Table 1) and Risk for the Procedure

Points	Pooled risk from four studies
0–5	1.6%
6–12	5.0%
13–25	16.0%
≥26	56.0%

^aThis profile may underestimate risk in particularly high-risk patients, such as those undergoing abdominal aortic aneurysm repair, by 30–50%.
Source: Modified from Braunwald E (ed). *Heart Disease*. 4th ed. 1991:1717.

   4. Conduction defects. ECG monitoring is, of course, appropriate for patients with heart block of any degree. However, with the exception of Mobitz II second-degree A-V block or complete heart block, transvenous pacing is not required for patients undergoing noncardiac surgery. Progression of first- or Lobitz I second-degree heart block is rare. If it should occur, it can usually be managed with external or transvenous pacing.

   The possibility that one or more of the functions of some of the sophisticated pacemakers, including total inhibition of the unit, can be induced by equipment used in operating rooms mandates that electrical equipment should be kept away from the pacing unit and conform to stringent electrical leakage and safety criteria.

   5. Atrial fibrillation. Because patients with atrial fibrillation are at increased risk, cardioversion before surgery is reasonable, if convenient, and implementable with appropriate precautions, including anticoagulation.

   Patients with a rapid ventricular response to atrial fibrillation and those with a very slow response require special attention. The former often have an underlying abnormality that should be corrected. Possibilities include a preexcitation syndrome (recognition is important because of the need to avoid agents such as digitalis, verapamil, diltiazem, and adenosine that block conduction at the AV node and can yield paradoxical cardioacceleration). A very slow ventricular response may reflect the sick sinus syndrome, with its risk for bradycardias and marked acceleration of ventricular rate in response to class 1A antiarrhythmic agents that reduce concealed conduction.

   6. Ventricular arrhythmias. Ventricular premature contractions rarely require treatment but should lead to a search for electrolyte imbalances, hypoxia, ischemia, or adverse effects of devices or inlying catheters that may be inducing or exacerbating the arrhythmia. Lidocaine is the drug of choice for prevention.

7. Pulmonary embolism. Patients with cardiovascular disease are at increased risk for pulmonary embolism and should be treated after surgery with subcutaneous heparin (5000 units every 12 hr) for prevention of deep venous thrombosis.

A. Complications

1. Acute myocardial infarction. Perioperative infarction is associated with a 30–35% mortality. However, its detection perioperatively is difficult. It had been thought most likely to occur on postoperative day 3 or during induction of anesthesia associated with hypotension; recently, however, it has been recognized commonly at the time of awakening after anesthesia. The astute clinician will recognize the possibility of ischemia or infarction whenever arrhythmias, hypotension, hypertension, or congestive heart failure appear. Increases in MB creatine kinase are associated with surgery, but substantial elevations are rare in the absence of a cardiac insult. Increased cardiac troponin I in plasma is helpful in the detection of perioperative infarction.

If recurrent episodes of ischemia or infarction occur, invasive intervention (catheterization with or without angioplasty or bypass surgery) may be needed. However, most often, arrhythmias and hemodynamic derangements can be managed medically.

2. Ischemia. Ischemia and infarction are treated similarly. In addition to aggressive treatment of arrhythmias and correction of hemodynamic derangements, anti-ischemic agents are often helpful. Intravenous nitroglycerin, diltiazem, and beta blockers can substitute for orally administered agents, but intravenous diltiazem and beta blockers may be deleterious if heart failure is present. The endpoint is elimination of episodes of ischemia. When this is not achievable, cardiac catheterization, angioplasty, or bypass surgery may be necessary. Because of the large fluid-volume shifts that occur in surgical patients, hypotension is common. It may be precipitated or exacerbated by anti-ischemic or vasodilating agents.

3. Congestive heart failure. Treatment is the same as that in the perioperative setting. Hemodynamic monitoring is often required because of fluid shifts that occur with surgery. Vasodilators will not improve forward cardiac output if preload is inadequate. Conversely, attempts to increase preload may fail if vasodilators are being given.

4. Supraventricular arrhythmias. Supraventricular arrhythmias (usually atrial fibrillation or flutter) are associated with high perioperative mortality (in Goldman's study, 49% with compared to 4% without) because they are often a marker of severe underlying heart disease, especially in patients over 70 years of age and in those with congestive heart failure, ischemia, or chronic lung disease. An aggressive search for underlying etiology is needed. Patients who are hemo-

dynamically unstable or have ischemia should undergo cardioversion on an emergency basis. Others can be managed with digitalis, verapamil, or diltiazem. Because atrial flutter is a more labile rhythm than atrial fibrillation, patients should not be left in atrial flutter, which can usually be converted to atrial fibrillation pharmacologically or by rapid atrial pacing.

5. Ventricular arrhythmias. Prelethal arrhythmias such as ventricular tachycardia should be treated with lidocaine. Underlying abnormalities should be identified. Alternatively, procainamide may be helpful.

SUGGESTED READING

Adams JE, Sicard G, Allen TB, et al. More accurate diagnosis of perioperative myocardial infarction with measurement of cardiac troponin I. N Engl J Med 1994; 330:670–674.

Eagle KA, Coley CM, Newell JB, et al. Combining clinical and thallium data optimizes perioperative assessment of cardiac risk before major vascular surgery. Ann Intern Med 1989; 110:859–866.

Goldman L, Caldera DL, Nassbaum SR, et al. Multifactorial index of cardiac risk in noncardiac surgical procedures. N Engl J Med 1977; 297:845–850.

Mangano DT, Hollenberg M, Fegert G, et al. Perioperative myocardial ischemia in patients undergoing noncardiac surgery—I. Incidence and severity during the 4 day perioperative period. J Am Coll Cardiol 1991; 17:843–850.

27

Preventive Cardiology

I. The Concepts of Prevention in Atherosclerotic Heart
   Disease   489
II. Evaluating the Coronary Risk Status of the Patient   490
III. Modifying Risk Factors   498
IV. Conclusions   508
   Suggested Reading   508

John C. LaRosa

I. THE CONCEPTS OF PREVENTION IN ATHEROSCLEROTIC HEART DISEASE

A. Primary Versus Secondary Prevention

Despite the dramatic declines in coronary mortality over the past 20 years, atherosclerosis of the coronary arteries continues to be the most common cause of death and disability in the United States and most western countries. A good deal is known about what factors promote atherogenesis in the coronary arteries and how that process can be prevented or at least retarded. Interventions to prevent or retard the *initial* appearance of clinical coronary disease are termed "primary" prevention. Interventions implemented *after* the onset of clinically apparent disease are termed "secondary" prevention.

Primary prevention is targeted against risk factors that reflect cause of coronary artery disease to prevent its initial occurrence. Primary prevention interventions must, of necessity, be applied to many people who are not actually destined to develop clinical coronary disease. The safety of such interventions, therefore, is of particular importance. For this reason, the emphasis in primary

489

prevention is usually on hygienic—that is, on nonpharmacological—interventions, including diet, exercise, and weight loss. Even so, in selected individuals, pharmacological interventions may be indicated.

The focus of secondary prevention is on patients who already have clinical manifestations of atherosclerosis. Without intervention, approximately 80% of individuals with clinically overt coronary disease are destined to die from it. Perhaps not surprisingly, it is easier to demonstrate the benefits of risk-factor interventions in patients with already established disease.

B. Compliance

Important considerations in any prevention strategy are those related to compliance. Patients are often resistant to lifestyle changes. As a result, physicians are unduly discouraged about preventive efforts. Poor compliance is apparent also with pharmacological interventions. It has been estimated, for example, that after 1 year, less than 50% of patients initially prescribed a lipid-lowering medication are still taking it. The most important element of successful patient compliance is *physician* commitment to the intervention. An intervention strongly endorsed by the physician and his or her staff is more likely to be successful than one to which the patient feels the physician is only casually committed. Regular monitoring of compliance to therapeutic regimens should be part of the follow-up process. It is a mistake to assume that whatever has been prescribed will automatically be utilized. Good compliance requires regular physician monitoring and reinforcement.

II. EVALUATING THE CORONARY RISK STATUS OF THE PATIENT

A. Special Aspects of the History

Family History

Both coronary disease and its antecedents occur in familial clusters. In evaluating the coronary risk status of a patient, therefore, it is important not only to gather information about the incidence of coronary disease in other family members but also the incidence of coronary risk factors such as smoking, high blood pressure, lipid abnormalities, weight and exercise patterns, and dietary habits. It should be remembered that familial clustering indicates not only genetic influences but also behavior patterns such as smoking and eating—habits that may also exhibit strong familial clustering.

A by-product of a careful family history may be family screening for risk factors. For example, a patient with clinical coronary disease and hypercholesterolemia, who is a candidate for secondary prevention, may lead to other family members with hypercholesterolemia but without manifest coronary disease who are candidates for primary prevention. An extended family history, then, is important not only for the patient but as a potential mechanism for detecting other candidates for prevention as well.

Dietary History

Many physicians unaccustomed to taking dietary histories find them both cumbersome and daunting. It is important to remember, however, that most of us eat relatively few different foods over a period of time. A good way of taking a dietary history, therefore, is to ask a patient what he or she eats on both a typical workday and a typical weekend or recreational day. Ask the patient to go through each meal, including between meals and evening snacks. Ask also about the time of day in which each meal is taken. Dietary history should include the number of times that the patient eats in restaurants or travels. Even on these occasions, most patients will generally exhibit repetitive eating habits, ordering the same kind of airplane meal, for example, or frequenting the same restaurants.

An important corollary of the dietary history is to ask about recent *changes* in diet as well as both recent and more long-term changes in weight patterns. The latter is of particular importance because substantial evidence indicates that weight deposited in the abdominal region is more likely to be associated with adverse changes in coronary risk factors, such as hypertension and dyslipoproteinemia, than weight gained in the hips and thighs. Abdominal weight gain is a characteristic of adult men in all their life stages but only in postmenopausal compared with other women. Premenopausal women are more likely to gain weight around their hips and thighs than around their abdomens.

Some evidence indicates that weight gained after reaching adulthood is more likely to be associated with adverse changes in risk factors than excess weight that has been present since childhood. Therefore, a good question to ask is how much a patient's weight has changed since the patient's midtwenties. Many people regard weight gain as an inexorable concomitant of aging and will not report it unless asked. For a variety of reasons, including a slowing of basal metabolic rate, the later in adulthood one gains weight, the more difficult it is to lose. Prevention of weight gain is an important focus in all patients but particularly in young adults.

Patterns of weight gain in family members may provide information relevant to the patient's propensity to gain weight and his or her attitudes about it. It is also important to ask the patient about personal attitudes about weight gain. Even today, in many cultures, weight gain is not viewed as a health problem but rather as an external manifestation of prosperity and well-being.

Exercise History

It is useful to ascertain how much a patient actually exercises in a day. Questions about regular, deliberate exercise such as walking, running, swimming, and so on and about how much exercise is required as part of the patient's ordinary day are helpful. Many patients have jobs that require considerable daily exercise. Like the dietary history, information should be solicited not only about working days but also about leisure days.

Tobacco, Alcohol, and Other Drug Use

Tobacco use of any kind, but particularly inhalation of smoke from burning tobacco products, is strongly related to increased risk of coronary disease. Therefore, it is important to elicit a careful history of both current and past tobacco use. Family history of tobacco use is important not only for gathering information about the patient's habits but also as a way of identifying family members who might be candidates for preventive interventions.

Alcohol may, in many instances, be protective against coronary disease. In other instances, however, it may aggravate dyslipoproteinemias, particularly hypertriglyceridemia, and actually contribute to coronary risk as a result. In addition, of course, alcohol contributes independently to myocardial disease and myocardial dysfunction, including arrhythmias. Therefore, a careful history of current as well as past use of alcohol is important in any assessment of coronary risk. It is important to ask specifically about wine, beer, and distilled spirits. Many patients regard only the last as having significant alcohol content and may dismiss beer and wine intake as inconsequential.

A careful history of current medicinal drug use is of importance. Drugs may have a cardiovascular protective *or* a risk-enhancing effect. Diuretics, for example, lower blood pressure but raise triglyceride and low-density lipoprotein (LDL) cholesterol. Beta-adrenergic–blocking agents (antihypertensive and antiarrhythmic) lower high-density lipoprotein (HDL) cholesterol and raise triglyceride levels.

Use of recreational drugs is of importance, although this history may be harder to obtain. Both amphetamines and cocaine, for example, have regularly been associated with cardiac arrhythmias and other manifestations of myocardial dysfunction.

Exogenous Steroid Use

Special attention should be paid in the history to use of exogenous steroidal hormones in oral contraceptives (OC), postmenopausal hormone replacement therapy (HRT), or anabolic steroids. In general, estrogens affect lipoproteins favorably and, more generally, coronary risk. Androgens, including both anabolic steroids and weakly androgenic progestins, have adverse effects.

Because specific estrogens or progestins differ in the potency of their effects on lipoproteins, it is important to know not only whether a patient is taking OC or postmenopausal HRT but also what specific compounds are involved.

Chronic Diseases

It is important to solicit information about the presence of chronic disease that may predispose to atherosclerosis such as diabetes mellitus, nephrosis, chronic renal failure, and hypothyroidism.

B. Special Aspects of the Physical Examination

Cardiac examination, including blood pressure measurement, is, of course, an essential part of any physical evaluation. Body weight and height should be measured, but so should body fat distribution. An easy way to do this is to estimate the ratio of the circumference of the waist (measured midway between the lower rib margin and the iliac crest) to the hips (measured at the greatest circumference over the greater trochanters). A waist-to-hip ratio above 0.9 in a female or 1.0 in a male is a rough index of increased abdominal girth and is associated with increased coronary risk through a variety of mechanisms.

Other aspects of the physical examination that may often be overlooked are those associated with dyslipoproteinemia. These include xanthomas, which may be eruptive, tuboeruptive, tuberous, tendinous, or planar. Xanthomas are found most often on extensor surfaces.

Eruptive xanthomas are isolated, small lesions that, like other xanthomas, are orange-red in color (Figure 1). They are not usually tender. These xanthomas are usually seen in conjunction with high levels of triglyceride, generally over 1000 mg/dL (11.36 mmol/L).

Tuboeruptive xanthomas (Figure 2)—eruptive xanthomas occurring in clusters—are generally over the elbows and knees. Unlike eruptive xanthomas, they may be tender and are usually indicative of elevations of intermediate density lipoprotein (IDL), that, in turn, is accompanied by elevations of both triglyceride and cholesterol. These are most often seen in dysbetalipoproteinemia (type III dyslipoproteinemia), a disorder, usually genetic in origin, in which IDL accumulates.

Tuberous xanthomas (Figure 3) are large subcutaneous collections of cholesterol ester seen most often over the elbows and knees, often in conjunction with underlying tendon xanthomas. Tuberous xanthomas are usually seen in patients with familial hypercholesterolemia, a disorder characterized by genetically determined deficiencies in LDL receptor activity and substantially elevated levels of circulating LDL.

Tendon xanthomas (Figure 4) are seen most often in the achilles tendon but also in the extensor tendons of the knees, elbows, fingers, and toes. Like tuberous xanthomas, they are generally a manifestation of familial hypercholesterolemia. Both tuberous and tendinous xanthomas are virtually diagnostic for familial hypercholesterolemia. They are not seen in other genetic or acquired disorders in which LDL accumulates.

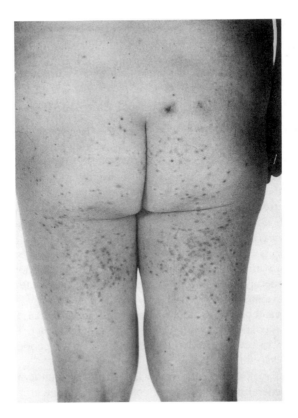

Figure 1   Eruptive xanthomas in a patient with severe hypertriglyceridemia.

Planar xanthomas (Figure 5) are flat lesions, larger than eruptive xanthomas. When seen in the webs of the fingers, they are usually associated with familial hypercholesterolemia. They may also be seen on the eyelids, in which case they are called xanthelasmas. Xanthelasmas may be associated with familial hypercholesterolemia, although they can occur in the absence of clearly defined genetic lipid abnormalities, particularly in individuals over age 50.

"Corneal arcus" refers to the presence of a silver-gray band just inside the corneal rim and surrounded by normal cornea. As it develops, arcus is visible first at the inferior and superior poles of the cornea. In later stages, it may circle the outer portion of the cornea entirely. Like xanthelasma, corneal arcus may be seen in older individuals without being associated with clearly defined dyslipoproteinemias. In individuals under age 50, however, the presence of corneal arcus is highly suggestive of LDL receptor deficiency or familial hypercholesterolemia.

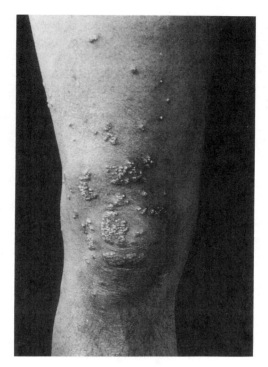

Figure 2   Tuboeruptive xanthomas in a patient with dysbetalipoproteinemia.

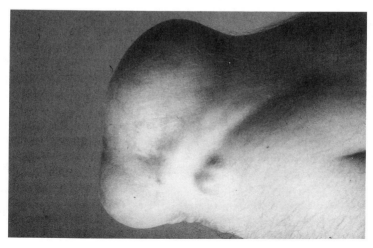

Figure 3   Tuberous xanthomas in a patient with familial hypercholesterolemia.

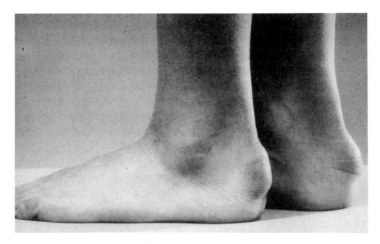

Figure 4   Tendon xanthomas in a patient with familial hypercholesterolemia.

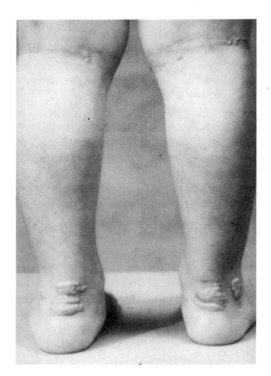

Figure 5   Planar xanthomas in a child with homozygous familial hypercholesterolemia.

Xanthomatous lesions are uncommon even in individuals with dyslipoproteinemias. Nevertheless, because their presence is often virtually diagnostic of dyslipoproteinemia, most frequently of genetic origin, it is important that every patient be examined for them.

C. Laboratory Evaluation

The U.S. National Cholesterol Education Program (NCEP) recommends that all individuals over age 20, male and female, have measurements of total cholesterol and HDL cholesterol to screen for those who may be at increased risk of coronary atherosclerosis as a result of dyslipoproteinemia. (The NCEP recommends total cholesterol screening in children with family histories of coronary disease or hypertriglyceridemia or with other coronary risk factors such as diabetes, obesity, or hypertension as well.)

Adults with cholesterol above 240 mg/dL (6.2 mmol/L) or, if two or more risk factors are present, above 200 mg/dL (5.2 mmol/L) are considered candidates for a "full" lipoprotein profile, consisting of total cholesterol, total triglyceride, HDL cholesterol, and LDL cholesterol (the last estimated by the formula LDL cholesterol = total cholesterol − the sum of HDL cholesterol + triglyceride ÷ 5). The risk factors that the NCEP considers important are summarized in Table 1.

Many other measurements, including apoprotein levels (apoproteins are the proteins that help to form the surface of lipoprotein particles), HDL subfractions, and lipoprotein(a) [Lp(a)] levels have been proposed to characterize coronary risk. There are two problems with these measurements, however. First, the epidemiological and clinical base that does exist to quantify risk for the more traditional lipoprotein measurements does not exist for these parameters. Until that database is in place, it is difficult to know how to use these measurements in an individual patient. Second, measures of total cholesterol, total triglyceride, HDL cholesterol, and estimated LDL cholesterol are reasonably well standardized across large U.S. laboratories, particularly those that subscribe to a Centers for Disease Control (CDC) standardization program. This is not the case for other proposed indexes.

Laboratory evaluation should include measurements of fasting blood glucose and thyroid as well as renal and liver function parameters. Diabetes, hyperthyroidism, and renal disease—including both nephrosis and chronic renal failure—may all contribute to dyslipoproteinemia and to coronary risk through this and other mechanisms.

More recently, it has been recognized that homocysteine and homocysteinuria may be independent risk factors for coronary disease, perhaps through direct injury to endothelium or by promoting platelet adhesiveness. It is difficult to justify routine measurements of homocysteine levels in blood or urine, however. At this point there are no clinical trials indicating that changing homocysteine levels changes risk.

Table 1 Risk Status Based on Presence of CHD Risk Factors Other than LDL Cholesterol

Positive risk factors[a]

    Age

        Men: ≥45 years

        Women: ≥55 years or premature menopause without estrogen replacement therapy

    Family history of premature CHD (definite myocardial infarction or sudden death before 55 years of age in father or other male first-degree relative or before 65 years of age in mother or other female first-degree relative)

    Current cigarette smoking

    Hypertension (≥140/90 mmHg[b] or on antihypertensive medication)

    Low HDL cholesterol (<35 mg/dL[b])

    Diabetes mellitus

Negative risk factor[c]

    High HDL cholesterol (≥60 mg/dL)

Abbreviations: CHD = coronary heart disease; LDL = low-density lipoproteins; HDL = high-density lipoproteins.

[a]High risk, defined as a net of two or more CHD risk factors, leads to more vigorous intervention. Age (defined differently for men and for women) is treated as a risk factor because rates of CHD are higher in the elderly than in the young and in men than in women of the same age. Obesity is not listed as a risk factor because it operates through other risk factors that are included (hypertension, hyperlipidemia, decreased HDL cholesterol, and diabetes mellitus), but it should be considered a target for intervention. Physical inactivity similarly is not listed as a risk factor, but it too should be considered a target for intervention, and physical activity is recommended as desirable for everyone.

[b]Confirmed by measurements on several occasions.

[c]If the HDL cholesterol level is ≥60 mg/dL, subtract one risk factor (because high HDL cholesterol levels decrease CHD risk).

Source: National Cholesterol Education Program. Second Report of the Expert Panel on Detection, Evaluation, and Treatment of High Blood Cholesterol in Adults (Adult Treatment Panel II). Circulation 1994; 89:1329–1445.

Resting and, in selected cases, exercise electrocardiography should be part of an evaluation of someone at risk for coronary disease. These examinations are discussed below.

III. MODIFYING RISK FACTORS

A. Review of Modifiable Risk Factors

Dyslipoproteinemia

The NCEP has issued guidelines for the detection, evaluation, and management of lipid disorders in adults (Table 2). The stimulus for these guidelines has been the overwhelming evidence that high levels of LDL cholesterol are a potent risk factor for coronary disease. Considerable evidence, moreover, indicates that lowering

Table 2 NCEP Guidelines for the Detection, Evaluation, and Management of Lipid Disorders in Adults Above Age 20

	Total cholesterol	LDL cholesterol	Triglycerides
Cholesterol and LDL Cutpoints (mg/dL) (mmol/L)			
High	≥240 (6.2)	≥160 (4.0)	>400 (4.5)
Borderline	200–239 (5.2–6.2)	130–159 (3.4–4.1)	200–399 (2.3–4.5)
Desirable	<200 (5.2)	<130 (3.4)	<200 (2.3)
Thresholds for drugs (after diet)			
		>200 (5.7) in men age <35 or premenopausal women	>400 (4.5) if CHD or other risk factors
		≥190 (4.9) in men age >35 or postmenopausal women	
		≥160 (4.1) in women if two or more risk factors	
		≥130 (3.4) if CHD present	
Therapeutic goals			
		<160 (4.1) if no CHD and no other risk factors	<200 (2.3)
		<130 (3.4) if no CHD and two or more risk factors	
		<100 (2.6) if CHD present	

LDL cholesterol prevents, arrests, or retards the development of coronary atherosclerosis and its clinical sequelae.

In patients with established coronary disease, the role of lipid lowering is well established. In clinical trials in which only very modest cholesterol lowering (in the 5–15% range) was achieved, there was, nevertheless, a dramatic fall in coronary morbid and mortal events. More recent studies of serial coronary angiograms have confirmed that LDL-cholesterol lowering and, to a lesser extent, raising of HDL-cholesterol can arrest the progression of atherosclerosis and in some cases even reverse it. In addition, it has been strongly demonstrated that favorable angiographic changes are correlated with declines in coronary event rates in the treated compared with the control groups. Thus, cholesterol lowering is an important intervention in patients with clinical coronary disease.

Cholesterol lowering in patients without clinical coronary disease is important also in preventing or delaying its occurrence. It has been difficult to demonstrate net declines in mortality in primary prevention trials, however. This is likely the result of the earlier stage of development of atherosclerosis in subjects included in such studies. Nevertheless, there is more debate about how vigorously to use *drug* therapy in patients with dyslipoproteinemia but without coronary disease than is the case in patients with clinically apparent coronary disease.

All patients with dyslipoproteinemia should be treated with hygienic interventions. These include changes in dietary composition to lower saturated fat and cholesterol content, low-calorie diets to lower body weight, and exercise to aid in weight loss or the prevention of weight gain as well for the benefits of regular exercise in retarding the onset of atheroslerosis.

The value of cholesterol-lowering drugs, however—while clearly apparent in patients with established coronary disease and probably indicated in all patients with high LDL cholesterol [over 160 mg/dL (4.1 mmol/L)] when such individuals also have other risk factors such as diabetes and/or hypertension—is less apparent in those without clinical coronary disease and with no other risk factors.

The NCEP guidelines suggest that in premenopausal women and men below 35 years of age, lipid-lowering drugs be considered only if LDL cholesterol stays above 220 mg/dL (5.7 mmol/L) (see Table 2). This conservative approach to the use of lipid-lowering medication is largely the result of the paucity of evidence that total mortality is affected by such interventions. On the other hand, completed primary prevention trials have been of relatively short duration (5 to 8 years) and were neither large enough nor long enough to demonstrate effects on total mortality.

HDL cholesterol is a very potent predictor of coronary disease. Some observers have suggested that the best single index of coronary risk is the ratio of either total cholesterol or LDL cholesterol to HDL cholesterol. Subgroup analysis in the Helsinki Study, a large primary prevention trial of gemfibrozil, a drug that primarily lowers triglycerides and raises HDL cholesterol, demonstrated that those individuals with the lowest HDL cholesterol and the highest triglycerides had the greatest benefit in prevention of first myocardial infarction. Some observers, however, have pointed out that such analyses are flawed because triglycerides, HDL cholesterol, and LDL cholesterol, as a result of their intertwining metabolism, are not independent variables. A good rule of thumb is that a drug should not be used in an individual solely to raise HDL cholesterol. On the other hand, in someone whose LDL cholesterol is high and whose HDL cholesterol is low, therapy directed at changing both markers may be of benefit.

The NCEP has issued guidelines for classifying patients with hyper-triglyceridemia (Table 2). It is more difficult to identify, among such patients, those who should be treated with drug therapy. As a general guideline, only those who have other lipoprotein abnormalities requiring drug interventions or who have personal or family histories of coronary disease indicating that their triglycerides are probably carrying atherogenic lipoprotein should be candidates for drug therapy, as opposed to hygienic interventions.

Hypertension

The Fifth Report of the United States Joint National Commission on Detection, Evaluation, and Treatment of High Blood Pressure (JNC V) has issued guidelines for detection and treatment of hypertension based on strong evidence that hypertension is a risk factor not only for coronary events but also for cerebrovascular disease and stroke. The JNC V definitions of hypertension are summarized in Table 3.

The benefit of blood pressure lowering in coronary disease, however, is slightly less certain. Coronary risk reduction in cholesterol-lowering trials has generally been that predicted from comparing population studies. Blood pressure lowering, however, has been demonstrated to lower coronary rates less than predicted from population studies. The reasons for this are not clear. It has been hypothesized (without much direct evidence) that it may be related to adverse effects that diuretics and beta-blocking agents, commonly used in blood pressure trials, have on lipoproteins. That is, the beneficial effects of blood pressure lowering on coronary disease are thought to be partially offset by the adverse effects on lipoproteins when these agents are used as blood pressure-lowering agents.

Because there are no clinical trials with cardiovascular or cerebrovascular endpoints using agents such as ACE inhibitors or calcium channel blockers to lower blood pressure, the JNC continues to recommend diuretics and beta blockers as drugs of first choice in the treatment of hypertension. However incomplete the effects on coronary disease, the lowering of blood pressure is clearly beneficial in terms of preventing stroke.

As in dyslipoproteinemia, hygienic interventions including low salt, low fat, low-calorie diets, and regular exercise are considered first lines of therapy, with drugs being used only when these interventions have failed to adequately control blood pressure. Unlike hypercholesterolemia, however, hypertension, when it is severe, may have *acute* cerebrovascular consequences, including stroke. Thus, greater sense of urgency exists to lower blood pressure than to lower cholesterol.

Table 3 Classification of Blood Pressure for Adults Age 18 Years and Older

Category	Systolic (mmHg)	Diastolic (mmHg)
Normal	<130	<85
High normal	130–139	85–89
Hypertension		
Stage 1 (Mild)	140–159	90–99
Stage 2 (Moderate)	160–179	100–109
Stage 3 (Severe)	180–209	110–119
Stage 4 (Very Severe)	≥210	≥120

Source: National Institutes of Health, National Heart, Lung, and Blood Institute. The Fifth Report of the Joint National Committee on Detection, Evaluation, and Treatment of High Blood Pressure. NIH Publication No. 93-1088, 1993.

Cigarette Smoking

The third major established risk factor for coronary atherosclerosis is cigarette smoking, although mechanisms responsible are still somewhat obscure. While per capita cigarette consumption has declined in the last 20 years (at the same time that the rate of coronary death has fallen), in some populations cigarette smoking is either unchanged or actually increasing. This is particularly true of women, especially young women.

Some have suggested that in order to achieve greater success, both with smoking prevention and smoking cessation programs among younger people, it is necessary to emphasize that the consequences of smoking as well as the benefits of quitting are quite immediate. For example, it has been demonstrated that young women who become convinced that smoking is unattractive and associated with unpleasant odors are more likely to stop than young women given messages about future adverse health effects.

Although it has not yet been possible to perform definitive clinical trials, results of observational studies indicate that individuals who have been smokers but who have stopped lower their risk of coronary disease toward the level of nonsmokers within a 2- to 5-year period. As a result, smoking cessation is a goal that should be pursued vigorously even among individuals who are initially unsuccessful. Smoking cessation rates *increase* with increasing age. The notion that at some age it is "too late" to stop and still gain benefits from smoking cessation is fallacious, at least as far as the risk of coronary disease is concerned.

Nicotine chewing gum, in conjunction with behavioral programs that encourage smoking cessation, is a useful adjunct for smoking cessation. Experience with such regimens is not long enough, however, to determine whether or not they have long-term beneficial effects on quit rates.

Diabetes Mellitus

Diabetes mellitus is a strong risk factor for atherosclerosis in general and coronary artery disease in particular. It is an even stronger risk factor in women than in men. This is true of older as well as younger women.

The reasons why diabetes is a stronger risk factor in women than in men are obscure. The effect is so dramatic, however, that diabetic men and women, unlike nondiabetic men and women, exhibit almost no difference in coronary disease risk, regardless of age. Thus, the strong protection that premenopausal women enjoy against atherogenesis is lost when diabetes is present.

The mechanism by which diabetes causes disease in medium- and large-sized vessels (as opposed to microangiopathy) is probably largely related to adverse changes in lipoproteins. In cultures in which dietary fat intake is low, as in rural China and Japan, diabetics develop microangiopathy but not atherosclerosis.

There is no direct evidence that tight control of diabetes lowers the risk of atherosclerosis, unlike microangiopathy, which is benefited by such tight control. Nor is there direct evidence in diabetics of the benefit of lipid lowering. Nevertheless, it is a reasonable assumption that both glycemic and lipidemic control is important as part of the therapeutic regimen needed to prevent accelerated atherosclerosis.

Diabetes appears to be aggravated by increased abdominal fat and increased body weight in general and is better controlled in the presence of a low waist-hip ratio, a low body mass index, and regular exercise.

Exercise

Although they have occasionally been attempted, definitive clinical trials of exercise are lacking because of the difficulty in maintaining control in treated groups with sufficient differences in exercise levels. Results of observational studies, however, strongly suggest that exercise lowers risk of both coronary and total mortality and makes management of body weight, blood lipids, and blood sugar easier.

For many individuals, however, regular exercise is not a daily part of normal activity. It must be specifically programmed into the daily routine. It requires the same sort of physician endorsement and prescription as other interventions. Particularly in patients over 40 years of age and in those with coronary disease, its intensity and duration must be regulated, based on findings of formal exercise testing. For most individuals, one-half hour a day of brisk walking (or its equivalent) is sufficient. Individuals should be encouraged to include as much exercise in daily activity as possible, including using stairs for one or two flights, deliberately parking at a distance from a building to be entered, and walking the halls to see a colleague instead of using the telephone.

Weight Control

Body mass index is a risk factor for atherosclerosis, and waist-to-hip ratio (the amount of abdominal fat present) is the best weight-related predictor of risk. It is necessary for patients to understand that weight gain is not an inexorable part of aging, that it can be prevented, and that the benefits—both in the immediate feeling or well-being and reduction of long-term morbidity and even mortality—are substantial.

The best way to deal with obesity is to prevent it. This is easier said than done. Because both men and women tend to gain weight in their twenties and beyond, prevention should begin early in life. Diets that are rich in fiber, low in fat, and low in calories are part but not all of the prescription for weight control. Regular exercise is also very important. The endorsement and supervision of the physician is essential.

B. Selecting the Appropriate Intervention

General Comments

Behavioral interventions are appropriate for all patients in need of coronary risk factor reduction. These include dietary interventions as well as exercise and weight loss. Those individuals with very high lipid or blood pressure levels (see Tables 2 and 3) may require pharmacological interventions, even in the absence of other risk factors.

Risk factors, however, are not merely additive. The presence of more than one risk factor usually results in an increase in risk greater than the sum of the parts. Moreover, risk factors commonly occur in clusters. It is more usual to find a patient with high blood pressure or high blood cholesterol who is also a smoker than one with only one risk factor.

Family history is an important risk factor because it may identify patients who are particularly susceptible to atherosclerosis. In fact, if those at particular risk because of such presumed susceptibility could be identified, risk factor interventions could be concentrated on such individuals and the need for general changes in population might be reduced. No screening tests have yet been devised, however. Thus, blood pressure and cholesterol interventions must be practiced on a large number of individuals in order to prevent relatively few from developing clinical coronary disease. As long as this involves only hygienic interventions, there is no particular harm. When a lifetime of drug taking is involved, however, the drugs used must be both effective and safe.

Dietary and Weight Change

Although such consultation would be ideal, it is not possible and probably not necessary for each patient who is to undergo dietary change to have instructions and supervision from a registered dietitian. There are simply not enough dietitians in the United States to perform such services.

A simple way of beginning with dietary change is to recognize that most patients eat in regularly repetitive food patterns. It is not necessary for them to learn an infinite variety of changes but simply to make the changes within their present eating patterns. For example, a patient who likes ice cream may be persuaded to eat low-fat frozen yogurt instead; a patient who enjoys pasta with meat sauce may be encouraged to try pasta with a vegetable-based sauce; and patients who enjoy snacks between meals may be encouraged to snack on air-popped popcorn and celery or carrot sticks instead of potato chips and candy bars.

Patients should be encouraged to spread their calories over the day, eating a good breakfast, usually composed of a high-fiber cereal and fruit juice, and a lunch consisting of a salad and/or another main dish. Regular, appetite-satisfying meals should be encouraged—rather than skimping on food all day and then eating one large meal at night, which does not provide the opportunity for the patient to burn calories after eating. Patients should be encouraged not to eat too late, so that time elapses between the completion of the meal and retiring for bed.

These maneuvers, coupled with the institution of regular daily exercise, will go a long way toward helping the patient to maintain or lose weight. It is probably true that most patients will not succeed in achieving a daily exercise program, but by *prescribing* it daily, the physician may encourage patients to aim for the goal and to exercise four or five times a week.

For patients who feel that the sacrifice is otherwise too great, it is important to allow them to *occasionally* (once every 2 or 3 weeks) stray from their diet. There is evidence, in fact, that such occasional straying does not materially affect cholesterol levels or interfere with weight reduction. There are several fine books that stress dietary fat reduction both as a way of lowering cholesterol levels and controlling weight by teaching the patient to count saturated fat calories during the day, probably the simplest and most practical way for patients to achieve both lower cholesterol levels and weight reduction.

It should be made clear to patients that they are unlikely to achieve real weight loss of more than a pound or two a week and that, in any weight-reduction program, there will be plateaus that, despite optimal adherence, may last as long as 2 to 3 weeks.

C. Pharmacological Interventions

Use of Hypolipidemic Drugs

The NCEP has established guidelines for the use of hypolipidemic drugs (Table 4) based on LDL-cholesterol levels that *remain* high after 3 to 6 months of dietary therapy. The NCEP recommends several drugs, including bile acid sequestrants (cholestyramine and colestipol), HMG-CoA reductase inhibitors or "statins" (lovastatin, pravastatin, simvastatin, and fluvastatin), gemfibrozil, and niacin. Details of pharmacology and side effects are described in the NCEP report.

The LDL goal suggested for patients with established coronary disease is quite low [< 100 mg/dL (2.6 mmol/L)], reflecting the critical importance of cholesterol lowering in preventing both recurrent infarction and coronary death.

To achieve LDL cholesterol levels this low will frequently require the combination of diet and one or more drugs (Table 4). Drug combinations consisting of bile acid sequentrants and one "systemic" drug (i.e., cholestyramine and pravastatin) can be used without increasing toxicity, since the bile acid sequestrants are not absorbed and are essentially without toxicity.

Combinations of two systemic drugs, however (i.e., lovastatin and gemfibrozil), must be used with more caution because the possibility of both hepatic toxicity and skeletal myositis is increased, the latter with an incidence as high

Table 4 NCEP Guidelines for Drug Selection in Hypocholesterolemia

	Single drug	Combination drug
Elevated LDL cholesterol and triglyceride levels <200 mg/dL	BAS HMG-CoA reductase inhibitor (statin) NA	BAS + statin BAS + NA Statin + NA[a]
Elevated LDL cholesterol and triglyceride levels 200–400 mg/dL	NA HMG-CoA reductase inhibitor Gem	NA + statin[a] Statin + Gem[b] NA + BAS NA + Gem

Abbreviations: BAS = bile-acid sequestrant; NA = nicotinic acid; and Gem = gemfibrozil.
[a]Possible increased risk of myopathy and hepatitis.
[b]Increased risk of myopathy; must be used with caution.
Source: National Cholesterol Education Program. Second Report of the Expert Panel on Detection, Evaluation, and Treatment of High Blood Cholesterol in Adults (Adult Treatment Panel II). Circulation 1994; 89:1329–1445.

as 5%. Patients on such combinations should have plasma alanine aminotransferase (ALT) assayed every 2–3 months. They should also be instructed to stop medications and contact their physician if any unusual muscle pain occurs. Unfortunately, regular monitoring of creatine kinase (CK), which rises only *after* the onset of pain, will not help to detect early myopathy, because symptoms precede the rise in CK levels.

Combinations of lipid-lowering agents may be used to achieve greater LDL cholesterol lowering; to achieve adequate LDL cholesterol lowering at lower doses at each medication, thus decreasing the possibility of side effects from individual medications; or to achieve multiple effects on lipoproteins. Triglyceride lowering and HDL cholesterol elevations as well as LDL cholesterol lowering, for example, may be achieved with a combination of colestipol plus gemfibrozil or niacin.

Use of Antihypertensive Agents

The JNC V guidelines suggest that diuretics and beta-blocking agents, because they have been demonstrated in clinical trials not only to lower blood pressure but also to lower cerebrovascular and coronary event rates, be the drugs of first choice in treating hypertension. Other drugs, like ACE inhibitors and calcium channel blockers, although equally effective in lowering blood pressure and without adverse effects on circulating lipoproteins, have not been studied in trials with morbidity or mortality as cardiovascular endpoints. Nevertheless, these agents are indicated in patients with demonstrated lipoprotein disorders in whom it is desirable to avoid aggravating lipid disorders that are already present.

Other Pharmacological Approaches to Coronary Disease Prevention

Aspirin   Aspirin reduces recurrent nonfatal events in men with coronary disease by about 40% and coronary death by about 20–25%. In primary prevention of myocardial infarction in men, results are more variable. Some studies show similar declines in first myocardial infarctions, similar to those in secondary trials. Aspirin dosage of one tablet every other day is probably adequate. None of these effects have been confirmed in women, although studies to assess their likelihood are currently under way.

There is a small increased risk of cerebral hemorrhage associated with regular aspirin use. As judged from current evidence of the benefit of regular use of aspirin in post–myocardial infarction patients, it is definitely indicated in male and probably in female patients. Its use in primary prevention in either men or women is less clear.

Beta-Adrenergic Blocking Agents   Despite the adverse lipid effects of some beta-adrenergic blocking agents, they lower death rates in at least the first year after infarction. Whether beta blockers are useful beyond 1 year is less certain. Unless specifically contraindicated, they should be used in all patients after a myocardial infarction.

ACE Inhibitors   In clinical trials of patients with congestive heart failure (CHF) secondary to coronary artery disease, ACE inhibitors not only prevent death from CHF but also reduce recurrent infarction rates. The question of whether ACE inhibitors have the same effect on recurrent infarction in the absence of CHF has not yet been resolved.

Antioxidants   In population studies, high intakes of vitamin E, beta carotene, and vitamin C in the diet or in dietary supplements have been associated with a lower risk of coronary disease. Because oxidized LDL is thought to be atherogenic, these agents may be useful for patients with established disease. Beneficial effects on coronary artery disease have not, however, been demonstrated in a clinical trial. Moreover, one recent trial demonstrated *excess* mortality from lung cancer in male smokers taking beta carotene. Although many practitioners recommend antioxidants to prevent progression of coronary atherosclerosis, their routine use cannot be generally justified at this time, either for primary or secondary prevention.

D. Encouraging Compliance

When measured, actual compliance to prevention regimens, either hygienic or pharmacological, is often substantially lower than hoped or expected. Several strategies can be used to increase compliance to medical regimens including:

1.   Making certain that instructions to patients are as simple and clear as possible.
2.   Providing a written prescription for a behavioral change is often helpful. This has the effect of attaching permanence and significance to a regimen that verbal instruction does not.
3.   Providing a written contract with a patient in which the patient agrees to a specific behavior change has a similar effect.
4.   Specifying specific intermediate goals in prescriptions, guidelines, or oral instructions. A 20-lb weight loss seems much more achievable when it is taken in 5-lb portions.
5.   Not assuming that filling a prescription is equivalent to taking the drug. Ask patients to bring in medications and do periodic "pill counts" to ascertain usage rates.
6.   If it is not economically detrimental, prescribing drugs in 2- to 4-month quantities so that there is an opportunity, particularly in the initial stages of therapy, to monitor compliance.

Many of these tactics can be carried out by nonphysician professionals, although they require clear and consistent endorsement by the supervising physician.

IV. CONCLUSIONS

Intervention targeted against coronary risk factors, both by behavior change and with drugs, can retard the progress of atherosclerosis. This is true both in those with and those without clinical evidence of coronary disease. Whatever intervention strategies are prescribed, success requires continual endorsement and involvement of the physician and staff who care for the patient.

SUGGESTED READING

Douglas PS. Cardiovascular Health and Disease in Women. Philadelphia: Saunders, 1993.
Goor R, Goor N. Eater's Choice: A Food Lover's Guide to Lower Cholesterol. 3d ed. Boston: Houghton Mifflin, 1992.
LaRosa JC, Cleeman JI. Cholesterol lowering as a treatment for established coronary heart disease. Circulation 1992; 85:1229–1235.
National Cholesterol Education Program. Second Report of the Expert Panel on Detection, Evaluation, and Treatment of High Blood Cholesterol in Adults (Adult Treatment Panel II). Circulation 1994; 89:1329–1445.
National Institutes of Health, National Heart, Lung, and Blood Institute. The Fifth Report of the Joint National Committee on Detection, Evaluation, and Treatment of High Blood Pressure. NIH Publication No. 93-1088, 1993.

Infective Endocarditis

I.	Definitions	509
II.	Clinical Presentations	510
III.	Diagnosis	511
IV.	Microbiology	512
V.	Treatment	514
VI.	Prophylaxis	517
	Sugested Reading	518

W. Kemper Alston and Christopher J. Grace

Despite dramatic advances in the diagnosis and treatment of infectious diseases, infective endocarditis (IE) remains threatening because of its diverse presentations, often obscure diagnosis, requirement for complex therapy, and often malignant course. As antimicrobial agents have evolved, so too have the pathogens. Prosthetic valves and the use of intravenous drugs are just two phenomena that have contributed to the changing epidemiology of the disorder.

I. DEFINITIONS

Simply defined, IE is an infection of the endocardium. Although the valve leaflets are the usual site of vegetations, other structures within the heart—such as the chordae tendineae, mural thrombi, or septal defects—can be involved. The traditional and now archaic classifications of acute and chronic endocarditis have been discarded because they fail to reliably distinguish pathogens or outcome. A virulent organism can seed an anatomically normal valve—for example, accompanying a nosocomial bacteremia. Relatively nonvirulent organisms act opportunistically, generally afflicting already damaged valves. Consideration of pathology, blood cultures, and features of the physical examination are helpful, but the salient features requiring definition are the organism isolated (e.g., *viridans* streptococci) and fundamental host factors, including the presence or absence of: (a) native valve endocarditis, (b) prosthetic valve endocarditis, and (c) intravenous drug use. In the antibiotic era, infective endocarditis is less commonly a sequela of uncontrolled infection (e.g., pneumonia) and more often an iatrogenic complication in an elderly or immunocompromised host. More cases are seen in elderly patients with degenerative heart disease and fewer in those with rheumatic heart disease. The incidence in the population at large is between 1 and 4 per 100,000 per year.

II. CLINICAL PRESENTATIONS

Although the confirmation of IE depends on identifying microorganisms in the blood, an astute clinician will suspect the diagnosis in any febrile patient with evidence of systemic inflammation. Key clinical manifestations of endocarditis are listed in Table 1. Although cultures should be obtained, therapy must often be initiated empirically while results are pending. A history of a recent procedure that could have caused bacteremia (dental, genitourinary, gastrointestinal) should be sought. Hallmarks of endocarditis—such as fever, murmur, splenomegaly, and anemia, seen with protracted endocarditis—may be blunted by host factors or previous treatment, obscuring the picture and delaying diagnosis. Except in the most debilitated hosts, fever is the most common clinical finding. Heart murmurs may reflect underlying pathology or a new valvular lesion and are detectable in nearly all patients with IE if careful, serial physical examinations are performed. In some patients the murmur will develop or change over time as the leaflet is destroyed.

Congestive heart failure is the most common cardiac manifestation and the most prominent cause of death. Splenomegaly is an important clue to the diag-

Table 1 Common Clinical Manifestations of Infective Endocarditis

Signs	Laboratory
Fever	Bacteremia
Heart murmur	Proteinuria
Congestive heart failure	Anemia
Splenomegaly	Elevated erythrocyte sedimentation rate
Petechiae	Immune complexes

nosis, especially in patients whose diagnosis has been elusive over weeks to months. Dermatological and mucosal lesions are less common presently because of the decline in the incidence of rheumatic heart disease and consequently chronic endocarditis. Petechiae, subungual splinter hemorrhages, Osler's nodes, Janeway lesions, and digital clubbing are nonspecific but suggestive signs. Retinal hemorrhages, or Roth spots, are rare and nonspecific but sometimes may suggest the diagnosis in a febrile patient. Myalgias and arthralgias, so common in a variety of infectious diseases, are typical also of infective endocarditis, either as a result of septic emboli or immune complex deposition. Renal abnormalities are present in nearly all patients and include glomerulonephritis and infarction.

Embolization is a serious complication and one that may occur after appropriate antimicrobial therapy has been initiated. Up to 50% of patients experience embolization from valvular vegetations. Visualization of such lesions by two-dimensional echocardiography may constitute a risk factor. Common sites of embolization include the spleen, kidney, brain, and eye. The diagnosis must be considered in any elderly patient presenting with focal neurological signs indicative of stroke, especially if fever is present. Intravenous drug users with right-sided vegetations frequently present with septic pulmonary emboli.

III. DIAGNOSIS

Cure of the infection requires prolonged, intensive, and appropriate antimicrobial therapy predicated on definitive and specific diagnosis. Because febrile systemic illnesses are so diverse, documentation of bacteremia with blood cultures is of paramount importance. Infective endocarditis is an intravascular infection resulting in nearly continuous bacteremia. Thus, culture-negative cases in the absence of antibiotics are unusual. All patients in whom the diagnosis is suspected must be queried about antimicrobial use that may have occurred before blood cultures were obtained. A bacteremia that persists over time is strong evidence for the diagnosis, especially in a patient with fever, a murmur, or evidence of embolization. The exact number and timing of blood cultures is less important than the need to obtain multiple sets over time before starting antimicrobials empirically. In unusual cases in which a clinical diagnosis cannot be confirmed with blood cultures, unusual pathogens may be involved (e.g., *Serratia* or fungi, among numerous other organisms).

Laboratory abnormalities (Table 2) include anemia (if the infection has been present for some time), an elevated erythrocyte sedimentation rate (ESR), and proteinuria. Leukocytosis alone is an insensitive criterion, especially with indolent endocarditis. When *Staphylococcus aureus* is isolated from urine, consideration should be given to bacteremia and endocarditis, because the organism is an unusual ascending urinary tract pathogen but may seed the kidney hematogenously. Immunological abnormalities can include cryoglobulinemia, elevated

Table 2 Laboratory Evaluation for Suspected Endocarditis

Blood cultures: three sets at intervals over 24 hr
Hematological profile
Urinalysis
Erythrocyte sedimentation rate
Renal function
Electrocardiogram
Echocardiography

rheumatoid factor, circulating immune complexes, and hypergammaglobulinemia all reflecting consequences of the near constant intravascular antigenemia.

All patients with suspected or proven infective endocarditis should be studied electrocardiographically to identify potential conduction disturbances that may indicate extension of the process beyond the leaflet into the valve ring. Complete heart block has long been associated with aortic valve infection. A baseline ECG should be followed by serial studies during the course of therapy.

Vegetations can frequently be identified on the downstream surface of regurgitant valves by Doppler echocardiography. Perhaps even more helpful in defining prognosis is assessment of valve function. Useful information regarding the site and distribution vegetations, involvement of multiple valves, presence of intracardiac abscess, and hemodynamic function can often be obtained. Transesophageal echocardiography (TEE) has high sensitivity and is especially useful when a prosthetic valve is in place.

IV. MICROBIOLOGY

Infective endocarditis is an appropriate name because infection can be caused not only by aerobic and anaerobic bacteria but also by chlamydiae, rickettsiae, mycoplasmas, mycobacteria, fungi, and perhaps even viruses. Most patients have bacterial endocarditis. Infective endocarditis can be categorized as infection occurring on native or prosthetic heart valves; infection in the absence of positive routinely acquired blood cultures (culture-negative); and infection in association with intravenous drug use.

A. Native Valve Endocarditis

Streptococcal species cause approximately 70% of native valve endocarditis (NVE), with *viridans* streptococci accounting for 40%, enterococci (now considered a separate genus) for 10%, and other streptococcal species for 20%. The *viridans* streptococci are normal inhabitants of the mouth (*S. mitus, S. sanguis, S.*

512

mutans, S. salivarius) and the bowel (*S. bovis*). They account for the vast majority of infections that occur in children and women with mitral regurgitation associated with mitral valve prolapse. *Streptococcus bovis* endocarditis is sometimes seen with carcinoma of the colon and other bowel lesions. Thus, diagnostic evaluation of the bowel is needed once the intracardiac infection has been documented and its treatment initiated. The enterococci (*E. faecium, E. faecalis*) are normal flora in the intestine and urethra. Endocarditis caused by these organisms is difficult to treat, in part because of their inherent drug resistance. Mortality is high.

Staphylococci cause approximately 20% of infections on native valves, with coagulase-positive staphylococci (*S. aureus*) accounting for most. *Staphylococcus aureus* is the most common pathogen (causing 47% of infections) in patients who present to community hospitals. Most are not intravenous drug users, have no underlying heart disease, and have an indeterminate source of bacteremia. Endocarditis caused by *S. aureus* frequently presents as an acute illness, sometimes with near catastrophic cardiac decompensation. It can be associated with valve ring abscess, purulent and fulminant pericarditis and tamponade, and metastatic abscesses. Early or immediate surgical intervention is required frequently.

Less common causes of endocarditis include aerobic gram negative bacilli (1–3%), fungi (2–4%), mixed organisms (1–2%), *Neisseria gonorrhoeae*, and the "HACEK" organisms. The acronym stands for *Hemophilus aphrophilus, Actinobacillus actinomycetemcomitans, Cardiobacterium hominis, Eikenella corrodans,* and *Kingella kingae*. HACEK bacteria are slow-growing, capnophilic (growing well in high-CO_2 environments) gram-negative bacilli that are normal oral flora.

B. Prosthetic Valve Endocarditis

Infection of mechanical or bioprosthetic heart valves (prosthetic valve endocarditis, or PVE) occurs in 2.5% of patients. Infection occurring within 60 days of surgery (i.e., early PVE) accounts for 31%. Late PVE accounts for 69%. Organisms causing early PVE usually infect the prosthesis during surgery. They gain access to the valve from the patient's or the surgical staff's skin or from the bypass pump intraoperatively. Postoperative bacteremia secondary to infected intravenous catheters, wound infections, or pneumonia contributes to early PVE as well.

The most common pathogens are *Staphylococcus epidermidis* (35%), *S. aureus* (17%), gram-negative bacilli (16%), corynebacteria (10%), and fungi (11%). Although fever is almost universal, less than 60% patients exhibit the classic signs of endocarditis (changing murmur, emboli, peripheral stigmata). One-year mortality exceeds 50%. Fungi, staphylococci, and gram-negative bacilli are most likely to be lethal.

Late PVE is caused by bacteremia with seeding of the valve. The microbiology is similar to that of NVE with *viridans* streptococci (25%), *S. aureus* (12%), and enterococci (9%) causing most infections. As with early PVE, many late infections are caused by coagulase-negative staphylococci (26%), gram-negative bacilli (12%), corynebacteria (4%), and fungi (4%). Clinical presentation is similar to that with early PVE, though mortality is lower.

C. Culture-Negative Endocarditis

Despite the generally excellent sensitivity of blood culture in identifying causative agents, up to 5% of patients with clinically suspected endocarditis will have negative cultures. The most common cause is treatment with antibiotics before culture. A week or two of use of noncurative antibiotics may transiently sterilize blood cultures for several weeks thereafter. Blood cultures are generally discarded after 7 days when there is no growth. Some bacteria, such as those in the HACEK group, may not grow for 3 weeks. Thus, blood cultures should be monitored for at least 4 weeks when culture-negative endocarditis is being considered. Certain less common pathogens, such as *Chlamydia*, *Coxiella*, *Mycoplasma*, *Legionella*, *Aspergillus*, nutritionally deficient streptococci, and *Brucellas* do not grow in routine blood culture media. Culturing in special media and serological diagnosis may be needed for diagnosis.

D. Endocarditis in the Injection Drug User

Because of altered normal skin flora, use of contaminated needles, overuse of nonprescription antibiotics and possible infection with human immunodeficiency virus (HIV), injection drug users (IDUs) have a high incidence of endocarditis caused by *S. aureus* (60%); gram-negative bacilli, especially *Pseudomonas* (13%); *Candida* species (13%); and polymicrobic agents (8%). The *S. aureus* infections are frequently right-sided and are becoming increasingly resistant to beta-lactam antibiotics.

Noninfectious causes of endocarditis exist, including marantic endocarditis, systemic lupus erythematosus, myxoma, rheumatic fever, Loeffler's endocarditis, carcinoid, and endocardial fibroelastosis. Any of these can cause endocarditis in an IDU as well as in nonusers.

V. TREATMENT

Cure of endocarditis requires penetration of an appropriate antibiotic into vegetations on heart valves with fibrin and platelet deposits encasing the microbes and protecting them from antibiotics in the blood. Penetration is generally limited. Because few white blood cells are present within vegetations, they are sites of relative immunocompromise. Numerous organisms are present in vegetations, but most are relatively inactive metabolically, thus reducing their susceptibility to drugs. Antibiotic therapy therefore must be bactericidal, with agents given intravenously in high doses and for prolonged periods of time. The minimal inhibitory concentration (MIC) should be determined for the isolated pathogen.

Streptococci are considered sensitive (MIC < 0.1 μg/mL) or resistant (MIC > 0.1 μg/mL) to penicillin (Table 3). Endocarditis caused by sensitive streptococci can be treated with a 4-week course of intravenous penicillin. An alternative regimen for patients with good renal function is 2 weeks of intravenous penicillin combined with gentamicin. Infections caused by resistant streptococci must be treated with two synergistic bactericidal antibiotics such as penicillin and an aminoglycoside. All enterococci are tolerant to penicillin and must be treated with intravenous penicillin or ampicillin and an aminoglycoside. Some enterococci are also highly resistant to aminoglycosides (MIC > 1000 μg/mL), making antibiotic synergy impractical and cure difficult.

Most *S. aureus* isolates are sensitive to nafcillin or oxacillin. For patients allergic to penicillin (without anaphylaxis), cefazolin is the best choice. Vancomycin should be reserved for patients with severe penicillin allergies or those with methicillin-resistant *Staphylococcus aureus* (MRSA). Infections in IDUs with right-sided *S. aureus* endocarditis can be treated with nafcillin and gentamicin for 2 weeks. Infections with aerobic gram-negative bacilli, including the

Table 3 Therapy for Native-Valve Endocarditis

Organism	First-Line Therapy	Alternative Therapy
Sensitive streptococci (MIC < 0.1 μg/mL)	A. Penicillin G 10–20 million units/day × 4 weeks B. Penicillin G 10–20 million units/day and gentamicin 1 mg/kg q8h × 2 weeks	A. Cefazolin 2 g q8h × 4 weeks B. Vancomycin 1g q12h × 4 weeks
Resistant streptococci (MIC > 0.1 μg/mL) and enterococci	A. Ampicillin 12 g/day and gentamicin 1 mg/kg q8h for 4–6 weeks B. Penicillin G 20 million units/day and gentamicin 1 mg/kg q8h × 4–6 weeks	A. Vancomycin 1g q12h and gentamicin 1 mg/kg q8h × 4–6 weeks
Staphylococcus aureus	Nafcillin or oxacillin 2 g q4h × 4–6 weeks ± gentamicin for first 3–5 days	A. Cefazolin 2 g q8h × 4–6 weeks B. Vancomycin 1 g q12h × 4–6 weeks
MRSA	Vancomycin 1 g q12h × 4–6 weeks	None
HACEK or other gram-negative bacilli	Third-generation cephalosporin × 6 weeks ± aminoglycoside	Aztreonam, ciprofloxacin

HACEK group, can be treated with high doses of a third-generation cephalosporin, aztreonam, or ciprofloxacin. Addition of an aminoglycoside is appropriate for *Pseudomonas* infections.

Outpatient treatment of endocarditis with intravenous antibiotics is becoming more common. The use of ceftriaxone, 2 g once daily for 4 weeks, to treat sensitive streptococcal endocarditis is effective. Careful selection of patients is required and close follow-up for complications from the IE and from the intravenous catheter is needed.

Therapy for PVE requires combinations of two and sometimes three antibiotics (Table 4). Surgery is frequently needed. The infections are extremely serious and difficult to treat despite the prolonged therapy (6 to 8 weeks) required.

Initial, empirical treatment for either NVE or PVE can be initiated with vancomycin and gentamicin. For IDUs, ceftazidime should be added until results of blood cultures become available.

Monitoring of antibiotic therapy with serum bactericidal titers (SBT) is time-honored but of unproven value. Weinstein and coworkers have suggested that a peak dilution of 1:64 and a trough dilution of 1:32 are predictive of bacteriological cure. Caution in interpretation is needed, however.

Mortality from IE is usually secondary to valvular regurgitation and progressive congestive heart failure. Systemic embolization of vegetations, uncon-

Table 4 Therapy for Prosthetic Valve Endocarditis

Organism	First-Line Therapy	Alternative Therapy
Coagulase-negative *Staphylococcus*	Vancomycin 1 g q12h and gentamicin 1 mg/kg q8h and rifampin 300 mg q8h PO × 6–8 weeks	None
Staphylococcus aureus	Nafcillin 2 g q4h IV and gentamicin 1 mg/kg q8h × 6–8 weeks	Cefazolin 2 gm q8h and gentamicin
MRSA	Vamcomycin 1 g q12h and gentamicin ± rifampin	None
Sensitive streptococci	Penicillin G 20 million units/day × 4–6 weeks and gentamicin × 2 weeks	Cefazolin 2 g q8h or Vancomycin 1 g q12h × 4–6 weeks and gentamicin 1 mg/kg q8h × 2 weeks
Resistant streptococci and enterococci	Penicillin G 20 million units/day and gentamicin × 6–8 weeks	Vancomycin 1 gm q12h and gentamicin 1 mg/kg 8qh × 6–8 weeks
Gram-negative bacilli	Third-generation cephalosporin and aminoglycoside × 6–8 weeks	Aztreonam or ciprofloxacin and aminoglycoside × 6–8 weeks

trolled infection including myocardial abscess formation, and resistant pathogens contribute to morbidity and mortality. Surgical intervention with debridement and valve replacement has greatly reduced mortality in high-risk patients. Indications for surgery include (a) poorly controlled congestive heart failure (CHF); (b) uncontrolled infection characterized by persistent fever or bacteremia; (c) signs of myocardial abscess formation such as bundle branch block; (d) repeated systemic emboli; (e) infection with fungi, gram-negative bacilli (except the HACEK group) and frequently *S. aureus*; (f) early PVE; and (g) late PVE except in the stable patient with a sensitive *viridans* streptococcal infection. Attempts to treat with antibiotics over prolonged intervals should not delay surgery.

VI. PROPHYLAXIS

Despite best medical and surgical treatment, endocarditis remains associated with high morbidity and mortality. Prevention is often possible but still underutilized. Endocarditis most often results from bacteremia with seeding of already damaged valvular endocardium. Therefore patients with underlying valvular abnormalities who undergo procedures that can cause bacteremia are at high risk. Prophylaxis is needed for those with prosthetic valves, previous endocarditis, valvular stenosis or regurgitation, ventricular septal defect, asymmetrical septal hypertrophy, patent ductus arteriosus, cyanotic congenital heart disease, previous intracardiac surgery, and mitral valve prolapse with regurgitation (MVP without regurgitation is considered low-risk for IE) (Table 5).

Table 5 Prophylaxis for Endocarditis

Procedure	First-Line Therapy	Alternative
Dental and upper respiratory tract surgery	Amoxicillin 3.0 g PO 1 hr prior; 1.5 g 6 hr later	Clindamycin 300 mg PO 1 hr prior; 150 mg PO 6 hr later
Genitourinary or gastrointestinal surgery	Amoxicillin 3.0 g PO 1 hr prior; 1.5 g 6 hr later	Ampicillin 2 g IV and gentamicin 1.5 mg/kg IV 1 hr prior and 8 hr postprocedure, or vancomycin 1 g IV and gentamicin 1.5 mg/kg IV 1 hr prior and 8 hr postprocedure
Any procedure in a high-risk patient (e.g., prosthetic heart valves previous IE)	Vancomycin 1 g IV and gentamicin 1.5 mg/kg IV 1 hr prior and 8 hr postprocedure	

SUGGESTED READING

Crane LR, Levine DP, Zervos MJ, Cummings G. Bacteremia in narcotic addicts at the Detroit Medical Center: I. Microbiology, epidemiology, risk factors, and empiric therapy. Rev Infect Dis 1986; 8:364–373.

Dinuble, M. Short course antibiotic therapy for right sided endocarditis caused by *Staphylococcus aureus* in injection drug users. Ann Intern Med 1994; 121:873–876.

Dinuble MJ, et al. Surgery in active endocarditis. Ann Intern Med 1982; 96:650–659.

Durack DT. Prevention of infective endocarditis. N Engl J Med 1995; 332:38–44.

Francioli PB. Ceftriaxone and outpatient treatment of infective endocarditis. Infect Dis Clin North Am 1993; 7:97–115.

King JW, Nguyen VQ, Conrad SA. Results of a prospective statewide reporting system for infective endocarditis. Am J Med Sci 1988; 295:517–527.

Sokil AB. Cardiac imaging in infective endocarditis. In: Kaye D, ed. Infective Endocarditis, 2d ed. New York: Raven Press, 1992:125–150.

Steckelberg JM, Melton LJ, Ilstrup DM, et al. Influence of referral bias on the apparent clinical spectrum of infective endocarditis. Am J Med 1990; 88:582–588.

Steckelberg JM, Murphy JG, Ballard D, et al. Emboli in infective endocarditis: The prognostic value of echocardiography. Ann Intern Med 1991; 114:635–640.

Terpenning MS, Buggy BP, Kauffman CA. Infective endocarditis: Clinical features in young and elderly patients. Am J Med 1987; 83:626–634.

Threlkeld MG, Cobbs CG. Infectious disorders of prosthetic valves and intravascular devices. In: Mandell GL, Bennett JE, Dolin R, eds. Principles and Practice of Infectious Disease, 4th ed. New York: Churchill Livingstone, 1995:783–793.

Tunkel AR. Evaluation of culture negative endocarditis. Hosp Pract 1993; 28(2A):59–62.

Von Reyn CF, Levy BS, Arbeit RD, et al. Infective endocarditis: An analysis based on strict case definitions. Ann Intern Med 1981; 94:505–518.

Wang K, Gobel F, Gleason DF, Edwards JE. Complete heart block complicating bacterial endocarditis. Circulation 1972; 46:939–947.

Wantanakunakorn C, Burkett T. Infective endocarditis at a large community teaching hospital, 1980–1990: A review of 210 episodes. Medicine 1993; 72:90–102.

Weinstein MP, Stratton CW, Ackley A, et al. Multicenter collaborative evaluation of a standardized serum bacteriocidal test as a prognositc indicator in infective endocarditis. Am J Med 1985; 78:262–269.

Yu LV, Fang GD, Keys TF, et al. Prosthetic valve endocarditis: Superiority of surgical valve replacement versus medical therapy only. Ann Thorac Surg 1994; 58:1073–1077.

518

Management of Patients with Antiarrhythmic Devices

I.	General Concepts	520
II.	Selection of Patients for ICDS	520
III.	Evaluation of ICD Shocks	521
IV.	Infection	522
V.	Management of Arrhythmias	523
VI.	Effects of Antiarrhythmic Drugs on ICD Performance	524
VII.	Perioperative Management	524
VIII.	Overall Perspective	525
	Suggested Reading	525

Bruce D. Lindsay

The implantable cardioverter defibrillator (ICD) plays an important role in the management of patients with life-threatening ventricular arrhythmias. Whether alone or in conjunction with antiarrhythmic drugs, therapy with ICDs has reduced the incidence of sudden death in high-risk subjects, which was once approximately 40%, down to about 6% over 4 years. The low operative mortality associated with implantation of nonthoracotomy lead systems and the effectiveness of ICDs in terminating ventricular arrhythmias have led to an exponential growth in the number of ICD systems implanted each year. Because of the growing number of patients with ICDs, physicians with diverse fields of interest encounter patients with these devices and may be required to make decisions that could be affected by the presence of such a system. Appropriate patient management requires an appreciation of the fundamental elements of an ICD system, the means by which it terminates an arrhythmia, and problems that patients with ICDs are prone to develop.

I. GENERAL CONCEPTS

An ICD system comprises a pulse generator and a lead system for pacing, arrhythmia sensing, and delivery of high-voltage shocks. The pulse generator of an ICD is approximately three to five times larger than that of a standard pacemaker and weighs 130 to 250 g, depending on the model. The expected life of the pulse generator is 3 to 4 years, and the need for replacement is determined in office visits by monitoring battery voltage or the time required to charge the high-voltage capacitors. Arrhythmia monitoring is accomplished with leads analogous to those in pacemaker systems, which can be implanted on the epicardium or inserted transvenously and positioned at the right ventricular apex. Separate leads are required to deliver high-voltage shocks for cardioversion or defibrillation. Epicardial lead systems can be implanted via a median sternotomy, a left lateral thoracotomy, or a subxiphoid incision. Nonthoracotomy lead systems commonly employ one or two leads inserted through the left subclavian vein, positioned at the right ventricular apex and superior vena cava. When a subcutaneous patch is required to reliably terminate ventricular fibrillation, it is typically positioned over the left lateral thorax. The pulse generator is usually implanted subcutaneously in the abdomen, but newer, smaller models can be positioned in the left pectoral region.

All ICDs have programmable arrhythmia detection criteria that require an arrhythmia to exceed a specified rate and duration. Syncope or near syncope may precede a shock from the defibrillator, because approximately 10 to 15 sec are needed for the ICD to detect an arrhythmia, charge its capacitors, and deliver a shock. Once an arrhythmia has been detected, it can be terminated by a high-voltage shock. Some ICD models are capable of terminating ventricular tachycardia with a burst of rapid pacing. The termination of an arrhythmia by a high-voltage shock is quite painful and causes the patient to jerk visibly. Fortunately, the pain caused by the shock is transient, followed by prompt recovery. In contrast, rapid bursts of antitachycardia pacing may not be recognized by the patient at all or associated only with a brief interval of light-headedness. When antitachycardia pacing fails to terminate an arrhythmia or causes it to accelerate, most ICDs deliver a therapeutic shock.

II. SELECTION OF PATIENTS FOR ICDS

ICDs are indicated for use in patients with life-threatening ventricular arrhythmias in whom antiarrhythmic drug therapy is judged to be inadequate. Most patients who have undergone implantation of a defibrillator system have survived at least one episode of ventricular fibrillation or hemodynamically unstable ventricular tachycardia. The use of ICDs has been extended to patients with recurrent ven-

520

tricular tachycardias that can be terminated by antitachycardia pacing. This approach may avoid the need for repeated admission to the hospital for cardioversion and prolonged monitoring on a telemetry unit while antiarrhythmic drug regimens are being modified.

ICDs are contraindicated for patients who have ventricular arrhythmias that are attributable to a reversible cause and are unlikely to recur. In patients who experience ventricular arrhythmias secondary to drug toxicity, electrolyte imbalances, hypoxia, sepsis, drowning, or electrocution, it is sufficient to treat the underlying condition. Patients who are resuscitated from ventricular fibrillation that occurs in the first 24–48 hr after acute myocardial infarction in the absence or cardiogenic shock are at low risk for subsequent sudden death and do not benefit from or require implantation of a defibrillator. ICDs are not indicated for patients with congestive heart failure refractory to medical therapy or other end-stage disorders associated with poor short-term prognosis.

III. EVALUATION OF ICD SHOCKS

One of the most common problems encountered in patients with ICDs is uncertainty about whether a shock delivered by the ICD was appropriate for treatment of a ventricular arrhythmia or inappropriate and provoked by supraventricular tachycardia or a sensing malfunction. Despite the safety and efficacy of ICDs, delivery of inappropriate shocks has posed a serious problem in long-term management. Approximately 66% of patients undergoing Holter or telemetry monitoring received shocks in response to sustained ventricular arrhythmias, 40% in response to supraventricular tachycardias, 10% while sinus or a paced rhythm prevails, and 4% in response to nonsustained ventricular tachycardia. Most newer ICDs divert shocks when ventricular arrhythmias terminate spontaneously; they also have the capacity to store intracardiac electrograms recorded at the time of occurrence of the arrhythmia that caused the ICD to deliver a shock. This property provides important diagnostic information, facilitating effective programming to avoid inappropriate discharges from the ICD.

When patients experience shocks delivered by an ICD, the inciting event may be obscure. With ventricular arrhythmias, severe symptoms precede the shock in 42% of patients. Prodromal symptoms are mild in 49% and absent in 30%. By contrast, only 2% of patients with supraventricular arrhythmias leading to a shock have severe symptoms, 39% have only mild symptoms, and 56% have no symptoms. Thus, severe symptoms are almost always associated with ventricular arrhythmias, but it is difficult to accurately differentiate initiators of shocks in patients with absent or mild symptoms.

A stepwise approach, as summarized in Table 1, may help to differentiate potential causes of inappropriate shocks. After a history of the event has been obtained, the ICD should be interrogated by a physician knowledgeable about its intricacies. Information obtained from the ICD can be used to determine whether

Table 1   Causes of Inappropriate
Shocks

Arrhythmias
   Sinus tachycardia
   Supraventricular tachycardia
   Atrial fibrillation
   Nonsustained ventricular tachycardia
Sensing abnormalities
   Sensing of pacemaker stimulus
   Double sensing of QRS
   T-wave oversensing
Compromised lead system
   Lead conductor fractured
   Lead insulation damaged
   Loose connection
   Lead dislodgment

the shock was delivered because of oversensing of T waves, interaction with a permanent pacemaker, artifact caused by a broken or dislodged sensing lead, or an arrhythmia. Devices that store R-wave intervals or electrograms preceding the shock provide valuable information that can facilitate such determinations. Stored electrograms are particularly helpful because the morphology of the signal may differentiate ventricular arrhythmias from supraventricular arrhythmias or electrical artifact caused by a broken lead. A chest x-ray may help to identify lead dislodgments or fractures that can lead to spurious sensing. When doubt remains regarding the initiation of frequent ICD shocks, recordings obtained by Holter or event monitors can usually identify the problem.

IV.   INFECTION

Despite advances in ICD technology, infection remains a major problem. Its incidence is 2.7% for epicardial lead systems and 1.3% for nonthoracotomy lead systems. Patients with serious infections may present with fever, chills, leukocytosis, and an elevated erythrocyte sedimentation rate. Although infection may be associated with obvious erosion at the site of the generator, in some cases the diagnosis may be difficult to confirm without opening the ICD generator pocket. In patients in whom the source of infection is occult, a gallium scan may show evidence of mediastinal inflammation. Computed tomography of the chest may show a collection of pericardial fluid. Although pericardial effusion is relatively common in the first month after surgery, its persistence in a patient with unexplained fever is a clue that infection may be present. In many patients, the diagnosis of infection can be established only by opening the generator pocket and ordering appropriate cultures. Although a patient with an infected generator can occasionally be treated by local debridement and topical antimicrobials, removal of the entire system is generally required.

V. MANAGEMENT OF ARRHYTHMIAS

Patients often seek medical attention after receiving a shock from an ICD. Those who experience a single shock with prompt resolution of symptoms do not require urgent evaluation. By contrast, patients who have symptoms that persist after a shock or those in whom multiple shocks are elaborated should be evaluated in an emergency room and admitted for observation. The major concern is that recurrent episodes of ventricular tachycardia or fibrillation, failure of the ICD to terminate the arrhythmia, or inappropriate shocks from other causes are occurring.

When patients have arrhythmias observed by paramedics, emergency room personnel, or those who provide care in an intensive care unit, the ICD usually detects and terminates the arrhythmia before any other intervention can be initiated. In some cases, antitachycardia pacing or the first shock delivered by the ICD may fail to terminate the arrhythmia. When the arrhythmia is associated with hemodynamic instability, external electrical cardioversion should be performed expeditiously if the ICD fails to terminate the arrythmia within 15 to 20 sec. Medical personnel who are touching the patient when an ICD delivers a shock may feel a slight tingling sensation but will not be injured. If transthoracic DC cardioversion or defibrillation is performed, the ICD will not be damaged provided that the defibrillation paddles are not positioned directly over its pulse generator.

ICDs may fail to detect a ventricular arrhythmia if the rate is below a programmed rate-detection criterion. If so, the arrhythmia should be treated as if an ICD had not been present. Alternatively, the ICD can be reprogrammed to detect and treat the arrhythmia if it is not associated with hemodynamic compromise and a programming device is readily available. This approach is appropriate for patients with arrhythmias easily terminated by antitachycardia pacing delivered by the ICD. Other causes of failure to detect an arrhythmia are fracture or dislodgment of the lead.

Occasionally patients are admitted because of repeated, physiologically inappropriate shocks from an ICD initiated by a supraventricular arrhythmia, nonsustained ventricular tachycardia, lead failure, or a sensing problem. Most ICDs can be deactivated temporarily by positioning a donut-shaped magnet over the pulse generator. Depending on the specific model of the ICD and the way it has been programmed, application of a magnet may temporarily suspend the detection algorithm or deactivate the device. The ICD's function should always be evaluated by experienced personnel as soon as possible afterwards to define the factors eliciting delivery of the shocks and to make certain that the ICD is functioning properly.

523

VI. EFFECTS OF ANTIARRHYTHMIC DRUGS ON ICD PERFORMANCE

Often antiarrhythmic drugs are used concomitantly with ICDs for the treatment of ventricular arrhythmias. They may be required for suppression of atrial fibrillation. The objective of antiarrhythmic drug therapy is to reduce frequent spontaneous arrhythmias that provoke shocks from the ICD. Although the use of antiarrhythmic drugs may be unavoidable, treatment should not be initiated without awareness that antiarrhythmic drugs can distort detection and termination of arrhythmias by an ICD. Antiarrhythmic drugs can be proarrhythmic, thereby increasing the number of shocks delivered by the ICD. They can cause ventricular tachycardia to occur at a slower rate and thereby fail to meet the rate detection criteria of the ICD. Antiarrhythmic drugs can affect the ability of the ICD to terminate an arrhythmia. They may make ventricular tachycardia more difficult to terminate by antitachycardia pacing. They can increase the energy required for defibrillation substantially, resulting in failure of the ICD to effectively defibrillate. For these reasons, whenever antiarrhythmic drugs are used, it is advisable to evaluate their effects on the capacity of the ICD to detect and terminate an arrhythmia.

VII. PERIOPERATIVE MANAGEMENT

When patients with ICDs undergo surgery for problems unrelated to cardiovascular disease, special precautions should be taken. Many patients with ICDs have coronary artery disease. Some have depressed left ventricular function for other reasons. Both of these factors can substantially affect surgical risk. Moreover, patients who are taking antiarrhythmic drugs may experience a sudden increase in arrhythmias when their drugs are discontinued in association with surgery. Intravenous formulations can be administered perioperatively to obviate this difficulty. If electrocautery is used intraoperatively, electromagnetic interference may cause an inappropriate shock to be delivered by an ICD. Alternatively, it may deactivate the ICD. Both can be avoided by deactivating the ICD and reactivating when the patient goes to the recovery room. Surgical personnel should be aware that the ICD is not active intraoperatively and that defibrillation may be necessary in the even that an arrhythmia occurs while the patient is unprotected.

A. Restriction of Activities

Most patients with ICDs can resume normal activities, limited only by the severity of their underlying heart disease. Those with good functional capacity can return to work and exercise as tolerated. In a few circumstances, electromagnetic interference in the workplace can pose a problem. An ICD can be affected in patients who work within a few feet of large transformers or power tools that require high currents. Thus, an electromagnetic field generated by an arch welder can affect the

524

performance of an ICD adversely by altering its programmed features, temporarily affecting sensing functions, or deactivating the device. Patients who travel should be advised that the ICD will be detected by airport security systems. Thus, a special identification card should be used. Exposure to standard appliances around the home or to microwave ovens is very unlikely to affect an ICD.

One of the problems that patients with ICDs face is whether to resume driving. A recurrence of ventricular tachycardia or fibrillation could result in syncope before termination of the arrhythmia by the ICD. Although most states have specific laws governing whether patients with seizure disorders can drive, relatively few impose restrictions on patients with arrhythmias. No studies provide definitive answers. In patients who have been resuscitated from sudden death and have been treated with ICDs or antiarrhythmic drugs, the 1-year recurrence rate of hemodynamically compromised arrhythmias is approximately 16.5%. The risk is especially high within the first few months after hospital discharge. Permanent restriction of driving would be harsh. When no legal guidelines exist in a patient's state of residence, the decision as to when to resume driving is a matter of judgment. As a general guideline, an interval of 6 to 12 months without presyncope, syncope, or a shock from an ICD is needed before the patient should resume driving. Patients should be advised not to swim for a comparable event-free interval because of the risk of drowning. They should resume swimming only in a closely supervised area. Shocks delivered by an ICD when the patient is immersed do not pose a danger to others in the water.

VIII. OVERALL PERSPECTIVE

ICDs reduce the risk of sudden death in patients with hemodynamically compromising arrhythmias not controlled by medications. Further study is needed to determine whether ICDs should replace antiarrhythmic drugs as primary therapy for ventricular arrhythmias. Limitations of antiarrhythmic drug therapy include the lack of reliable therapeutic endpoints needed in evaluating drug efficacy, toxicity of antiarrhythmic medications, the need for high compliance, and long-term costs. ICDs are effective. Implantation procedures have been facilitated by development of nonthoracotomy lead systems. Operative mortality has been reduced to < 1%. Nevertheless, the risk of infection remains approximately 2%, and lead dislodgments occur in another 2%. Although ICDs are expensive, costs will decline as technical advances increase the longevity of pulse generators.

SUGGESTED READING

Akhtar M, Avitall B, Jazayeri M, et al. Role of implantable cardioverter defibrillator therapy in the management of high-risk patients. Circulation 1992; 85(suppl I):I-131–I-139.

Grimm W, Flores BF, Marchlinski FE. Symptoms and electrocardiographically documented rhythm preceding spontaneous shocks in patients with implantable cardioverter-defibrillator. Am J Cardiol 1993; 71:1415–1418.

Hauser RG, Kurschinski DT, McVeigh K, et al. Clinical results with nonthoracotomy ICD systems. PACE 1993; 161:41–148.

Hook BG, Callans DJ, Kleiman RB, et al. Implantable cardioverter-defibrillator therapy in the absence of significant symptoms: Rhythm diagnosis and management aided by stored electrogram analysis. Circulation 1993; 87:1897–1906.

Kelly PQ, Cannom DS, Garan H, et al. The automatic implantable cardioverter-defibrillator: Efficacy, complications, and survival in patients with malignant ventricular arrhythmias. J Am Coll Cardiol 1988; 11:1278–1286.

Kuppermann M, Luce BR, McGovern B, et al. An analysis of the cost-effectiveness of the implantable defibrillator. Circulation 1990; 81:91–100.

Lehman MH, Steinman RT, Schuger CD, Jackson K. The automatic implantable cardioverter defibrillator as antiarrhythmic treatment modality of choice for survivors of cardiac arrest unrelated to acute myocardial infarction. Am J Cardiol 1988; 62: 803–805.

Nisam S, Mower MM, Thomas A, Hauser R. Patient survival comparison in three generations of automatic implantable cardioverter defibrillators: Review of 12 years, 25,000 patients. PACE 1993; 16:174–178.

Singer I, Guarnieri T, Kupersmith J. Implanted automatic defibrillators: Effects of drugs and pacemakers. PACE 1988; 11:2250–2261.

Strickberger SA, Cantillon CO, Friedman PL. When should patients with lethal ventricular arrhythmia resume driving? An analysis of state regulations and physician practices. Ann Intern Med 1991; 115:560–563.

Winkle RA, Mead RH, Ruder MA, et al. Long-term outcome with the automatic implantable cardioverter-defibrillator. J Am Coll Cardiol 1989; 13:1353–1361.

MEDICATIONS

Judicious use of pharmacological agents and devices in the medical management of patients with heart disease requires not only knowledge of the specific properties and characteristics of each agent and device but also knowledge of pathophysiological mechanisms targeted by each therapeutic moiety and the nature of interactions between the therapeutic agent and the pathophysiological target. Reliance on a definitive knowledge base is a far from trivial requirement. The use of certain antiarrhythmic agents that held sway for years declined when it became clear from the results of studies that a disparity existed between suppression of arrhythmogenesis and the anticipated impact on survival. Thus, in the CASS trial, type IC antiarrhythmic agents suppressed ventricular ectopy but increased mortality. Similarly, many treatment modalities that are fashionable in one decade fall by the wayside in another as more extensive information becomes available. The early dietary management of patients with type II diabetes mellitus that relied on limitation of carbohydrate intake with a disproportionate augmentation of fat intake became obsolete when it was learned that such a regimen might exacerbate rather than retard atherogenesis.

In practice, the astute clinician will fully understand mechanisms of action of drugs in specific classes and frequently will refresh memory by referring to definitive pharmacological texts, journals, and other clinical literature. In this part no effort is made to provide a comprehensive synopsis of cardiovascular therapeutics. What is presented is a compilation and brief description of salient features of selected therapeutic approaches and agents referred to extensively in the preceding four parts of the book. It is hoped that the presentation of medical regimens in a somewhat telegraphic form will benefit the clinician faced with implementation or modification of a therapeutic regimen in a particular setting.

In contrast to much of the preceding material, the content of this part is, by definition, in a state of flux. It has been said that the half-life of medical therapeutics is approximately five years in the sense that new entries become established and preceding approaches become obsolete with remarkable rapidity. It is only by constantly considering therapeutic modalities in the context of the pathophysiological mechanisms that they modify and on the basis of their properties, pharmacokinetics, pharmacodynamics, and impact on specific pathophysiological mechanisms that the clinician can fulfill the responsibilities of providing patients with current and optimal treatment.

Use of Common Medications in the Treatment of Patients with Heart Disease

I.	Beta-Adrenergic Blockers	529
II.	Calcium Channel Blockers	532
III.	Angiotensin-Converting Enzyme (ACE) Inhibitors	534
IV.	Nitrates	535
V.	Nitroprusside	536
VI.	Agents Used for Sedation and Neuromuscular Blockade in an Intensive or Coronary Care Unit Setting	537
VII.	Agents Used for Neuromuscular Blockade	542
VIII.	Other Classes of Agents	546
IX.	Drug Interactions	550

Robyn A. Schaiff, Paul R. Eisenberg, and Burton E. Sobel

Specific therapeutic regimens have been delineated and discussed throughout this book. In the material to follow, several classes of drugs are considered in general terms, and several highly selected practical aspects of pharmacology pertinent to their use are covered.

I. BETA-ADRENERGIC BLOCKERS

Beta-adrenergic blocking agents (Table 1) are commonly used for treatment of hypertension and ischemic heart disease. They decrease mortality after myocar-

Table 1   Beta-adrenergic Blocking Agents

Drug	Beta$_1$-selective	Intrinsic sympathomimetic activity	Initial dose
Atenolol	Yes	No	50 mg qd
Betaxolol	Yes	No	10 mg qd
Bisoprolol[a]	Yes	No	5 mg qd
Metoprolol	Yes	No	50 mg bid
			XL 50–100 mg qd
Acebutolol[a]	Yes	Yes	200 mg bid
Carteolol[a]	No	Yes	2.5 mg qd
Penbutolol	No	Yes	20 mg qd
Pindolol	No	Yes	5 mg bid
Nadolol	No	No	40 mg qd
Propranolol	No	No	40 mg bid
			SR 80 mg qd
Timolol	No	No	10 mg bid
Labetalol	No	No	100 mg bid
	Alpha blocker		

[a]Dosage adjustment is required in patients with renal dysfunction.

dial infarction. Thus, all patients who have sustained an acute myocardial infarction and who do not have an absolute contraindication to their use—such as severe bradycardia, significant obstructive airway disease, and overt heart failure—can benefit. Decreased left ventricular ejection fraction per se in the absence of clinically evident heart failure is not a contraindication.

The antihypertensive effect of beta blockers remains incompletely understood. Although cardiac output is decreased (through negative inotropic and chronotropic effects) immediately after intravenous dosing, the blood pressure frequently remains unchanged initially. With long-term use, magnitude of the hypotensive effect correlates only poorly with the magnitude of the decrease in cardiac output. Decreased sympathetic outflow from the central nervous system to peripheral vessels and decreased renin release because of beta-adrenoreceptor blockade appear to contribute to the hypotensive effect.

Cardioselective beta blockers such as metoprolol, atentolol, and betaxolol have higher affinity for the beta$_1$ as compared with beta$_2$ receptors. They are less likely to produce beta$_2$-mediated side effects such as bronchospasm, claudication, and hyperglycemia and are the agents of choice if beta blockers are required in patients with chronic obstructive airway disease (COAD), peripheral vascular disease, or diabetes mellitus. However, cardioselectivity declines or is lost as dosage is increased.

Acebutolol and pindolol exhibit intrinsic sympathomimetic activity (ISA) and partial agonist activity at all dosages. Their effect on resting heart rate and blood pressure varies with the prevailing level of sympathetic activation in a given patient. Generally, they do not decrease resting heart rate and resting blood pressure markedly. Instead, they blunt the rise associated with exercise. Beta blockers with ISA may be less effective than others in severe angina because they lower myocardial oxygen demand less. They have not been shown specifically to decrease mortality after myocardial infarction.

Labetalol, a nonselective beta-adrenergic blocker, also blocks peripheral alpha receptors. Thus, this agent is useful for management of hypertension in some circumstance. The combination of arterial vasodilation plus negative inotropic and chronotropic effects make labetalol especially useful in the management of hypertension in patients with aortic aneurysm. Labetalol has also been shown to be relatively safe in the management of hypertensive emergencies, even those occurring during pregnancy.

A. Clinical Considerations

Beta-blocking agents should be initiated at low dosage because of the variation in levels of prevailing sympathetic tone present in different patients. When they are used orally, dose should be increased at 1- to 2-week intervals until resting heart rate is decreased to 50 to 60 beats/min and heart rate during exercise does not exceed 100 beats/min. When used long-term, agents that can be given once daily (atenolol, betaxolol, metoprolol XL) are often taken more regularly. If symptoms occur at the end of a dosing interval, either the dose can be increased or the frequency of dosing increased to twice daily.

When beta blockers are administered intravenously, negative inotropic and chronotropic effects are manifest rapidly. Effects on blood pressure are less predictable, again because of the influence on adrenergic tone. Esmolol is very short-acting (half-life = 9–10 min). In contrast, the duration of action of propranolol, metoprolol, and atenolol is 1–2, 4–6, and 12–24 hr respectively. Thus, esmolol may be the initial agent of choice in selected patients at high risk of hemodynamic compromise to assess tolerability before switching to a longer-acting agent. When beta-adrenergic blockade is required for patients who are unable to take oral medications, bolus doses of metoprolol administered at 4–6 hr intervals are effective and generally well tolerated.

B. Adverse Effects

Adverse effects are mostly extensions of pharmacological properties and include bradycardia, hypotension, and exacerbation of heart failure. Beta$_2$ blockade can cause claudication, hyperglycemia, or bronchospasm in predisposed subjects. If beta blockade is required in a patient with diabetes mellitus or chronic obstructive pulmonary disease, a cardioselective agent is preferable. Monitoring for adverse drug reactions should be thorough.

Long-term use of beta blockers increases plasma triglyceride concentrations and decreases HDL cholesterol. However, mortality benefits after myocardial infarction outweigh hypothetical adverse effects of those changes.

With excessive doses, severe bradycardia, decreased contractility, and even circulatory collapse can occur. Immediate artificial pacemaker placement and use of a nonadrenergic positive inotropic agent such as amrinone can be lifesaving. Although glucagon can increase contractility independent of the beta receptor, its dose requirement is high. Glucagon should be reserved for patients who continue to exhibit severely decreased cardiac output despite the use of amrinone and pacing.

Toxic doses of beta blockers (such as propranolol) with membrane-stabilizing effects can elicit seizures. Supportive treatment is usually sufficient.

II. CALCIUM CHANNEL BLOCKERS

Currently available calcium channel blockers (Table 2) include verapamil, diltiazem, and numerous dihydropyridines. The three subclasses differ in the degree of calcium channel blockade in cardiac nodal tissue, myocardium, and vascular smooth muscle. Verapamil, a phenylalkylamine, and diltiazem, a benzothiazepine, are effective in the management of (PSVT) and control of ventricular rate with atrial fibrillation or flutter. They slow sinus rate, decrease atrioventricular nodal conduction, decrease cardiac contractility, and induce systemic and coronary arterial dilation.

Table 2 Calcium Channel Blockers

Drug	Nodal blockade	Negative inotropic effects	Initial dose
Verapamil	+ +	+ + +	80 mg tid SR 120 mg qd
Diltiazem	+ +	+ +	30 mg qid CD 180 mg qd
Nifedipine	−	+ +	10 mg tid XL 30 mg qd
Nicardipine	−	+	20 mg tid SR 30 mg bid
Isradipine	−	+	2.5 mg bid
Felodipine	−	sl	5 mg qd
Amlodipine	−	sl	5 mg qd

Because of the effects on the conduction system and their negative inotropic effects, verapamil and diltiazem should be avoided in patients being given beta blockers and in those with left ventricular dysfunction.

Used intravenously, verapamil's efficacy for treatment of PSVT and control of ventricular rate with atrial fibrillation is similar to that with adenosine or diltiazem. However, because verapamil produces more marked systemic vasodilation, diltiazem may be better tolerated in patients with borderline low blood pressure. Both agents can elicit hemodynamic compromise when administered to patients with ventricular tachycardia.

Verapamil and diltiazem may be useful in the management of symptoms of heart failure in patients with well-preserved systolic function but impaired diastolic function. A special case in point is the patient with hypertrophic cardiomyopathy.

Dihydropyridine (DHP) agents include nifedipine, nicardipine, isradipine, felodipine, and amlodipine. They have negligible effects on the cardiac conduction system in vivo and are powerful systemic arterial dilators and potent antihypertensives. Nifedipine exhibits the most marked (yet still modest) negative inotropic effects in vivo. Felodipine and amlodipine exhibit the least. Initially, negative inotropic effects may be offset by afterload reduction, but deterioration of ventricular performance can occur when nifedipine or nicardipine is administered to patients with left ventricular dysfunction. In general, avoidance of all DHP agents is prudent in patients with moderate or severe left ventricular systolic dysfunction.

Nicardipine is available in injectable form for management of hypertension. Despite a long elimination of half-life, its duration of action is determined largely by distribution (50% if the effect is lost in 30 min). Accordingly, continuous infusion is necessary. Because the solution is extremely irritating, a central venous route is preferred. Side effects are similar to those of other arterial dilators and include flushing, reflex tachycardia, and coronary steal. Nicardipine may be helpful when nitroprusside is not well tolerated.

A. Adverse Effects

Adverse effects seen with long-term use of verapamil and diltiazem include hypotension and bradycardia. To decrease constipation seen with verapamil, increased fiber and fluid intake is useful. Side effects seen with dihydropyridines include flushing, hypotension, reflex tachycardia, and peripheral edema.

When ingested in large quantities, calcium channel blockers can induce hypotension (all), bradycardia (verapamil, diltiazem), and decreased cardiac output. Management includes circulatory support with pacing, inotropic agents, and pressors as needed. Intravenous calcium (e.g., 2 g calcium gluconate) is often an effective adjunct.

Table 3 Angiotensin-Converting Enzyme Inhibitors

Drug	Usual initial dose	Usual maximum dose	Dosage adjustment in renal dysfunction
Benazepril (Lotensin)	10 mg PO qd	20 mg PO bid or 40 mg PO qd	Yes
Captopril (Capoten)	25 mg PO bid-tid	100 mg PO qid	Yes
Enalapril (Vasotec)	5 mg PO qd, or 1.25 mg IV q6h	20 mg PO bid, or 5 mg IV q6h	Yes
Fosinopril (Monopril)	10 mg PO qd	80 mg PO qd or 40 mg PO bid	No
Lisinopril (Zestril, Prinivil)	10 mg PO qd	40 mg PO qd or 20 mg PO bid	Yes
Quinapril (Accupril)	10 mg PO qd	80 mg PO qd or 40 mg PO bid	Yes
Ramipril (Altace)	2.5 mg PO qd	20 mg PO qd or 10 mg PO bid	Yes

III. ANGIOTENSIN-CONVERTING ENZYME (ACE) INHIBITORS

The ACE inhibitors (Table 3) are helpful in the management of patients with hypertension, congestive heart failure, and diabetic nephropathy. They decrease mortality in patients with NYHA class 2–4 CHF and decrease the risk of overt heart failure in patients with asymptomatic left ventricular dysfunction. They decrease the risk of left ventricular dilation, heart failure, recurrent myocardial infarction, and death in patients who have suffered acute myocardial infarction.

Inhibition of conversion of angiotensin I to angiotensin II results in arterial and venous dilation. Other mechanisms contributing to afterload reduction include decreased degradation of bradykinin and increased production of the vasodilatory prostaglandins I2 and E2. Intracardiac effects of ACE inhibition may include reduced angiotensin-mediated postsynaptic norepinephrine release and diminished ventricular ectopy and left ventricular hypertrophy (presumably related to attenuation of trophic effects of angiotensin). Coronary blood flow may be increased. Restoration of baroreceptor function may diminish sympathetic stimulation. Antiatherogenic effects have been reported.

A. Clinical Considerations

The ACE inhibitors are potentially helpful in all patients with left ventricular dysfunction unless absolute contraindications exist, including bilateral renal artery stenosis or a history of ACE-inhibitor-induced angioedema or renal failure. Patients with preexisting renal dysfunction may tolerate ACE inhibitors if initial doses are low and serum creatinine is monitored closely. Patients being given nonsteroidal anti-inflammatory drugs and those who are volume-depleted are at increased risk for nephrotoxicity. Despite their utility as antihypertensive agents in long-term treatment, ACE inhibitors are not particularly useful in the initial management of hypertensive emergencies.

Several prospective studies have established the efficacy of ACE inhibitors in reduction of morbidity, particularly heart failure and mortality after acute myocardial infarction. Accordingly, they should be administered beginning early after infarction regardless of the decision to treat with thrombolytic agents, aspirin, and beta blockers.

B. Adverse Effects

The ACE inhibitors can induce hypotension, decreased glomerular filtration rate, angioedema, and a nonproductive cough (presumably mediated by kinins). The risk of hypotension can be minimized by initiating therapy with low doses and caution when volume depletion or renal dysfunction is present. ACE inhibitors decrease glomerular filtration rate in predisposed individuals by blocking angiotensin II–mediated constriction of the efferent arteriole in the nephron. Renal blood flow is increased, but glomerular filtration pressure may fall. These effects are generally reversible when the drug is discontinued. Hyperkalemia is encountered with ACE inhibitors when renal function is severely impaired or concomitant treatment with potassium-sparing diuretics or potassium supplements is involved.

ACE inhibitor–induced angioedema is rare and life-threatening. Patients who develop it with one ACE inhibitor should avoid all agents in the class. Cough (annoying but not necessarily physiologically threatening) occurs in 20% of treated patients with all ACE inhibitors. Symptomatic treatment with a cough suppressant may permit continuation of the ACE inhibitor.

IV. NITRATES

Pharmacological effects of organic nitrates include venous dilation, arterial dilation (when administered in higher doses intravenously), and prevention or reversal of coronary arterial spasm. The nitrates in a multitude of formulations are a mainstay in the management of patients with angina pectoris. In patients with unstable angina or acute myocardial infarction, they decrease pain and sometimes decrease infarct size. Intravenous nitrates are useful in the management of hypertensive emergencies. Nitroglycerin is a preferred initial agent in treatment of such events in patients with coronary artery disease because it is less likely than nitroprusside to induce coronary steal.

Tachyphylaxis to hemodynamic effects occurs with intravenous nitroglycerin, oral isosorbide dinitrate, and transdermal nitroglycerin. Mechanisms include depletion of sulfhydryl groups in the vascular wall and neurohormonal upregulation. Long-term administration of nitrates that includes a regular 10–12 hr nitrate-free interval decreases the incidence of tachyphylaxis. Coadministration with an ACE inhibitor may diminish tachyphylaxis by preventing neurohormonal compensation. Tachyphylaxis occurring during the course of intravenous infusions of nitroglycerin to control unstable angina may require escalation of dose and addition of other agents.

Adverse effects of nitrates include hypotension and headache. Hypotension reflects primarily venodilation and responds quickly to decreased dose and volume expansion. Patients with intravascular volume depletion or right ventricular infarction are at particular risk. Headache is common during the first few days of treatment. With continued therapy, it usually abates. Acetaminophen is helpful in decreasing its severity.

V. NITROPRUSSIDE

Nitroprusside, a direct-acting arterial and venous dilator, is the drug of choice for treatment of most hypertensive emergencies because of its efficacy and short half-life, permitting titration. Patients with coronary artery disease may benefit instead from intravenous nitroglycerin. If nitroprusside is required, low initial doses and cautious titration to avoid reflex tachycardia are essential.

Because nitroprusside contains cyanide (5 per molecule), treatment leads to release of cyanide rapidly into the bloodstream, followed by metabolism in the liver, mediated by rhodanese to thiocyanate, which is cleared by the kidney (half-life 3 days, but 7 days with end-stage renal disease). Cyanide toxicity can result with high doses or hepatic dysfunction. Decreased responsiveness to nitroprusside, metabolic acidosis, and central nervous system depression may appear. Accumulation of thiocyanate is a potential consequence of prolonged administration of nitroprusside in proportion to cumulative dose. Manifestations include paresthesias, mental status changes, and seizures. Patients with renal dysfunction given nitroprusside should be monitored with serum thiocyanate determinations after 72 hr. Those with normal renal function do not generally require such determinations unless treatment continues beyond 5 days. Serum thiocyanate levels should be kept below 10 mg/dL. Hemodialysis may be required in symptomatic patients.

Other antihypertensive agents, many of which are vasodilators, and their conventional dosage are listed in Table 4.

536

Table 4 Additional Antihypertensive Agents

Alpha$_1$-adrenergic blockers	Initial dose	Adjusted dose
Doxazosin (Cardura—Roerig)	1 mg qd	Peak effect, 2–6 hr
Prazosin (Minipress—Pfizer)	1 mg bid-tid (1st dose at bedtime)	
Terazosin (Hytrin—Abbott/BW)	1 mg qd (1st dose at bedtime)	Peak effect, 2–3 hr
Centrally Acting		
Clonidine (Catapres—BI)	0.1 mg bid	7-day adj
Clonidine patch (Catapres TTS)	TTSI per week (equiv. to 0.1 mg bid release)	Weekly adj
Guanfacine (Tenex—Robins)	1 mg qd (HS)	Titrate after 3–4 weeks
Guanabenz (Wyeth)	4 mg bid	Weekly adj
Methyldopa (Aldonmet—Merck)	250 mg bid PO/IV	48-hr adj
Antiadrenergic		
Reserpine (various)	0.1 mg qd	1-wk adj
Guanethidine (Ismelin—CIBA)	10 mg qd	1-wk adj
Guanadrel (Hylorel—Fisons)	5 mg bid	1-wk adj
Direct Vasodilators		
Hydralazine (Apresoline—CIBA)	10 mg qid PO 20 mg q 6 hr IV	1-wk adj Peak effect, 20–80 min
Minoxidil (Loniten—Upjohn)	5 mg qd	1-wk adj

VI. AGENTS USED FOR SEDATION AND NEUROMUSCULAR BLOCKADE IN AN INTENSIVE OR CORONARY CARE UNIT SETTING

Continuous infusions of sedatives are frequently required in intensive care units to increase patient comfort, minimize risk in highly instrumented patients, and facilitate effective circulatory and ventilatory support. Adequate sedation is vital in patients undergoing pharmacological neuromuscular blockade, frequently required to facilitate mechanical ventilation. Agents used for this purpose and given

Table 5 Pharmacology of Frequently Used Sedatives and Analgesics

	Sedative agents (bolus dosing)	Analgesic and sedative agents sometimes given by continuous infusion	Sedative agents (continuous infusion)
	DIAZEPAM (Valium)	**FENTANYL (Sublimaze)**	**MIDAZOLAM (Versed)**
Dose / Dilution	Dose: 2.5–10 mg q3–6h	Dilution: 1250 µg/250 mL NS	Dilution: 50 mg/50 mL NS
Bolus dose		Bolus dose: 50–100 µg (until desired effect)	Bolus dose: 1–5 mg (until desired effect)
Maintenance		Maintenance: 50–100 µg/hr (max 500 µg/hr)	Maintenance: 1–4 mg/hr (max 10 mg/hr)
Drip increment		Drip increment: 50 µg/hr (after rebolus)	Drip increment: 1–2 mg/hr (after rebolus)
Daily cost	$5–15	$5–20	$60–300
Comments	Quick onset (1–2 min); duration 2–4 hr after single dose; effects prolonged in renal and hepatic failure; may accumulate upon repeated doses; may cause hypotension with rapid injection; do not dilute	Minimal histamine releasing effects; sedative effects prolonged in hepatic and renal failure	Minimal additional benefits seen from doses above 10 mg/hr; sedative effects prolonged in hepatic and renal failure
	LORAZEPAM (Ativan)	**MORPHINE**	**PROPOFOL (Diprivan)**
Dose / Dilution	Dose: 2–8 mg q4–8h	Dilution: 50 mg/50 mL NS or D5W	Dilution: 500 mg/50 ml 10% lipid
Concentration		Concentration: 1 mg/mL	
Bolus dose		Bolus dose: 10–15 mg (until desired effect)	Bolus dose: 0.5 mg/kg (optional)
Maintenance		Maintenance: 1–4 mg/hr (max 50 mg/hr)	Maintenance: 1–3 mg/kg/hr (max 7 mg/kg/hr)
Drip increment		Drip increment: 2–5 mg/hr (after rebolus)	Drip increment: 0.5 mg/kg/hr (after rebolus)
Daily cost	$15–100	$1–10	$80–550 per 70 kg
Comments	Slow onset (20–40 min); intermediate duration (4–6 hr after single dose); not appropriate for acute agitation due to slow onset; may accumulate upon repeated doses	Hypotension may occur upon rapid injection due to histamine release; sedative effects prolonged in hepatic and renal failure	May cause hypotension (especially with boluses); monitor triglycerides; adjust lipid in TPN as necessary
	HALOPERIDOL (Haldol)		
Dose	Dose: 2–5 mg (double dose every 20 min until desired effect, then 1/2 of effective bolus dose q4hr)		
Daily cost	$5–20		
Comments	Slow onset (10–15 min); intermediate duration (3–6 hr after single dose); extrapyramidal effects rarely seen with IV doses; monitor QRS. QT intervals; should not exceed 80 mg/dose		

Table 6 Considerations Involved and Agents Used for Neuromuscular Blockade

Therapeutic paralysis	Neuromuscular blocking agents[b]	
Indication for continued neuromuscular blockade:	**PANCURONIUM** (Pavulon)	
Poor oxygenation or patient-ventilator interaction which persists despite adequate sedation	Dilution	50 mg/50 mL undiluted
	Loading dose	0.08 mg/kg
	Maintenance	0.02–0.04 mg/kg/hr
	Drip increment	1 mg/hr
Guidelines for Therapeutic Paralysis	Daily cost	$5–15 per 70 kg
1. Adequate sedation (Ramsay 4-5) and analgesia must be achieved before starting paralytic agent	Comments	May cause mild tachycardia; paralytic effects prolonged in renal and hepatic failure
2. Dosage should be monitored by peripheral nerve stimulator at least every 4 hours (usual goal is 1 out of 4 twitches)	**VECURONIUM** (Norcuron)	
	Dilution	50 mg/50 mL NS or D5W
	Loading dose	0.1 mg/kg
3. Paralysis should be stopped daily (4 out of 4 twitches) to ensure adequate sedation and continued need for paralysis	Maintenance	0.02–0.04 mg/kg/hr
	Drip increment	1 mg/hr
	Daily cost	$100–200 per 70 kg
4. Discontinue paralysis as soon as clinically possible	Comments	Paralytic effects prolonged in renal and hepatic failure
Using the Peripheral Nerve Stimulator	**ATRACURIUM** (Tracrium)	
1. Place electrodes along ulnar nerve	Dilution	500 mg/100 mL NS or D5W
2. Attach alligator clips	Loading dose	0.4 mg/kg
3. Hold fingers down; observe only the thumb for twitch response	Maintenance	0.4 mg/kg/hr
	Drip increment	0.1 mg/kg/hr
4. Press Train of Four (TOF) once to administer stimuli	Daily cost	$300–1000 per 70 kg
5. If no response, administer 5–10 sec tetany	Comments	Nonenzymatic decomposition; remains "short acting" in renal and hepatic failure, increased dose requirements over time
6. Repeat TOF		
Interpreting Train of Four Twitches		
4/4 <75% blocked		
3/4 75% blocked		
2/4 80% blocked		
1/4 90% blocked		
0/4 100% blocked[a]		

[a]In patients with 0 out of 4 twitches, TOF response should return postetany. If not, patient is significantly over blocked, and the drug should be discontinued until twitches return
[b]Concurrent use of corticosteroids or aminoglycosides may increase risk of myopathy.

Table 7 Intravenously Administered Agents Used in an Intensive Care Setting

Drug	Dilution (concentration)	Loading dose	Initial maintenance dose	Comments
Amrinone (Inocor)	200 mg/100 mL NS[a] (2 mg/mL)	0.75 mg/kg over 2–3 min	5 μg/kg/min (Max 10 μg/kg/min)	Inotrope with vasodilating properties; may cause hypotention and thrombocytopenia; $t_{1/2}$ 3–4 hr.
Bretylium (Bretylol)	2 g/500 mL NS or D5W (4 mg/mL)	5 mg/kg (followed by 10 mg/kg × 3 if needed)	1–4 mg/min	Initial ↑ BP followed by hypotension; may exacerbate arrhythmias and underlying hypotension.
Diltiazem (Cardizem)	125 mg/125 mL NS or D5W (1 mg/mL)	0.25 mg/kg (followed by 0.35 mg/kg if needed)	5–10 mg/hr (Max 15 mg/hr)	May cause hypotension; cost 20 times more than verapamil.
Dobutamine (Dobutrex)	500 mg/250 mL NS or D5W (2000 μg/mL)	—	2 μg/kg/min (Max 20 μg/kg/min)	Selective inotropic (β) effect; may cause tachycardia and arrhythmias.
Dopamine (Intropin)	400 mg/250 mL NS or D5W (1600 μg/mL)	—	Dopa 1–3 μg/kg/min β 3–10 μg/kg/min α 10–20 μg/kg/min	Clinical response is dose and patient dependent; may cause arrhythmias and tachycardia.
Epinephrine	5 mg/500 mL NS or D5W or 4 mg/100 mL NS or D5W	—	1–4 μg/min[b]	Mixed α and β effects; use central line; may cause tachycardia and hypertension.
Esmolol (Brevibloc)	2.5 g/250 mL NS or D5W (10 mg/mL)[a]	500 mcg/kg/min × 1 minute (optional)	50 μg/kg/min (Max 300 μg/kg/min)	Selective β_1 blocker; 9 minute $t_{1/2}$; not elminated by hepatic or renal routes; may cause hypotension.
Heparin	25000 units/250 mL NS or D5W (100 units/mL)	50–100 units/kg	15–25 units/kg/hr	Obtain PTT every 4–6 hours until PTT is 1.5–2.0 times control may cause thrombocytopenia.
Isoproterenol (Isuprel)	2 mg/500 mL NS or D5W (4 μg/mL)	—	2–10 μg/min[b]	Pure β effects; may cause myocardial ischemia, tachycardia, and hypotension.

Drug	Preparation	Loading dose	Rate	Comments
Lidocaine	2 g/500 mL D5W[a] (4 mg/mL)	1 mg/kg (may repeat × 2)	1–4 mg/min	Dose should be decreased in patients with hepatic failure, acute MI, CHF, or shock.
Nitroglycerin (Tridil)	50 mg/250 mL D5W (200 µg/mL)	—	5–20 µg/min[b]	Use cautiously in right-sided MI.
Nitroprusside (Nipride)	50 mg/250 mL D5W* (200 µg/mL)	—	0.25–0.50 µg/kg/min (Max 10 µg/kg/min)	Signs of nitroprusside toxicity include metabolic acidosis, tremors, seizures, and coma; thiocyanate may accumulate in renal failure.
Norepinephrine (Levophed)	8 mg/500 mL D5W (16 µg/mL)	—	2–10 µg/min[b]	Potent α effects; mainly β_1 effects at lower doses; use central line.
Phenylephrine (Neosynephrine)	10 mg/250 mL NS or D5W (40 µg/mL)	—	10–100 µg/min[b]	Pure α effects; use central line; may cause reflex bradycardia and decreased cardiac output.
Procainamide (Pronestyl)	2 g/500 mL NS (4 mg/mL)	17 mg/kg (@ 20 mg/min)	1–4 mg/min	Monitor serum procainamide (4–8 mg/L) and NAPA (10–20 mg/L) levels, and QTc; NAPA may accumulate in renal failure.
Prostaglandin E$_1$ (Alprostadil)	1000 µg/100 mL NS (10 µg/mL)	—	0.01 µg/kg/min[b]	Pulmonary selectivity lost at higher doses.
Theophylline	800 mg/500 mL D5W[a] (1.6 mg/mL)	5–6 mg/kg over 30 minutes	0.2–0.9 mg/kg/hr	Monitor serum levels (5–20 mg/L); decrease dose in hepatic failure or CHF; may cause tachyarrhythmias, nausea, vomiting, and seizures.

[a]Only recommended diluent
[b]Variable dosage range; titrate to desired effect.

by continuous infusions include midazolam, fentanyl, and propofol. Several general principles apply.

Underlying causes of agitation must be addressed before initiating pharmacological sedation. Examples include an improperly positioned or partially obstructed endotracheal tube, unrelieved pain, pneumothorax, hypoxia, myocardial ischemia, shock, and improper mechanical ventilator settings.

Frequent titration (at least once every 8 hr) to minimum effective dose is essential. Continued use of all sedatives can lead to tachyphylaxis. All except propofol can accumulate with repeated or continuous administration, leading to markedly prolonged effects. Accumulation and tachyphylaxis can occur simultaneously, making it impossible to predict whether dose requirements in a given patient will increase or decrease with time.

Initial control of agitation must be achieved with boluses of sedatives before initiation of a maintenance regimen. The dose required initially is generally larger than that required for maintained sedation. If a continuous infusion is used in an acutely agitated patient without initial boluses, control of agitation can be delayed. When it is finally achieved, if the infusion rate is not lowered to maintenance levels, accumulation of the agent and oversedation are likely.

For maintenance of sedation, bolus regimens should be used unless contraindicated or documented to be ineffective. Because their use permits evaluation of the patient before additional drug is administered, they decrease the risk of both oversedation and delayed recovery from sedation.

Some patients may require continuous infusion, including those who experience high peak airway pressures, exhibit marked hypoxia, or experience severe myocardial ischemia with agitation. Patients receiving neuromuscular blockers may be best treated with continuous infusions of sedatives. When they become agitated, sedation should be accomplished with bolus doses of the sedative followed by small increases in maintenance rate.

The pharmacology of some sedatives and analgesics used frequently is summarized in Table 5.

VII. AGENTS USED FOR NEUROMUSCULAR BLOCKADE

Neuromuscular blocking drugs are often needed in an intensive care setting to decrease oxygen consumption, improve ventilation, and prevent injury. They should be used only when such indications are present despite adequate sedation.

Potential complications of continuous neuromuscular blockade include prolonged paralysis because of accumulation of the drug at the neuromuscular junction (preventable by monitoring and adjusting dose according to results of analysis of peripheral nerve stimulation and conduction), development of myopathy (reported with all neuromuscular blockers with risk increased by concomitant use of corticosteroids), and failure to detect concurrent conditions because of

Table 8 Lipid-Lowering Drugs

Drug	Dose range	LDL	HDL	Triglycerides
Cholestyramine[a]	4–24 g/day qd	↓ 15–35%	↑ 3–8%	↑ 5–30%
Colestipol	5–30 g/day 2–3 dd	↓ 15–35%	↑ 3–8%	↑ 5–30%
Niacin[a]	2–6 g/day 2–3 dd	↓ 15–35%	↑ 10–20%	↓ 20–40%
Lovastatin	20–80 mg/day qd	↓ 20–45%	↑ 2–10%	↓ 20–30%
Pravastatin	10–40 mg/day qd	↓ 20–45%	↑ 2–10%	↓ 20–30%
Simvastatin	5–40 mg/day qd	↓ 20–45%	↑ 2–10%	↓ 20–40%
Gemfibrozil[a]	1200 mg/day 2 dd	↓ 5–20%	↑ 10–20%	↓ 30–60%

[a]Documented to decrease cardiovascular mortality.

Table 9 Agents Used for Prevention and Treatment of Episodes of Rejection of Heart Transplants

Drug	Mechanism	Routes of administration	Side effects
Azathioprine (Immuran)	Suppresses T-cell formation by antagonizing purine metabolism	IV, PO	Bone marrow suppression, nausea, pancreatitis, hepatotoxicity
Corticosteroids	Inhibition of IL-1 release from macrophages; others	IV, PO	Growth retardation, osteoporosis, adrenal suppression, hyperglycemia, cataracts, ? GI ulceration
Cyclosporine (Sandimmune)	Blocks release of IL-2 and other cytokines from T-helper cells; others	IV, PO	Nephrotoxicity, hypertension, tremor, seizures, headache, hyperkalemia, gingival hyperplasia
Tacrolimus (FK-506, Prograf)	Inhibits cytotoxic and helper T-cells by inhibiting IL-2, 3, 4, TNF, and gamma interferon; inhibits B-cell activation	IV, PO	Tremors, headache, seizures, nephrotoxicity, insomnia
Antithymocyte globulin	T-cell depletion	IV	Fever, chills, leukopenia, thrombocytopenia, serum sickness, anaphylaxis, erythema, urticaria
Orthoclone OKT3, Muromonab CD3	T-cell depletion	IV	Fever, chills, dyspnea, wheezing, pulmonary edema, aseptic meningitis

543

Table 10 Features of Selected Plasminogen Activators and Anticoagulants

Agent	Approximate $t_{1/2}$ of clearance (min)	Currently used or favored IV dosage	Salient advantages/disadvantages
Nonfibrin-Selective Plasminogen Activators			
Streptokinase	25–80	1.5 million units IV over 1 hr	Not fibrin selective; immunogenic; reduced patency rates; inexpensive; fibrinogen degradation products persist for 24 to 48 hr
Urokinase	15	1.5 million units bolus followed by 1.5 million units over 1 hr	Not fibrin selective; nonimmunogenic; patency like SK; expensive
Anisoylated plasminogen streptokinase activator complex (APSAC Anistreplase, Eminase)	100	30 mg IV bolus	Amenable to bolus administration; not fibrin selective; expensive
Reteplase (r-PA)		10 MU/IV 1 30 min × 2	Not fibrin selective
Fibrin-Selective Plasminogen Activators			
Tissue-type plasminogen activator (t-PA)	5	15 mg IV bolus, 50 mg over first 30 min; and 35 mg over next 60 min	Fibrin selective; nonimmunogenic; high patency rates
Single-chain urokinase-type plasminogen activator (scu-PA)	5	20 mg IV bolus, 60 mg over the next 1 hr	Fibrin selective
Staphylokinase (STA [bacterial origin] or STAR [recombinant])	1–2	2 mg bolus followed by 18 mg over 30 min	Fibrin selective but immunogenic

Plasminogen Activators Under Development[a]
Vampire bat-PA (a congener of t-PA that is clot selective)
Other t-PA variants (domain deletion or substitution mutants such as TNK-t-PA [fibrin selective])
Chimeric plasminogen activators
Antibody-targeted plasminogen activators

Novel Anticoagulants

Low-molecular-weight heparin	2500–5000 U b.i.d. s.c.	Clearance is substantially prolonged compared with that of standard heparin	See Table 11 for potential advantages
Hirudin	0.1 to 0.6 mg/kg bolus followed by 0.1 to 0.2 mg/kg/hr for 96 hr (safety not yet established but under investigation)	Clearance is prolonged compared with that of heparin	A direct-acting antithrombin that does not require interaction with ATIII (heparin cofactor III) or heparin cofactor II

[a]Additional characteristics are not listed for agents in this category because of limited experience with them to date.

Table 11 Low-Molecular-Weight Heparin Compared with Standard Heparin

Diminished effects on platelets (PF4 release and thrombocytopenia)
Less bleeding in relation to therapeutic efficacy (IIa inhibition is less than that of Xa compared with that seen with standard heparin)
Diminished induction of osteoporosis (less osteoclast activation)
Less likelihood of increased vascular permeability (less endothelial cell binding)
Greater absorption and decreased clearance
Greater bioavailability (less protein binding)
Less need for monitoring (after pTCA, after thrombolysis, with initiation of coumadin)
Greater utility in pregnancy (less monitoring required)
Greater potential for inhibition of tumor angiogenesis (greater inhibition of basic FGF binding)

paralysis (e.g., failure to detect peritonitis because of absent detectable abdominal tenderness or guarding).

A brief list of neuromuscular blockers and some of their properties is shown in Table 6.

VIII. OTHER CLASSES OF AGENTS

Antiarrhythmic drugs are discussed in preceding sections of this book dealing with treatment of specific arrhythmias and are not discussed further here. Analgesics are considered in sections dealing with painful conditions such as acute myocardial infarction. Antimicrobials are considered in chapters dealing with infectious disease, including endocarditis and rheumatic heart disease. Agents given intravenously and used in an intensive care setting to increase cardiac performance, suppress ventricular arrhythmias or reduce the risk of recurrent ventricular fibrillation, induce anticoagulation, or reduce pulmonary arterial vasoconstriction or bronchospasm and their dosage are shown in Table 7. Lipid-lowering drugs are summarized in Table 8. Agents used in the prevention and treatment of episodes of rejection in heart transplant recipients are listed in Table 9. Fibrinolytic and anticoagulant agents are discussed in Chapters 11 and 13, dealing with coronary thrombosis and pulmonary thromboembolism. In view of recent developments in anticoagulation and fibrinolysis, some established agents and some novel ones are delineated in Table 10. Compared with standard heparin, the recently developed low-molecular-weight heparins (Table 10) exhibit relatively greater inhibition of factor Xa than inhibition of thrombin. In contrast to direct-acting antithrombins (such as hirudin, Table 10), they combine, as does standard heparin, with heparin cofactor III (antithrombin III) and heparin cofactor II. Some of their properties are indicated in Table 11.

Table 12 Interactions Between Commonly Used Agents

Medication	Increases level or effect of:	Decreases level or effect of:	Potentiates side effect or toxicity of:
Acetazolamide	Quinidine		Phenytoin
Allopurinol	Azathioprine, cyclophosphamide, 6-mercaptopurine, warfarin		Ampicillin
ACE inhibitors	Potassium salts		
Aminoglycosides	Neuromuscular blocking drugs		Loop diuretics
Amiodarone	Digoxin, quinidine, warfarin, cyclosporine, phenytoin, procainamide		
Anabolic steroids	Warfarin		
Antacids	Quinidine	Cimetidine, iron salts, isoniazid, quinolone antibiotics, salicylates, tetracycline	
Antithyroid agents		Warfarin	
Aspirin	Methotrexate	ACE inhibitors	
Bactrim (See co-trimoxazole)	Warfarin		
Barbiturates	CNS depressants	Chloramphenicol, beta antagonists, corticosteroids, estrogens, oral contraceptives, quinidine, theophylline, tricyclic antidepressants, warfarin	
Benzodiazepines	CNS depressants		
Beta antagonists	Chlorpromazine, epinephrine (pressor effect)		
Cefamandole	Warfarin		
Cefoperazone	Warfarin		
Cefotetan	Warfarin		
Cefoxitin	Warfarin		
Carbamazepine	Isoniazid, lithium	Theophylline, warfarin, tricyclic antidepressants	
Chloral hydrate	Ethanol, warfarin		
Chloramphenicol	Barbiturates, phenytoin, oral hypoglycemic agents		
Chlorpromazine	Beta antagonists		

Table 12 Continued

Medication	Increases level or effect of:	Decreases level or effect of:	Potentiates side effect or toxicity of:
Cimetidine	Benzodiazepines, beta antagonists, CNS depressants, felodipine, procainamide, quinidine, theophylline, tricyclic antidepressants, verapamil, warfarin	Antacids	
Clofibrate	Oral hypoglycemics, warfarin		
Clarithromycin			Astemizole, terfenidine, cisapride
Clonidine			Beta antagonists
CNS depressants	Anticonvulsants, barbiturates, benzodiazepines, beta antagonists, cimetidine, ethanol, MAO inhibitors, opiate analgesics, phenothiazines		Lithium, muscle relaxants
Co-trimoxazole	Warfarin		
Digoxin	Amiodarone		
Diltiazem	Cyclosporin, theophylline		
Disulfiram	Phenytoin, warfarin		
Erythromycin (macrolides)	Carbamazepine, cyclosporine, theophylline, warfarin		Astemizole, terfenidine, cisapride
Fluoxetine	Phenytoin, tricyclic antidepressants		
Furosemide (loop diuretics)			Digoxin
Griseofulvin		Warfarin	
HMG-CoA reductase inhibitors			Gemfibrozil
Iron		Quinolones	
Isoniazid	Phenytoin, carbamazepine		
Ketoconazole	Warfarin		Astemizole, terfenidine, cisapride
Lidocaine			Phenytoin

Table 12 Continued

Medication	Increases level or effect of:	Decreases level or effect of:	Potentiates side effect or toxicity of:
Lovastatin			Gemfibrozil
MAO inhibitors	CNS depressants, oral hypoglycemic agents, sympathomimetics		Meperidine
Methotrexate		Vaccines	
Methyldopa	Lithium, MAO inhibitors		
Metronidazole	Disulfiram, warfarin		
Muscle relaxants	CNS depressants		
Nicardipine	Cyclosporine		
NSAIDs	Lithium, methotrexate	ACE inhibitors, diuretics, beta antagonists	Triamterene, warfarin
Phenytoin		Quinidine, theophylline, warfarin (first 1–2 weeks)	Warfarin (after 1–2 weeks)
Probenecid	Penicillins, methotrexate, zidovudine (AZT)		
Propafenone	Beta antagonists, digoxin, warfarin		
Propoxyphene	Carbamazepine		
Prophylthiouracil	Warfarin		
Quinidine	Dextromethorphan, digoxin, neuromuscular blocking drugs, warfarin		
Quinolone antibiotics	Theophylline, warfarin		
Rifampin		Beta antagonists, benzodiazepines, calcium blockers, cyclosporine, digoxin, disopyramide, methadone, oral contraceptives, oral hypoglycemics, phenytoin, quinidine, theophylline, warfarin	
Salicylates	Acetazolamide, methotrexate, oral hypoglycemics, warfarin		
Sertraline	Tricyclic antidepressants		
Spironolactone	Digoxin		

Table 12 Continued

Medication	Increases level or effect of:	Decreases level or effect of:	Potentiates side effect or toxicity of:
Sucralfate	Aluminum salts	Digoxin, ketoconazole, phenytoin, quinolones, quinidine, warfarin	
Sulfonamides	Oral hypoglycemics, methotrexate, phenytoin, warfarin		
Theophylline		Adenosine, lithium	
Thiazide diuretics	Lithium, digoxin		
Thyroid hormone	Warfarin		
Trazodone		Clonidine	
Triamterene	NSAIDs, potassium		ACE inhibitors
Tricyclic antidepressants	Catecholamines	Clonidine	
Verapamil	Beta antagonists, carbamazepine, cyclosporine, digoxin, quinidine, theophylline		
Zidovudine (AZT)			Ganciclovir

Compiled by Robyn A. Schaiff, Pharm.D., and Lesley Ann Watson, R.Ph.

IX. DRUG INTERACTIONS

The use of the multitude of pharmacological agents constituting the cardiovascular therapeutic armamentarium requires not only extensive knowledge but also wisdom. The risk of adverse drug interactions is profound. Skilled clinicians are those who are particularly attuned to what can happen and are therefore sufficiently sensitive to what does happen to institute prompt corrective action. Some important, sometimes life-threatening interactions that require a particularly high index of suspicion are shown in Table 12.

Index

Abnormal pulsations, 97-99
  arterial pulsations, 97-98
  venous pulsations, 98-99
Accessory pathway-mediated tachycardia, 318-329
  electrocardiographic characteristics, 321-326
  Mahain fibers, 320-321
  management, 326-329
  manifest and concealed accessory pathways, 318
  mechanism underlying tachycardia, 318-320
Acebutolol, 530
Acetazolamide, 544
Acne in adults with congenital heart disease, 470
Acute aortic regurgitation, chronic aortic regurgitation versus, 249
Acute myocardial infarction, 189-219
  as cause of pericarditis, 272
  as complication of noncardiac surgery with ischemic heart disease, 486
  diagnosis of, 190-195
    cardiac-specific enzymes and proteins, 192-194
    characteristic symptoms, 190
    electrocardiographic findings associated with acute infarction, 191-192
    noninvasive cardiac imaging in patients with suspected MI, 194-195
  initial management of patients with, 195-207
    general measures, 195-196
    risk stratification, 196-207

[Acute myocardial infarction]
  management of bradyarrhythmias and conduction abnormalities in, 212-214
  management of tachyarrhythmias and ventricular arrhythmias in patients with, 214-217
    asymptomatic arrhythmias, 216-217
    electromechanical dissociation, 214-215
    life-threatening ventricular arrhythmias, 214
    symptomatic but non-life-threatening arrhythmias, 215-216
  pulmonary artery catheterization and management of hemodynamic subsets, 207-212
    bedside catheterization with balloon-tipped catheter, 208
    common indications, 207
    guidelines in interpreting hemodynamic measurements, 209
    hemodynamic subsets characterized by catheterization, 209-211
    measurements obtained, 208-209
    recognition and management of complications of invasive procedures, 211-212
  rehabilitation and secondary prevention after MI, 217-218
    activity counseling, 217
    counseling, 217-218
    risk stratification after MI, 218
    secondary prevention, 218
Acute pericarditis, 270-271

Acute pulmonary embolisms, 54-55
Acute ventricular septal defect (VSD), shock as
    cause of, 155-156
Adenosine, 76
    during pregnancy, 445, 451
Adrenal cortical enzyme deficiencies, 131
Adrenal hypertension, 127-133
    adrenal cortical enzyme deficiencies, 131
    aldosteronism, 129-130
    coarctation of the aorta, 132-133
    Cushing's syndrome, 130-131
    hyperparathyroidism, 132
    ingestion of licorice, 132
    oral contraceptive hypertension, 131-132
    pheochromocytoma, 127-129
Adults with congenital heart disease, 467-
    480
    activity and, 479-480
    anatomic defects (shunt lesions), 471-474
        atrial septal defects, 472-473
        basic principles, 471-472
        patent ductus arteriosus, 473-474
        ventricular septal defects, 473
    associated abnormalities, 468-470
        acne, 470
        bleeding diathesis, 469
        erythrocytosis, 468-469
        gallstones, 469
        hemoptysis, 470
        hyperuricemia/gout, 469
        noncardiac surgery, 470
        paradoxic emboli, 469
    associated defects, 474, 478
    cyanosis and, 467-468, 480
    endocarditis and, 478-479
    management of, 471
    management of hypoxemia in acquired heart
        disease, 470-471
    mechanism of cyanosis and age of onset,
        467-468
    postoperative congenital heart disease, 474
    pregnancy and, 479
    surgical procedures for, 475-477
Alcohol usage:
    in evaluating patient's coronary risk status,
        492
    hypertension and, 133-134

Aldosteronism, 129-130
    screening test for, 120
Allergic reactions associated with thrombolytic
    agents, 33
Allopurinol, 544
Ambulatory ECG monitoring:
    in detection of myocardial ischemia, 19
    in detection of palpitations, 68
Aminoglycosides, 544
Aminophylline, 456
Amiodarone, 544
    in pregnancy, 445, 450
Amiodipine, 532
Anemia, management of unstable angina and,
    183
Angina pectoris, 4-35, 169-187
    associated symptoms, 7-8
    cardiac risk factors, 9
    characteristics of, 5-7
    chest pain: physical findings in patients with
        angina pectoris, 14-16
    chest radiography, 16
    differential diagnosis, 9-14
        chest pain attributable to gastrointestinal
            disease, 12-13
        neuromuscular-skeletal causes of chest
            discomfort, 13
        psychogenic causes of chest pain, 11
        pulmonary causes of chest pain, 14
    electrocardiography and, 16
    management of inoperable coronary disease
        and frequent unstable symptoms, 187
    management of patients, 184-186
        angina and diabetes mellitus, 185
        angina and hypertension, 184-185
        angina and lung disease, 185
        angina and poor left ventricular function,
            185
        angina and valve disease, 185-186
        atypical stable angina, 186
    noninvasive testing for detection of
        myocardial ischemia, 17-21
        ambulatory ECG recordings, 19
        coronary arteriography, 21
        exercise ECG, 18-19
        positron emission tomography, 20
        radionuclide ventriculography, 20-21

[Angina pectoris]
stress echocardiography, 21
stress myocardial perfusion scintigraphy, 20
other tests likely to be helpful in patients with chest pain, 17
patients requiring revascularization, 181-182
pharmacological management of stable angina, 171-176
antiplatelet agents, 176
beta blockers, 174-175
calcium channel antagonists, 173-174
nitrates, 171-173
pharmacological management of unstable angina, 176-181
anticoagulation and thrombolysis, 178-179
antiplatelet agents, 178
beta blockers, 177-178
calcium channel antagonists, 177
nitrates, 176-177
support of circulation with intraaortic balloon pump, 179-180
selection of patients for angiography, 180-181
stable angina, 180
unstable angina, 180-181
specific management issues, 182-184
high-risk ECG patients with unstable angina, 183
non-Q-wave myocardial infarction, 184
"syndrome X," 182-183
unstable angina and hypertension or anemia, 183
unstable angina and poor left ventricular function, 183
stable angina pectoris,169-171
terminology, 4-5
unstable angina, 186-187
with ST-segment elevation, 22-34
Angioplasty, thrombolytic therapy compared with, 29-30
Angiotensin-converting enzyme (ACE) inhibitors, 507, 534-535, 544
adverse effects, 535
for CHF therapy, 231
clinical considerations, 534-535

[Angiotensin-converting enzyme (ACE) inhibitors]
for initial management of myocardial infarction, 201, 203
Anomalous pulmonary venous connection, dyspnea caused by, 56
Antiarrhythmic devices. See Implantable cardioverter defibrillator (ICD)
Antiarrhythmic drugs in pregnancy, 446-452
class I, 446-449
disopyramide, 444. 447
flecainide, 448
lidocaine, 444, 447-448
mexiletine, 444, 448
phenytoin, 444, 448
procainamide, 444, 447
propafenone, 445, 448-449
quinidine, 444, 446-447
class II, 449
class III, 449-450
amiodarone, 445, 450
sotalol, 445, 450
class IV, 450-451
diltiazen, 451
verapamil, 445, 450-451
other antiarrhythmic drugs, 451-452
adenosine, 445, 451
digoxin, 445, 451-452
Anticoagulants:
in initial management of myocardial infarction, 201, 204
for pulmonary hypertension, 236
Antihypertensive agents, 506, 536, 537
See also Hypertension, antihypertensive therapy
Antioxidants, 507
Antiplatelet agents:
in management of stable angina, 176
in management of unstable angina, 178
Antithymocyte globulin, 543
Aorta, coarctation of, 132-133
screening test for, 120
Aortic dissection, 10
Aortic regurgitation, 248-251
acute versus chronic aortic regurgitation, 249
functional manifestations, 249-250
laboratory results, 250-251

[Aortic regurgitation]
management of, 251
management of angina and, 185-186
mixed aortic stenosis and, 242-243
Aortic stenosis:
causes of, 241-242
functional consequences of, 242
laboratory findings, 245-247
management of, 247-248
management of angina and, 185
mixed aortic stenosis and aortic regurgitation, 242-243
physical findings, 244-245
shock as cause of, 154
signs and symptoms of, 243-244
treatment, 248
Arrhythmias:
asymptomatic, 216-217
in COPD, 456-458
management of specific arrhythmias, 458-460
management in pregnancy of, 442-453
class I drugs, 446-449
class II drugs, 449
class III drugs, 449-450
class IV drugs, 450-451
management of specific arrhythmias, 452-453
nonpharmacological management, 452
other antiarrhythmic drugs, 451-452
pharmacological management, 443-446
shock and, 158-159
See also Bradyarrhythmias; Palpitations; Supraventricular arrhythmias; Tachyarrhythmias; Ventricular arrhythmias; other types of arrhythmias
Arterial blood gases, measurement of, 46-47
Arterial dilators for CHF therapy, 231-233
Arterial pulsations, abnormal, 97-98
Artificial heart valve, management in pregnancy of, 439
Aspartate transaminase (AST), 17
Aspirin, 31, 507, 544
in management of myocardial infarction, 201, 203
in management of stable angina, 176
in management of unstable angina, 178

Asymptomatic arrhythmias, 216-217
Atenolol, 530
Athletes:
cardiac arrhythmias in, 427
management of specific arrhythmias in, 427-431
bradyarrhythmias, 430-431
premature beats, 428
supraventricular arrhythmias, 428-429
ventricular arrhythmias, 429-430
preparticipation screening of, 431
Athletic heart syndrome, 423-426
Atrial fibrillation, 305-311
additional therapeutic considerations, 310-311
electrocardiographic manifestations, 306
initial treatment of, 306-308
long-term therapy for, 308-310
in patients with dilated cardiomyopathy, 464
Atrial flutter, 303-305
Atrial premature depolarizations (APDs), 290-293
characteristics, 290-292
epidemiology, 292
etiology, 292
pathophysiology, 290
treatment for, 293
Atrial septal defects:
in adults, 472-473
dyspnea caused by, 56
Atrioventricular (AV) conduction abnormalities, 380-387
electrocardiographic diagnosis, 383-384
management of, 395-397
role of electrophysiology study, 384-385
symptoms, 382
Atrioventricular (AV) nodal reentrant tachycardia, 313-317
antiarrhythmic drugs for, 316-317
electrocardiographic characteristics, 312-314
management strategies, 314-315
nonpharmacological therapies, 317
pathology, 311-312
Atypical angina pectoris, 6
Atypical stable angina, 186
Automatic atrial tachycardia, 293, 294
management strategies, 295

Autonomic testing for survivor of cardiac arrest, 410
Azathioprine, 543
AZT (zidovudine), 547

Basic life support (BLS) for cardiac arrest, 397
usual component of, 398-399
Bedside pulmonary artery catheterization with balloon- tipped catheter, 208
Benazepril, 534
Beta-adrenergic blocking agents, 32, 506, 529-532, 544
adverse effects, 531-532
clinical considerations, 531
in initial management of myocardial infarction, 201, 203
in management of stable angina, 174-175
in management of unstable angina, 177-178
in pregnancy, 445, 449
in management of supraventricular tachycardia, 76
Beta mimetic agents, 456
Betaxolol, 530
Bisoprolol, 530
Bleeding associated with thrombolytic agents, 33-34
Bleeding diathesis, 469
Borderline hypertension, management of, 110-111
Brady-asystolic arrest, 400-401
Bradyarrhythmias:
management in pregnancy, 453
in patients with acute myocardial infarction, 212-214
Bradycardias, 373-395
abnormalities of impulse formation, 373-392
cardiac pacing for bradycardia, 387-392
carotid sinus syndrome, 377-379
disturbances of atrioventricular conduction, 380-387
malignant vasovagal syncope, 379-380
sinus node dysfunction, 374-376
athletes with, 430-431
cardiac pacing for, 387-392
mode of pacing, 388-389
permanent pacing, 387-388
rate-adaptive pacing, 389-390

[Bradycardias]
rate hysteresis, 390
temporary pacing, 390-392
intraventricular conduction abnormalities, 393-395
in patients with myocardial infarction, 212-214
shock and, 158-159
Bronchial provocation testing, 48-49
Bronchodilator drugs, arrhythmogenicity of, 455-456

Calcium channel blockers, 32, 532-534
adverse effects, 533
for CHF therapy, 231-232
in management of stable angina, 173-174
in management of unstable angina, 177
Calcium intake, hypertension and, 133
Captopril, 534
Carbamazepine, 544
Cardiac and pulmonary arrest, 397-401
basic life support for, 397, 398-399
brady-asystolic arrest, 400-401
pulseless electrical activity, 400
ventricular fibrillation, 399-400
ventricular tachycardia, 399
See also Survivor of cardiac arrest
Cardiac catheterization:
dyspnea and, 49-50
pericardial disease and, 276-277
for survivor of cardiac arrest, 412-413
Cardiac pacing:
for bradycardias, 387-392
mode of pacing, 388-389
permanent pacing, 387-388
rate-adaptive pacing, 389-390
rate hysteresis, 390
temporary pacing, 390-392
indications for permanent pacing in IV conduction block, 395
Cardiac shock, 146
Cardiac-specific enzymes and proteins released into plasma due to myocardial infarction, 192-194
Cardiac tamponade, 274-276
hemodynamic assessment of, 277
Cardiogenic shock, 152-154
primary pump failure, 152-153

[Cardiogenic shock]
   therapeutic considerations, 153-154
Cardiopulmonary exercise testing, 47
Cardiopulmonary resuscitation (CPR), 397
Cardiovascular evaluation of the hypertensive
   patient, 116, 117, 120-122
Carotid sinus massage (CSM), 377-379
   in evaluation of syncope, 88-89
Carotid sinus syndrome, 377-379
   carotid sinus massage, 377-379
   management of, 379
   symptoms, 377
Carteolol, 530
Cathedral ceiling, syndrome, 82
Chest asymmetry, 99-100
Chest pains of cardiac origin. *See* Angina
   pectoris
Chest radiography, 16, 84
   for shock evaluation, 151
   suspicions of cardiovascular disease raised
      by, 161-162
Chlorpromazine, 544
Cholesterol evaluation in determining coronary
   risk status, 497-498
Cholestyramine, 543
Chronic aortic regurgitation, acute aortic regurgitation versus, 249
Chronic atrial fibrillation, 310
Chronic diseases in evaluating coronary risk
   status, 493
Chronic obstructive pulmonary disease (COPD),
   455-460
   arrhythmias in, 456-458
      multifocal atrial arrhythmias, 457-458
   arrhythmogenicity of bronchodilator drugs,
      455-456
      aminophylline/theophylline, 456
      beta mimetic drugs, 456
      digitalis, 456
   management of specific arrhythmias, 458-
      460
Cigarette smoking:
   as coronary risk factor, 492, 502
   hypertension and, 134
Cimetidine, 545
Clonidine, 545
Clubbing, 99-100

Coarctation of the aorta, 132-133
   screening test for, 120
Colestipol, 543
Congenital complete heart block, athletes with,
   431
Congenital heart disease:
   dyspnea and, 56
   management in pregnancy, 438, 440
   See also Adults with congenital heart disease
Congestive heart failure (CHF), 221-233
   clinical presentation, 227
   as complication of noncardiac surgery with
      ischemic heart disease, 486
   definition of terms, 221-223
   evaluation, 227-229
   left ventricular systolic dysfunction, 225
   predominantly diastolic dysfunction, 223-225
      evaluation, 224
      management, 224-225
   treatment of, 229-233
      arterial dilators, 231-233
      goals of therapy, 229-231
Conjunctive agents, 31-32
Constrictive pericarditis, 281-284
   differential diagnosis, 283-284
   management, 284
   noninvasive diagnostic studies, 283
   physical examination, 282-283
Coronary arteriography in detection of myocardial ischemia, 21
Coronary artery bypass graft surgery, 182
   for unstable angina, 186-187
Coronary artery disease, ventricular tachycardia
   associated with, 347-359
Coronary risk status, evaluation of. *See* Preven-
   tive cardiology, evaluating coronary
   risk status of patient
Coronary vasospasm with chest pain, 22-23
Corticosteroids, 543
Cough, 59-60
Creatine kinase (CK), 192-193
Culture-negative endocarditis, 514
Cushing's syndrome, 130-131
   screening test for, 120
Cyanosis, 99-100
   in adults with congenital heart disease, 467-
      468, 480

[Cyanosis]
maternal complications during pregnancy due to, 440
Cyclosporine, 543

Degenerative arthritis, 13
Diabetes mellitus:
as coronary risk factor, 502-503
management of angina and, 185
Diaphoresis, 7
Diastolic hypertension, 104-105
Dietary history in evaluating coronary risk status, 491
Digitalis, 456
Digoxin, 545
during pregnancy, 445, 451-452
in management of pulmonary hypertension, 235
in management of supraventricular tachycardia, 76-77
Dilated cardiomyopathy (DCM), 464-465
atrial fibrillation in, 464
ventricular arrhythmias in, 335, 464-465
Diltiazem, 532
during pregnancy, 451
Direct-current cardioversion, 74-75
Disopyramide, 444, 447
Distributive shock, 146, 147-148
Disulfiram, 545
Diuretics:
in management of pulmonary hypertension, 235-236
thiazide, 547
Drug-related syncope, 83
Drugs:
abuse of
endocarditis in injection drug user, 514
in evaluating coronary risk status, 492
unstable chest pain in patients with history of, 24
interactions between commonly used drugs, 544-547, 548
See also Antiarrhythmic drugs; Medications; names and types of drugs
Dyslipoproteinemia as coronary risk factor, 498-500
Dyspnea, 37-57

[Dyspnea]
congenital heart disease and, 56
distinction of cardiovascular causes from pulmonary causes of, 41-42
initial diagnostic tests, 43-46
key physical findings, 42-43
as manifestation of pulmonary vascular disease, 51-55
primary pulmonary hypertension, 51-54
pulmonary embolism, 54-55
onset and pattern of, 38-41
specialized diagnostic tests, 46-50
strategies for management, 50-51
as symptom of angina pectoris, 8

Echocardiography:
in evaluation of suspected myocardial infarction, 195
in shock evaluation, 151
stress echocardiography, 21
in study of survivor of cardiac arrest, 407-408
suspicions of cardiovascular disease raised by, 164-165
Ectopic atrial tachycardia, 293-296
characteristics of the electro- cardiogram, 294-295
electrophysiological studies, 295
multifocal atrial tachycardia, 294, 295
pathophysiology, 293-294
specific management strategies, 295-296
Eisenmenger's syndrome, maternal complications during pregnancy due to, 441
Electrical cardioversion in management of supraventricular tachycardia, 77
Electrocardiography:
in detection of chest pain, 16
in detection of dyspnea, 45-46
in detection of palpitations, 68
in shock evaluation, 151
suspicions of cardiovascular disease raised by, 162-164
Elevated blood pressure. See Hypertension
Enalapril, 534
Endocarditis:
in adults with congenital heart disease, 478-479
See also Infective endocarditis

Erythrocytosis, 468-469
Erythromycin, 545
Essential hypertension compared with
secondary hypertension, 103
Exercise:
as coronary risk factor, 503
electrophysiological changes during 424
hypertension and, 134
Exercise history in evaluating coronary risk
status, 491-492
Exercise testing:
in detection of myocardial infarction, 18-19
in detection of palpitations, 68-69
in study of survivor of cardiac arrest, 408-
409
Exogenous steroid use in evaluating coronary
risk status, 492

Failed thrombolysis, 34
Faintness, 7
Family history in evaluating coronary risk
status, 490-491
Fatigue, 7
Felodipine, 532
Fibrinolytic agents, 28, 30-31
Flecainide, 448
Fosinopril, 534

Gallstones, 469
Gastrointestinal disease, chest pain attributable
to, 12-13
Gemfibrozil, 543
Gout, 469

Heart rhythm during palpitation, 65-69
ambulatory electrocardiographic monitoring,
68
electrocardiogram and rhythm strip, 68
electrophysiological studies, 69
exercise testing, 68-69
Heart transplant rejection, agents used for prevention and treatment of, 543, 548
Hemopytsis, 470
Heparin:
in management of myocardial infarction, 201,
203
in management of unstable angina, 178-179

Herpes zoster, 13
High resolution computed tomography (HRCT),
50
Holter monitoring for survivor of cardiac arrest,
409-410
Hydralazine, 231
Hyperparathyroidism, 132
Hypertension, 101-144
adrenal hypertension, 127-133
adrenal cortical enzyme deficiencies, 131
aldosteronism, 129-130
coarctation of the aorta, 132-133
Cushing's syndrome, 130-131
hyperparathyroidism, 132
ingestion of licorice, 132
oral contraceptive hypertension, 131-132
pheochromocytoma, 127-129
antihypertensive therapy, 133-137, 138-139
alcohol, 133-134
changes in lifestyle, 133
exercise, 134
obesity, 133
pharmacological agents, 134-137, 138-139
sodium, potassium, calcium, and
magnesium intake, 133
"stepped care" treatment algorithm, 135,
136
stress, 134
consequences of elevated blood pressure,
103-107
as coronary risk factor, 500-501
definitions, 101-103
diagnostic studies for secondary
hypertension, 123-127
hypertension emergencies and urgencies,
137-142
pathology of malignant hypertension, 137-
142
management of angina and, 183, 184-185
management of the hypertensive patient, 107-
123
borderline hypertension, 110-111
patient evaluation, 113-123
rationale for treatment, 107-110
systolic hypertension, 111-112
therapeutic goals, 112-113
types of, 104-105

[Hypertension]
    ventricular arrhythmias in patients with, 335-336
    See also Primary pulmonary hypertension; Secondary pulmonary hypertension
Hypertrophic cardiomyopathy (HCM), 461-464
    management of "high-risk" patients, 463-464
    management in pregnancy, 438
    supraventricular arrhythmias, 461-462
    ventricular arrhythmias, 334-335, 462-463
Hyperuricemia, 469
Hypolipidemic drugs, 505-506
Hypotension associated with thrombolytic agents, 33
Hypovolemic shock, 146, 148-149
Hypoxemia, 470-471

Implantable cardioverter defibrillator (ICD), 519-526
    effect of antiarrrhythmic drugs on ICD performance, 524
    evaluation of ICD shocks, 521-522
    general concepts, 520
    infection, 522-523
    management of arrhythmias, 523
    overall perspective, 525
    perioperative management, 524-525
    selection of patients, 520-521
    for survivor of cardiac arrest, 416, 417-418
Infection caused by ICDs, 522-523
Infectious pericarditis, 272-273
Infective endocarditis (IE), 509-518
    clinical presentations, 510-511
    definitions, 508-510
    diagnosis, 511-512
    microbiology, 512-514
        culture-negative endocarditis, 514
        endocarditis in the injection drug user, 514
        native valve endocarditis, 512-513
        prosthetic valve endocarditis, 513-514
    prophylaxis, 517
    treatment, 514-517
Injection drug users (IDUs), endocarditis in, 514
Inoperable coronary artery disease, 187
Intraaortic balloon pump in management of unstable angina, 179-180

Intraatrial reentrant arrhythmias, 299-311
    atrial fibrillation, 305-311
    atrial flutter, 303-305
    intraatrial reentrant tachyardia, 300-301
Intraventricular conduction abnormalities, 393-395
Ischemic chest pain not due to coronary atherosclerosis, 7
Ischemic heart disease, noncardiac surgery and, 481-487
    complications, 486-487
    evaluation, 481-483
    recommended evaluation, 483
Isoniazid, 545
Isradipine, 532
Joint National Committee on Detecting, Evaluation and Treatment of Hypertension (JNC V), 101-102
    "stepped care" treatment algorithm of, 135, 136

Jugular vein pulse, 64
Junctional escape beats, 296-297
Junctional premature depolarization, 296-297

Ketoconazole, 545

Labetalol, 530
Lactate dehydrogenase (LDH), 17, 193
Left ventricular function, management of angina and, 183, 185
Left ventricular systolic dysfunction, 225
    pathophysiology of congestive heart failure related to, 225-227
Lesions affecting the aortic valve, 241-248
    causes of aortic stenosis, 241-242
    definitive measures, 248
    functional consequences of aortic stenosis, 242
    laboratory findings, 245-247
    management, 247-248
    mixed aortic stenosis and aortic regurgitation, 242-243
    physical findings, 244-245
    signs and symptoms, 243-244
Licorice, ingestion of, 132
Lidocaine, 32, 545
    in pregnancy, 444, 447-448

Lifestyle changes, as antihypertensive therapy, 133

Life-threatening ventricular arrhythmias, 214

Lipid disorders as coronary risk factor, 498-500

Lipid-lowering drugs, 543, 547-548

Lisinopril, 534

Lone atrial fibrillation, 308-309

Lovastatin, 543, 545

Lung disease, management of angina and, 185

Magnesium intake, hypertension and, 133

Magnetic resonance imaging (MRI), 408-409

Mahaim fibers, 320-321

Malignant hypertension, 137-142

Malignant vasovagal syncope (MVVS), 379-380

MAO inhibitors, 546

Marfan's syndrome, maternal complications during pregnancy due to, 440

Medications, 529-548
   agents used for neuromuscular blockade, 539, 542-547
   agents used for sedation and neuromuscular blockade, 537-542
   agents used for prevention and treatment of heart transplantation rejection, 543, 548
   angiotensin-converting enzyme (ACE) inhibitors, 534-535
      adverse effects, 535
      clinical considerations, 534-535
   for antihypertensive therapy, 133-137, 138-139
   beta-adrenergic blockers, 529-532
      adverse effects, 531-532
      clinical considerations, 531
   calcium channel blockers, 532-534
      adverse effects, 533
   drug interactions, 544-547, 548
   lipid-lowering drugs, 543, 547-548
   nitrates, 535-536
   nitroprusside, 536
   other antihypertensive agents, 537

Methotrexate, 546

Methyldopa, 546

Metoprolol, 530

Mexiletine, 444, 448

Mitral regurgitation, 255-258
   functional manifestations, 255-256
   laboratory findings, 256-257
   management, 257-258
   shock as cause of, 154-155

Mitral stenosis:
   functional consequences of, 252-253
   management in pregnancy of, 437

Mitral valve disease, 251-255
   functional consequences of mitral stenosis, 252-253
   laboratory findings, 253-254
   management, 254-255

Mitral valve prolapse, 11
   management in pregnancy of, 437-438
   ventricular arrhythmias in, 335

Monomorphic ventricular tachycardia, 354-359

Multifocal atrial tachycardia (MAT), 294, 295
   management strategies, 296
   in patients with COPD, 457-458

Myocardial infarction (MI):
   initial evaluation of patients with ST-segment elevation and, 25-26
   non-Q-wave, 184
   reperfusion in patients with ST-segment elevation and, 26-27
   selection of fibrinolytic and conjunctive agents, 30-34
   selection of patients, 27-30
      age-related risk-versus-benefit of different strategies, 28
      thrombolytic therapy compared with primary angioplasty, 29-30
      timing of reperfusion, 27-28
      treatment of patients with hypertension, 28-29
   ventricular arrhythmias after, 334
   See also Acute myocardial infarction

Myocardial ischemia:
   chest pain due to, 15
   noninvasive testing for, 17-21
      ambulatory ECG recordings, 19
      coronary arteriography, 21
      exercise ECG, 18-19
      positron emission tomography, 20
      radionuclide ventriculography, 20-21
      stress echocardiography, 21

[Myocardial ischemia]
stress myocardial perfusion scintigraphy, 20
Myocardial rupture, shock and, 158
Myocarditis with chest pain 23-24

Nadolol, 530
Native valve endocarditis, 512-513
therapy for, 515
Nausea, 7
Neoplastic pericarditis, 273
Neuromuscular blocking drugs, 539, 542-547
used in intensive or coronary care units, 537-542
Neuromuscular-skeletal causes of chest pain, 13
Niacin, 543
Nicardipine, 532, 546
Nifedipine, 532
Nitrates, 535-536
for congestive heart failure therapy, 230-231
in initial management of myocardial infarction, 203-204
in management of stable angina, 171-173
in management of unstable angina, 176-177
Nitroglycerin, 32
Nitroprusside, 536
Nonanginal chest pain, 6
Noncardiac surgery:
for adults with congenital heart disease, 470
for patients with ischemic heart disease, 481-487
Nonischemic chest pain of cardiac origin, 9
Noninvasive testing for myocardial ischemia, 17-21
ambulatory ECG recordings, 19
coronary arteriography, 21
exercise ECG, 18-19
positron emission tomography, 20
radionuclide ventriculography, 20-21
stress echocardiography, 21
stress myocardial perfusion scintigraphy, 20
Nonparoxysmal AV junctional tachycardia, 298
electrocardiographic characteristics of, 298-299
epidemiology, 299
management, 299

Non-Q-wave myocardial infarction, 184
Nonsustained ventricular tachycardia, 462-463
therapy for, 348-352
Normal sinus rhythm (NSR), 286
NSAIDs, 549

Obesity:
as coronary risk factor, 503
hypertension and, 133
Obstructive shock, 146-147
Oral contraceptive hypertension, 131-132
Organic heart disease:
atrial fibrillation and, 309
ventricular tachycardia in patients without, 364-367
Orthoclone OKT3, 543
Orthopnea, 40

Palpitations, 61-78
documentation of heart rhythm during, 65-69
initial assessment of heart rhythm, 69-74
initial management of sustained arrhythmias, 74-78
medical history, 61-63
functional and emotional consequences, 63
precipitating factors, 62-63
presence and types of arrhythmias, 62
physical examination, 63-65
arterial pulse, 64-65
heart sounds, 65
jugular vein pulse, 64
Paradoxic emboli, 469
Paroxysmal nocturnal dyspnea (PND), 40
Patent ductus arteriosus, 473-474
Penbutolol, 530
Percutaneous transluminal coronary angioplasty (PTCA), 181-182
for unstable angina, 187
Pericardial disease, 267-284
anatomy and pathophysiology, 267-268
cardiac catheterization, 276-277
cardiac tamponade, 274-276
with chest pain, 7, 23
constrictive percarditis, 281-284
differential diagnosis, 283-284

[Pericardial disease]
management, 284
noninvasive diagnostic studies, 283
physical examination, 282-283
differential diagnosis, 272-273
acute myocardial infarction, 272
infectious pericarditis, 272-273
neoplastic pericarditis, 273
evaluation, 271-272
hemodynamic assessment of pericardial effusions, 277
management, 273-274, 277-281
noninvasive diagnostic procedures, 276
pathophysiology, 269-270
pericardial functions, 269
physiological properties of the normal pericardium, 268
primary disease of the pericardium, 270-271
acute pericarditis, 270-271
Peripartum cardiomyopathy:
management in pregnancy, 438-439
with residual left ventricular dysfunction, 441
Phenytoin, 546
in pregnancy, 444, 448
Pheochromocytoma, 127-129
screening test for, 120
Physical exercise. *See* Exercise
Pindolol, 530
Platypnea, 40
Polymorphic ventricular tachycardia:
associated with long QT intervals, 367-370
therapy for, 359
Poor left ventricular function, management of angina and, 185
Positron emission tomography (PET), 20
Postoperative atrial fibrillation, 310
Postoperative congenital heart disease, 474
surgical procedures used in, 475-477
Potassium intake, hypertension and, 133
Pravastatin, 543
Predominantly diastolic dysfunction, 223-225
evaluation of, 224
management of, 224-225
Pregnancy, 433-453
management of arrhythmias in, 442-453
class I antiarrhythmic drugs, 446-449
class II antiarrhythmic drugs, 449

[Pregnancy]
class III antiarrhythmic drugs, 449-450
class IV antiarrhythmic drugs, 450-451
management of specific arrhythmias, 452-453
nonpharmacological management, 452
other antiarrhythmic drugs, 451-452
pharmacological management, 443-446
management of cardiac disease in, 434-441
cardiac evaluation, 434-435
cardiac physiology associated with pregnancy, 434
congenital heart disease, 438, 440
hypertrophic cardiomyopathy, 438
laboratory findings, 435
medical conditions associated with increased risk to the mother, 439-441
mitral stenosis, 437
mitral valve prolapse, 437-438
patients with prosthetic valves, 439
peripartum cardiomyopathy, 438-439
reasons for cardiac consultations in pregnant subjects, 435-436
valvular heart disease, 437
maternal risks associated with congenital heart disease, 479
Premature beats:
athletes with, 428
management in pregnancy, 452
Presumed cardiac syncope, 90
Presyncope. *See* Syncope and presyncope
Preventive cardiology, 489-508
concepts of prevention in atherosclerosis heart disease, 480-490
evaluating coronary risk status of patient, 490-498
laboratory evaluation, 497-498
special aspects of history, 490-493
special aspects of physical examination, 493-497
modifying risk factors, 498-508
cigarette smoking, 502
diabetes mellitus, 502-503
dyslipoproteinemia, 498-500
encouraging compliance, 507-508
exercise, 503
hypertension, 500-501

[Preventive cardiology]
    pharmacological interventions, 505-507
    selecting appropriate intervention, 504-
       505
    weight control, 503
Primary aldosteronism, screening test for, 120
Primary pulmonary hypertension, 235-237
   anticoagulants for, 236
   digoxin for, 235
   diuretics for, 235-236
   dyspnea and, 51-54
   maternal complications during pregnancy due
      to, 440-441
   prostacyclin for, 236-237
   vasodilators for, 236
Probucol, 543
Procainamide, 77
   in pregnancy, 444, 447
Propafenone, 546
   in pregnancy, 445, 448-449
Prophylaxis for endocarditis, 517
Prophylthiouracil, 546
Propranolol, 530
Prostacyclin, 236-237
Prosthetic heart valves:
   management in pregnancy, 439
   in management of valvular heart disease,
      264-265
Prosthetic valve endocarditis, 513-514
   therapy for, 516
Psychogenic cause of chest pain, 11
Pulmonary arrest. *See* Cardiac and pulmonary
      arrest
Pulmonary artery catheterization in management
      of acute myocardial infarction, 207-212
   bedside catheterization with balloon-tipped
      catheter, 208
   common indications, 207
   guidelines in interpreting hemodynamic
      measurements, 209
   hemodynamic subsets characterized by
      catheterization, 209-211
   measurements obtained, 208-209
   recognition and management of
      complications of invasive procedures,
      211-212
Pulmonary causes of chest pain, 14

Pulmonary embolism:
   dyspnea and, 54-55
   with chest pain, 24
Pulmonary regurgitation, 261-263
   functional manifestations, 262
   laboratory findings, 262-263
   management, 263
Pulmonary stenosis, 263-264
Pulmonary vascular disease:
   dyspnea as manifestation of, 51-55
   See also Primary pulmonary hypertension;
      Secondary pulmonary hypertension
Pulseless electrical activity, 400

Quinapril, 534
Quinidine, 546
   in pregnancy, 444, 446-447
Quinolone antibiotics, 546

Radionuclide ventriculography (RVG), 20-21
Ramipril, 534
Reentrant arrhythmias, 340
Reflexive syncope. *See* Syncope and pre-
      syncope
Reflux esophagitis, 12
Rejection of heart transplant, agents used for
      prevention and treatment of, 543, 548
Renal artery stenosis, screening test for, 120
Renal evaluation of the hypertensive patient,
      123
Renal parenchymal disease, 123-124
   screening test for, 120
Renovascular hypertension, 124-127
Retinal examination of the hypertensive patient,
      117-119
Rifampin, 546

Salicylates, 546
Secondary pulmonary hypertension, 237
   diagnostic studies for, 123-127
     renal function tests, 124
     renal parenchymal disease, 123-124
     renovascular hypertension, 124-127
   essential hypertension compared with, 103
   screening tests for, 120
Sedation, agents used in intensive or coronary
      care units for, 537-542

Septicemia, 147-148
Serum glutamic-oxaloacetic transaminase
    (SGOT), 17
Sestamibi scintigraphy, 195
Shock, 145-159
    arrhythmias and, 158-159
    cardiogenic shock, 152-154
        primary pump failure, 152-153
        therapeutic considerations, 153-154
    distributive shock, 147-148
    hemodynamics of, 146-147
    hypovolemic shock, 148-149
    initial considerations using physical findings,
        149-151
    myocardial rupture, 158
    noninvasive studies, 151-152
    right venticular dysfunction secondary to
        ischemia, 156-158
    secondary to cardiac dysfunction, 154-156
        acute ventricular septal defect, 155-156
        aortic stenosis, 154
        mitral regurgitation, 154-155
Shocks due to ICDs, evaluation of, 521-522
Shortness of breath. *See* Dyspnea
Shunt lesions in adults with congenital heart
    disease, 471-474
Sick sinus syndrome (SSS). *See* Sinus node
    dysfunction
Signal-averaged electrocardiography, 410-412
Simvastatin, 543
Sinus node dysfunction, 374-376
    athletes with, 430
    electrocardiographic diagnosis, 374-376
    management, 376
    role of electrophysiology study, 376
    symptoms, 374
Sinus node reentry, 288-290
    clinical characteristics and treatment, 290
    electrocardiographic manifestations, 289
    pathophysiology, 288-289
Sinus rhythms, 286
Sinus tachycardia, 286-288
    electrocardiographic characteristics, 287-288
    management, 288
Situational syncope. *See* Syncope and pre-
    syncope
Sodium intake, hypertension and, 133

Sotalol, 445, 450
Spirometry in detecting dyspnea, 46
Spironolactone, 546
Stable angina pectoris. *See* Angina pectoris
"Stepped care" treatment algorithm for hyper-
    tension, 135, 136
Stress, hypertension and, 134
Stress echocardiography, 21
Stress myocardial perfusion scintigraphy, 20
Sucralfate, 546
Sulfonamides, 547
Supraventricular arrhythmias, 285-331
    accessory pathway-mediated tachycardia,
        318-329
    athletes with, 428-429
    atrioventricular and reentrant tachycardia,
        311-317
    as complication of noncardiac surgery with
        ischemic heart disease, 486-487
    intraartrial reentrant arrhythmias, 299-311
    management of patients with cardiac
        arrhythmias, 286-297
        atrial premature depolarizations, 290-293
        ectopic atrial tachycardia, 293-296
        junctional escape beats and junctional
            premature depolarizations, 296-297
        sinus node reentry, 288-290
        sinus rhythm, 286
        sinus tachycardia, 286-288
    management in pregnancy, 452-453
    in patients with hypertrophic
        cardiomyopathy, 461-462
    therapy for, 75-77
Survivor of cardiac arrest, 403-420
    evaluation of, 406-407
    invasive laboratory studies, 412-416
        cardiac catheterization, 412-413
        electrophysiological evaluation, 413-416
    noninvasive studies, 407-412
        autonomic testing, 410
        echocardiography, 407-408
        exercise testing and nuclear imaging, 408-
        409
        Holter monitoring, 409-410
        signal-averaged electrocardiography, 410-
        412
    therapeutic approach, 416-420

Symptomatic (but non-life-threatening)
  arrhythmias, 215-216
Syncope and presyncope, 79-93
  athletes with, 431
  diagnostic yields and implications, 90-92
  presentation of the patient, 80-85
    chest x-ray, 84
    electrocardiogram, 84
    history, 80-83
    immediate, 80
    initial data and tentative diagnosis, 80
    laboratory abnormalities, 84-85
    late, 80
    physical examination, 83-84
  presumed cardiac syncope, 90
  situational/reflexive syncope, 85-89
    carotid sinus massage. 88-89
    stress tests, 89
    time frame, 89
    workup and the decision tree, 85-88
  subsequent evaluation after tentative
    diagnostic evaluation, 85
Syndrome X, 182-183
Systolic hypertension, 105
  management of, 111-112

Tachyarrhythmias:
  in patients with myocardial infarction, 214-
    217
    asymptomatic arrhythmias, 215-217
    electromechanical dissociation, 214-215
    life-threatening ventricular arrhythmias,
      214
    symptomatic but non-life-threatening
      arrhythmias, 215-218
Tachycardia:
  shock and, 158-159
  See also types of tachycardias
Tacrolimus, 543
Technetium 99m pyrophosphate, 195
Theophylline, 547
  as cause of arrhythmias in chronic obstructive
    pulmonary disease, 456
Thiazide diuretics, 547
Thoracic outlet syndrome, 13
Thrombolytic therapy:
  angioplasty compared with, 29-30

[Thrombolytic therapy]
  complications associated with, 33-34
  monitoring of, 33
Tietze's syndrome, 13
Timolol, 530
Tobacco:
  as coronary risk factor, 492, 502
  hypertension and, 134
Torsades de pointes, 399
Trepopnea, 40-41
Triamterene, 547
Tricuspid regurgitation, 258-260
  functional manifestations, 259
  laboratory findings, 259-260
  management, 260
Tricuspid stenosis, 260-261
Tricyclic antidepressants, 547
Troponin, 193-194
Two-dimensional echocardiography, 195
Type 1 second-degree atrioventricular block,
  431
Type 2 second-degree atrioventricular block,
  431
Typical angina pectoris, 6

Unstable angina pectoris. See Angina pectoris

Vagal stimulation in treatment of
  supraventricular tachycardia, 76
Valvular heart disease, 239-265
  aortic regurgitation, 248-251
  lesions affecting the aortic valve, 241-248
  management in pregnancy, 437
  mechanical and surgical interventions
    required in management of, 264-265
  mitral regurgitation, 255-258
  mitral valve disease, 251-255
  pulmonary regurgitation, 261-263
  pulmonary stenosis, 263-264
  tricuspid and pulmonary valve disease, 258-
    260
  tricuspid stenosis, 260-261
Variant (Prinzmetal's) angina, 101
Vasodilators:
  for congestive heart failure, 230
  for pulmonary hypertension, 236
Venous pulsations, abnormal, 98-99

Ventilation-perfusion scanning, 49
Ventricular arrhythmias, 333-371
    as complication of noncardiac surgery with
        ischemic heart disease, 487
    management in pregnancy, 453
    in patients with dilated cardio- myopathy,
        464-465
    in patients with hypertension, 335-336
    in patients with hypertrophic
        cardiomyopathy, 334-335, 462-465
    in patients with myocardial infarction, 214-
        217, 334
        asymptomatic arrhythmias, 215-217
        electromechanical dissociation, 214-215
        life-threatening ventricular arrhythmias,
            214
        symptomatic but non-life-threatening
            arrhythmias, 215-218
Ventricular fibrillation, 399-400
Ventricular premature complexes (VPCs), 333-
    342
    electrocardiography, 336-338
    epidemiology, 334-336
    mechanism, 338-340
    treatment, 340-342
Ventricular septal defect, 473

Ventricular tachycardia (VT), 343-370, 399
    athletes with, 429-430
    electrocardiographic features, 345-347
    pathophysiologic basis, 344-345
    specific types of VT, 347-370
    therapy for, 77, 347-370
Verapamil, 78, 532, 537
    during pregnancy, 445, 450-451
    in management of supraventricular
        tachycardia, 76
Vomiting, 7

Weight control as factor in preventive
    cardiology, 503
Wide QRS complex tachycardia, 72-74
    therapy for, 77-78
Wolff-Parkinson-White (WPW) syndrome, 318-
    329
    electrocardiographic characteristics, 321-
        326
    management, 326-329
    Mahain fibers in, 320-321
    mechanisms underlying tachycardia, 318-
        320

Zidovudine (AZT), 547

About the Editor

BURTON E. SOBEL is Amidon Professor and Chair of the Department of Medicine at The University of Vermont College of Medicine, Burlington, and Physician-in-Chief, Fletcher Allen Health Care—Medical Center Hospital of Vermont Campus, Burlington, Vermont. The editor, with Désiré Collen, of *Coronary Thrombolysis in Perspective* (Marcel Dekker, Inc.) and the author or coauthor of over 630 articles and book chapters, he has lectured at universities and conferences throughout the world. He has served as Editor of the journals *Circulation*, *Coronary Artery Disease*, and *Current Opinion in Cardiology*, and as an Associate Editor and editorial board member of, among many others, the *Journal of Clinical Investigation*, *Annals of Internal Medicine*, *Circulation Research*, and the *American Journal of Physiology: Heart and Circulatory Physiology*. He is a Fellow of The Royal Society of Medicine in the U.K., the American College of Cardiology (which he served as Governor), and the American College of Physicians, and he is a member of numerous societies, including the American Society for Clinical Investigation, the Americn Physiological Society, the Society for Experimental Biology and Medicine, and the Association of Professors of Cardiology. Dr. Sobel received the A.B. degree (1958) from Cornell University, Ithaca, New York, and the M.D. degree (1962) magna cum laude from Harvard Medical School, Boston, Massachusetts.